1 Los efectos del manejo ante mortem a los [illegible] rendimientos y calidad de las canales porcinas
2 Consideraciones del tratamiento post-mortem a la calidad de la carne
2 El papel de la carne en la dieta humana [illegible]

1 Rendimiento en carne

3 Otras interacciones de carne - grasa [illegible]
4 Bacterias patógenas asociadas a la ca[illegible]

MEAT AND HEALTH

ADVANCES IN MEAT RESEARCH, VOLUME 6

CONTENTS OF VOLUME 5—EDIBLE MEAT BY-PRODUCTS

MEAT AND HEALTH

ADVANCES IN MEAT RESEARCH
VOLUME 6

Edited by

A. M. PEARSON

Department of Animal Science,
Brigham Young University, Utah, USA

and

T. R. DUTSON

Agricultural Experiment Station,
Oregon State University, Oregon, USA

ELSEVIER APPLIED SCIENCE
LONDON and NEW YORK

ELSEVIER SCIENCE PUBLISHERS LTD
Crown House, Linton Road, Barking, Essex IG11 8JU, England

Sole Distributor in the USA and Canada
ELSEVIER SCIENCE PUBLISHING CO., INC.
655 Avenue of the Americas, New York, NY 10010, USA

WITH 110 TABLES AND 56 ILLUSTRATIONS

British Library Cataloguing in Publication Data

Meat and health.
1. Man. Health. Effects of meat
I. Pearson, A. M. (Albert Marchant) *1916–*
II. Dutson, T. R.
III. Series
613.2′8

Library of Congress Cataloging-in-Publication Data

LC card number 86-655182

ISBN 1-85166-452-1
ISSN 0885-2405

Printed in Great Britain by Galliard (Printers) Ltd, Great Yarmouth

Preface

In recent years a great deal of negative press has been devoted to so-called problems in human health from eating meat and other animal products. Much of the information presented has been distorted and sensationalized with little attempt being made to focus upon both the advantages and disadvantages of meat, poultry and fish in the human diet. Thus, the topic *Meat and Health* was chosen as the central theme for this book, with the aim of presenting both the rationale for eating meat and any negative aspects of such consumption.

The authors of the various chapters are leaders in their field, with many of them being recognized for their contributions to nutritional research. As has been the custom for other volumes in this series, each chapter has been subjected to a peer review by an expert in the respective field covered by the topic. Although the Editors have attempted to bring continuity to the various chapters, the opinions of the authors were held inviolate.

Chapter 1 provides an introduction to the topic of meat and health by briefly reviewing some of the health concerns and also some of the advantages of meat in the human diet. Chapters 2 and 3 discuss the interrelationships between fat, cholesterol and different fatty acids in meat and their probable relation to coronary heart disease and stroke. Chapter 4 focuses on the possible relationship between meat consumption and cancer. Chapters 5, 6 and 7 discuss toxic compounds produced during cooking and meat processing, chemical and pesticide residues in meat, and meat pathogens, respectively. Most of the remaining chapters discuss the nutritional contributions or lack of contributions from meat, such as iron (Chapter 8), zinc (Chapter 9), copper, cobalt, manganese, and magnesium

(Chapter 10), calcium, phosphorus, sodium and potassium (Chapter 11), protein and essential amino acids (Chapter 12), the fat-soluble vitamins A, E, D and K (Chapter 13), thiamin, riboflavin, niacin and pantothenic acid (Chapter 14), and finally vitamin B_6, vitamin B_{12}, and folate acid (Chapter 15). The last two chapters (16 and 17) are devoted to the rationale for including meat in the human diet (Chapter 16), and some new methods of processing and ways for reducing the fat content of meat and meat products (Chapter 17). It is believed that in all this book presents a balanced discussion on the role of meat in the human diet and its relationship to human health.

A. M. PEARSON
T. R. DUTSON

Contents

List of Contributors

the late GEORGE M. BRIGGS

Department of Nutritional Sciences, 119 Morgan Hall, University of California, Berkeley, California 94720, USA

L. S. DARNELL

University of Texas Medical Branch, Preventive Medicine and Community Health, 301 University Boulevard, Keiller 136, Rt. F-17 Galveston, Texas 77550, USA

J. I. GRAY

Department of Food Science and Human Nutrition, Michigan State University, East Lansing, Michigan 48824, USA

R. GAURTH HANSEN

Department of Nutrition and Food Sciences, Utah State University, Logan, Utah 84322-8700, USA

JOSEPH H. HOTCHKISS

Institute of Food Science, Stocking Hall, Cornell University, Ithaca, NY 14853, USA

PHYLLIS E. JOHNSON

USDA, ARS, Human Nutrition Research Center, PO Box 7166, University Station, Grand Forks, North Dakota 58202, USA

Njeri Karanja
Oregon Health Sciences University, Division of Nephrology and Hypertension, 3181 SW Sam Jackson Park Road, Portland, Oregon 97201, USA

David Kritchevsky
The Wistar Institute of Anatomy and Biology, 3601 Spruce Street, Philadelphia, Pennsylvania 19104, USA

Talash A. Likimani
Oregon Health Sciences University, Division of Nephrology and Hypertension, 3181 SW Sam Jackson Park Road, Portland, Oregon 97201, USA, Present address:
University of Nairobi, Department of Food Science and Nutrition, Faculty of Agriculture and Veterinary Science, PO Box 29053, Kabete, Kenya

David A. McCarron
Oregon Health Sciences University, Division of Nephrology and Hypertension, 3181 SW Sam Jackson Park Road, Portland, Oregon 97201, USA

Donald J. McNamara
Department of Nutrition and Food Science, University of Arizona, Tucson, Arizona 85721, USA

Elaine R. Monsen
Nutritional Sciences/Medicine, University of Washington, Seattle, Washington 98195, USA

Forrest H. Nielsen
USDA, ARS, Human Nutrition Research Center, PO Box 7166, University Station, Grand Forks, North Dakota 58202, USA

Robert S. Parker
Division of Nutritional Sciences, Savage Hall, Cornell University, Ithaca, New York 14853, USA.

A. M. Pearson
Department of Animal Science, Brigham Young University, 355 WIDB, Provo, Utah 84602, USA

PETER L. PELLETT
Department of Human Nutrition, University of Massachusetts at Amherst, Amherst, Massachusetts 01003, USA

MICHAEL M. PULLEN
Department of Large Animal Clinical Sciences, College of Veterinary Medicine, University of Minnesota, St. Paul, Minnesota 55108, USA

RAYMOND REISER
Department of Biochemistry and Biophysics, Texas Agricultural Experiment Station, Texas A&M University System, College Station, Texas 77843-2128, USA

H. H. SANDSTEAD
University of Texas Medical Branch, Preventive Medicine and Community Health, 301 University Boulevard, Keiller 136, Rt. F-17 Galveston, Texas 77550, USA

HOWERDE E. SAUBERLICH
Department of Nutrition Sciences, University of Alabama at Birmingham, Birmingham, Alabama 35294, USA

the late BERNARD S. SCHWEIGERT
Department of Food Science and Technology, 126 Cruess Hall, University of California, Davis, California 95616, USA

F. B. SHORLAND
School of Biological Sciences, Victoria University of Wellington, Wellington, New Zealand

JOHN EDGAR SMITH
Nutrition Department, Henderson Building South S-128A, Pennsylvania State University, University Park, Pennsylvania 16802, USA

L. B. SMITH
Department of Food Science and Nutrition, University of Minnesota, St. Paul, Minnesota 55108, USA

J. C. WALLWORK
University of Texas Medical Branch, Preventive Medicine and Community Health, 301 University Boulevard, Keiller 136, Rt. F-17 Galveston, Texas 77550, USA

CAROL T. WINDHAM
Department of Nutrition and Food Sciences, Utah State University, Logan, Utah 84322-8700, USA

BONNIE WORTHINGTON-ROBERTS
Nutritional Sciences/Epidemiology, University of Washington, Seattle, Washington 98195, USA

BONITA W. WYSE
Office of the Dean, College of Family Life, Utah State University, Logan, Utah 84322-2900, USA

VERNON R. YOUNG
Clinical Research Center and Laboratory of Human Nutrition, School of Science, Massachusetts Institute of Technology, Cambridge, Massachusetts 02139, USA

E. A. ZOTTOLA
Department of Food Science and Nutrition, University of Minnesota, St. Paul, Minnesota 55108, USA

1

An Overview of Meat in the Diet

THE LATE GEORGE M. BRIGGS
Department of Nutritional Sciences, University of California, Berkeley, California, USA

AND

THE LATE BERNARD S. SCHWEIGERT
Department of Food Science and Technology, University of California, Davis, California, USA

I. INTRODUCTION

This volume is about meat and its relationship to health. Meat, as we eat it, is the cooked (generally) flesh or organs of animals and fowls.

In this volume, as in the food marketing trade, the term 'meat' generally refers to red meats (that of cattle, pigs, and sheep), but occasionally comparisons are made with the meat of poultry (chickens, turkeys, ducks, and geese). Technically, however, the term meat also includes the meat of wild animals such as rabbits, possums, deer, moose, caribou, bear, wild game birds and many other animals abundant in various parts of the world. Also, the edible flesh of ocean and freshwater fish, seafood, shellfish, and invertebrates is 'meat' including that of tuna, salmon, trout, bass, catfish, etc., and shellfish, such as clams, squid, crabs, and shrimp. The meat of seals, polar bears, and walruses, where not protected, is normally eaten by Eskimos throughout the world including those in Alaska and Canada. In some foreign countries, including third world countries, the meat of the horse, camel, buffalo, goat, dog, and many other species including rodents is eaten. The meat of wild animals and marine foods, however, is not covered to any extent in this volume.

The meat of all mammals, when adjusted for fat, has reasonably similar nutritive values although their sensory properties differ.

II. MEAT AS A FOOD

Our hominid ancestors starting in the Stone Age have consumed meat for several millions of years making meat a 'time honored' food (Eaton and Konner, 1985; Abrams, 1987). Human beings, going back at least 30 000 years have consumed meat, primarily from wild animals until the practice of domestication of animals gradually developed. With the growth of urban centers, a meat marketing trade developed with increasing dependence on farmers and ranchers raising domestic animals for sale or barter. Thus, meat has always been considered a highly valued food (Harris, 1986; Lauwerier, 1986).

A. Preservation Methods

Our rural ancestors, before the advent of electricity and modern refrigeration, have for centuries developed different methods of preserving the meat they obtained by hunting or from growing domesticated animals and fowls. The methods utilized for preservation include drying, smoking, sausage making, salting and, in northern climates, using ice and cold temperatures. According to Stewart and Amerine (1973) canning of meat was developed about 1795 by Nicholas Appert for preserving food for the French Army, even before the discovery of microorganisms and their role in food spoilage. These preservation methods are the forerunners of today's modern processing and packaging methods, which make it possible to have the meat of many species available to consumers the year around in any climate.

B. Meat and Health

In the past 20 years or so, the consumption of red meats on a *per capita* basis has declined from previous record levels. This is the result of changes in eating habits and life styles, the widespread availability of relatively lower cost poultry, and as a result of recommendations by various public health agencies and consumer activists to eat less fat and to consume less red meat in order to prevent cardiovascular disease and cancer (US Senate Select Committee on Nutrition and Human Needs, 1977). Today, contrary to this last point, there is strong agreement, often from the same agencies, that the regular consumption of moderate amounts of lean red meats is a desirable healthful practice (Schweigert *et al.*, 1985; American Dietetic Association, 1986; Hansen *et al.*, 1986; Cronin *et al.*, 1987; Iacono, 1987; Cronin and Shaw, 1988; Mullis and Pirie, 1988; Surgeon General's Report on Nutrition and Health, 1988; Watts *et al.*, 1988; Frantz *et al.*, 1989). Apparently, many health educators and mass media personnel have not 'caught up' with the more recent recommendations.

As a result of what we would call anti-red meat advice, a modified 'new vegetarianism' is popular with about 5–10% of the American public, who avoid consuming red meat, even when it is lean, but do consume poultry, fish, and dairy products. Another problem for an understanding of meat as a food is that animal fats are often equated with 'saturated fats'. This is false and misleading because there are no 'saturated fats' as such in nature but *only fats* with *different proportions* of *saturated* and *unsaturated fatty acids* (Hansen *et al.*, 1986; Moore, 1986; Briggs, 1987). Pork fat (lard) has about 40% of saturated fatty acids and beef fat (tallow) has around 43–50% of saturated fatty acids, depending to some extent on the part of the animal body from which it is derived. When calculated as the percent of total lipids, including the glycerol molecule, phospholipids, etc. in fats, rather than as the percent of the total fatty acids, the percentages become about 10% lower (Breidenstein, 1987). The levels of saturated fatty acids in animal fats are similar to the amounts of saturated fatty acids, including *trans* fatty acids, in many commercial hydrogenated vegetable fats used for shortenings and margarines (see Chapter 2). The outdated advice and short-cut nomenclature in the popular press and even in scientific journals on 'saturated fats' has resulted in huge financial harm to the nation's farmers and to the animal and tropical oil (coconut and palm oil) industries. This misinformation also has resulted in daily meals of lower nutritive value (i.e. less proteins, minerals and vitamins) as well as lesser enjoyment of tasty meals.

The overall purpose of this book is to give the latest possible reliable information on the relationship of meat and health in all of its aspects. This information should prove of value not only to researchers in the field but also to the many nutrition, health, dietetic, medical, and food professionals who give advice to health agencies and to the public. This includes nutrition educators, food editors, and mass media personnel. The book would be useful also as a reference to informed members of the general public.

It is fortunate that this book is published now at the peak of the confusion over the health aspects of red meat. The meat industry is at a crossroads and, although it seems certain that people will always eat meat regardless of negative caveats, the future availability of meat to the population of the world is of current concern.

III. MEAT COMPOSITION

A. Water

The major component of fresh meat is intra- and inter-cellular water, some of which is lost in cooking. Cooked meats average about 58–64% of water (see Table 1-1) which is a major factor in its palatability, and storage ability. Cooked fish is somewhat higher in water content.

B. Protein and Fat

As shown in Table 1-1, other than water, lean cooked meat consists of protein (24–31%) and fat (6–14%). These values are higher than the protein and fat content of lean meat when uncooked because of the loss of moisture during cooking. Meats in general, unlike fruits, root vegetables, legumes, and grains, contain less than 1% of carbohydrates (minor amounts of sugars and glycogen). No starch or fiber (plant types) are present. This is because animals store energy as fat rather than as carbohydrates as plants do.

The protein content of meat is roughly the same as beans or other dried legumes. However, the nutritional quality of meat protein is generally superior to the protein in cooked legumes due to a better balance of amino acids. In mixed diets these differences are generally obscured (Chapter 12). Cooked beans and other legumes provide about the same amount of fat as lean meats, although the fat of beans and legumes when not hydrogenated contains higher levels of monounsaturated and polyunsaturated fatty acids. Of course, there is considerable variation in the fat content of different meat products.

C. Vitamins

All meat provides important amounts of vitamins but in small amounts—less than 0·1% of the total composition, which is not shown in Table 1-1. Meats are important sources of all the B-complex vitamins, including thiamin, riboflavin, niacin activity, biotin, vitamins B_6 and B_{12}, pantothenic acid, and folacin, which is especially abundant in liver (Chapters 14 and 15). Liver and certain other organs supply appreciable amounts of vitamins A, D, E, and K (Chapter 13).

TABLE 1-1

APPROXIMATE COMPOSITION OF VARIOUS MEATS READY-TO-EAT (COOKED) AND FAT-TRIMMED[a]

Type of meat	*Amount per 100 g of cooked lean meat*							
	Kcalories (%)	*Moisture*[b] (*water*) (%)	*Protein* (%)	*Carbo-hydrates* (%)	*Ash*[c] (*minerals*) (%)	*Total fat* (%)	*Saturated fatty acids* (%)	*Cholesterol* (*mg*)
Beef—round (broiled)	190	66	27	<1	1·4	6·2	2·2	84
Pork—leg (broiled)	220	62	26	<1	1·1	11·0	3·8	94
Lamb—shank (roasted)	180	64	28	<1	1·1	6·7	1·8	87
Chicken—breast (roasted—no skin)	170	64	31	<1	1·0	4·3	1·3	79
Chicken—dark (fried with skin)	240	59	26	<1	1·0	14·0	4·2	88
Turkey—dark (roasted with skin)	200	58	29	<1	1·0	11·8	3·5	79
Fish (salmon) (broiled)	160	68	24	<1	1·5	6·2	1·1	47

[a] Adapted from Briggs and Calloway (1984) and Breidenstein (1987) and based on USDA *Handbook 8* values.
[b] The moisture (water) values are rounded off and calculated by subtracting values for protein, fat, and ash from 100.
[c] Values for ash (total minerals) of meat other than the first three items are estimated.

D. Minerals, including Trace Elements

Unprocessed cooked meats, without bones, contain only very minor amounts of calcium and low levels of sodium, with about 60–90 mg per serving (Chapter 11). Meat contributes significant amounts of magnesium (about 25–30 mg per serving), phosphorus (200 to 250 mg per serving), and potassium (about 220–360 mg per serving) (Breidenstein, 1987; also see Chapter 11).

Meats are excellent sources of trace elements such as iron, copper, zinc, and manganese and the newer 'ultra trace elements' (Chapters 8, 9, and 10). These minerals are not easily obtained from daily meals in sufficient amounts in diets without meat. Meats, as is true with all foods, contain traces of many non-essential elements.

E. Other Nutrients and Non-nutrients

Essential nutrients that are low in, or missing, in cooked muscle meats include vitamin C, calcium, plant fibers, fat soluble vitamins, and carbohydrates, which are easily provided in the usual daily menu from a variety of foods consumed, in moderation, and chosen from the well known food groups. Only carnivorous animals, such as members of the feline species, depend nearly entirely on the consumption of animal tissues.

Meat contains cholesterol, but in relatively moderate amounts generally falling in the range of 70–90 mg/100 g for cooked meat (Table 1-1). The relationship between cholesterol intake and blood cholesterol is covered in Chapter 3 and as pointed out, dietary cholesterol is probably of relatively little importance to most consumers. Many of the fatty acids and amino acids in meat are not essential nutrients. However, they are 'nutrients' in that they contribute energy and have metabolic functions in the body (Chapters 2 and 12).

F. Species Differences

The values presented in Table 1-1 do not show the usually small but important differences in composition of meat and its components from the various cuts and species of meat animals. The small differences within and between species are determined largely by the genetic background of the animal, by the type of feed eaten and feeding and finishing practices, by age, by differences in the environment, and by processing, storage, and marketing practices. One important species difference is that pork muscle contains much greater quantities of thiamin (vitamin B_1) than beef or lamb muscle cuts or organ meats. The composition, flavor, and cooking characteristics of the unsaturated fatty acids from monogastric species can be particularly affected by the composition of the fatty portion of the animal's diet. The common practice of using standardized feeding and rearing methods in the nutrition of domestic animals and poultry generally prevent any major differences in flavour from occurring. However, major differences in the fat content of meat can occur due to feeding and management, especially for beef, lamb, and pork.

The meat resulting from so called 'natural' or 'organic' rearing practices does not provide any more nutritional or health-providing benefits than that from conventionally raised animals. However, aside from generally being leaner the meat of chickens or pigs reared in open pens or fields may have a different flavor, since grass, weeds, insects, manure, soil, etc. are freely available to the free-ranging animals.

G. Additional Compositional Information

Recent values for the nutrient content of various retail cuts of Canadian beef and pork are given by Stewart and Wood (1987) and Wood *et al.* (1988). A series of fourteen reports on the composition of Australian pork, poultry, beef, lamb, rabbits, etc. were recently published by Greenfield (1987). Many other reports are available in the recent literature on meat composition from different countries, but no attempt is made to cite these herein. In the United States, the basic source for meat and processed meat composition is found in the revised *Handbooks 8* (nos. 7, 10, and 13) available from the US Government Printing Office.

IV. MEAT CONSUMPTION

In the United States we eat an average of about 220 lb (100 kg) of red meats and poultry per person per year based on 'disappearance' figures (USDA, 1988). This is roughly about 14% of our total food intake, and after adjusting for fat trimming, cooking losses, and plate waste, amounts to about 16% of our total energy intake (National Live Stock and Meat Board, 1984; Rathje and Ho, 1987). The National Live Stock and Meat Board (1984) has estimated that we consume only about 66% of ready-to-eat edible meat from retail cuts due not only to losses in fat during cooking but also to the types of wastage mentioned above along with discarded bones. There is more wastage in pork than in beef. Of course, losses exist for all types of meat, as well as for fruit, vegetables, and carbohydrate foods, after trimming, cooking, and plate waste are taken into account.

Meat intake varies with social, economic, political, and geographical

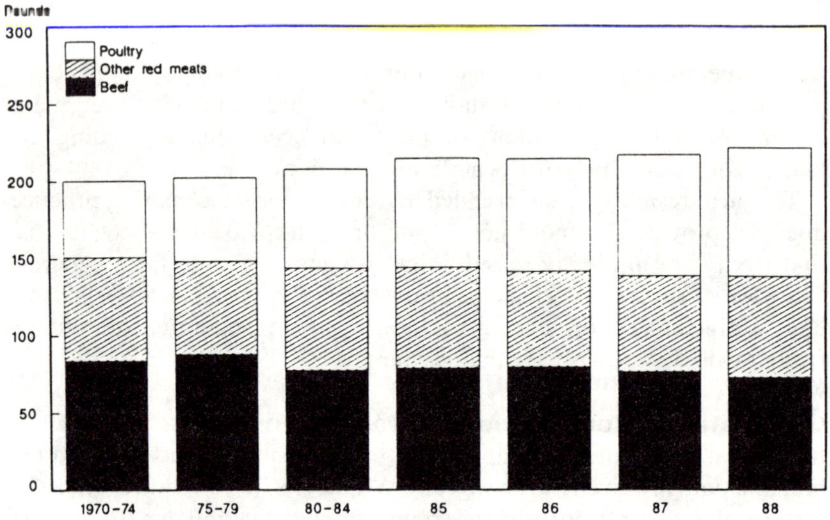

FIG. 1-1. US and world meat and poultry production from 1980 to 1988 by species (USDA, 1988).

differences on a world wide basis. Certain South American countries, for instance (such as Argentina and Uruguay), and New Zealand and Australia consume more red meat on a *per capita* basis than the United States, Canada, and most European countries. In economically deprived parts of the world meat intake is considerably less.

About 150 million metric tons of meat (red meats and poultry) are produced annually on a world wide basis. The United States produces about 27 million metric tons per year or about 18% of the world's total production (Fig. 1-1—USDA, 1988). The total amount of all meat produced world wide increases each year—especially pork and poultry—due to increases in the world population and as a result of improved production practices.

A. Meat Consumption in United States

Figure 1-2 shows detailed trends of meat intake since 1970–74 in the United States. There has been a slow, but inconsistent, decline in beef consumption since the 1975–79 peak period to the current figure of about 70 lb (32 kg) per person per year based on retail meat availability statistics. Poultry has, on the other hand, surpassed beef in consumption—up to a total consumption

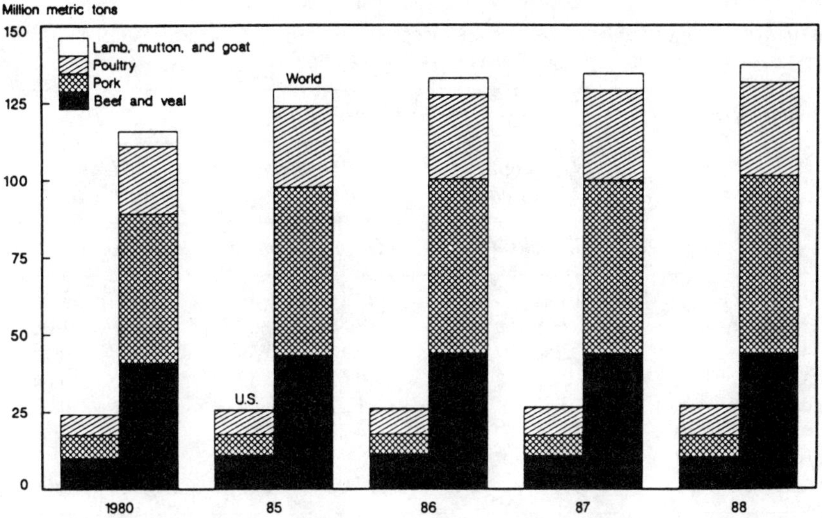

FIG. 1-2. *Per capita* meat and poultry consumption (disappearance data) in United States by species for selected years between 1970 and 1988 (USDA, 1988).

of about 78 lb (35 kg) *per capita* in 1988. In comparison, total lamb disappearance is now about only 1·1 lb (0·5 kg) *per capita* per year, while total fish is up to about 15 lb (7 kg) *per capita* in 1985 and is still gaining (National Research Council, 1988). Turkey consumption comprises about 19% of the total poultry figure.

As is well known, 'averages' can be misleading when dealing with any heterogenous populations of various ages, culture, meat consumption habits, and with social–economic differences. Table 1-2 provides estimated daily intake data for cooked red meats in the US diet for 1984. These values are based on a telephone survey of 1211 individuals made for the National Live Stock and Meat Board (Breidenstein and Williams, 1987; National Research Council, 1988). The values are broken down by different habits of meat consumption and are corrected for cooking losses and trimmable and discarded fat. The table shows the average *per capita* consumption by 'light' consumers of meat is 41 g (1·45 oz) per day, by 'moderate' consumers amounts to 117 g (4·14 oz) per day, and 'heavy' consumers eat 216 g (7·66 oz) per day. The values include beef, ground beef, pork, lamb, veal, and processed meats.

TABLE 1-2

ESTIMATED AVERAGE DAILY CONSUMPTION OF COOKED RED MEATS FOR LIGHT, MODERATE AND HEAVY MEAT EATERS IN US FOR 1984[a,b]

Red meat	*Consumption level*					
	Light meat eaters		*Moderate meat eaters*		*Heavy meat eaters*	
	Grams	*Ounces*	*Grams*	*Ounces*	*Grams*	*Ounces*
Beef	16·31	0·57	42·16	1·49	67·44	2·38
Ground beef	7·89	0·28	17·50	0·62	30·14	1·06
Pork	2·80	0·10	11·17	0·39	21·99	0·78
Lamb	0·32	0·01	0·62	0·02	1·23	0·04
Veal	0·63	0·02	1·22	0·04	2·41	0·09
Processed meat	13·18	0·47	44·33	1·56	93·11	2·38
Total red meat ingested	41·14	1·45	117·00	4·14	216·31	7·66

[a] The values are reconciled from data on total amounts of red meat available for consumption in the United States. (The values are corrected for cooking losses and for amounts of trimmable fat discarded by consumers, assuming that no meat spoiled.)
[b] Adapted from Breidenstein and Williams (1987).

The nutrients contributed by these amounts of meat consumed by the different segments of meat eaters are shown in Table 1-3 (National Research Council, 1988). These are useful figures and serve as background information for many of the following chapters.

Table 1-4 shows trends in consumption between 1977 and 1985 in red meats, poultry, organ meats, processed meats, and fish and shellfish (National Academy of Sciences, 1988). Values are given for the actual amount of meat consumed for any one day rather than averages for longer periods. They are broken down for children ages 1–5, females ages 19–50, and males ages 19–50. Such data are very useful in the undertaking and evaluation of nutritional surveys, of nutrition education programs, and of nutrition research.

B. Factors Affecting Meat Consumption

Many factors determine meat consumption practices—or in other words, consumer demand and supply ratios. A summary of these factors include individual tastes based on cultural and social differences, geographical differences (i.e. differences between Eskimos and Midwestern farmers,

TABLE 1-3

NUTRIENT CONTRIBUTION OF TOTAL COOKED RED MEAT BY CONSUMPTION LEVELS IN THE US DIET FOR 1984[a,b,c,d]

Nutrient	*Consumption levels*			*Total ingested by average user*	*RDA (%)*[b]
	Light	*Moderate*	*Heavy*		
Total red meat[c] (g)	41·14	117·00	216·31	118·89	
Total red meat (oz)	1·45	4·13	7·63	4·19	
Calories (kcal)	117·5	334·9	618·1	340·1	17·0
Cholesterol (mg)	33·4	92·2	167·8	93·2	—
Lipids (g)	8·48	24·46	45·55	24·95	—
Protein (g)	9·47	26·33	47·57	26·44	47·2
Vitamins					
Niacin (mg)	1·751	4·911	9·062	4·998	27·8
Riboflavin (mg)	0·063	0·189	0·372	0·198	12·4
Thiamin (mg)	0·091	0·302	0·605	0·317	22·7
Vitamin B_{12} (μg)	0·830	2·207	3·899	2·200	73·3
Minerals					
Iron (mg)	0·91	2·49	4·44	2·50	25·0
Sodium (mg)	160·9	526·4	1 086·4	568·4	17·2–51·7
Zinc (mg)	1·77	4·75	8·27	4·71	31·4

[a] The values are reconciled from data on total amounts of red meat available for consumption in the United States. (The values are corrected for cooking losses and for amounts of trimmable fat discarded by consumers, assuming that no meat spoiled.)

[b] This column represents the percentage of recommended dietary allowances (RDAs) for males aged 23–50 except for lipids, cholesterol, calories, and sodium entries. There are no RDAs for lipids and cholesterol. The calorie percentage is based on 2000 kcal mean energy needs of a 154-lb sedentary US adult male or active female. The sodium percentage is based on a 1100–3300-mg range of estimated safe and adequate daily intake for adults (National Research Council, 1980).

[c] Red meat is beef, veal, pork, and lamb. In this case, the category also includes processed meats.

[d] Adapted from Breidenstein and Williams (1987).

people in large urban centers, coastal and island dwellers, etc.); religious beliefs, cost of production and economic factors; perceived or actual health and food safety concerns (including microbial contamination); food advertising and nutrition education; convenience and fast food factors, packaging factors; availability of refrigeration; a desire for variety in one's own food selections, and many other reasons. A number of research studies have been conducted to examine some of these factors (Breidenstein, 1988).

TABLE 1.4
TRENDS IN CONSUMPTION AND MEAN INTAKE OF MEAT, POULTRY, AND FISH[a,b,c]

Group and food	Number of survey participants		Mean intake (g/day)		Percent consuming	
	1977	1985	1977	1985	1977	1985
Children, 1–5	690	548				
Beef			21	14	29·1	17·5
Pork			7	7	20·5	16·2
Lamb, veal and game			—[b]	1	0·3	1·4
Organ meats			—[b]	—[b]	0·7	0·3
Frankfurters, sausages, and luncheon meats			15	12	33·1	28·2
Chicken			17	16	17·0	19·6
Fish and shellfish			5	5	7·0	8·1
Mixtures[a]			45	45	34·7	32·0
Females, 19–50	2 228	1 503				
Beef			49	27	34·9	23·1
Pork			18	14	24·0	20·5
Lamb, veal and game			1	1	1·3	1·0
Organ meats			1	1	0·9	1·0
Frankfurters, sausages, and luncheon meats			16	13	25·1	24·6
Chicken			22	19	16·1	16·8
Fish and shellfish			11	13	9·8	11·5
Mixtures[a]			65	88	33·2	37·1
Males, 19–50	1 778	1 134				
Beef			80	52	42·0	28·3
Pork			28	26	28·2	25·3
Lamb, veal and game			3	1	1·9	0·5
Organ meats			2	1	1·4	0·4
Frankfurters, sausages and luncheon meats			32	27	35·7	31·4
Chicken			28	23	14·0	13·3
Fish and shellfish			14	21	8·5	11·4
Mixtures[a]			105	110	39·0	39·7

[a] Mixtures are mainly meat, poultry, or fish.
[b] Values are less than 0·5 but more than 0·0.
[c] Adapted for women 19–50 years and their children 1–5 years, 1 day, 1985 (USDA, 1986).

V. MEAT, MEAT FAT, AND CHRONIC DISEASES

A. Meat versus Vegetarianism

While lean meat is one of the most popular foods in the diet, today excessive meat fat is not acceptable in developed countries. Lean meat is 'nutrient dense' since it provides a greater proportion of the required amounts of major nutrients (proteins, vitamins, and minerals) in relation to the calories it supplies. For this and other reasons, there is general agreement on the value of lean meat in the diet by most private and public agencies who give dietary guidelines to the general public (Schweigert *et al.*, 1985; American Dietetic Association, 1986; Hansen *et al.*, 1986; Cronin *et al.*, 1987; Iacono, 1987; Cronin and Shaw, 1988; Mullis and Pirie, 1988; Surgeon General's Report on Nutrition and Health, 1988; Watts *et al.*, 1988).

There are exceptions to this positive advice for meat by such groups as those with religious beliefs against the eating of meat, and by those persons making up the 'new vegetarians'. Persons in the latter group do not eat red meat because of their concern over 'animal rights' or animal welfare. Still other non-meat consumers have a concern over the perceived presence of toxic substances from the use of 'chemicals', hormones, growth promotants, and possible contaminants in the raising of animals. Chapter 6 discusses residues in the meat.

With these exceptions, the most recent dietary guidelines by public and private groups in the United States, Canada, and in many other countries consistently recommend consumption of lean red meat, poultry (with the skin removed), and fish (Schweigert *et al.*, 1985; Schweigert, 1986; Iacono, 1987; Cronin and Shaw, 1988; Lewis, 1988; Mullis and Pirie, 1988; National Research Council, 1988; Surgeon General's Report on Nutrition and Health, 1988; McGinnis and Nestle, 1989).

B. Meat Fat and Fatty Acids

Eating the fat of meat and advice related to doing so, however, is another matter and not without great differences of opinion. The excessive intake of any fats, including plant and vegetable fat and oils and hydrogenated fats, is not recommended by anyone except for otherwise healthy persons who have insufficient energy intake or insufficient intake of essential fatty acids. In fact, it is well accepted that the intake of excessive fat, over one's caloric needs, is an important risk factor in cardiovascular disease, hypertension, stroke, diabetes, obesity, and/or specific types of cancer (Cronin and Shaw, 1988; Lewis, 1988; Surgeon General's Report, 1988; National Research Council, 1988; McGinnis and Nestle, 1989). When not eaten in excess of one's caloric needs, in an otherwise nutritionally balanced diet, the evidence that moderate amounts of animal fats are harmful is sparse (Cliff, 1987; Stehbens, 1989).

Since the 1950s it has been clear that dietary fatty acids, and hence fats, differ rather markedly in affecting blood cholesterol and other blood lipid levels. Advice to individuals today generally limits intake of saturated fatty acids to not more than 10% of one's caloric intake, which translates to 22 g (0·77 oz) per day in a 2000 kcalorie diet. Current recommendations for intake of polyunsaturated fatty acids are also to limit them to 10% of calories but for a different reason—the possibility of increased cancer risk and oxidative destruction of nutrients and food flavors. Monounsaturated fatty acids make up the rest of the recommended 30–35% of calorie intake (American Heart Association, 1988; Kris-Etherton *et al.*, 1988). More details on the effects of various fatty acids is discussed in Chapters 2 and 3.

The ratio of polyunsaturated fatty acids to saturated fatty acids (P/S ratio) has been commonly used in research experiments on diets as they relate to blood lipid levels. The P/S ratio, however, is outmoded because of recent studies on genetic and other types of biological variation among people in response to changes in dietary fatty acid intake. Also, it is now clear that there are many differences from the effects of different fatty acids within and beyond these categories. For instance, the higher polyunsaturated fatty acids found in fish oils are known to be metabolized differently than linoleic acid, the common essential fatty acids with two double bonds (Becker *et al.*, 1983; Herold and Kinsella, 1986).

Another example, stearic acid, one of the common saturated fatty acids found in many animal fats in relatively large amounts, is converted in the body to oleic acid, the most abundant monounsaturated fatty acid. Hence, stearic acid behaves in the diet as a monounsaturated fatty acid (Bonanome and Grundy, 1988). In fact, Grundy (1989) has recently proposed that 'new flexibility' is needed in giving dietary advice 'for improved adherence by the public'. Grundy (1989) has suggested a diet with a maximum of 7% of calories from both polyunsaturated fatty acids and saturated fatty acids (other than stearic acid), and from 10–25% of calories from monounsaturated fatty acids. This makes a total of 24–39% of calories from fat (or 53–87 g in a 2000 kcalorie diet) which is more in accord with 'traditional American eating habits' (Grundy, 1989). This is a liberal departure from the more restrictive dietary advice being offered by some current dietary guidelines, but still a convincing approach. Future studies should be watched with interest. For more information on the metabolic behavior of different fatty acids, readers are referred to Chapter 2.

Because of the significant differences in the fatty acid content of various types of animal fats, it is not difficult to see why a number of scientists in this area feel it is too early to make restrictive recommendations for animal fat intake by the entire population (Hansen *et al.*, 1986; Cliff, 1987; Goldbourt, 1987; McNamara *et al.*, 1987; Oliver, 1987; Palumbo, 1988; Stehbens, 1989). It is essential that still better controlled experiments in humans and improved epidemiological studies be made to get better information on this important topic. It is becoming more evident, for instance, that when caloric intake is controlled fats have no more effect on cancer incidence than carbohydrates (Simopoulos, 1987). Discussion of this topic is reviewed in Chapter 4.

With so much debate going on over dietary cholesterol and fat in the diet it is interesting to note that Taylor *et al.* (1987) concluded that:

> For persons aged 20 to 60 years who are at low risk, we calculate a gain in life expectancy of 3 days to 3 months from a lifetime program of cholesterol reduction. For persons who are at high risk the calculated gain ranges from 18 days to 12 months.

The topic of dietary cholesterol and its relationship to coronary vascular disease is discussed in Chapter 3.

It is time that dietary guidelines for the public and nutrition education programs take a more positive approach to the development of eating habits. Eating should be an enjoyable experience for normal persons with low chronic disease risk factors and with moderate eating habits, normal weights, and regular exercise habits. We can still eat well and include in our diets within caloric limitations moderate amounts of such foods as red meats, luncheon meats, sausages, pork rind, which is said to be a favorite snack of President Bush, bacon, smoked meats, and a piece of pecan pie, chocolate or 'rich' cake on special occasions.

VI. NUTRIENTS IN MEAT AND HEALTH

Meat is a complex, natural biological material designed by nature as the major structural and temperature regulating protein source in the animal or human body. Muscle has many physiological functions. The chapters that follow discuss the various classes of nutrients in meat and their relationship to health—fat and fatty acids (Chapters 2 and 3), minerals (Chapters 8, 9, 10 and 11), protein (Chapter 12) and essential fatty acids (Chapter 2), and vitamins (Chapters 13, 14 and 15). Carbohydrates are not discussed since such small amounts are present. Thus, carbohydrates do not serve as significant sources of energy in meat, with the exception of glycogen in lean muscle and liver, which provides a limited source of energy for short periods. Although many other carbohydrates are present in small amounts, they are all made in the body and, hence, are not essential nutrients.

Meat contains small amounts of essential trace elements not covered in this book such as iodine, molybdenum, chromium, selenium, nickel, and vanadium.

VII. NON-NUTRIENTS IN MEAT

Meat, including cured meats, literally contains thousands of different compounds many of which contribute to or are the result of normal metabolism in muscle. Some, no doubt, remain unidentified. Because they do not play a direct dietary role in the health of people these non-nutrients are not generally discussed in this volume on meat and health. For instance, among the many cellular metabolites and components of muscle tissue are many enzymes, proteins, non-dietary essential coenzymes, peptides, nucleic acids, nucleosides and nucleotides, purines and pyrimidines, pigments, volatile and non-volatile flavors, phenolics, natural hormones and hormone-like compounds, other steroids including cholesterol, hundreds of natural nitrogen and non-protein containing compounds (i.e. amines, polyamines, nitrates, carnitine, creatinine, most phospholipids, choline, lipoic acid, taurine, etc.), non-essential minerals, and many environmental contaminants present at insignificant levels just as is the case in vegetables, fruits, and grains (Briggs and Calloway, 1984). Meat also contains collagen which, when present in large enough amounts, can serve as a source of bulk in the diet functioning in absorption of water similar to dietary fiber (Pearson, 1987).

VIII. OTHER HEALTH CONCERNS

Chapter 17 covers newer methods of meat processing, packaging, and marketing which affect the nutritive value of meat and meat products. When most any food is over-cooked (including meats, poultry, fish, and legumes) mutagens and mutagen-like substances can be formed depending on the length of time and the temperature, which is reviewed in Chapter 5.

There is no evidence that the trace amounts of these mutagens in normal food products provide a significant risk to human health.

The subject of meat standards, new government meat grades and how they affect fat levels and quality of meats has been briefly covered in Chapter 16. The subject of meat pathogens as they may affect health is discussed in Chapter 7.

IX. SUMMARY

Meat has been used as a food by human beings throughout recorded history. Preservation of meat by drying, smoking, salting and canning plus the use of low temperature storage (refrigeration and freezing) has made meat products available throughout the year. Thus, meat has played an important role in meeting nutrient needs of human beings.

Although research has shown meat is not only a flavorful product that provides protein, essential minerals, including trace elements, and vitamins (especially B vitamins), in recent years meat has been attacked as contributing to the degenerative diseases, including cardiovascular disease (heart attacks), stroke and cancer. As a result, vegetarianism has become increasingly more popular among some segments of the population, especially among young adults, who may not receive adequate amounts of minerals and vitamins on strict vegetarian diets. The subject of animal fats and the terms saturated and unsaturated fatty acids are clarified and discussed to set the stage for discussion on the role of animal fats and fatty acids on the health and well being of those that are regular consumers of meat or meat products. Cholesterol and its presence and concentration in various meat items is also discussed to introduce the chapter dealing with the relationship between dietary and blood cholesterol.

The contributions of red meat and poultry meat in providing essential minerals and vitamins is briefly introduced to allow development of a number of chapters dealing with the functions of essential minerals and trace elements, vitamins and proteins to the health and well being of man. The introduction is intended to lay a foundation for discussion of the metabolic function(s) of each essential nutrient and the contribution or lack of contribution that meat makes to requirements. It also introduces discussion of the effects of meat processing upon the various nutrients.

Ground work is also laid for discussion of toxic compounds produced during meat processing and the probable hazards to human health from meat pathogens and various residues in meat and poultry products. Such concerns are important and are the basis for further discussion in the chapters covering these topics.

This chapter covers not only an introduction to the specific nutrients in meat and poultry products but also discusses problems with which meat producers and nutrition scientists should be aware in order to assure the health and well being of consumers. Overall, the discussion concludes that meat is a nutrient-dense food and provides a number of essential nutrients that are important to the health and well being of mankind.

X. REFERENCES

ABRAMS, H. L., JR (1987). The preference for animal protein and fat: A cross-cultural survey. In *Food and Evolution, Toward a Theory of Human Food Habits* (M. Harris and E. B. Ross, Eds), p. 207. Temple University Press, Philadelphia.

AMERICAN DIETETIC ASSOCIATION (1986). The American Dietetic Association's nutrition recommendations for women. *J. Am. Diet. Assoc.* **86,** 1663.

AMERICAN HEART ASSOCIATION (1988). Dietary guidelines for healthy American adults. *Arteriosclerosis* **8**, 218A.

BECKER, N., ILLINGWORTH, D. R., ALAUPOVIC, P., CONNOR, W. E. and SUNDBERG, W. E. (1983). Effects of saturated, monounsaturated, and omega-6 polyunsaturated fatty acids on plasma lipids, lipoproteins and apoproteins in humans. *Am. J. Clin. Nutr.* **37**, 355.

BONANOME, A. and GRUNDY, S. M. (1988). Effect of dietary stearic acid on plasma cholesterol and lipoprotein levels. *New Engl. J. Med.* **318**, 1244.

BREIDENSTEIN, B. C. (1987). Nutrient value of meat. *Food & Nutrition News* **59**(2), 43.

BREIDENSTEIN, B. C. (1988). Changes in consumer attitudes toward red meat and their effect on marketing strategy. *Food Technol* **82**(1), 112.

BREIDENSTEIN, B. C. and WILLIAMS, J. C. (1987). *Contributions of Red Meat to the US Diet.* National Live Stock and Meat Board, Chicago, Illinois.

BRIGGS, G. M. (1987). The red meat controversy. *Sci. Food Agric.* **5**(2), 2.

BRIGGS, G. M. and CALLOWAY, D. H. (1984). *Nutrition and Physical Fitness.* Holt, Rinehart and Winston, New York.

CLIFF, W. J. (1987). Coronary heart disease: Animal fat on trial. *Pathology* **19**, 325.

CRONIN, F. J. and SHAW, A. M. (1988). Summary of dietary recommendations for healthy Americans. *Nutr. Today* **23**(6), 26.

CRONIN, F. J., SHAW, A. M., KREBS-SMITH, S. M., MARSLAND, P. M. and LIGHT, L. (1987). Developing a food guidance system to implement the dietary guidelines. *J. Nutr. Educ.* **19**, 281.

EATON, S. B. and KONNER, M. (1985). Paleolithic nutrition: A consideration of its nature and current implications. *New Engl. J. Med.* **312**, 283.

FRANTZ, I. D., JR, DAWSON, E. A., ASHMAN, P. L., GATEWOOD, L. C., BARTSCH, G. E., KUBA, K. and BREWER, E. R. (1989). Test of effect of lipid lowering by diet on cardiovascular risk. *Arteriosclerosis* **9**, 129.

GOLDBOURT, U. (1987). High risk versus public health strategies in primary prevention of coronary heart disease. *Am. J. Clin. Nutr.* **45**, 1185.

GREENFIELD, H. (Ed.) (1987). The nutrient composition of Australian meats and poultry. *Food Technol. Australia* **39**(5), 181.

GRUNDY, S. M. (1989). Grundy proposes new, more palatable cholesterol dietary strategy. *Food Chem. News* **30**(47), 55.

HANSEN, R. G., WINDHAM, C. T., WITTWER, C. T. and WYSE, B. W. (1986). Placing the role of meat in human nutrition in perspective. *J. Anim. Sci.* **62** (Suppl. 1), 7.

HARRIS, M. (1986). The 100 000-year hunt. *The Sciences 1986* (Jan.), 22.

HEROLD, P. M. and KINSELLA, J. E. (1986). Fish oil consumption and decreased risk of cardiovascular disease: A comparison of findings from animal and human feeding trials. *Am. J. Clin. Nutr.* **43**, 566.

IACONO, J. M. (1987). Dietary intervention studies to reduce risk factors related to cardiovascular diseases and cancer. *Prev. Med.* **16**, 516.

KRIS-ETHERTON, P. M., KRUMMEL, D., RUSSELL, M. E., DREON, D., MACKEY, S., BORCHERS, J. and WOOD, P. D. (1988). The effect of diet on plasma lipids, lipoproteins, and coronary heart disease. *J. Am. Diet. Assoc.* **88**, 1373.

LAUWERIER, R. C. G. M. (1986). The role of meat in the Roman diet. *Endeavour* **10**(4), 208.

LEWIS, C. (1988). New guidelines for high blood cholesterol: Summary of the 1987 report of the Adult Treatment Panel of the National Cholesterol Education Program. *Clin. Nutr.* **7**, 232.

MCGINNIS, J. M. and NESTLE, M. (1989). The surgeon general's report on nutrition and health: Policy implications and implementation strategies. *Am. J. Clin. Nutr.* **49**, 23.

MCNAMARA, D. J., KOLB, R., PARKER, T. S., BATWIN, H., SAMUEL, P., BROWN, C. D. and AHRENS, E. H., JR (1987). Heterogeneity of cholesterol homeostasis in man. *J. Clin. Invest.* **79**, 1729.

MOORE, T. (1986). All clear for beef fat? *Lancet* (Feb. 15), 389.

MULLIS, R. M. and PIRIE, P. (1988). Lean meats make the grade—A collaborative nutrition intervention program. *J. Am. Diet. Assoc.* **88**, 191.

NATIONAL LIVE STOCK AND MEAT BOARD (1984). *Red Meat in the Diet: A new look.* National Live Stock and Meat Board, Chicago, Illinois.

NATIONAL RESEARCH COUNCIL (1980). *Recommended Dietary Allowances.* National Academy Press, Washington, DC.

NATIONAL RESEARCH COUNCIL (1988). *Designing Foods, Animal Product Options in the Marketplace.* National Academy Press, Washington, DC.

OLIVER, M. F. (1987). Dietary fat and coronary heart disease: There is much more to learn. *Cardiology* **74**, 22.

PALUMBO, P. J. (1988). National Cholesterol Education Program: Does the Emperor have any clothes? *Mayo Clin. Proc.* **63**, 88.

PEARSON, A. M. (1987). Summary of collagen as a food symposium. *Advances in Meat Research Vol. 4.* Elsevier Science Publishers, London, p. 377.

RATHJE, W. L. and HO, E. E. (1987). Meat fat madness: Conflicting patterns of meat fat consumption and their public health implications. *J. Am. Diet. Assoc.* **87**, 1357.

SCHWEIGERT, B. S. (1985–86). Human nutrition dietary guidelines and their future significance. *J. Anim. Sci.* **62** (Suppl. 1), 16.

SCHWEIGERT, B., KAMIN, H., KRITCHEVSKY, D., OLSON, R. E., SALANS, L., LEY, R., MILLER, S. A., STERN, J. S. and STARE, F. J. (1985). Dietary Guidelines for Americans. *Home and Garden Bulletin No. 232* 2nd edn, US Dept of Agriculture, Washington, DC.

SIMOPOULOS, A. P. (1987). Calories and energy expenditure in carcinogenesis: Conference report. *J. Am. Diet. Assoc.* **87**, 92.

STEHBENS, W. E. (1989). Diet and atherogenesis. *Nutr. Reviews* **47**(1), 1.

STEWART, G. F. and AMERINE, M. A. (1973). *Introduction to Food Science and Technology*. Academic Press, New York.

STEWART, L. M. and WOOD, D. F. (1987). Physical composition and cooking yields of retail cuts of Canadian beef and pork. *J. Can. Diet. Assoc.* **48**(2), 103.

SURGEON GENERAL'S REPORT ON NUTRITION AND HEALTH (1988). Summary and Recommendations. *Nutr. Today* **23**(5), 22. (Full report from Supt of Documents, US Govt Printing Office, Washington, DC, GPO Stock No. 017-001-00465-1.)

TAYLOR, W. C., PASS, T. M., SHEPARD, D. S. and KOMAROFF, A. L. (1987). Cholesterol reduction and life expectancy. *Annals Intern. Med.* **106**, 605.

USDA (1986). Nationwide Food Consumption Survey, Continuing Survey of Food Intakes by Individuals. Human Nutrition Information Service. Rpt No. 85-3. US Department of Agriculture, Washington, DC.

USDA (1988). Meat and livestock production. In *1988 Agricultural Chartbook; Agricultural Handbook No. 673*. p. 21. US Dept of Agriculture, Washington, DC.

US SENATE SELECT COMMITTEE ON NUTRITION AND HUMAN NEEDS (1977). Dietary Goals for US. Index. No. 052-070-04376-8. US Government Printing Office, Washington, DC.

WATTS, G. F., AHMED, W., QUINEY, J., HOULSTON, R., JACKSON, P., ILES, C. and LEWIS, B. (1988). Effective lipid lowering diets including lean meat. *Brit. Med. J.* **296**, 235.

WOOD, D. F., STEWART, L. M. and CAMPBELL, C. A. (1988). Nutrient composition of 21 retail cuts of Canadian beef. *J. Can. Diet. Assoc.* **49**(1), 29.

2

Meat Fats and Fatty Acids

RAYMOND REISER

*Department of Biochemistry and Biophysics,
Texas Agricultural Experiment Station, Texas A&M University System,
Texas, USA*

AND

F. B. SHORLAND

*School of Biological Sciences,
Victoria University of Wellington, Wellington,
New Zealand*

'The stone that the builders rejected has become the chief corner stone'
(Psalms 118:22)

I. INTRODUCTION

During the past 25 years, and with increasing emphasis, dietary fat has been getting a bad press. It has replaced starches and other carbohydrates as the reputed major contributor to obesity. Dietary fats are said to promote, and possibly initiate, breast and colon cancer, although meat fats to a lesser degree than polyunsaturated vegetable oils. The latter are said to have other undesirable characteristics: they form deleterious in-vivo peroxides, free radicals, polymers, and ceroids. They also increase the vitamin E requirement. More recently linoleic acid has been implicated in blood platelet adhesiveness and thrombosis. It was for those reasons that the recommendation in favor of a high level of linoleic acid was reduced to the same low 10% of calories as for saturated fatty acids; but one does not hear the same unremitting castigations against them. In moderation all fats are healthy foods. There is a biochemical balance in omnivorous animals, especially in man, for the metabolism of dietary plant, terrestrial animal, and fish fats.

The most severe charge against dietary saturated fat, especially meat fat, in addition to its high calorie content is that it is a major contributor to the development of atherosclerosis and coronary heart disease (CHD). In view of these concepts, the National Cholesterol Education Program (NCEP) (1988) has recommended that everyone limit fat consumption to less than 30% of total calories and increase carbohydrates to about 50 or 60%. However, there is concern that changes in plasma glucose, insulin, triglycerides, and lipoproteins, which can accompany such high carbohydrate diets, can actually increase the risk of CHD and induce diabetes in susceptible people (Houtsmuller, 1975; Reaven, 1988).

Within the past few years new data on human biochemical responses to dietary fats and oils are prompting reassessment of the diet:heart theory. Dietary oleic and stearic acids, previously considered as having no effect on blood cholesterol (or stearic acid as being included among the hypercholesterolemic saturated acids) were found to produce lower plasma cholesterol than complex carbohydrates to which they were compared. It has also been found that the *n*-3 fatty acids of fish oils control the level of plasma triglycerides and also inhibit cyclooxygenase activity, thus constraining the level of thromboxane $A_2(TXA_2)$, which is responsible for blood platelet adhesiveness and the resultant thrombosis and CHD. These new observations are resulting in revision of the controversial saturated (meat) fat:CHD theory. The chapter will review and critically examine the data and rationalization of the evolution of the diet:heart theory, revised by the American Heart Association (AHA) (1986) and the National Cholesterol Education Program (NCEP) (1988). It will also discuss the impact on the diet:heart theory of the new observations outlined above, and suggest how the composition of the fat of meat animals may be modified to take advantage of the new knowledge.

II. NUTRITIVE VALUES OF FATS

A. Meat Fats and Vegetable Oils

Over the years excesses and deficiencies of fats, carbohydrates, and proteins have each, in turn, been accused of being the cause or a contributing factor to various diseases. A potential drawback of authoritative recommendations to limit or increase consumption of a food constituent is that the advice can assume the force of a proscription or prescription and lead to unbalanced diets. With little justification, the usual level of American dietary fat, about 40% of total calories, has been accused of being the major cause, directly or indirectly, of obesity, diabetes, cancer, suppression of the immune response, etc., as well as of CHD.

Besides being present in natural foods, fats and oils are necessary constituents of, or adjuncts to, spreads, shortenings, gravies, dressings, and sauces and to many if not most prepared foods, and, if not naturally present, must be added. Almost all baked goods, i.e. cakes and cookies, crackers, and most breads, would be unacceptable, if not impossible to make, without the addition of fat. For many of these functions vegetable oils have advantages over animal fats, explaining their popularity and why they quickly replaced animal fat after development of technical processes for their production. Many resist oxidation better because of constituent antioxidants, have a better flavor, and are high in most fat soluble vitamins. The charge that *trans* acids of partially hydrogenated oils are hypercholesterolemic has been overstated and is probably not true at all (Reiser, 1981). In some foods, animal fats are equal to or superior to vegetable oils. Butter makes almost any food taste better than substitutes, especially in baked goods, while lard is said to make better pie and other flaky crusts than vegetable oil substitutes. Chicken fat is a favorite in the cuisine of some cultures.

The charges that 'saturated fats' are sources of excessive and harmful calories and are hypercholesterolemic and thus atherogenic, has unreasonably instilled qualms, if not actual phobias, against meat fat. Although the dietary recommendations (NCEP, 1988) are that total dietary fat should not exceed one-third each of saturated, monounsaturated, and polyunsaturated fatty acids, conventional wisdom has translated 'saturated fatty acid' to mean 'saturated fat', and that meat fat is all saturated. It is actually so described in the AHA Nutrition Committee's defence of its dietary recommendations (Nutrition Committee, 1982).

Since every fatty acid has its own metabolic pathway, meat fatty acids elicit physiological and biochemical responses similar to those of vegetable oils with some quantitative differences. There are enough essential fatty acids in meat animal tissues, even of ruminants, to meet nutritive requirements when included in normal diets, but they do not contain the potentially deleterious high levels present in many vegetable oils. Due to their high oleic acid content meat fats cause an increase in the desirable high density lipoprotein (HDL). Meat tissue lipids contain eicosanoid *n*-3 fatty acids and the essential nutrient, choline, which is mostly removed from vegetable oils by refining. Hydrogenation of vegetable oils to remove nutritionally desirable but potentially unflavorable n-3 α-linolenic acid and reduce polyunsaturation in general, or to obtain semisolid fats, produces fatty acid isomers of questionable health significance.

As explained below, the fatty acid composition of meat fats does not suggest that their consumption will increase blood cholesterol from normal to atherogenic levels. On the contrary, they have been shown not to increase blood cholesterol when included in practical diets (Lasier, 1972; O'Brien and Reiser, 1980; Flynn *et al.*, 1981, 1982; Reiser *et al.*, 1985).

In meeting the challenge of red meat and their fats as possible contributors to CHD, it is pertinent to point out their positive contribution to the beneficial and possibly essential n-3 polyunsaturated fatty acids. Recent investigations, as reviewed by Shorland (1988), indicate that humans are not efficient in synthesizing n-3 C_{20} and C_{22} acids from α-linolenic acid. However, this may not be true of meat animals. Although Hubbard and Pocklington (1968) have pointed out that beef and sheep fats have negligible concentrations of C_{20} and C_{22} polyunsaturated fatty acids, this may be due to the analytical extraction process, which tends not to include phospholipids, and to the excess of C_{16} and C_{18} fatty acids. In contrast, Crawford *et al.* (1969) found that the lean muscle fatty acids of seven species of wild ruminants contained 0·9–2·1% of C-20:5 n-3 and 1·2–4·1% of C-22:5 n-3 compared with 0·9% for C-20:5 n-3 and 0·6% of C-22:5 n-3 found in United Kingdom beef. The data suggest that the meat from wild ruminants contains more C_{20-22} polyunsaturated acids than that of domesticated animals. The result, however, may be obscured by the relatively high levels of triglycerides in the lean of domesticated animals. Provisional data from the Meat Industry Research Institute of New Zealand, confirm the UK values for beef, lamb, and mutton fatty acids, which were found to contain respectively, 0·9, 1·4, and 0·7% of C-20:5 n-3; 0·3, 0·5, and 0·4% for C-22:5 n-3; and 0·05, 0·14, and 0·17% for C-22:6 n-3 (Meat Industry Research Institute of New Zealand, Inc., unpublished data).

C_{20-22} polyunsaturated fatty acids occur in lipoprotein phospholipids in cell membranes. Detailed analyses of the phospholipid fatty acids of rumen and abomasum tissues of adult (1–2 year old) Romney ewes (Body and Shorland, 1974) showed that the phosphatidyl ethanolamine (PE) and phosphatidyl choline (PC) fractions, which comprise approximately 25 and 45% of the total phospholipids, were rich in C_{20-22} polyunsaturated fatty acids. The main components in the PE fraction were 4·3% of C-20:5 n-3; 7·1% of C-22:5 n-3; 3·1% of C-22:6 n-3; and 8·4% of C-20:4 n-6 when expressed as percent of total fatty acids. The high levels of n-3 fatty acids are ascribed to the fact that the animals were pasture-fed, the main dietary fatty acid being linolenic. However, in the absence of α-linolenic acid the levels of *n*-3 acids may become negligible. Shorland *et al.* (1981) showed that the fatty acids of the total phospholipids of the *l. dorsi* muscle of veal calves (receiving as their total fat supplement either corn or coconut oil in which linolenic acid is absent) contained only 0·4% of C-20:5 *n*-3 as the total *n*-3 contribution, the main C_{20-22} polyunsaturated fatty acids being made up of 8·0% of C-20:4 *n*-6 and 0·5–1·6% of C-20:3 *n*-9. This suggests that corn-fed animals may lack *n*-3 polyunsaturated C_{20-22} acids. The data suggest that the meat from wild ruminants contains more *n*-3 C_{20-22} polyunsaturated acids than does that of domesticated animals. Thus, the levels of *n*-3 polyunsaturated C_{20-22} fatty acids appear to be dependent on the presence of adequate amounts of α-linolenic acid in the diet.

Fats give texture, taste, and flavor to foods, an important food science subject by itself. In some populations and at various times, fatter meat has been considered as having a better texture and taste than very lean meat, and some people have been, and are, willing to pay more for the fatter grades. This subject is discussed in Chapters 16 and 17 and by Smith and Carpenter (1976) and by Savell and Cross (1988).

B. Dietary Fats and Obesity

Some physiological attributes of dietary fat can help in control of obesity. It has a high satiety value which signals one to stop overeating, and it slows the emptying time of the stomach and absorption rate from the intestines, delaying hunger. Carbohydrates have the opposite effects, due, in part, to rapid emptying of the stomach and to the hunger response from hypoglycemia following their ingestion. Before the current attack on fat as being the cause of obesity, it was attributed to starches and sugars. A low fat, high carbohydrate diet may be more caloric and difficult to handle biochemically than a more evenly balanced low carbohydrate one. Low fat, high carbohydrate regimens can effect enhanced triglyceridemia and possibly, hyperinsulinemia (Houtsmuller, 1975; Reaven, 1988). It is a common observation that obesity is more prevalent among the less advantaged, high carbohydrate consuming subcultures in the United States than among the affluent high meat consuming groups.

Some studies on the effects of the fat to carbohydrate ratio on body weight have concluded that high calorie-dense diets from fat result in more weight gain than low calorie-dense diets. The phenomenon was recently reexamined by Dreon *et al.* (1988), and that conclusion was found to be overly simplistic. A study by Jiang and Hunt (1983) showed that it is the distribution of time of food intake and size and frequency of meals that are related to obesity and that non-obese subjects show no relationship between body weight and energy consumption. Dreon *et al.* (1988) concluded that although percent body fat is correlated positively with g/1000 kcal intake of total saturated and monounsaturated fatty acids and negatively with carbohydrates and plant proteins, nevertheless, the total calories, number of meals, and distribution of calories were unrelated to body fat. These authors quoted several other reports demonstrating that calorie intake of obese persons may be less than that of the non-obese. Leveille and Clouthier (1987) in a recent review concluded that 'the composition of the diet with respect to the proportions of the major nutrients—protein, fat, and carbohydrate—has a profound and variable effect on the efficiency of food energy use...'. It was noted by Dreon *et al.* (1988) that the multivarient analysis of nutrient intake is not possible because of statistical limitations due to 'imprecision in estimated nutrient intake', and that 'colinearity among variables precludes an assessment of their independent effects'.

One can only conclude that obesity, like plasma cholesterol, is a complex phenomenon which differs between individuals because of variation in a number of genetically controlled biochemical factors. The relative amounts of fat, carbohydrate, and protein ingested may be utilized variously by different individuals. Thus, to the best of current knowledge, excess calorie consumption and overweight in the United States and other western countries floating in a plethora of good tasting food cannot be laid to the door of either fat, carbohydrate, or protein alone. What is to blame is excess food (calories) consumption. In societies where gourmet food is held in high regard and is consumed as a social function, overeating is common. On the other hand, energy is the number one food requirement in shortest supply, not only in developing countries, but also among the poor everywhere. A little more fat in the surplus foods distributed to such people would be an advantage. Caution must be utilized in limiting fat consumption by children.

Nevertheless, the present preoccupation in the United States with thinness and avoiding 'obesity' has resulted in recommendations to shun fat, especially from meat. This was encouraged by the National Institutes of Health consensus development statement (1985) and the NCEP (1988) which recommend fat intakes as low as 20% of total calories for persons with over 240 mg/dl of plasma cholesterol who are not able to reduce that level by limiting total fat to 30%. However, the NCEP (1988) contradicted itself by the following statement:

'However, very low fat intakes have low satiety value and are often not well accepted. Recent evidence indicates that a marked reduction in dietary fat is not required for satisfactory lowering of plasma low density lipoprotein (LDL) cholesterol provided that saturated fatty acids levels are reduced and the remaining fat is mainly unsaturated. In other words, a decrease in total fat to below 30% of calories may not be needed for the sole purpose of lowering plasma cholesterol level.'

Similarly, it has not been proven that reducing total fat calories from 40% to 30% will have a beneficial effect. Thus, the recommendation against either animal or vegetable fats at the levels normally consumed in order to control either obesity or blood cholesterol, must be seriously questioned. It has not been demonstrated that fat at the usual 40% of calories is unhealthful. In fact the natural Eskimo diet has an estimated fat content approaching 50% of total calories (Bang *et al.*, 1980) but is associated with an absence of chronic diseases (Lancet Editorial, 1983). None of the above should be interpreted as meaning that fat, either vegetable or animal, can be consumed in unlimited amounts.

Ironically, the rejected stones, stearic and oleic acids, in the light of their newly claimed negative cholesterolemic effects (Grundy, 1986a, b; Bonanome and Grundy, 1988) and the thrombotic:antithrombotic concept of the *n*-6/*n*-3 fatty acid ratio as described below, may turn out to be the chief corner stones. Adipose and other meat tissues contain adequate amounts of essential fatty acids which are needed only at about 1% of total calories. In this regard, they are superior to the potentially excessive amounts of some vegetable oils as had been recommended but more recently deprecated because of suspected carcinogenicity (NRC, 1982) and in-vivo peroxidation. They also form free radicals leading to potentially deleterious polymers and increase the vitamin E requirements.

C. Fish Oils and Thrombosis

The fats of plants, land animals, and fish are a major source of energy for omnivorous animals which have developed a complementary balance for the biochemical utilization of the three different kinds of fats. There is a mechanism by which linoleic acid effects a reduction in the amounts of atherogenic LDL cholesterol, lessening the chance of CHD. Perversely, however, in the process the *n*-6 linoleic acid is converted, by way of the essential arachidonic acid, to TXA_2 in the blood platelets leading to their aggregation, and thus to thrombosis, the ultimate cause of CHD. On the other hand the *n*-3 fatty acids of fish oils, eicosapentaenoic acid (EPA) and docosahexaenoic acid (DHA) balance that effect by inhibiting TXA_2 formation, thus reducing its level. They also produce inactive TXA_3 in the platelets and the antiaggregatory PGI_3 in the arterial endothelium (Dyerberg *et al.*, 1978). An additional paradox, but an important part of the balance in the metabolism of the different kinds of dietary fatty acids, is the conversion of arachidonic acid to prostacyclin (PGI_2) in the endothelial cells, aiding in the inhibition of platelet aggregation and thrombosis. It may be that the saturated fatty acids of animal origin somehow balance and control the deleterious effects of excess linoleic acid. The balancing effects of the *n*-6 and *n*-3 fatty acids on the thrombotic:antithrombotic ratio have been excellently analyzed by Budowski (1988) and by Crawford (1987).

It has been suggested by Taylor *et al.* (1979) that the rapid rise of CHD during this century may have been due to a 65% increase in the consumption of linoleic acid in the form of vegetable oil, margarines, and cooking and salad oils, which has been made available through technological advances in their production (Rizek *et al.*, 1983). This has greatly increased the *n*-6/*n*-3 ratio in western diets. Even though linoleic acid may decrease the risk of CHD by decreasing atherosclerosis, it may increase CHD more by increasing thrombosis. It is possible that the recent decrease in incidence of deaths due to CHD is more the result of advances in treating thrombosis than in reducing atherosclerosis by diet. This concept is supported by a National Center for Disease Control (CDC) (1989) report which stated that while deaths from ischemic heart disease have declined 20% since 1968 the rate of hospitalization from heart disease has risen. This is discussed in more detail below in the Public Health versus High Risk Approach. The above information suggests an explanation for the anomaly that the curves representing the relationships between plasma cholesterol concentrations and total CHD and CHD death incidences differ more at concentrations above 220 mg/dl than at concentrations below 220 mg/dl (Pooling Project Research Group, 1978; Stamler *et al.*, 1986). That is, CHD deaths may be more easily prevented in patients with low levels of plasma cholesterol than in those with high levels. This might be explained if the attacks in persons with high plasma cholesterol concentrations are due to both atherosclerotic and nonatherosclerotic TXA_2 thrombi but the attacks in persons with low levels are due to TXA_2 thrombi alone and the latter are more easily and completely treated with thrombolytic drugs, such as streptokinase and tissue plasmalogen activator.

Recent work thus indicates that CHD is mainly a thrombotic event that takes place against an atherosclerotic–hypercholesterolemic background induced by TXA_2 synthesized from linoleic acid in the platelets. Hyslop and York (1980) found that cholesterol enriched platelets produced twice as much TXA_2 as did their controls. The data of Shattil and Cooper (1976) suggest that this is due to a decrease in membrane fluidity associated with an increased platelet cholesterol/phospholipid ratio. Clearly, hypercholesterolemia has direct implications in both atherosclerosis and thrombosis. On the other hand, Sinzinger *et al.* (1979) have shown that healthy arterial tissues generate anti-aggregatory prostacyclin nearly twice as rapidly as those with atherosclerosis. Such a condition not only suggests the need for an *n*-6/*n*-3 balance, and the threat of thrombosis, even without atherosclerosis, when the *n*-6/*n*-3 ratio is too high, but also that clotting time would be adversely affected in atherosclerotic arteries.

The above concepts are thought to explain the low incidence of CHD in fish eating populations such as the Greenland Eskimos (Simopoulos *et al.*, 1986). The *n*-3 EPA and DHA can readily be incorporated into swine and poultry tissues in desirable amounts by feeding menhaden oil (Brown, 1931). Incorporation into cattle tissue presents the problem of rumen hydrogenation. This subject is discussed later under Modification of Meat Fat Fatty Acids.

III. BLOOD CHOLESTEROL RESPONSES TO MEAT FAT

A. Background

The concept that animal fats are positively cholesterolemic and, *ipso facto*, atherosclerotic and a risk factor for CHD, originated during attempts to determine whether humans are like rabbits in their response to dietary cholesterol. During the first four decades after the observation that egg consumption causes high blood cholesterol and atherosclerosis in rabbits (Ignatowski, 1908) attempts to demonstrate that phenomenon in humans were mainly negative. The first interpretation of the hypercholesterolemic and atherosclerotic effect of eggs in rabbits was that the egg protein was responsible (Ignatowski, 1908). However, in a review Weiss and Minot (1933) concluded there was no evidence that meat consumption is related to the condition. One study was on Eskimos ‘living almost entirely on animal tissues’ but among whom there was little renal or vascular disease (Thomas, 1927). Recently the role of the various polyunsaturated fatty acids of fish oils on CHD among Eskimos has been recognized (Lancet Editorial, 1983).

Weiss and Minot (1933) also made reference to the observations of Ruffer (1921) who studied 800 autopsies on vegetarian Mohammedan pilgrims and found that arterial disease was as prevalent among them as among Europeans. Ruffer (1921) also compared the arteries of Egyptian mummies with modern Egyptians and concluded: 'my experience in Egypt and the Far East has not strengthened the theory that meat eating is the cause of arterial disease'. Donnison (1929), who studied natives of Kenya, Africa 'whose food habits include a generous consumption of meat', found no clinical evidence of atherosclerosis and reported that postmortem examination demonstrated that atheromas were infrequent occurrences.

B. Genesis of the Saturated Fat:CHD Theory

During the 1920s, even though it was the protein of meat and not its fat that was being tested, the entire meat, fat included, was exonerated. Furthermore, epidemiological data gathered after World Wars I and II (Katz and Stamler, 1953) supported the earlier observations on individuals (Luden, 1917). In those countries where animal products were in short supply there was a significant drop in CHD incidence. The incidence increased to former levels after the wars. This observation revived credence in the cholesterol hypothesis and stimulated belief in a fatty acid role in CHD. There are many other factors, however, such as mal- and undernutrition which could account for the phenomenon. Nordoy and Simonsen (1987) have referred to a 3–4 times increase in fish consumption in Europe during the war, which alone could account for much of the decrease in CHD mortality.

The diet fat:CHD theory did not at first distinguish between vegetable and animal fat (Keys, 1953), but Kinsell *et al.* (1953) announced that formula diets containing 'large amounts' of vegetable oils (amounts and kinds not given) consistently resulted in a major fall in serum cholesterol and phospholipids in patents with myxedema and other hormonal problems. The subjects were kept on metabolic wards and given liquid formula diets. The reduction in serum cholesterol went to below 100 mg/dl. Ahrens *et al.* (1954) then compared serum cholesterol responses of healthy subjects consuming diets containing butter to responses of those consuming a vegetable margarine and obtained a 20% higher concentration of serum cholesterol with the butter diet. This study, like the Kinsell study (1953), was conducted in a metabolic ward but with a solid basal diet supplemented with liquid formulas. These initial studies stimulated investigations on the relationships between blood cholesterol levels and dietary fats and fatty acids. The consensus at that time was that dietary cholesterol did not play a serious role in the matter, if any. It is beyond the objectives of this report to detail the steps which identified the roles of individual and classes of fatty acids, but they eventually led to the identification of lauric, myristic, and palmitic acids as the only ones which were significantly and positively cholesterolemic, and the polyunsaturates as being negatively cholesterolemic (Keys *et al.*, 1957a, b, 1965).

In the evaluation of the cholesterolemic properties of fatty acids it seems necessary to consider the nature of the fatty acids produced following their absorption. This applies especially to coconut oil, which contains some 45% lauric, 20% myristic, and 10% palmitic acids and has been used extensively as evidence relating to the saturated fat theory concerning meat. As shown by Shorland and Czochanska (1970) chickens fed coconut oil produced depot fats similar in fatty acid composition to that of the dietary fat, but in humans and mammals generally only limited amounts of lauric acid appear in the depot fats. The evidence suggests (Shorland *et al.*, 1981) that lauric acid is chain extended to form increased levels of myristic and palmitic acids. Thus, the cholesterolemic properties of the medium chain lauric and myristic acids may be due to the increased levels of palmitic acid which they produce.

The campaign against the fat in red meat began because of a perceived higher content of cholesterol in red meat than in fish or poultry. When it was realized that such is not necessarily so, and that dietary cholesterol is a minor risk factor, the anti-meat recommendations then changed to the equally questionable faulting of its energy and saturated fatty acid levels. Since the amount of adiposity in meat animals can be reasonably controlled and has, for good economical reasons, already been adjusted in swine and to some degree in cattle, it has been found easier to adjust to the anti-high fat vogue than to fight it. Some factors involved will be discussed in Chapters 16 and 17.

Human fat resembles the meat fat of other monogastric animals. One might wonder if the dietary animal fat:atherosclerosis theory is correct, why animals, including humans, permeated with their own animal fat, do not uniformly develop spontaneous atherosclerosis. Some, such as poultry, do, but not for that unbiological reason (Roberts and Straus, 1965).

(i) Oleic and stearic acids

As determined by the relative cholesterolemic responses to various fats and fat mixtures and use of multiregression equations, as well as by comparison with low fat, high carbohydrate diets (Ahrens *et al.*, 1954; Keys *et al.*, 1965), it was concluded that oleic and stearic acids are neutral in regard to their effects on blood cholesterol. However, recent direct comparisons with low fat, high carbohydrate diets have suggested that oleic acid may be as potent a negatively cholesterolemic diet factor as linoleic (Mattson and Grundy, 1985; Mensink and Katan, 1987; Baggio *et al.*, 1988). There is also an indication that stearic acid may be negatively cholesterolemic (Bonanome and Grundy, 1988). This appears reasonable since stearic acid is the metabolic precursor of oleic acid. But that logic is defeated by the fact that palmitic acid is the precursor of stearic and if any acid is positively cholesterolemic it is palmitic. Further confusing the issue is evidence that by blocking desaturation of stearic acid with cyclopropene fatty acids, oleic acid may be synthesized from lauric by an alternative route (Raju and Reiser, 1969). The answer may lie somewhere in the facts that palmitic is the end product of the fatty acid synthetase system, being elongated to stearic by alternative elongation systems, and that vaccenic acid, which constitutes up to 10% of beef fat and 25% of beef phospholipids (Wood, 1983), is derived from palmitic acid by way of palmitoleic. All this must be involved in answer to the question asked previously as to why, being ourselves permeated with animal fat, we do not spontaneously develop hypercholesterolemia and atherosclerosis. Obviously, the interrelated system is under complex homeostatic controls and only those persons with aberrant controls develop hypercholesterolemia, whether from endogenous or exogenous influences. More simply stated, animal fat may be positively cholesterolemic, depending upon to what it is being compared, but it is not hypercholesterolemic. It does not increase plasma cholesterol from normal to pathological (abnormal) levels, at least not in normal people.

C. Epidemiology

Most of the evidence of a positive relationship between fat intake, plasma cholesterol and CHD is epidemiological or otherwise indirect and not experimental, and much of the epidemiological evidence is negative. Most dietary intervention trials with humans, as well as clinical trials, have been negative (Multiple Risk Factor Intervention Trial Research Group, 1981), questionable (Authoritative Comments, 1984), and called flawed by the AHA's Nutrition Committee (1982) itself. Epidemiological data relating the thinness of low fat consuming and other thin peoples to their low incidence of CHD do not demonstrate a cause and effect relationship for the disease and can be misleading. Many such populations have other characteristics or problems which can explain the relationship, such as genetics and under- and malnutrition. The validity of the epidemiological evidence for the dietary fat:blood cholesterol:CHD relationships is examined below. There is no direct relationship between degrees of overweight and plasma cholesterol concentrations, and only indirect relationships between obesity and CHD. However, obesity is deleterious for those indirect relationships as well as numerous other reasons, such as its relation to non-insulin-dependent diabetes.

Epidemiological relationships between populations are based on statistical data and may reflect the response of only a percentage of the number of persons in the groups being compared, such as the Japanese who moved to Hawaii versus those who remained in Japan. A statistically significant difference between plasma cholesterol levels can be caused by a minority of cohorts in either or both of the groups being compared. Additionally, a statistically significant difference does not prove a pathologically significant difference between groups. Both values may be well within benign levels. It is often overlooked that the measure for statistical significance is an arbitrary number ($P < 0{\cdot}05$), and not a matter of life or death.

As stated above, the most persuasive evidence relating consumption of animal depot fat to blood cholesterol and CHD has been epidemiological, by comparing countries, sections of countries, and towns differing in their consumption of animal and vegetable products. An example is a study of three regions of Yugoslavia: (1) an area of high fat, mainly pork, consumption, (2) an area where the people consume little fat of any kind, and (3) an area where the people use olive oil and small amounts of animal products (Brozek *et al.*, 1957). Many of the latter are also fishermen and, therefore, fish eaters. On average the serum cholesterol concentration of the men eating pork was 238 mg/dl in the 3rd through 6th decades of life. It was 214 mg/dl in the plasma of the men on the low fat regimen, and 198 mg/dl of the men in the olive oil and fish area. However, there were other variables between the three groups besides their diets which could account for the differences in serum cholesterol. The men in the low fat diet were the smallest and 'lightest' and those in the pork eating group were the largest and heaviest. The latter group may also have been the most sedentary while those in the olive oil consuming group were farmers and fishermen. No data are offered relative to the numbers of smokers. It is quite possible that the differences in serum cholesterol could have been due not only to differences in their energy demanding occupations, diets, and life styles in general, but also to ethnic differences, common to various areas of Yugoslavia, which was suggested by differences in the anthropometric measurements of the men in the three areas. The differences could also be due to variation in the relative percentage of non-responders, and/or differences in degrees of responsiveness between them. Thus, the difference in plasma cholesterol between the three groups could be due to variation in the indigenous peoples and general life styles and not to differences in the fats of their diets other than fish oils.

Another, and more recent, epidemiological comparison between peoples differing in the nature of their diets was one in which the relative amounts of dietary saturated, monoenoic, and linoleic acids were compared for blood cholesterol levels (Daughtery *et al.*, 1987). The subjects were in Italy, Finland, and the United States. The sources of the food fats, which were classified as animal tissue, dairy, or vegetable, are not given, although it was said that dietary records were kept. One hint is a statement in the discussion that the relatively high level of saturated fatty acids in the Finnish diet 'can be attributed to the high intake of fat-rich dairy products and fatty meat and sausages', and the high level of monounsaturated acids in the Italian diet to a high consumption of olive oil. Nothing is said about the food of the Americans, which traditionally, is also high in dairy and meat products. Although the individual dietary fatty acids were said to have been analyzed, only the total amount of saturates is recorded, along with the percentages of oleic and linoleic. It was apparently assumed that all saturated fatty acids are biochemically equal and make the same contribution to the level of blood lipids. This is puzzling since the incorporation of individual saturated fatty acids into cholesterol esters and phospholipids of red blood cells and blood platelets was a major objective of the study. The results are summarized in Table 2-1. The authors were puzzled by the statistically significant lower plasma cholesterol concentration of the Americans relative to that of the Italians which they attributed to the higher linoleic

TABLE 2-1

PERCENT OF TOTAL CALORIES OF THE DIETARY FAT AND FATTY ACIDS, AND THE CORRESPONDING LEVELS OF PLASMA TOTAL CHOLESTEROL IN AN EPIDEMIOLOGICAL STUDY[a]

	(% of total calories)		
	Italy	*Finland*	*USA*
Total fat	32	40	32
Saturated	10·7	22·6	14·0
Oleic	17·8	11·7	15·4
Linoleic	2·4	2·4	7·3
Plasma cholesterol (mg/dl)[b]	213 ± 7[c]	242 ± 11[c]	191 ± 6[c]

[a] From Daughtery *et al.* (1987).
[b] All three plasma cholesterol concentrations were significantly different from each other.
[c] Standard deviation.

acid content, 7·3 versus 2·4% of calories. The three groups were different in ethnic origins and life styles. One can conclude that there are more genetically high plasma cholesterol responders among Finns than among Italians, a phenomenon similar to the fact that there are more lactase deficient people in Southern than in Northern Europe.

Perhaps the most referenced epidemiological study of the relationship of dietary saturated fatty acids to blood cholesterol and to CHD incidence and mortality is the Seven Country Report (Keys, 1970). The study involved about 12 000, 40–59-year-old men initially free of CHD. They were from 18 cities in 7 different countries, with as few as 509 in Tanushimaru, Japan and as many as 2571 US railroad workers. The relationships between the percentages of total calories from saturated fatty acids, serum cholesterol concentration, and incidence of CHD of 14 of the 18 locales were given in graphic form and presented as demonstrating a continuum in the relation between the percentages of dietary saturated fatty acids and CHD incidence and deaths. The values of those factors, as best can be estimated from the graphs, are given in Table 2-2. Total CHD incidence is used here because the incidence of CHD deaths involve other factors as explained elsewhere in this chapter.

Although Table 2-2 indicates there was an increase in serum cholesterol level with an increase in the proportions of saturated fatty acids consumed the increase is not in a straight line relationship but is curvilinear or in steps. Between 6 and 13% of saturated fatty acid calories, the serum cholesterol level remains reasonably constant at about 200 mg/dl, with the 160 mg/dl for Velikà Krona, Yugoslavia being indicated as questionable. At some point between 13 and 18% of dietary saturated fatty acids, the homeostatic mechanism described below appears to break down and serum cholesterol increases with each additional concentration of fatty acids, which was not true between 6 and 13%. Although the blood cholesterol concentration increases with each step above 18% saturated fatty acids the ratio decreases, which is evidence for the functioning of the complex homeostatic mechanism. That tendency is also shown by the high serum cholesterol/saturated fatty acid ratio of the Japanese and low corresponding values of the American, Dutch, and Finish subjects. However, other factors are also different between low and high saturated fatty acid diets and the people who eat them. Diets low in the percentage of saturated fatty acids are probably high in negatively cholesterolemic vegetable matter also. The nature and amounts of proteins and carbohydrates can also vary drastically. Furthermore, life styles involving other risk factors are very different in Yugoslavia, Italy, and Greece to those in Holland, Finland, and

TABLE 2-2

PERCENT TOTAL CALORIES CONSUMED AS SATURATED FATTY ACIDS, SERUM CHOLESTEROL CONCENTRATIONS, AND INCIDENCE OF CORONARY HEART DISEASE IN SEVEN COUNTRY STUDY[a]

Location	*Dietary saturated fatty acids (% of calories) (A)*	*Serum cholesterol (mg/dl) (B)*	*(B)/(A)*	*Incidence*[b]
Tanushimaru, Japan	2	170	85	—[c]
Corfu, Greece	6	200	33	0·3
Velika Krsna, Yugoslavia	8	160(?)	20	0·2
Crete, Greece	9	200	25	0·3
Montegiorgia, Italy	9	195	22	0·9
Dalmatia, Yugoslavia	9	185	21	0·4
Crevelcore, Italy	10	190	19	1·2
Zrenjanin, Yugoslavia	10	210	21	0·4
Belgrade, Yugoslavia	12	215	18	0·8
Slavonia, Yugoslavia	13	190	15	0·8
United States	18	235	13	1·7
Zutphen, Holland	19	230	12	1·4
West Finland	19	250	13	1·4
East Finland	22	265	12	2·4

[a] From Keys (1970).
[b] Percent per year CHD among men at risk.
[c] Rate for Tanushimaru not indicated in the graphs.

the United States. These data were obtained before the effects of fish oils were realized, a factor which could help to explain the Japanese data.

Note that the dietary levels of saturated fatty acids of the Italians and Finns in the seven countries studied and their corresponding total blood cholesterol levels (Table 2-2) agree reasonably well with those in the Italian, Finnish, US study (Table 2-1), which speaks well for the confidence one may have in the two studies. The occupations, diet, and blood cholesterol levels of the US subjects were different in the two studies and the differences are reflected in the data, so much so that they actually could have been from two different countries. The US railroad workers in the seven countries study were switchmen (875), 'sedentary' (1305), and 'other' (391). The Americans in the Italian, Finnish, and US study were farmers from near Washington, DC. Thus, contrary to current interpretation, the Seven Countries data offer evidence against rather than in support of the saturated fat theory as well as against Key's equation for calculation of changes in blood cholesterol with changes in three groups of diet fatty acids (Keys *et al.*, 1965), at least under 18% of total calories from saturated fatty acids. The equation ignores other variables such as homeostatic mechanisms, the many dietary constituents known to have positive or negative cholesterolemic effects, the effects of monoenoic acids, unknown differences between the individual fatty acids within the three fatty acid groups, *n*-3 fatty acids, exercise, alcohol, and many others. It is a truism that epidemiological data can only show relationships and be suggestive. Important as they are, they should not be depended on for scientific truth or to urge 230 million Americans to, perhaps unnecessarily, give up or seriously limit desirable and nutritious food.

These examples are reasonably representative of the pitfalls of designing and interpreting epidemiological studies. It is not possible to control all the factors, environmental, genealogical as well as dietary, which may affect statistically significant differences in plasma cholesterol and CHD between test groups. Conclusions and recommendations with respect to diet composition based on such epidemiological studies should be recognized as mostly suggestive and not conclusive with respect to cause and effect. As discussed above for the Yugoslavia studies, differences in relative numbers of responders (non-adaptors) to diet constituents between ethnic groups and/or degrees of responsiveness of the responders, could explain much of the statistically significant differences in response to diet. That is, the people were different in genetically controlled homeostatic mechanisms.

D. Public Health versus High Risk Approach

The probability that about one man in 200 of a large group of men with an average plasma cholesterol concentration of 225 mg/dl or less will have a CHD in any given year does not mean that each individual in that group has 0·5% chance of having an attack. The statistics, based on averages, do not apply to individuals '... because of the intra- and inter-variability...and because the magnitude of a difference in cholesterol for a given dietary change tends to be related to the characteristic serum-cholesterol level of the individual' as stated by Keys *et al.* (1957a, b). The recommendations are made to the entire population as a unit but can only be followed by individuals with different genes. Why apply to everyone what is true only for the few who effect averages in statistics? The AHA (1986), NIH (1985), and the Surgeon General (1988) make recommendations to the masses. As public health agencies they are interested in statistics. They are preoccupied with the concept that if everyone in the US above 20 years of age could be induced to conform to the recommendations, *maybe* the statistics for CHD in this country would improve. One should note that a significant number of the people on panels such as the Consensus Report of the National Institutes of Health (1985) or the NCEP (1988), are not hands-on-scientists of diet, blood chemistry, and CHD but administrators and public policy experts. The panels can only arrive at a consensus of their own groups. It is misleading, unfair, and potentially dangerous to ask all the American people to limit eggs and red meat below their customary levels if statistically significant differences in a study are due to a small percentage of metabolically abnormal participants. Unfortunately, the data, as given, do not show the distribution of the responders and non-responders to dietary cholesterol.

In a dietary study often quoted to demonstrate the validity of the diet–heart theory and the public health approach (Dayton *et al.*, 1969), more CHD deaths occurred in an animal fat control group than in a vegetable oil test group, but total mortality was the same in both groups. Similarly, in a test in which reductions in plasma cholesterol and CHD deaths were both reduced by cholestyramine, total mortality was the same in control and test groups (Lipid Research Clinics Program, 1984). However, all aspects—design, statistics, and interpretation of the data of the latter study have been severely criticized (Authoritative Comments, 1984).

The current NCEP (1988) efforts to screen everyone for their blood cholesterol level to find those who need treatment is the correct approach, although too long delayed. The claim that the lack of a simple assay method made screening too expensive cannot be defended. If only a part of the funds spent on the failed attempts to demonstrate a population-wide diet-to-blood cholesterol relationship had been spent screening the public (even by the then current methods) for high (whether 220 mg/dl or 240 mg/dl) blood cholesterol the hypercholesterolemics would long ago have been found and treated. The corollary of the above stated objective of the NCEP (1988) is to find those who do not need treatment. It, therefore, defeats its purpose by continuing to ask everyone to follow the same dietary advice. To what end does the NCEP (1988) recommend that persons with blood cholesterol in the 'desirable' levels below 200 mg/dl conform to the dietary recommendations?

The public health approach of the dietary recommendations to the public for prevention of coronary heart disease is based on two false assumptions:

1. There is a straight line relationship between blood cholesterol concentrations and risk of CHD at all levels.

2. The corollary to 1: statistically significant differences between blood cholesterol levels always indicate significant health differences.

These two false assumptions also lead to misinterpretation of experimental data.

E. Blood Cholesterol Homeostasis

Cholesterol is a normal blood constituent and like all normal blood constituents has a normal range of concentrations, maintained by a number of biochemical controls, both exogenous and endogenous. Dietary cholesterol may be at least partially inhibited from absorption by the presence of phytosterols in the diet. Bile acids in the intestine are bound by dietary pectins and gums, with the chelate being excreted. That phenomenon breaks the enterohepatic cycle, allowing more blood cholesterol to be catabolized and excreted as bile acids. Endogenously, the function of the LDL receptors is to maintain a low maximum concentration of blood LDL cholesterol by transporting it into liver and other cells where it inhibits cholesterol synthesis and stimulates its conversion to bile acids. Further stabilizing the homeostatic mechanism is a series of events by which dietary fatty acids are involved in the synthesis of lipoproteins. Most of those mechanisms are under genetic control, and in most people the controls are adequate to maintain the lipoproteins and their constituent cholesterol fractions within normal, i.e. benign, limits. Individuals who lack those controls have a disease, hypercholesterolemia, analogous to the hyperglycemia of diabetics. As with diabetes, only people with the disease should be treated. Currently (NCEP, 1988) everyone is asked to treat themselves as hypercholesterolemics. The homeostatic mechanisms, even of normal people, can be overwhelmed. Thus, in one test of response to egg cholesterol 7–19 egg yolks were administered intragastrally to six prisoners by Connor *et al.* (1961). Serum cholesterol increased by 34–94% over the control diet. Because of individual variations in the homeostatic mechanisms, we are confronted with the questions of the upper limit of normality and the beginning of abnormality, i.e. the diseased state.

The criteria of the normal range for levels of plasma cholesterol are data relating concentrations to incidence of CHD (Pooling Project Research Group, 1978; Stamler *et al.*, 1986). Currently there is a tendency to relate concentrations of plasma cholesterol to the incidence of death, as represented by the Stamler *et al.* (1986) and MRFIT (1981) data, rather than to the incidence of the disease. However, the difference between the incidence of the disease and the incidence of death due to the disease varies with the quality of treatment, which varies from place to place and time to time, whereas the diet to blood cholesterol to incidence of CHD relationships involves basic cause and effect phenomena.

As was stated above, the CDC (1989) has reported that although deaths from CHD have been declining, hospital admissions due to the disease have been increasing. It was suggested that the decrease in deaths may reflect improvement in medical care. Past announcements in the news media of decreases in CHD deaths have misleadingly been accredited to following of dietary recommendations. If that is true, it should lead to fewer CHD hospitalizations as well as fewer deaths. As was theorized for the rise in CHD incidence during this century (Taylor *et al.*, 1979), the current increase in the incidence of CHD could be attributed to the dietary recommendations, resulting in too high n-6/n-3 polyunsaturated fatty acid ratio, thus increasing TXA_2 and thrombosis. Efforts to follow the low total fat, low saturated fatty acid, low cholesterol, low calorie, high complex carbohydrate dietary recommendations can, predictably, lead to unbalanced diets and their multiple deleterious sequelae. The NIH (1985) Consensus Report and later the NCEP (1988) both made estimates from the data of the relationships between cholesterol concentrations and CHD (or CHD deaths) that there is minimum risk (desirable level) of coronary heart disease at concentrations below 200 mg/dl of cholesterol, and moderate risk between 200 and 240 mg/dl. Thus, considering differences between individuals and groups and the errors in obtaining such data (including the plasma cholesterol assay), it is conservative to consider 220 mg/dl as a rule of thumb in dividing 'normal' from abnormal plasma cholesterol concentrations. Using that criterion, it is a fair approximation that around 65–75% of American men of middle age (LRCPEC, 1979) have normal or non-threatening plasma cholesterol concentrations. Individuals with normal blood cholesterol concentrations who suffer from CHD probably have some other risk factor such as TXA_2 triggered thrombosis. The concept that any level of blood cholesterol is a greater risk for CHD than any level below it, at all levels, such as 166 versus 140 mg/dl (Sachs, 1988), is an absurdity. A straight line connecting accepted levels of risk between 250 mg/dl and 200 mg/dl if extended would intercept zero risk at about 150 mg/dl! It would also mean that diet and blood cholesterol levels are the only causes of CHD. At another level, it is unbiological and unreasonable that an essential blood constituent should be toxic at all levels, teleological as that rationalization may be. Yet in most epidemiological, retrospective, prospective, and research studies, it has been usually incorrectly assumed when there is a statistically significant difference between the blood cholesterol responses that there is also a difference in risk, regardless of the absolute cholesterol levels. Data from the Framingham study (Cornfield, 1962; Kannel and Gordon, 1982) which have been quoted to demonstrate a continuous gradient, had too few subjects, especially at the lower levels, from which to generalize. More correctly, the effect of any factor on risk should be measured not by any change in plasma cholesterol, but by changes from normal levels (less than 220 mg/dl) to abnormal ones (greater than 220 mg/dl) or from one abnormal level to a higher one. Guidelines for change in risk could also be the NCEP (1988) classification of risk levels.

The anomaly that the curves relating plasma cholesterol concentration to total CHD incidence and CHD deaths are different at high levels of concentration but similar at low levels (Grundy, 1986b) appears to have been unnoticed. Possibly the thrombi at the higher levels of blood cholesterol are atherosclerotic-based; while those at the lower levels, such as below 220 mg/dl, are mainly or solely TXA_2 triggered, and thus, are more successfully treated by clot dissolving drugs as was suggested above in connection with the nutritive value of fish oils and the *n*-6/*n*-3-thrombotic: antithrombotic ratio. This concept is supported by a study (Steering Committee of the Physicians Health Study Research Group, 1989) which showed that one aspirin (325 mg) every other day effected a reduction of 44% in coronary heart attacks in male physicians over 50 years of age, *mostly in those with low levels of plasma cholesterol.* Aspirin inhibits the formation of TXA_2.

Do meat fats overwhelm cholesterol homeostatic mechanisms? The fact is that, except for the uncertain and questionable epidemiological comparisons, animal fats, other than fish oils and butter, have rarely been tested on humans. Butter fat, which is not a meat fat, has consistently shown statistically significant higher plasma cholesterol levels than carbohydrates or polyunsaturated vegetable oils (Shepard *et al.*, 1980). However, all such data should be reevaluated to determine whether the differences were within normal limits and to separate the hyper-responders (non-adapters) from the normal subjects. The results could turn the interpretations around. Butter fat ingestion may result in statistically higher plasma cholesterol concentration than a vegetable margarine, but does it increase risk? It does not do so unless it can be shown to increase plasma cholesterol from one NCEP (1988) risk level to the next or from one high risk level (greater than 220 mg/dl) to a still higher level. Butter may not effect (Shepard *et al.*, 1980) or may actually decrease (Rossouw *et al.*, 1981) the LDL cholesterol/HDL cholesterol ratio.

F. Diet Cholesterol

When it became realized that there is approximately as much cholesterol in poultry and fish as in beef, the emphasis on the dangers of cholesterol in red meat waned. Little effort is being made to change the amounts in meats although efforts to reduce it in eggs are continuing. The current interest in cholesterol in red meat is for the determination of its concentrations in various tissues, and for the differences effected by the amounts of fat and by cooking. Thus, Rhee *et al.* (1982) analyzed longissimus muscle from beef steaks of eight levels of marbling from 'moderately abundant' to 'practically devoid'. Seven of the eight marbling level groups contained the same amount of cholesterol on the fresh basis, only 'practically devoid' contained less (60–65 mg/100 g versus 51 mg/100 g). There was no difference between the samples on the dry basis, 200 mg/100 g to 229 mg/100 g. The low cholesterol fresh steak had more water, which accounted for its low level. After cooking the steaks to an internal temperature of 60 or 75°C, all contained essentially the same amount of cholesterol, 77–87 mg/100 g at 60°C and 86–90 mg/100 g at 75°C.

Hoelscher *et al.* (1988) determined the cholesterol content of the membranes and the intracellular components of muscle and of the adipocytes of raw and cooked longissimus beef steaks. Three grades and three subcutaneous fat trim levels were examined. The membranes had 60–80% of the muscle cholesterol and the 'storage component' the remainder. The reverse was true for the adipocyte, the membrane containing 8–12% and the storage fraction 88–92% in all quality grades.

The stimulus for research on the quantities and distribution of cholesterol in meat is the dietary recommendation of NCEP (1988) and the earlier AHA series that no one consume more than 300 mg of cholesterol per day. Since an egg contains about 210–250 mg that allows very little from any other source if one egg is eaten in any form. Any meat tissue (lean or adipose) contains about 75 mg/100 g on the fresh basis. Thus, about 3 oz (85 g) of meat and one egg contain the recommended level of 300 mg of cholesterol per day. That the 300 mg/day restriction is unrealistic has been convincingly expressed. The Framingham study (Dauber, 1982) in an analysis of its data on 912 men over many years concluded:

> that within the range of egg intake of this population differences in egg consumption were unrelated to blood cholesterol or to CHD incidence.

Graham and Vaupel (1980) of The Institute of Policy Sciences and Public Affairs of Duke University after a study of all aspects of the subject concluded that:

> Recommendations to the general public calling for reduced egg consumption are inappropriate and may be counter-productive to health objectives.

The Food and Nutrition Board (1980) of the National Research Council, National Academy of Science has stated:

> No significant correlation between cholesterol intake and serum cholesterol concentration has been shown in free-living persons in this country. For these reasons the Board makes no specific recommendations about dietary cholesterol for the healthy person.

With respect to saturated fatty acids the Food and Nutrition Board (1980) further added:

> It does not seem prudent at this time to recommend an increase in the dietary P/S ratio except for individuals in the high risk categories.

Increase in CHD risk may conservatively be considered as at least a 20 mg/dl increase in plasma cholesterol from below 220 mg/dl to greater than 220 mg/dl as a rule-of thumb. An increase from greater than 220 mg/dl to a still higher concentration by over 10% might also be considered as an increase in risk. By those criteria, out of a total of 70 men consuming three eggs per day in three separate studies (Slater *et al.*, 1976; O'Brien and Reiser, 1980; O'Brien and McMurray, 1988) only 8, or about 10% of the subjects, could be said to have increased their risk. Several subjects in those studies actually lowered their plasma cholesterol by over 10% on eating three eggs a day, a demonstration of normal variation and homeostatic control.

McNamara *et al.* (1987) tested the effect of three eggs per day for six weeks on the blood lipoproteins and total cholesterol of 25 men consuming 35% of total calories as a polyunsaturated vegetable oil or as dairy fat diets. Only two of the 25 men experienced a significant (more than 10%) increase in plasma cholesterol from 'borderline' (NCEP, 1988) to 'high' risk while eating the eggs with the vegetable oil. Three men (none the same as the above) increased their risk from 'high' to higher risk while consuming the dairy fat (McNamara, unpublished data). Considering intra-individual variability, the numerous potentials for experimental errors in such tests, the fact that the tests were made only once, and the arbitrary limit of 10% estimated for the sum of those variables, it is possible that none of the 95 men in the above reviewed studies experienced a change in risk by the consumption of three eggs per day. (Slater *et al.*, 1976; O'Brien and Reiser, 1980; McNamara *et al.*, 1987; O'Brien and McMurray, 1988).

The NCEP (1988) presents no evidence for limiting total cholesterol for everyone to less than 300 mg/day. On the contrary it states:

> ... high intake of cholesterol in humans rarely causes striking rises in the plasma cholesterol level... The degree of rise varies from person to person... Overall excess(?) of dietary cholesterol *appears to contribute* to the high LDL cholesterol levels seen in high risk patients and thus *may* add to CHD risk.

(Emphasis and question mark added by the present authors.) The 'excess' is an individual matter experienced by the 10% who develop it, as shown above, and as was discussed in the description of the homeostatic control mechanisms. This is not a public health but an individual problem for those who lack the controls and have hypercholesterolemia.

The subject of dietary cholesterol and its relationship to blood cholesterol levels is discussed in more detail in Chapter 3 of this volume. Readers are referred to it for further information on this topic.

G. Experimental Trials of Cholesterolemic Responses to Meat and Meat Fats and Coconut Oil

Meat fats have seldom been specifically tested under controlled conditions for their effects on human blood lipids and lipoproteins, either alone or with attendant meat. Measures of aberrant responses have been epidemiological as described above, or by extrapolation from data on trials with coconut oil or butter under the assumption that all three are 'saturated' and, therefore, equally cholesterolemic. But even here, the criterion has been differences in levels of plasma cholesterol not differences in risk levels. Coconut oil has been shown in experimental (Reiser *et al.*, 1985) studies to be positively cholesterolemic, but within low normal levels. Epidemiological data suggested that fatal and non-fatal CHD rates in the test populations were fewer than in the controls (Prior *et al.*; 1966, 1981; Shorland *et al.*, 1969).

Gradually, in the mind of the 'man on the street' the term 'saturated fats' has come to be associated with animal fats and an increased risk of CHD. Thus, meat fats have been condemned by association, contrary to the data of controlled trials. In a trial carried out by Reiser *et al.* (1985), 19 approximately 26-year-old men consumed beef fat, coconut oil and safflower oil at 21% of total dietary calories (60% of the total 35% fat calories). The approximate ratios of the percentages of saturated (excluding stearic) to one half of the monounsaturated plus polyunsaturated fatty acids in the beef fat was 28:28 or 1:1 and approximately 10% each of total calories. The results of the study are summarized in Table 2-3. Results

TABLE 2-3

RESPONSES OF PLASMA LIPIDS AND LIPOPROTEINS FOR 26-YEAR-OLD MEN TO THEIR HABITUAL DIETS AND TO TEST DIETS OF 21% OF TOTAL CALORIES FROM FAT (60% OF 35% TOTAL FAT CALORIES) AS BEEF FAT, COCONUT OIL, AND SAFFLOWER OIL FOR FIVE WEEKS[a,b]

Diets	*Number persons*[b]	*(mg/dl ± SEM)*			
		Total cholesterol[c]	*HDL cholesterol*[d]	*LDL cholesterol*[c]	*Tri-glycerides*[c]
Habitual[c]	19	156 ± 7·0	44 ± 3·0	97 ± 7·9	84 ± 8·7
Test					
Beef fat (BF)	17	155 ± 3·0	36 ± 1·2	98 ± 4·5	89 ± 3·5
Coconut oil (CO)	16	168 ± 3·0	44 ± 1·1	110 ± 4·1	75 ± 3·6
Safflower oil (SO)	17	141 ± 3·1	40 ± 1·2	90 ± 4·7	80 ± 3·7
		P values[e]			
BF vs CO		0·01	0·01	0·08	0·01
BF vs SO		0·01	0·07	0·24	0·06
CO vs SO		0·01	0·02	0·01	0·39

[a] From Reiser *et al.* (1985).
[b] Twelve men completed all three diets, two the beef fat and safflower oil diets, and three the coconut oil and safflower oil diets; 17 completed the beef fat diet, 17 the coconut oil diet, and 16 the safflower oil diet.
[c] Average after fourth and fifth weeks on the diets. There was no significant difference between the two.
[d] There was no significant difference between the habitual pre-beef fat, coconut oil, or safflower oil diet plasma values.
[e] P values $> 0·05$ are not significantly different.

demonstrated that beef fat in the diet did not cause any significantly different concentration of plasma LDL or HDL cholesterols or triglycerides than an equal amount of high linoleic acid safflower oil. The total cholesterol concentration was significantly higher ($P < 0·05$) for the men fed beef fat compared to sunflower oil (155 mg/dl versus 141 mg/dl), but both at the same low risk level. Although the beef fat diet was, thus, positively cholesterolemic with respect to the safflower oil, it was not hypercholesterolemic. NIH (1985) defines hypercholesterolemia as 'an abnormally high blood cholesterol' which must mean above normal risk levels or above 220 mg/dl. None of the responses to beef fat differed from the control values. As pointed out above, statistically significant differences are not necessarily disease threatening.

A study by Lasier (1972) compared responses of beef fat and corn oil to each other and to a typical Canadian dietary regimen. The typical Canadian diet consisted of meat, whole milk, and eggs as well as butter, mayonnaise, lard, and vegetable oil shortening. The test diets were designed to resemble the above but with textured soy protein replacing meat as the protein source for 'beef' stew, 'meat' balls, 'pork' casserole, and 'meat' loaf. The test diet fats were either beef tallow or corn oil, which constituted 95% of the total fat of 35% of calories. The study appears to have been well designed and carried out. However, there were only five subjects, approximately 26-year-old males. The subjects consumed the control diet for 6 days, the beef tallow diet for 21 days, followed by a free choice diet period of 15 days and a second control period of 6 days, and finally the corn oil diet for another 21 days. The average serum cholesterol concentrations at the beginning and end of each of the above periods were: first control diet period, 188 and 191 mg/dl; beef tallow, 171 and 171 mg/dl; the free choice meal, 171 and 192 mg/dl; second control diet period, 192 and 190 mg/dl; and the corn oil diet period, 140–141 mg/dl, respectively. The three critical values are: control, 190 mg/dl; beef fat, 171 mg/dl; and corn oil, 141 mg/dl. Thus, the beef fat at 27% of total calories of a 35% total calories from fat diet resulted in 20 mg/dl lower serum cholesterol than a typical Canadian meal. That the level was higher than that effected by corn oil has no CHD significance and, therefore, the beef fat diet was not hypercholesterolemic.

A study by O'Brien and Reiser (1980) compared red meats to fish and poultry, each with or without three eggs per day. The subjects were 29 healthy male university scientists between 30 and 60 years of age. The men were divided into two groups of 15 (Group I) and 14 (Group II). The two groups ate the four diets in reverse order. A minimum of 6 oz (170 g) of flesh (meat, fish, or poultry) were eaten each day. The data are summarized in Table 2-4. There was no significant difference between the levels of plasma cholesterol in the red meat diet compared to the fish and poultry diet, either with or without eggs. The highest average plasma cholesterol response to the red meat was 206 mg/dl even with eggs. There were statistically significant differences between the egg and no egg diets accompanying both meat diets in Group II but not in Group I. The highest plasma cholesterol level reached was 217 mg/dl in the men of Group II consuming fish and poultry with eggs, but this compared to only 200 mg/dl in the men in Group I consuming the same diet. One must assume that the 17 mg/dl difference is a combination of normal variations and experimental error, but of no health significance. In any event it was associated with the eggs, not the meat.

Two similar studies have since been published, with the first by Flynn *et*

TABLE 2-4

SERUM CHOLESTEROL CONCENTRATIONS OF 30 TEXAS A&M MALE PROFESSORS 30–60 YEARS OF AGE[a,b]

	Red meat diet (mg/dl)	*Fish and poultry diet (mg/dl)*
Three eggs/day		
Group I	204 ± 47[c]	200 ± 43
Group II	206 ± 34[d]	217 ± 30[d]
No eggs		
Group I	195 ± 38	200 ± 41
Group II	193 ± 24	195 ± 26

[a] From O'Brien and Reiser (1980).
[b] All participants were on all four diets for six weeks each.
[c] Standard deviation.
[d] Statistically greater ($P < 0{\cdot}05$) than no eggs. Group I started with egg diets in January, Group II in June.

al. (1981) involving 74 men and 55 women between 23 and 70 years of age who had normal serum lipid levels while consuming standard American diets. The subjects were divided into two groups. They were allowed normal self-selected diets except that they contained either one egg and at least 5 oz (142 g) of beef daily or one egg and 5 oz (142 g) of poultry and fish. The diets were reversed after three months and continued for an additional three months. There was no significant difference between the blood lipid levels during the two dietary regimens except for the triglycerides of the women. Total plasma cholesterol levels for the women were 204 and 226 mg/dl during the first and second periods on the fish and poultry diet and 199 and 226 mg/dl on the two beef periods. The corresponding plasma cholesterol values for the men were 212 and 225 mg/dl while eating fish and poultry and 208 and 217 mg/dl while consuming beef. A similar study by the same group (Flynn *et al.*, 1982) used pork as the meat. Again there was no significant effect on blood lipids.

Thus, no statistical or health difference in blood lipids and lipoproteins has been found to be produced by consumption of beef, pork, or fish and poultry in experimental studies. It is unfortunate that epidemiological and public health groups have spent hundreds of millions of dollars on uncontrolled and inconclusive mass dietary intervention studies such as the Multiple Risk Factor Intervention Trial (1981) and Lipid Research Clinics (1984) Coronary Primary Prevention Trial, but have eschewed controlled experiments. The Nutrition Committee (1982) of the American Heart

Association has itself declared all intervention trials 'flawed in one or another aspect of experimental design', but has not given credence to controlled tests, such as those described above.

There is evidence that ingested lauric, myristic, and palmitic acids produce higher levels of blood cholesterol than low fat control diets and are positively cholesterolemic (Keys *et al.*, 1965). Since both coconut oil and animal fats have high levels of these fatty acids, though in widely different amounts, it is understandable why researchers have used coconut oil as a model for animal fats. Furthermore, coconut oil is easy to obtain, inexpensive, liquid, stable, and mixes readily in dry diets. Most edible animal fats are relatively expensive, solid and quickly become rancid, especially when added to a feed or food mixture, and when cold they are difficult to mix in diets. Lard and beef tallow offered for sale for human consumption have been rearranged and otherwise treated to meet certain physical characteristics. Such treatments no doubt influence their cholesterolemic characteristics. However, the differences do not stop there. Although both coconut oil and meat fats are 'high' in lauric, myristic, and palmitic acids, they differ greatly in the absolute and relative amounts and in the rest of their constituent fatty acids. Various meat fats differ greatly from each other in their fatty acid composition, as can be seen from Table 2-5, so they cannot be ranked together. It is obvious that if the kinds and relative amounts of fatty acids play any role at all, extrapolation cannot be made from the effects of coconut oil to meat fats, such as beef and mutton tallows (Table 2-5). Using data from Table 2-5 and assuming that

TABLE 2-5

BLOOD CHOLESTEROL RELEVANT GROUPS OF FATTY ACIDS OF COCONUT OIL AND MEAT-ANIMAL FATS[a,b]

Fats	*PCE*[c] (%)	*Stearic*[d] (%)	*Monoenoic* (%)	*Polyenoic* (%)	*PCL*[e] / *PCE*[c]
Coconut	70	2·8	5·8	1·8	0·07
Beef	30	19	42	4·0	0·83
Mutton	25	20	41	8·0	1·14
Lard	25	14	45	11	1·34
Chicken	22	6·0	45	21	1·98

[a] From USDA *Handbook No. 8-4* (USDA, 1979).
[b] Rounded to two significant numbers.
[c] PCE = plasma cholesterol elevating fatty acids: lauric, myristic, palmitic.
[d] Assumed neutral.
[e] PCL = plasma cholesterol lowering fatty acids: linoleic + 1/2 monoenoic.

monoenoic acid is half as negatively cholesterolemic as polyunsaturated, as explained below, and stearic is neutral, the ratios of cholesterol lowering to cholesterol elevating acids (linoleic (lauric + myristic + palmitic)) of coconut oil and beef, mutton, lard, and chicken fats are 0·07, 0·83, 1·14, 1·34 and 1·98, respectively. Thus, even from the fatty acid theory viewpoint, only coconut oil, of the saturated fats, should tend to elevate plasma cholesterol and the meat fats tend to be neutral or tend to lower it. Coconut oil even when consumed at 80% of fat calories in real life situations has been found to be associated with normal blood cholesterol concentrations with little evidence of atherosclerosis or CHD (Prior *et al.*, 1966, 1981; Shorland *et al.*, 1969).

Finally, in evaluating the effects of fatty acids on hypercholesterolemia it is important to consider the nature of the fatty acids produced following ingestion of dietary fat, which applies especially to coconut oil. Coconut oil fed to chickens produces depot fats that have a similar fatty acid composition to that of dietary fat containing high levels (*c.* 50%) of lauric acid (12:0). In humans, however, as in other mammals, lauric acid appears in the depot fats to only a limited extent (Shorland and Czochanska, 1970), with enhanced levels of myristic (14:0) and palmitic (16:0) acids being present. As shown by experiments on veal calves by Shorland *et al.* (1981), coconut oil significantly increases the levels of myristic (14:0) and of palmitic (16:0) acids but not of stearic acid (18:0), indicating that the chain extension process is confined to the first two acids only. Coconut oil may thus be regarded as a palmitic acid contributor without invoking lauric acid *per se* as the factor in hypercholesterolemia. As is well known, medium chain (8:0, 10:0) fatty acids have been used in parenteral nutrition (Jennifer *et al.* (1988) as immediately available sources of energy to spare protein and do not appear in the depot fats. To a lesser extent this would apply also to lauric acid.

IV. MODIFICATION OF MEAT FAT FATTY ACIDS

The unremitting attack on meat fat as the major source of ‘saturated’ fat and fatty acids as well as a source of cholesterol and excess calories, and consequently, the primary dietary contributor to CHD, whether real or overstated, has stimulated the meat industry and meat animal scientists to meet the charges. The industry had already, in recognition of the economic waste of fat in swine, slimmed down that meat animal by both genetic selection and dietary means. In the relatively recent past, cattle had been bred and fed to meet the demand for the more expensive fatty grades, so techniques to reverse the process are readily available.

Animals generally do not differ appreciably in the fatty acid composition of their endogenous fat (Reiser, 1954; Anderson *et al.*, 1970a, b) although they may differ in the arrangement of the fatty acids in the glyceride molecule, as is the case for swine (Anderson *et al.*, 1970a). However, commercial monogastric meat animal tissue fatty acids can vary pronouncedly, depending on the composition of the fats in their diets. This is not simply a dilution effect, although that is an important factor which can be utilized in tailor-making of animal fats. There are numerous potential modifying mechanisms. The very presence of exogenous fat inhibits lipogenesis, the effect being greatest for polyunsaturated dietary fatty acids (Hill *et al.*, 1958; Reiser *et al.*, 1963b). The ingestion of cyclopropene fatty acids of gossypium plants, especially cottonseed and its oil, inhibits stearic acid desaturase resulting in an increase in stearic acid and a decrease in the oleic acid content of the animal tissues (Reiser and Raju, 1964). It is not unreasonable to seek to control the palmitate:stearate:oleate ratios by shifting the elongation reactions to the right, thus, reducing palmitate and increasing oleate, the reverse of cyclopropene acid inhibition. Perhaps some application can be made of the observation of the alternate route to oleic acid synthesis from laurate which by-passes palmitate and stearate (Raju and Reiser, 1969).

Reiser (1951) and Reiser and Reddy (1956) demonstrated that the high level of stearic and low level of polyunsaturated acids of ruminant fat is due to biohydrogenation in the rumen. A more detailed description of the rumen fatty acid products of pasture linolenic acid was elucidated by Shorland *et al.* (1957). Rumen hydrogenation was considered to be unfortunate for beef eaters at a time in which diet:heart theorists were touting polyunsaturated fatty acids as the panacea for CHD. Cook and Scott (1970) showed that it is possible to circumvent the rumen hydrogenation process by feeding formaldehyde-treated polyunsaturated vegetable oil–protein particles to beef and dairy cattle, and thus were able to produce polyunsaturated meat and dairy products. However, there were flavor and economic problems with producing and selling the products so that when the potential deleterious effects of large amounts of dietary polyunsaturated fatty acids were realized, the efforts to produce polyunsaturated beef and dairy products were discontinued.

Until recently, little attention has been paid to dietary oleic acid levels or its possible role in the balance between dietary saturated and polyunsaturated acids in the development of CHD. No one seemed concerned with oleic acid levels in meat fats or how its quantities might be altered, or why it should be, until Mattson and Grundy (1985) and Grundy (1986a) showed that oleic and stearic acids produce negative cholesterolemic responses. These reports have stimulated efforts to increase oleic acid, and if possible, to lower the palmitic acid content of meat fats by feeding high oleic acid oils such as high oleic sunflower, canola (high oleic acid rapeseed), and olive oils. Since oleic acid is the end product of fatty acid synthesis it accumulates in the tissues when fed (Tove and Smith, 1960).

Modification of pig fat was stimulated by the soft pork problem which was due to the excessive feeding of peanuts and soybeans. The older work on soft pork and its prevention was reviewed by Hilditch and Williams (1964) in their classical book on natural fats. The data in Table 2-6, taken from Hilditch and Williams (1964), though very old and obtained by antiquated technology, is a classic example of how pork fat may be modified to meet today's demand. Brown (1931) showed that the pig can deposit the C_{20} and C_{22} fatty acids of menhaden oil, and Garton *et al.* (1952) demonstrated that pigs can absorb and deposit whale oil. Soybean oil, which is high in linoleic acid, greatly increases the linoleic acid content of lard at the expense of the other fatty acids. The linolenic acid effect on pig fat fatty acids by feeding soybeans to swine was observed by Ellis and Isbell (1926). Cottonseed oil has an anomalous effect. As reported by Harrington and Adriance (1893) earlier, Ellis *et al.* (1931) could not account for the decrease in oleic and increase in stearic acids in swine after cottonseed oil

TABLE 2-6
MODIFICATION OF PORK FAT BY DIETARY OILS[a]

	Pig back fat			
	Palmitic (%)	*Stearic* (%)	*Oleic* (%)	*Linoleic* (%)
Diet oils				
Low fat	25	14	50	9
Soybean	14–17	8–10	40	38–40
Cottonseed[b,c]	14	26	32	27

[a] From Hilditch and Williams (1964).
[b] Fed at 12% by weight.
[c] Although the linoleic acid of the adipose tissue fat of the cottonseed oil fed pig is high the fat has a high melting point due to its low oleic and high stearic acid contents, the effect of the inhibition of stearic acid desaturase by the constituent cyclopropene fatty acids, sterculic and malvalic, of cottonseed oil (Reiser *et al.*, 1963a; Raju and Reiser, 1967).

consumption. Hilditch and Williams (1964) postulated that the pig was simply diluting pig fat with cottonseed oil. It has since been shown that cottonseed oil contains the cyclopropene fatty acids (malvalic and sterculic) which, on ingestion, inhibit tissue desaturation of stearic to oleic acid (Reiser *et al.*, 1963b; Raju and Reiser, 1967), thus resulting in high stearic and low oleic acids both in the body fat from pigs and in eggs from chickens.

A recent attempt by St. John *et al.* (1987) to produce high oleic and low palmitic acid fat in beef by feeding rapeseed to steers was unsuccessful due to the apparent lack of digestibility of the rapeseed, which replaced 20% corn in the rations. In the same report swine were fed 10 or 20% canola oil diets or a control corn–soybean meal diet. The canola oil contained 64% oleic acid. Treatment was started at approximately 35 days of age or about 20 kg body weight and ended at about 100 kg after 80 days on the trial. The fat was sampled from five depot areas. There was no significant difference in composition between the fat samples from the different body areas. However, the stearic acid concentration in the adipose tissue of the control and in the 10, and 20% canola oil fed pigs were 12·9, 7·3, and 4·3%, respectively. The corresponding palmitic acid contents were 25·6, 16·7, and 10·8%; the oleic acid 46·9, 52·7, and 56·1%; and the linoleic acid 11·5, 17·2, and 21·5%. Thus, by substituting 10% and 20% canola oil for corn and soybean meal, the study clearly achieved its objective of reducing palmitic acid by 43 and 56%, stearic acid by 43 and 66%, and increasing oleic acid by 12 and 20% and linoleic acid by 46 and 87%, respectively.

Casper *et al.* (1988) compared the composition of the butter fat from ten Holstein cows fed concentrates containing either high oleic acid or high linoleic acid sunflower seeds or corn–soybean meal. The fatty acid compositions of the resultant butters were 21, 20, and 29% palmitic; 13, 12, and 8% stearic; 34, 37, and 21% oleic; and 1·9, 3·5, and 2·2% linoleic acids, respectively. Both oils thus greatly reduced the palmitic acid and increased the stearic and oleic acid contents of the butter.

The fatty acid composition of ruminant animals is difficult to modify and several reviewers of the subject have found no truly meaningful variations due to diet. Shorland (1955) reviewed early studies which showed that feeding liberal allowances of highly unsaturated oils to steers for 260 days had no effect on mean unsaturation of body fat. More recently, Christie (1979) concluded that the only way to modify the depot or skeletal muscle fatty acids of beef is through by-passing the rumen. There have been a few reports of minor variation in the composition of the body fats of beef cattle but they do not appear to be of any practical significance (Edwards *et al.*,

1961; Cabezas *et al.*, 1965; Church *et al.*, 1967; Skelley *et al.*, 1973; Thompson *et al.*, 1986). The study of Thompson *et al.* (1986) is of special interest in that it is relatively recent and canola oil was used. However, no effect on the monoenoic fatty acids in body fat was found.

Modern molecular biology opens the possibility for modifying rumen microorganisms in order to reduce their hydrogenation capabilities and permit passage of unchanged oleic acid through the rumen. However, the basic conditions in the rumen can be changed but little. It might prove practical to introduce small amounts of the *n*-3 C_{20} and C_{22} acids of fish oil into cattle tissue by the protective method instead of using larger amounts of *n*-6. Since very small amounts would be needed it might be practical to introduce encapsulated protected fish oil preparations by mouth. There are many opportunities for research in these areas. By introducing fish oil, such as menhaden, into meat animals, consumption of their meat would have the same low plasma triglyceride and antithrombotic effects as the consumption of fish itself (Simopoulos *et al.*, 1986). It would require trial and error experimentation to determine the proper relationship between the quality and quantity of exogenous dosages and between methods of administration and tissue fat quality. However, as discussed above in the section on the Nutritive Values of Fats, meat fats are not devoid of *n*-3 long chain polyunsaturated fatty acids produced from dietary α(*n*-3) linolenic acid and may supply a nutritionally significant amount. It may be possible to extend this principle to significantly increase the EPA and DHA in ruminant animal tissues.

V. SUMMARY

Since about 1965, dietary fats have been said to be responsible for a growing number of metabolic diseases, leading to recommendations that the public severely restrict fat consumption, especially so called ‘saturated fat’. Previously recommended high linoleic acid-rich diets are now also disapproved of but their numerous deleterious effects are not so highly propagandized. The charges against the fats and cholesterol of red meat, eggs, and dairy products can lead to underconsumption of essential minerals, vitamins and high quality protein. Fats and oils serve many important functions, biochemical, culinary, and gustatory and their responsibility for obesity is overstated. There are biochemical mechanisms to balance the metabolism of the mixed fatty acids of plant, terrestrial animal, and fish fats normally consumed by omnivorous humans. Saturated fatty acids increase the beneficial HDL cholesterol and balance some of the untoward effects of linoleic acid. Linoleic acid helps control LDL cholesterol concentration, but develops into thrombus-producing TXA_2. The *n*-3 fatty acids of animal tissue lipids, especially fish oils, help control plasma triglycerides as well as the levels of TXA_2. A high ratio of the *n*-6 linoleic acid to *n*-3 acids in the diet favors TXA_2 formation and thus, in spite of being anti-atherosclerotic, may be responsible for the high CHD rate of this century, especially at low plasma cholesterol levels, rather than the saturated fatty acids from meat. That and the thrombolytic drugs may explain why the incidence of CHD deaths at low plasma cholesterol levels is little less than total CHD incidence whereas the incidences of CHD and CHD deaths at high plasma cholesterol levels are very different but probably involve both atherosclerotic and non-atherosclerotic TXA_2 thrombi.

The dietary cholesterol and saturated fat theory of hypercholesterolemia is simplistic, ignoring normal (non-pathological) variations in levels of plasma cholesterol and misusing the term 'hypercholesterolemia'. It misinterprets to the public the statistics of epidemiological and research data as applying to all members of a population, but which, in fact, apply to only a small genetically aberrant minority. Epidemiological data are susceptible to alternative interpretations and mass trials, such as the LRC–CPPT (1984) have been charged with being faulty in design and interpretation (Authoritative Comments, 1984). Recognition of the above, along with present knowledge of eicosanoid metabolism increasingly makes it clear that the current diet:heart concept and the dietary recommendations built on it are outdated. Controlled experimental trials of meat, meat fat, coconut oil, and eggs have shown that few individuals increase their blood cholesterol level from normal to pathological or from one pathological level to a higher one as a result of consumption of those foods. Those who do are abnormal. It should be more generally recognized that hypercholesterolemia (levels above 220 mg/dl) is a metabolic disease comparable to hyperglycemia and only those who have the disease should be treated, even by dietary manipulation. Normally there are genetically controlled mechanisms which maintain plasma cholesterol homeostasis. The concept that there is a straight line relationship between blood cholesterol concentration and risk of CHD at all levels is an absurdity. The practice of crediting the recent reduced incidence of CHD deaths to the effectiveness of the dietary recommendations is not only incorrect in principle but disproven by the CDC report (1989) that although CHD deaths are being reduced by improved medical treatment, CHD hospitalizations are increasing.

To meet the current objections that meat is too fat, producers are breeding and feeding leaner animals, and processors and merchants are drastically trimming carcasses and various cuts. The subject is discussed in detail in Chapters 16 and 17. Techniques are also available to increase unsaturation and decrease saturation of the fatty acids of meat fat, especially in non-ruminant animals. Examples in nature are the *n*-3 fatty acids of the microflora eaten by fish and up the food chain to sea mammals and humans. Long time experience with food-producing animals fed peanuts, soybeans, and cottonseed oil-containing products has shown that the fat in the tissues of pigs and chickens can be altered by diet.

The oldest nutritional advice is still the most practical and the best. Diets should consist of a variety of animal products including beef, pork, chicken, and fish in conservative size portions, as well as eggs and dairy products. The diet also should contain a variety of fruits, vegetables, and grains. Such diets would make it unnecessary to attempt the impractical, if not impossible, task of counting calories from saturated, monounsaturated, and polyunsaturated fatty acids and complex carbohydrates, of estimating and limiting daily cholesterol to 300 mg, and to thus run the risk of malnutrition. People should first learn if they are hypercholesterolemic and, if so, treat the disease. If they are normal they need not then feel guilty for eating eggs for breakfast and beef for dinner, but enjoy the pleasure and benefits of their high biological value protein, minerals, and B vitamins. They need not treat themselves for a disease they do not have.

Financially interested segments of the food industry, and opportunists self styled as 'nutritionists', have seized upon the well meaning but over-interpreted reports and advice from the AHA and NIH and capitalized on them, often with gross exaggeration. The propaganda has misled not only the general public but also clinicians and qualified dieticians who justifiably trust and depend on the prestigious medical societies and governmental agencies, and then apply and propagate the misleading disinformation.

VI. ACKNOWLEDGEMENT

The authors are indebted to Dr Gary C. Smith, Department of Animal Sciences of Texas A&M University for his reading of the manuscript and for his constructive comments.

VII. REFERENCES

AHRENS, E. H., BLANKENHORN, D. H. and TSALTAS, T. T. (1954). Effect on serum lipids of substituting plant for animal fat in diet. *Proc. Soc. Exptl Biol. Med.* **86**, 872.

AMERICAN HEART ASSOCIATION (AHA) (1986). A statement for physicians and health professionals by the Nutrition Committee of the American Heart Association. *Dietary Guidelines for Healthy Americans*. Publication No. 71-003-C. American Heart Association, Dallas, Texas.

ANDERSON, R. E., BOTTINO, N. R. and REISER, R. (1970a). Animal endogenous triglycerides: I. Swine adipose tissue. *Lipids* **5**, 161.

ANDERSON, R. E., BOTTINO, N. R. and REISER, R. (1970b). Animal endogenous triglycerides: II. Rat and chicken adipose tissue. *Lipids* **5**, 1656.

AUTHORITATIVE COMMENTS (1984). Diet and heart disease, responses to LRC–CPPT findings. *Nutrition Today* **19**(5), 22.

BAGGIO, G., PAGNAN, A., MURACA, M., MARTINI, S., OPPORTUO, A., BONANOME, A., AMBROSIO, G. B., FERRARI, S., GUARINI, P., PICCOLO, D., MANZATO, E., CORROCHER, R. and CREPALDI, G. (1988). Olive-oil enriched diet: Effect on serum lipoprotein levels and biliary cholesterol saturation. *Am. J. Clin. Nutr.* **47**, 960.

BANG, H. O., DYERBERG, J. and SINCLAIR, H. M. (1980). The composition of Eskimo food in Northwestern Greenland Coast Eskimos. *Am. J. Clin. Nutr.* **33**, 2657.

BODY, D. R. and SHORLAND, F. B. (1974). The fatty acid composition of the main phospholipid fractions of the rumen and abomasum tissues of foetal and adult sheep. *J. Sci. Food Agric.* **25**, 197.

BONANOME, A. and GRUNDY, S. M. (1988). Effect of dietary stearic acid on plasma cholesterol and lipoprotein levels. *N. Engl. J. Med.* **318**, 1244.

BROWN, J. B. (1931). The nature of highly unsaturated fatty acids stored in lard from pigs fed on menhaden oil. *J. Biol. Chem.* **90**, 133.

BROZEK, J., BUZINA, R., MILIC, F., HORVAT, N., ZABER, M. and RAO, M. M. (1957). Population studies on serum cholesterol and dietary fat in Yugoslavia. *Am. J. Clin. Nutr.* **5**, 279.

BUDOWSKI, P. (1988). *n*-3 fatty acids in health and disease. *Wld Rev. Nutr. Diet.* **57**, 214.

CABEZAS, M. T., HENTGES, J. F., JR, MOORE, J. E. and OLSON, J. A. (1965). Effect of diet on composition of body fat of steers. *J. Anim. Sci.* **24**, 57.

CASPER, D. P., SCHINGOETHE, D. J., MIDDAUGH, R. P. and BEER, R. J. (1988). Lactational response of dairy cows to diets containing regular and high oleic acid sunflower seeds. *J. Dairy Sci.* **71**, 1267.

CHRISTIE, W. W. (1979). The effects of diet and other factors on the lipid composition of ruminant tissues and milk. *Prog. Lipid Res.* **17**, 245.

CHURCH, D. C., RALSTON, A. T. and KENNICK, W. H. (1967). Effect of diet or diethylstilbesterol on fatty acid composition of bovine tissue, *J. Anim. Sci.* **26**, 1296.

CONNOR, W. E., HODGES, R. E. and BLEILER, R. E. (1961). The serum lipids in men receiving high cholesterol and cholesterol free diets. *J. Clin. Invest.* **40**, 894.

COOK, L. J. and SCOTT, T. W. (1970). Protection of dietary polyunsaturated fatty acids from ruminal microbial hydrogenation. *Proc. Austral. Biochem. Soc.* **3**, 393.

CORNFIELD, J. (1962). Joint dependence of risk of coronary heart disease on serum cholesterol and systolic blood pressure: A discriminant function analysis. *Fed. Proc.* **21**, 58.

CRAWFORD, M. A. (1987). The requirements of long chain *n*-6 and *n*-3 fatty acids for the brain. I. In *Polyunsaturated Fatty Acids and Eicosanoids.* (W. E. M. Land, Ed.), p. 207. Am. Oil Chem. Soc., Champaign, IL, USA.

CRAWFORD, M. A., GALE, M. M. and WOODFORD, M. H. (1969). Linoleic and linolenic elongation products in muscle tissue of *Syncerus caffer* and other ruminant species. *Biochem. J.* **115**, 25.

DAUBER, R. T. (1982). Eggs, serum cholesterol, and coronary heart disease. *Am. J. Clin. Nutr.* **36**, 617.

DAUGHTERY, R. M., GALLI, C., FERRO-LUZZI, A. and IACONO, J. M. (1987). Lipid and phospholipid fatty acid composition of plasma, red blood cells, and platelets and how they are effected by dietary lipids: A study of normal subjects from Italy, Finland, and the USA. *Am. J. Clin. Nutr.* **45**, 443.

DAYTON, S., PEARCE, M. L., HASHIMOTO, S., DIXON, W. J. and TOMIYASU, U. (1969). A controlled clinical trial of a diet high in unsaturated fat in preventing complications of atherosclerosis. *Circulation* **40** (suppl. 11), 1.

DONNISON, C. P. (1929). Blood pressure in the African native, its bearing upon the aetiology of hyperpiesia and atherosclerosis. *Lancet* **i**, 6.

DREON, D. M., FREY-HEWITT, B., ELLSWORTH, N., WILLIAMS, P. T., TERRY, R. B. and WOOD, P. D. (1988). Dietary fat:carbohydrate ratio and obesity in middle-aged men. *Am. J. Clin. Nutr.* **47**, 995.

DYERBERG, J., BANG, H. O., STOFFERSON, E., MONCADA, S. and VANE, J. R. (1978). Eicosapentaenoic acid and prevention of thrombosis and atherosclerosis. *Lancet* **i**, 117.

EDWARDS, D. L., TOVE, S. B., BLUMER, T. N. and BARRICK, E. R. (1961). Effects of added fat on fatty acid composition of fattening steers. *J. Anim. Sci.* **20**, 712.

ELLIS, N. R. and ISBELL, H. S. (1926). Soft pork studies II. Influence of the character of the ration on the composition of the body fat of hogs. *J. Biol. Chem.* **69**, 239.

ELLIS, N. R., ROTHWELL, C. S. and POOL, W. O. (1931). The effect of the ingestion of cottonseed oil on the composition of body fat. *J. Biol. Chem.* **92**, 385.

FLYNN, M. A., NEWMANN, H. D., NOLPH, G. B., NAUMANN, H. D., PARISI, E., BALL, D., KRAUSE, G., ELLERSIECK, M. and WARD, S. S. (1981). Serum lipids in humans fed diets containing beef or fish and poultry. *Am. J. Clin. Nutr.* **34**, 2734.

FLYNN, M. A., NAUMANN, H. D., NOLPH, G. B., KRAUSE, G. and ELLERSIECK, M. (1982). Dietary 'meats' and serum lipids. *Am. J. Clin. Nutr.* **35**, 935.

FOOD AND NUTRITION BOARD (1980). *Toward Healthful Diets.* National Research Council, National Academy of Sciences, Washington, DC.

GARTON, G. A., HILDITCH, T. P. and MEARA, M. L. (1952). The composition of the depot fat of a pig fed on a diet rich in whale oil. *Biochem. J.* **50**, 517.

GRAHAM, J. D. and VAUPEL, J. W. (1980). *The Impact of Egg Consumption on Coronary Heart Disease. A Policy Perspective.* Center for the Study of Policy Analysis. Institute of Policy Sciences and Public Affairs. Duke University, Durham, NC.

GRUNDY, S. M. (1986a). Comparison of monounsaturated fatty acids and carbohydrates for lowering plasma cholesterol. *N. Engl. J. Med.* **314**, 745.

GRUNDY, S. M. (1986b). Cholesterol and coronary heart disease. *JAMA.* **256**, 2849.

HARRINGTON, H. H. and ADRIANCE, D. (1893). Effects of cotton seed and cotton seed meal on butter, beef tallow, lard, and sheep suet. *Texas Agri. Expt. Sta. Bull.* **29**, 347.

HILDITCH, T. P. and WILLIAMS, P. N. (1964). *The Chemical Constitution of Natural Fats*, 4th edn. John Wiley & Sons, Inc., New York.

HILL, R., LINAZASARO, J. M., CHEVALLIER, F. and CHAIKOFF, I. L. (1958). Regulation of hepatic lipogenesis: The influence of dietary fats. *J. Biol. Chem.* **233**, 305.

HOELSCHER, L. M., SAVELL, J. W., SMITH, S. B. and CROSS, H. R. (1988). Subcellular distribution of cholesterol within muscle and adipose tissues of beef loin steaks. *J. Food Sci.* **53**, 718.

HOUTSMULLER, A. J. (1975). The role of fat in the treatment of diabetes mellitus. In *The Role of Fats in Human Nutrition* (A. J. Vergroesen, Ed.) p. 231. Academic Press, New York.

HUBBARD, A. W. and POCKLINGTON, W. D. (1968). Distribution of fatty acids as an aid to identification of animal tissues. Part 1. Bovine, porcine, ovine, and some avian species. *J. Sci. Food Agric.* **19**, 571.

HYSLOP, P. A. and YORK, D. A. (1980). Membrane fluidity and adenyl cyclase activity in genetically obese mice. *Biochem. Biophys. Res. Comm.* **92**, 819.

IGNATOWSKI, A. I. (1908). On the influence of animal food on the tissues of the rabbit. *Reports of the Imperial Military Medical Academy. St. Petersburg* **16**, 1154. Cited by Dock (1958). Research in arteriosclerosis. The first fifty years. *Ann. Int. Med.* **49**, 699.

JENNIFER, M. F., WAN-TIEW, C., BABAYAN, V. K. and BLACKBURN, C. L. (1988). Invited comment: Lipids and the development of immune dysfunction and infection. *J. Parenter. Enter. Nutr.* **12**, 438.

JIANG, C. L. and HUNT, J. N. (1983). The relation between freely chosen meals and body habits. *Am. J. Clin. Nutr.* **38**, 32.

KANNEL, W. B. and GORDON, T. (1982). The search for an optimum serum cholesterol. *Lancet* **ii**, 374.

KATZ, L. N. and STAMLER, J. (1953). *Experimental Atherosclerosis.* Charles C. Thomas, Springfield, IL.

KEYS, A. (1953). Atherosclerosis: A problem in newer public health. *J. Mt Sinai Hospital* (New York City) **20**, 118.

KEYS, A. (1970). Coronary heart disease in seven countries, *Circulation* (Suppl) **XLI**, A53.

KEYS, A., ANDERSON, J. T. and GRANDE, F. (1957a). Serum cholesterol response to dietary fat. *Lancet* **i**, 787.

KEYS, A., ANDERSON, J. T. and GRANDE, F. (1957b). Prediction of serum-cholesterol responses of man to changes in fats in the diet. *Lancet* **ii**, 959.

KEYS, A., ANDERSON, J. T. and GRANDE, F. (1965). Serum cholesterol responses to changes in the diet. IV. Particular saturated fatty acids in the diet. *Metabolism* **14**, 776.

KINSELL, L. W., MICHAELS, G. D., PARTRIDGE, J. W., BOLING, L. A., BALCH, H. E. and COCHRANE, G. C. (1953). Effect upon serum cholesterol and phospholipids of diets containing large amounts of vegetable fat. *J. Clin. Nutr.* **1**, 224.

LANCET EDITORIAL (1983). Eskimo diets and diseases. *Lancet* **i**, 1139.

LASIER, M. C. (1972). Comparison of the effect of beef tallow and corn oil on serum lipid patterns in young men. PhD Thesis. University of Manitoba, Saskatchewan, Manitoba, Canada.

LEVEILLE, G. A. and CLOUTHIER, D. T. (1987). Isocaloric diets: Effects of dietary changes. *Am. J. Clin. Nutr.* **45**, 158.

LIPID RESEARCH CLINICS PROGRAM (1984). The lipid research clinics coronary primary prevention trial results. 1. Reduction in incidence of coronary heart disease. *JAMA* **251**, 351. 2. The relationship of reduction in incidence of coronary heart disease to cholesterol lowering. *JAMA* **251**, 365.

LIPID RESEARCH CLINICS PROGRAM EPIDEMIOLOGIC COMMITTEE—LRCPEC (1979). Plasma lipid distributions in selected North American populations: The lipid research clinics prevalence study. *Circulation* **60**, 1979.

LUDEN, G. (1917). Studies on cholesterol. IV. Experiments concerning the relation of the diet, the blood cholesterol and the 'lymphoid disease' *Lab. Clin. Med.* **3**, 141. Quoted by Weinhouse, S. (1943). *The Blood Cholesterol Arch. Path.* **35**, 438.

MATTSON, F. H. and GRUNDY, S. M. (1985). Comparison of effects of dietary saturated, monounsaturated, and polyunsaturated fatty acids in plasma lipids and lipoproteins in man. *J. Lipid Res.* **26**, 194.

MCNAMARA, D. J., KOLB, R., PARKER, T. S., BATWIN, H., SAMUEL, P., BROWN, C. D. and AHRENS, E. A., JR (1987). Heterogeneity of cholesterol homeostasis in man. *J. Clin. Invest.* **79**, 1729.

MENSINK, R. P. and KATAN, M. B. (1987). Effect of monounsaturated fatty acids versus complex carbohydrates on high-density lipoproteins in healthy men and women. *Lancet* (Jan. 17), 122.

MULTIPLE RISK FACTOR INTERVENTION TRIAL RESEARCH GROUP (1981). The multiple risk factor intervention trial (MRFIT). R. C. Beneari and R. Sherwin, Eds. *Preventive Medicine 10*, 387.

NATIONAL CENTER FOR DISEASE CONTROL (CDC) (1989). Hospitalization rates for ischemic heart disease—United States, 1970–1986 Chronic disease reports: Coronary heart disease mortality—United States, 1986. *Morbidity and Mortality Weekly Report.* **38**, 275–85.

NATIONAL CHOLESTEROL EDUCATION PROGRAM—NCEP (1988). Report of the National Cholesterol Education Program expert panel on detection, evaluation, and treatment of high blood cholesterol in adults. *Arch. Intern. Med.* **148**, 36.

NATIONAL INSTITUTES OF HEALTH (NIH) (1985). Lowering blood cholesterol to prevent heart disease. *Atherosclerosis* **5**, 404.

NATIONAL RESEARCH COUNCIL—NRC. (1982). Committee on diet, nutrition, and cancer, assembly of life sciences. *Diet, Nutrition, and Cancer* National Academy Press, Washington, DC 20418.

NORDOY, A. and SIMONSEN, T. (1987). Dietary *n*-3 fatty acids, experimental thrombosis, and coronary heart disease in man. In *Polyunsaturated Fatty Acids and Eicosanoids* (W. E. M. Lands, Ed.) p. 25. Am. Oil Chem. Soc., Champaign, IL.

NUTRITION COMMITTEE (1982). Rational of the diet–heart statement of the American Heart Association. *Circulation* **65**, 839A.

O'BRIEN, B. C. and REISER, R. (1980). Human plasma lipid responses to red meat, poultry, fish, and eggs. *Am. J. Clin. Nutr.* **33**, 2573.

O'BRIEN, B. C. and MCMURRAY, D. N. (1988). Human plasma lipid and immunological responses to eggs and ascorbic acid. *Nutr. Res.* **8**, 353.

POOLING PROJECT RESEARCH GROUP (1978). Relationship of blood pressure, serum cholesterol, smoking habit, relative weight, and ECG abnormalities to incidence of major coronary events: Final report of the Pooling Project. *J. Chronic Dis.* **31**, 201.

PRIOR, I. A., HARVEY, H. P. B., NEAVE, M. N. and DAVIDSON, F. (1966). The health of two groups of Cook Island Maoris. N.Z. *Department of Health Special Report Series* **26**, 1.

PRIOR, I. A., DAVIDSON, F., SALMUND, C. E. and CZOCHANSKA, Z. (1981). Cholesterol, coconuts, and diet on Polynesian Atolls: A natural experiment: the Pukapuka and Tokelau Island studies. *Am. J. Clin. Nutr.* **34**, 1552.

RAJU, P. K. and REISER, R. (1967). Inhibition of fatty acid desaturase by cyclopropene fatty acids. *J. Biol. Chem.* **242**, 379.

RAJU, P. K. and REISER, R. (1969). Alternate route for the biosynthesis of oleic acid in the rat. *Biochim. Biophys. Acta* **176**, 48.

REAVEN, G. M. (1988). Looking at the world through LDL–cholesterol-colored glasses. *J. Nutr.* **116**, 1143.

REISER, R. (1951). Hydrogenation of polyunsaturated fatty acids by the ruminant. *Fed. Proc.* **10**, 236.

REISER, R. (1954). The influence of dietary fat on the glyceride structure of animal fat. *J. Am. Oil Chem. Soc.* **31**, 625.

REISER, R. (1981). Nutrition and metabolism of trans fatty acids. *La Rivista Italiana della Sostange Grasse* **LVIII**, 565.

REISER, R. and RAJU, P. K. (1964). The inhibition of saturated fatty acid dehydrogenation by dietary fat containing sterculic and malvalic acids. *Biochem. Biophys. Res. Comm.* **17**, 8.

REISER, R. and REDDY, H. A. R. (1956). The hydrogenation of dietary unsaturated fatty acids by the ruminant. *J. Am. Oil Chem. Soc.* **33**, 155.

REISER, R., PARECH, C. K. and MEINKE, W. W. (1963a). The metabolism of cyclopropenyl fatty acids. In *Biochemical Problems of the Lipids* (A. C. Frazer, Ed.) BBA Library, Vol. 1, p. 251. Elsevier Publishing Co., Amsterdam.

REISER, R., WILLIAMS, M. C., SORRELS, M. F. and MURTY, H. L. (1963b). Biosynthesis of fatty acids and cholesterol as related to diet fat. *Arch. Biochem. Biophy.* **102**, 276.

REISER, R., PROBSTFIELD, J. L., SILVERS, A., SCOTT, L. W., SHORNEY, M. L., WOOD, R. D., O'BRIEN, B. C., GOTTO, A. M., JR and INSULL, W. (1985). Plasma lipid and lipoprotein response of humans to beef fat, coconut oil, and safflower oil. *Am. J. Clin. Nutr.* **42**, 190.

RHEE, K. S., DUTSON, T. S., SMITH, G. C., HOSTETLER, R. L. and REISER, R. (1982). Cholesterol content of raw and cooked beef longissimus muscles with different degrees of marbling. *J. Food Sci.* **47**, 716.

RIZEK, R. L., WELSH, S. D., MARSTON, R. M. and JACKSON, E. M. (1983). Levels and sources of fat in the US food supply and in diets of individuals. In *Dietary Fats and Health* (E. G. Perkins and W. J. Visek, Eds), p. 13. American Oil Chemists Society, Champaign, IL.

ROSSOUW, J. E., BURGER, E. M., VAN DER VYVER, P. and FERREIRO, J. J. (1981). The effect of skim milk, yogurt and full cream milk (3·3%) on human serum lipids *Am. J. Clin. Nutr.* **34**, 351.

ROBERTS, J. C. and STRAUS, R. (1965). *Comparative Atherosclerosis.* Hoeber Medical Division, Harper & Row, New York.

RUFFER, M. A. (1921). *Studies in the Paleopathology of Egypt*, Universal Press, Chicago. Quoted by Weiss and Minot (1933).

SACHS, F. H. (1988). Letter to the Editor. *N. Engl. J. Med.* **314**, 1090.

SAVELL, J. W and CROSS, H. R. (1988). The role of fat in the palatability of beef, pork, and lamb. In *Designing Foods: Animal Product Options in the Marketplace*, p. 345. Committee on Technical Options to Improve Nutritional Attributes of Animal Products, Board of Agriculture, National Research Council. National Academy Press, Washington, DC.

SHATTIL, S. J. and COOPER, R. A. (1976). Membrane microviscosity and human platelet function. *Biochemistry* **15**, 4832.

SHEPARD, J., PACKARD, C. J., GRUNDY, S. M., YESHURUN, D., GOTTO, A. M., JR and TAUNTON, O. D. (1980). Effects of saturated and polyunsaturated fat diets on the chemical composition and metabolism of low density lipoproteins in man. *J. Lipid Res.* **21**, 91.

SHORLAND, F. B. (1955). Formation of animal fat. In *Progress in the Chemistry of Fats and Other Lipids*, Vol. 3 (R. T. Holman, W. O. Lundberg and T. Malkin, Eds). Pergamon Press, London and New York, p. 275.

SHORLAND, F. B. (1988). Is our knowledge of human nutrition soundly based? *Wld Rev. Nutr. Diet.* **57**, 126.

SHORLAND, F. B. and CZOCHANSKA, Z. (1970). The fatty acid composition of the depot fats of hens fed on coconut meal. Differences in fat metabolism between birds and mammals. *Austral. J. Sci.* **32**, 330.

SHORLAND, F. B., WEENINK, R. O., JOHNS, A. T. and MCDONALD, I. R. C. (1957). The effect of sheep-rumen contents on unsaturated fatty acids. *Biochem. J.* **67**, 328.

SHORLAND, F. B., CZOCHANSKA, Z. and PRIOR, I. A. M. (1969). Fatty acid composition of adipose tissue and blood lipids of Polynesians. *Am. J. Clin. Nutr.* **22**, 124.

SHORLAND, F. B., IGENE, J. O., PEARSON, A. M., THOMAS, J. W., MCGUFFY, R. K. and ALDRIDGE, A. E. (1981). Effects of dietary fat and vitamin E on the lipid composition and stability of veal during frozen storage. *J. Agric. Food Chem.* **29**, 863.

SIMOPOULOS, A. P., KIFER, R. R. and MARTIN, R. E. (Eds) (1986). *Health Effects of Polyunsaturated Fatty Acids of Seafoods.* Academic Press, New York.

SINZINGER, H., FEIGEL, W. and SILBERBAUER, K. (1979). Prostacyclin generation in atherosclerotic arteries. PGI_2 lower in atherosclerotic than in normal tissue. *Lancet* **ii**, 469.

SKELLY, G. C., STANDFORD, W. C. and EDWARDS, R. L. (1973). Bovine fat composition and its relation to animal diet and carcass characteristics. *J. Anim. Sci.* **36**, 576.

SLATER, G., MEAD, J., DHOPESHWARKAR, G., ROBINSON, S. and ALFIN-SLATER, R. B. (1976). Plasma cholesterol and triglycerides in man with added eggs in the diet. *Nutr. Repts Intern.* **14**, 249.

SMITH, G. C. and CARPENTER, Z. L. (1976). Eating quality of meat animal products and their fat content. In *The Fat Content and Composition of Animal Products*, p. 183. Proc. Symp., National Research Council, National Academy of Sciences, Washington, DC.

STAMLER, J., WENTWORTH, D. and NEATON, J. D. (1986). Is relationship between serum cholesterol and risk of premature death from coronary heart disease continuous and graded? *JAMA* **256**, 2823.

STEERING COMMITTEE OF THE PHYSICIANS HEALTH STUDY RESEARCH GROUP (1989).

Final report on the aspirin component of the ongoing physician's health study. *New Engl. J. Med.* **321**, 129.

St. John, L. C., Young, C. R., Knabe, D. A., Thompson, L. D., Schelling, G. T., Grundy, S. M. and Smith, S. B. (1987). Fatty acid profiles and sensory and carcass traits of tissues from steers and swine fed an elevated monounsaturated fat diet. *J. Anim. Sci.* **64**, 1441.

Taylor, T. G., Gibney, M. J. and Morgan, J. B. (1979). Haemostatic function and polyunsaturated fatty acids. *Lancet* **iii**, 1378.

The Surgeon General's Report on Nutrition and Health (1988). US Department of Health and Human Services. DHHA (PHS) Publication no. 88-50210, Superintendent of Documents, US Government Printing Office, Washington, DC 20402.

Thomas, W. A. (1927). Health of a carnivorous race, a study of the Eskimo. *JAMA* **88**, 1559.

Thompson, L. D., Schelling, G. T., Byers, F. M. and Greene, L. W. (1986). Effect of feeding whole canola rapeseed on the fatty acid composition of depot fat in steers. *J. Anim. Sci.* **63** (Suppl. 1), 66.

Tove, S. B. and Smith, F. H. (1960). Changes in fatty acid composition of the depot fat of mice induced by feeding oleate and linoleate. *J. Nutr.* **71**, 264.

USDA (1979). Science and Education Administration. *Composition of Foods, Fats, and Oils, Raw, Processed, Prepared. Handbook No. 8-4.* United States Department of Agriculture, Washington, DC.

Weiss, S. and Minot, G. R. (1933). Nutrition in relation to arteriosclerosis. In *Arteriosclerosis* (E. V. Cowdry, Ed.), p. 235. McMillan Co., New York.

Wood, R. D. (1983). Geometrical and positional monoene isomers in beef and several processed meats. In *Dietary Fats and Health* (E. G. Perkins and W. J. Visek, Eds), p. 341. American Oil Chemists Society, Champaign, IL.

3

Relationship Between Blood and Dietary Cholesterol

DONALD J. MCNAMARA

Department of Nutrition and Food Science, University of Arizona, Tucson, Arizona, USA

I. INTRODUCTION

A. Heart Disease Mortality and Morbidity in the USA

Cardiovascular diseases (CVD) accounted for 48% of all deaths in the USA in 1985 with over 900 000 Americans dying of heart attacks, strokes and other blood vessel diseases. As the leading cause of mortality and morbidity in the USA, elucidation of the causative factors and development of effective preventive approaches are high priorities for the biomedical community. Numerous epidemiological studies have defined multiple metabolic and life-style risk factors for CVD which independently, and in combination, play major roles in the development and progression of this disease. Over the years intervention trials have indicated that risk factor reduction can effectively decrease CVD incidence so that current public health policy has been aimed at reducing those risk factors for which interventions have been shown to be effective. The advances made in clinical care of patients with CVD and the diagnosis and effective intervention of CVD risk factors have resulted in a steady decline in CVD mortality and morbidity in the United States during the last twenty years (Gillum *et al.*, 1984).

B. Heart Disease Risk Factors

Genetics is no doubt a major determinant of an individual's own CVD risk profile, which is why a family history of premature CVD is considered a major risk factor, as are increasing age and male sex that are risk factors not amiable to intervention and thus preclude reduction. The life-style factors, which are major primary risk factors for CVD, include cigarette smoking, high blood pressure, and a high blood cholesterol level (Stamler *et al.*, 1986). Other risk factors include obesity, a sedentary life style and a Type A personality (Hopkins and Williams, 1981). A number of secondary risk factors for CVD, which arise from an independent metabolic or clinical disorder, have also been defined (Hopkins and Williams, 1981) and include glucose intolerance, renal disease, endocrine disorders and others.

While CVD is known to develop from a variety of causes, and clearly has a multiple etiology, this review will concentrate on the significance of an elevated plasma cholesterol level in determining an individual's risk for CVD and the potential role of dietary cholesterol in elevating plasma cholesterol levels, and CVD risk. The role of dietary fat quality and quantity in determining plasma cholesterol levels and CVD risk are discussed in some detail in Chapter 2.

II. BLOOD CHOLESTEROL AND HEART DISEASE RISK

A. Evidence for Relationship

There is little doubt that an elevated plasma cholesterol level is related to an increased risk for CVD. Cross-cultural studies have shown that the higher the average plasma cholesterol in a population, the higher the mortality rate from CVD (Simons, 1986). Data from both the Framingham Study (Kannel *et al.*, 1979) and the Multiple Risk Factor Intervention Trial (Stamler *et al.*, 1986) have clearly established the relationship between elevated plasma cholesterol levels and an increased CVD risk. There have been arguments pro and con regarding the existence of a threshold level of plasma cholesterol relative to CVD risk, and the actual level of plasma cholesterol above which CVD risk is increased remains a point of some controversy. What is clear is that an elevated plasma cholesterol is an independent risk factor for CVD and that interventions to reduce an elevated level constitute a reasonable approach to reducing the incidence of CVD in the population.

B. Interaction with Other Risk Factors

An elevated plasma cholesterol level not only has a significant impact on CVD risk in its own right but also exacerbates the effects of other risk factors. As shown by data from both the Framingham Study and MRFIT, the presence of an elevated plasma cholesterol level along with cigarette smoking, high blood pressure, or both of these major risk factors results in a

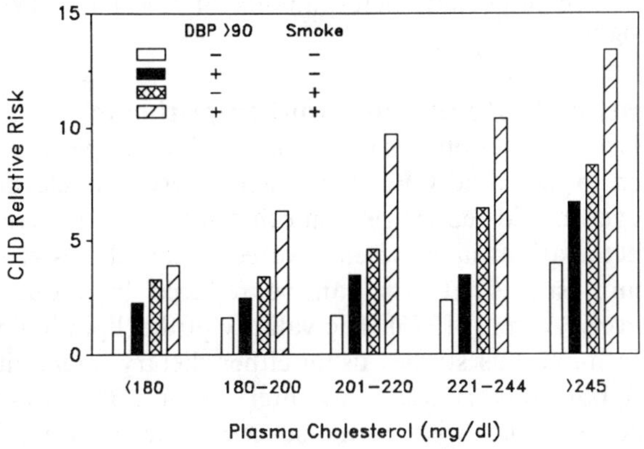

FIG. 3-1. Interactions between plasma cholesterol, hypertension, and cigarette smoking on coronary heart disease risk. CHD relative risk as a function of plasma cholesterol levels in the absence and presence of hypertension (diastolic blood pressure (DBP) > 90), cigarette smoking, and hypertension plus cigarette smoking. CHD risk relative to plasma cholesterol level < 180 mg/dl in normotensive, non-smoker = 1·0. Data from the Multiple Risk Factor Intervention Trial (Stamler *et al.*, 1986).

pronounced increase in CVD risk (Fig. 3-1). In the presence of a high plasma cholesterol level, the effects of cigarette smoking and hypertension on CVD risk are greatly enhanced and the combination of all three of these major CVD risk factors results in a 13-fold increase in CVD risk. Based on these types of data it can be clearly seen that attempting to reduce an elevated plasma cholesterol level has the potential to be a significant CVD risk reducing modality, especially when combined with cessation of cigarette smoking and treatment of high blood pressure.

It should be kept in mind that measurement of plasma total cholesterol levels provides only a partial evaluation of the CVD risk profile since plasma cholesterol levels are determined by various types of lipoproteins, which have both atherogenic (low density lipoproteins, LDL) and anti-atherogenic (high density lipoproteins, HDL) effects (Gordon *et al.*, 1977). An individual with a low total cholesterol level may be at increased CVD risk due to a high LDL/HDL ratio while another individual with an elevated plasma cholesterol level may actually be at low risk by virtue of having a low LDL/HDL ratio (Abbott *et al.*, 1988). In addition to the importance of the LDL/HDL ratio in determining CVD risk, recent studies have indicated that a number of lipid related measures, such as apolipoprotein levels, are important determinants of CVD risk (Wallace and Anderson, 1987).

C. Intervention Tests of the 'Lipid Hypothesis'

The 'Lipid Hypothesis' proposes that since an elevated plasma cholesterol level is related to increased CVD risk, then lowering an elevated plasma cholesterol level should reduce risk; in other words, that there is a direct cause and effect relationship between elevated plasma cholesterol levels and CVD incidence, such that risk can be reduced by reducing plasma cholesterol levels (Ahrens, 1976). The validity of the 'lipid hypothesis' has been tested in numerous studies using either dietary interventions, drug treatments or both dietary and drug interventions. The results of these various studies have met with partial success in determining the validity of the lipid hypothesis when aggressive drug interventions are used to lower an elevated plasma cholesterol level (Multiple Risk Factor Intervention Trial Group, 1982; Lipid Research Clinics Program, 1984a, b; Canner *et al.*, 1986; Blankenhorn *et al.*, 1987; Frick *et al.*, 1987; Manninen *et al.*, 1988). Reviews of lipid-lowering clinical trials by Tyroler (1987) and Bilheimer (1988) emphasize the validity of identification and treatment of high-risk hypercholesterolemic individuals to reduce CVD risk and the rationale of treating the hypercholesterolemic patient with dietary modifications prior to initiation of drug therapy.

D. Risk Classification

The National Cholesterol Education Program (National Cholesterol Education Program Expert Panel, 1988) has defined CVD risk relative to plasma cholesterol levels in three groups: (1) low risk at plasma cholesterol levels less than 200 mg/dl, (2) moderate risk at cholesterol levels between 200 and 240 mg/dl, and (3) high risk for cholesterol levels greater than 240 mg/dl. While there may be some disagreement regarding the levels chosen, whether too high or too low, this debate is not under consideration here. What this risk classification means is that, when based solely on plasma cholesterol levels, approximately 50% of the American population is classified as having low risk, 25% at moderate risk and 25% at high risk. Thus half the American population exists above the average risk cut-off of 200 mg/dl and would receive the recommendation to alter their diet to a lower saturated fat and cholesterol intake, a dietary change which would result in a substantial alteration in the overall food consumption pattern in this country. The major questions raised regarding dietary recommendations to the public to decrease dietary saturated fat and cholesterol consumption deal with the efficacy and safety of such changes and the potential benefits to be gained in terms of reducing CVD morbidity and mortality.

III. DIETARY CHOLESTEROL EFFECTS ON BLOOD CHOLESTEROL

A. Cholesterol Metabolism in Humans

The average American has a dietary cholesterol intake of approximately 450 mg/day. Absorption of dietary cholesterol averages 60% in the population with individual values ranging from 20–80% (McNamara, 1987). Endogenous cholesterol synthesis ranges between 11–13 mg/day per kg body weight, so a 70 kg male will produce approximately 770–910 mg/day. Assuming a synthesis of 840 mg/day and an absorbed dietary cholesterol input of 270 mg/day (60% of 450 mg), the total amount of cholesterol the body must handle equals 1110 mg/day; 24% from diet and 76% from synthesis. Some 20–30% of this cholesterol is used for bile acid synthesis and small amounts are needed for steroid hormone production and tissue repair. Since the body has no mechanisms to degrade steroids, the majority of this daily input must be excreted as unabsorbed bile acids and biliary cholesterol. Under steady state conditions the fecal excretion of cholesterol and bile acids equals the sum of endogenous cholesterol synthesis plus dietary cholesterol (McNamara, 1987).

Plasma cholesterol transport by the lipoproteins represents a complicated network of lipoproteins involved in exogenous and endogenous fat transport, lipoprotein uptake by body tissues, and transport of cellular cholesterol, obtained by uptake of plasma lipoprotein cholesterol and by endogenous synthesis in the cell, back to the liver for catabolism and excretion (Hamsten, 1988). There are a limited number of studies investigating the effects of dietary cholesterol on in-vivo lipoprotein metabolism in man (McNamara, 1987) and the results have been highly variable.

B. Epidemiological Evidence for a Relationship between Dietary and Plasma Cholesterol Levels

Epidemiological evidence for a relationship between dietary cholesterol intakes and plasma cholesterol levels is weak at best and confounded by the association of dietary cholesterol with saturated fat intake. Analysis of the data in a recent review of the Seven Countries Study data by Hegsted and Ausman (1988) indicates that deletion of the two countries with the lowest dietary cholesterol intakes (Japan and Italy) reduces the linear correlation between CHD and dietary cholesterol from 0·63 ($n = 18$, $P < 0{\cdot}01$) to 0·48 ($n = 16$, $P > 0{\cdot}05$). Since there exists a strong relationship between saturated fat and dietary cholesterol intakes, the relationship between CVD and dietary cholesterol is very difficult to validate. The relationship between dietary cholesterol intake and CHD incidence is marginal and may relate more to numerous cultural differences than to dietary effects on plasma cholesterol levels. Epidemiological studies in the USA have been unable to document a consistent relationship between dietary cholesterol consumption and CVD incidence. However, one study, the Western Electric Study, has reported a significant relationship between dietary cholesterol and CVD incidence (Grundy *et al.*, 1988). It should be noted that in this study the relationship between saturated fat intake and CVD incidence, which has been found in a number of studies, was not significant. Why this single study found a significant relationship between dietary cholesterol intake and CVD incidence, when it would be expected that the fractional absorption of dietary cholesterol would be highly variable in the study population, is not clear and is inconsistent with other epidemiological data within the population.

C. Dietary Cholesterol Studies: Physiological versus Pharmacological

Studies of the effects of dietary cholesterol on plasma cholesterol levels can be classified into two broad categories, physiological and pharmacological. These definitions are based on whether a study uses amounts of dietary cholesterol which result in a dietary cholesterol input less than (physiological) or greater than (pharmacological) the body's own production rate. Almost any dietary constituent given in excess of the body's ability to metabolize the compound can result in a toxic response; however, this is not necessarily evidence that the dietary constituent in question is toxic at all levels.

Assuming an average of 60% absorption of dietary cholesterol and an endogenous synthesis rate of 12 mg/kg-day, it is obvious that a dietary cholesterol challenge of 2000 mg/day to a 70 kg man would result in a net dietary cholesterol input of 1200 mg/day, an amount which exceeds his daily endogenous synthesis rate (840 mg/day) by 360 mg. Assuming our theoretical patient has an ideal feedback mechanism, which is capable of totally suppressing endogenous synthesis, he will continue to have a net excess input of 360 mg/day of cholesterol. Under this condition it is not surprising that an increase in plasma cholesterol is observed. If, on the other hand, our study subject is challenged with 800 mg of cholesterol per day, the net daily input from diet would be 480 mg or 57% of the daily synthesis rate, an amount which could be compensated for by a reduction in endogenous cholesterol synthesis if effective feedback control mechanisms are operational. For the purpose of this review, dietary cholesterol studies using test amounts of 1000 mg/day or less will be classified as physiological while those testing intakes greater than 1000 mg/day will be considered pharmacological.

While it could be argued that this classification system is arbitrary, such a classification has significance in consideration of the recommendations that the dietary cholesterol intake of the population be reduced from an average of 450 mg/day to less than 300 mg/day. Rarely do individuals consume more than 1000 mg on any given day, let alone daily over an extended time period. In consideration of the data to support or refute such a recommendation it is essential that the evidence be considered on the basis of 'real life' situations and not solely on the basis that if a massive dose is very bad, then a small dose must be judged equally harmful.

(i) Evidence of a relationship

The effects of dietary cholesterol on plasma cholesterol levels and endogenous cholesterol and lipoprotein metabolism have been the subject of studies for over three decades yet the question remains a hotly debated topic. Numerous review articles have been written on the subject (McGill, 1979; Grundy, 1979, 1983; Beynen *et al.*, 1987; McNamara, 1987; Quintao and Sperotto, 1987; Grundy *et al.*, 1988) and the reader is referred to these reviews for detailed analysis and the various rationales of the pro and con arguments. Interpretation of the available data in the literature is complicated due to the wide spectrum of study designs and subjects which have been utilized to study the relationship between dietary cholesterol intake and plasma cholesterol levels: solid food versus formula diets; metabolic ward versus controlled dietary intake versus free-living population studies; variations in dietary fat quality and/or quantity; normolipidemic versus hyperlipidemic study subjects; feeding crystalline cholesterol versus natural food sources such as eggs; variations in body weights of the study populations, which affects the relationship between absorbed dietary cholesterol and endogenous cholesterol synthesis; and duration of the test diets. In addition, a major flaw in most studies is the use of a single plasma determination of cholesterol levels during each phase of the feeding trial. Studies have shown that the average physiological variance from week to week in plasma cholesterol levels averages 5% (Hegsted and Nicolosi, 1987; Rotterdam *et al.*, 1987), a level which for many studies is equal to or greater than the potential dietary cholesterol induced change in the plasma level. Finally, the intra-individual variability in dietary cholesterol absorption, which ranges between 20 and 85% (McNamara, 1987) adds a significant inter-individual variable since the vast majority of studies quantitate the amount of cholesterol fed not the actual amount of cholesterol that a subject absorbs. The combination of intra-individual variance in plasma cholesterol levels and inter-individual variance in cholesterol absorption may in part account for the conflicting conclusions reported in the literature and for the failure to clearly establish whether dietary cholesterol does or does not have a significant impact on plasma cholesterol levels.

In an attempt to evaluate the available literature regarding the relationship between dietary cholesterol intake and plasma cholesterol levels, 68 studies, carried out between 1961 and 1987, are summarized in Table 3-1. These studies represent analysis of the effects of dietary cholesterol on plasma cholesterol levels in 1490 study subjects, use a wide range of baseline and challenge cholesterol levels, and vary in terms of dietary fat quality and quantity. Even with these numerous variables it is surprising to find that the data indicate a fairly consistent dietary cholesterol induced increase in plasma cholesterol levels as presented in Fig. 3-2 and a significant relationship between the change in dietary cholesterol intake and the change in plasma cholesterol levels ($r = 0{\cdot}64$, $P < 0{\cdot}001$, $n = 68$). However, extrapolation of a statistically significant correlation to a biologically important effect are not necessarily one and the same thing. The slope of the relationship between the change in dietary cholesterol intake and change in plasma cholesterol levels is relatively small (0·018 mg/dl per mg dietary cholesterol added) and indicates that a change in dietary cholesterol intake of 100 mg/day would result in a change in the plasma cholesterol level of 1·8 mg/dl. If these 68 studies are normalized to compare the change in the plasma cholesterol level per 100 mg increment in dietary cholesterol fed, the results of these various studies are fairly consistent (Fig. 3-2) with an average change in plasma cholesterol of 2·3 mg/dl ($\pm 0{\cdot}2$ SEM, $n = 68$) for each 100 mg/day increment in dietary cholesterol intake. Based on this analysis one would predict that an average 70 kg adult with a baseline plasma cholesterol of 210 mg/dl would increase his/her plasma level by 1·1% when dietary cholesterol intake is increased by 100 mg/day; a value one-fifth of the week-to-week normal physiological

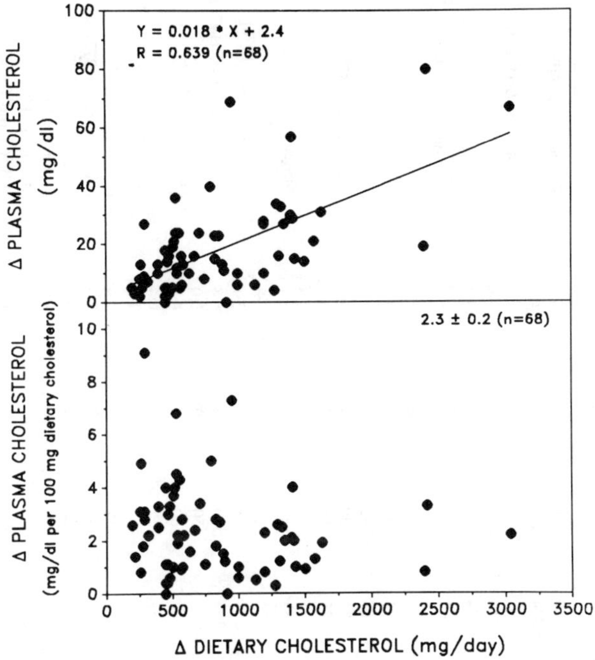

FIG. 3-2. Relationships between changes in dietary cholesterol intake and plasma cholesterol levels. The data represent 68 clinical studies in 1490 subjects. The upper graph represents the correlation between the increment in dietary cholesterol intake (mg/day) and the average change in plasma cholesterol levels (mg/dl). The correlation is significant at $P<0{\cdot}001$ with a slope of 0·018 mg/dl change per mg increment in dietary cholesterol. The lower figure presents the same data where the change in plasma cholesterol is normalized per 100 mg/day increment in dietary cholesterol. The mean change per 100 mg/day increase equals 2·3 mg/dl ($\pm 0{\cdot}2$, $n=68$).

cholesterol variance, and therefore, virtually undetectable. Considering that a 100 mg/day increase in dietary cholesterol mediates this small increment in plasma cholesterol levels it is not surprising that in only a limited number of studies, those studies feeding very large amounts of dietary cholesterol, have significant differences been reported (McNamara, 1987).

The data presented in Table 3-1 can be used to address a number of unresolved questions regarding the relationship between dietary and plasma cholesterol levels. As presented in Table 3-2, a number of permutations in study designs have been evaluated to determine their

TABLE 3-1

SUMMARY OF DIETARY CHOLESTEROL STUDIES

Study	No. patients	Average wt (kg)	Dietary fat		Dietary cholesterol (mg/day)		Plasma cholesterol (mg/dl)		Cholesterol		Change mg/dl per 100 mg increase in cholesterol	Reference
			%cal	P/S	Low	High	Low	High	Change diet[a] (mg/day)	Change plasma (mg/dl)		
1	6	70	40	0·8	0	950	191	260	950	69	7·3	Connor *et al.* (1961a)
2	6	70	40	0·8	0	2 400	205	224	2 400	19	0·8	
3	6	75	40	1·0	0	2 592	167	247	2 419	80	3·3	Connor *et al.* (1961b)
4	22	70	44	1·6	50	520	196	210	470	14	3·0	Grande *et al.* (1965)
5	22	70	40	1·3	49	1 449	194	224	1 400	30	2·1	
6	22	70	44	1·6	50	1 403	196	223	1 353	27	2·0	
7	22	70	8	0·5	47	1 550	205	219	1 503	14	0·9	
8	22	70	40	0·1	49	1 449	228	257	1 400	29	2·1	
9	22	70	44	1·6	520	1 403	210	223	883	13	1·5	
10	14	70	39	0·3	0	793	158	198	793	40	5·0	Mattson *et al.* (1972)
11	13	70	39	0·3	0	530	157	181	530	24	4·5	
12	14	70	39	0·3	0	265	162	175	265	13	4·9	
13	5	75	43	0·1	493	789	192	197	276	5	1·8	Nestel *et al.* (1975)
14	5	75	43	1·0	520	796	169	177	258	8	3·1	
15	12	70	35	4·7	3	291	122	130	288	8	2·8	Anderson *et al.* (1976)
16	12	70	35	0·3	3	291	158	167	288	9	3·1	
17	9	66	40	1·9	240	740	268	304	530	36	6·8	Nestel and Poyser (1976)
18	15	70			340	790	170	170	450	0	0·0	Slater *et al.* (1976)
19	46	70			340	600	198	200	260	2	0·8	
20	21	70	43		250	715	251	253	465	2	0·4	Kummerow *et al.* (1977)
21	40	70	30	2·5	500	965	261	266	465	5	1·1	
22	114	75	38		301	536	223	226	219	3	1·4	Porter *et al.* (1977)
23	7	69	40	2·0	250	3 250	282	349	3 043	67	2·2	Quintao *et al.* (1977)
24	6	62			80	1 080	180	186	1 129	6	0·5	Whyte *et al.* (1977)
25	116	70	38		260	800	196	206	540	10	1·9	Flynn *et al.* (1979)
26	9	22		2·0	135	585	272	287	1 432	15	1·0	Martin and Nestel (1979)
27	29	83			250	1 000	194	204	633	10	1·6	O'Brien and Reiser (1980)
28	16	74	33	0·4	350	900	205	226	520	21	4·0	Chenoweth *et al.* (1981)
29	16	74	33	1·0	180	800	185	198	586	13	2·2	
30	12	70	49	0·5	400	1 400	170	176	1 000	6	0·6	Flaim *et al.* (1981)
31	5	67	40	0·4	375	1 250	171	171	914	0	0·0	Ginsberg *et al.* (1981)
32	37	74	41		520	2 020	190	219	1 419	29	2·0	Mistry *et al.* (1981)
33	14	74	41		480	1 230	190	214	709	24	3·4	

34	16	67	40		196	728	219	243	556	24	4·3	Roberts *et al.* (1981)
35	40	73			412	975	158	170	540	12	2·2	Buzzard *et al.* (1982)
36	6	80	31	1·0	215	1 715	178	194	1 313	16	1·2	Nestel *et al.* (1982)
37	6	70	40	0·8	300	1 500	175	202	1 200	27	2·3	Schonfeld *et al.* (1982)
38	11	70	40	0·3	300	1 500	164	192	1 200	28	2·3	
39	6	70	40	2·5	300	1 500	141	151	1 200	10	0·8	
40	6	70	40	2·5	300	750	141	143	450	2	0·4	
41	11	70	40	0·3	300	750	170	188	450	18	4·0	
42	6	70	40	0·8	300	750	175	180	450	5	1·1	
43	12	51	49	1·0	160	450	238	251	398	13	3·3	Stein *et al.* (1982)
44	12	51	35	1·5	160	450	234	244	398	10	2·5	
45	11	42	40	1·0	160	450	172	188	483	16	3·3	
46	11	42	35	1·5	160	450	169	172	483	3	0·6	
47	13	58		2·0	50	1 400	277	308	1 629	31	1·9	Maranhao and Quintao (1983)
48	4	82	31	1·0	215	1 715	176	180	1 280	4	0·3	Nestel and Billington (1983)
49	4	79	31	0·3	215	1 715	198	231	1 329	33	2·5	
50	7	64	38	0·2	180	1 470	197	254	1 411	57	4·0	Packard *et al.* (1983)
51	23	70		0·6	400	1 400	182	192	1 000	10	1·0	Quig *et al.* (1983)
52	9	70	40	0·8	137	1 034	184	195	897	11	1·2	Applebaum-Bowden *et al.* (1984)
53	17	70	31	0·6	97	418	175	182	321	7	2·2	Sacks *et al.* (1984)
54	6	71	33	0·5	207	1 803	167	188	1 574	21	1·3	Beynen and Katan (1985)
55	8	54	20	0·7	0	1 000	113	147	1 296	34	2·6	McMurry *et al.* (1985)
56	21	83	39	0·5	256	938	193	209	575	16	2·8	Oh and Monaco (1985)
57	54	71	38	0·3	256	938	193	209	672	16	2·4	Flynn *et al.* (1986)
58	41	70	41	0·2	106	673	202	207	567	5	0·9	Katan *et al.* (1986)
59	32	70	41	0·2	129	989	199	222	860	23	2·7	
60	94	69	41	0·2	121	625	203	222	511	19	3·7	
61	6	70	31	1·6	190	940	149	157	750	8	1·1	Nestel (1986)
62	161	70	30	0·7	135	330	210	215	195	5	2·6	Edington *et al.* (1987)
63	32	79	35	0·3	290	860	243	248	505	5	1·0	McNamara *et al.* (1987)
64	39	76	35	1·7	190	820	218	224	580	6	1·0	
65	9	63	31	0·6	130	875	154	169	828	15	1·8	Zanni *et al.* (1987)
66	9	63	31	2·1	130	875	136	159	828	23	2·8	
67	4	77	33	0·4	179	504	151	178	295	27	9·1	Bowman *et al.* (1987)
68	6	77	46	0·4	207	504	164	163	270	−1	−0·4	
X	22	69	37	1·0	208	1 028	190	208	840	18	2·3	
±SEM	3	1	1	0·1	18	68	4	5	68	2	0·2	
(*n*)	68	68	60	57	68	68	68	68	68	68	68	

[a] Normalized per 70 kg body weight.

TABLE 3-2

ANALYSIS OF DIETARY CHOLESTEROL STUDIES

N	*Wt* (*kg*)	*Dietary fat*		*Dietary cholesterol*		*Plasma cholesterol*		*Cholesterol*		*Change mg/dl per 100 mg dietary cholesterol*	(*n*)
		% cal	*P/S*	*Low*	*High*	*Low*	*High*	*Change diet*[a]	*Change plasma*		
Composite data:											
22	69	37	1·0	208	1 028	190	208	840	18	2·3	(68)
±3	±1	±1	±0·1	±18	±68	±4	±5	±68	±2	±0·2	
Effect of dietary cholesterol mass:											
26	67	38	1·2	225	562	186	194	359	8	2·3	(22)
±8	±2	±1	±0·2	±32	±41	±8	±8	±21	±2	±0·4	
28	71	38	0·8	217	903	191	209	677	18	2·8	(24)
±6	±1	±1	±0·1	±29	±39	±6	±7	±31	±3	±0·4	
12	68	36	1·0	180	1 632	194	220	1 497	27	1·7	(22)
±2	±3	±2	±0·2	±31	±116	±9	±10	±103	±4	±0·2	
Effect of fat P/S ratio:											
21	71	37	0·4	181	1 004	182	201	826	19	2·6	(33)
±5	±1	±1	±0·03	±24	±85	±4	±5	±86	±3	±0·4	
14	65	38	1·7	197	1 096	198	217	955	19	2·1	(24)
±2	±3	±1	±0·2	±30	±143	±10	±11	±139	±4	±0·3	
Effect of fat calories:											
21	69	31	1·1	171	917	181	195	744	14	2·2	(21)
±5	±2	±1	±0·2	±25	±108	±8	±8	±96	±2	±0·4	
22	70	41	0·8	218	1 098	192	214	880	21	2·5	(39)
±4	±1	±1	±0·1	±25	±99	±5	±6	±99	±3	±0·3	
Effect of initial dietary cholesterol:											
21	65	36	1·0	93	898	188	209	871	21	2·8	(35)
±5	±2	±1	±0·2	±12	±92	±6	±7	±95	±3	±0·3	
23	73	39	0·9	329	1 167	193	207	837	14	1·8	(33)
±5	±1	±1	±0·1	±17	±95	±6	±7	±96	±2	±0·2	
Effect of initial plasma cholesterol:											
16	70	38	0·9	210	1 023	173	191	810	18	2·3	(48)
±3	±1	±1	±0·1	±22	±71	±3	±4	±66	±3	±0·3	
35	66	37	1·1	203	1 041	233	250	910	17	2·2	(20)
±9	±3	±2	±0·2	±31	±157	±6	±8	±166	±3	±0·3	

[a] Normalized per 70 kg body weight.

effects on plasma cholesterol levels. The results of analysis of all 68 studies are presented under Composite Data for comparison to analysis of the effects of dietary cholesterol mass, fat polyunsaturated to saturated (P/S) ratio, fat calories, initial dietary cholesterol levels, and initial plasma cholesterol levels. In each case the average numbers of patients in each study are presented (N); average body weights; dietary fat calories and P/S ratio; dietary cholesterol intakes and plasma cholesterol levels during the low and high intake periods; changes in dietary cholesterol intake and plasma cholesterol levels; the change, in mg/dl, of plasma cholesterol levels per 100 mg dietary cholesterol fed; and the number of studies in each classification.

In the first analysis of the data in Table 3-1, the studies were divided into three groupings, dependent upon the increment in dietary cholesterol intake: (1) studies feeding increments of less than 500 mg/day, and (2) studies feeding between 500–1000 mg/day, both representing physiological studies, and (3) studies using dietary challenges in excess of 1000 mg/day, a pharmacological dietary cholesterol challenge. As the average increment of dietary cholesterol increased from 359 to 677 to 1497 mg/day, plasma levels increased 8, 18 and 27 mg/dl. However, the increase per 100 mg dietary cholesterol remained fairly constant at $2{\cdot}3 \pm 0{\cdot}4$ ($n = 22$), $2{\cdot}8 \pm 0{\cdot}4$ ($n = 24$) and $1{\cdot}7 \pm 0{\cdot}2$ ($n = 22$) mg/dl per 100 mg. The decreased value in the greater than 1000 mg/day group may be accounted for by a decreased fractional absorption of cholesterol when intakes exceed 1500 mg/day (Quintao *et al.*, 1971). What does seem apparent is that at all levels of dietary cholesterol intake there is a minimal increase in the average plasma cholesterol level. The finding of an average change in the plasma cholesterol level of 2·3 mg/dl per 100 mg dietary cholesterol is quite different from the calculated changes using the formulas of Keys *et al.* (1965) and Hegsted *et al.* (1965) which predict average changes of 6·8 and 9·6 mg/dl, respectively, for a 100 mg/day increment in dietary cholesterol intake.

There have been a number of studies which suggest that the quality of dietary fat effects the response to a dietary cholesterol challenge (Schonfeld *et al.*, 1982). However, other studies have suggested that the response to a dietary cholesterol challenge is independent of dietary fat quality (Bowman *et al.*, 1987; McNamara *et al.*, 1987; Zanni *et al.*, 1987). Analysis of the data in Table 3-1, based on dietary fat quality with P/S ratios of less than 1·0 versus equal to or greater than 1·0, indicate that the change in plasma cholesterol levels per 100 mg dietary cholesterol are the same for 33 studies with an average P/S ratio of 0·4 and an incremental increase in plasma cholesterol of $2{\cdot}6 \pm 0{\cdot}4$ ($n = 33$) mg/dl per 100 mg dietary cholesterol, and 24 studies of average P/S ratio of 1·7 and plasma cholesterol increases of 2·1 ± 0·3 ($n = 24$) mg/dl per 100 mg fed (Table 3-2). It should be noted in this comparison that the mean values for virtually all other variables are equivalent and that fat quality is the only test variable. These data provide evidence that the P/S ratio of the dietary fat does not affect the plasma cholesterol response to a dietary cholesterol challenge.

Even though the quality of dietary fat has no effect on the plasma cholesterol response to dietary cholesterol, it is possible that dietary fat quantity does. Analysis of the data in Table 3-1, based on the percent of calories from dietary fat, of less than 35% versus equal to or greater than 35%, indicate that dietary fat quantity also fails to effect the response to a dietary cholesterol challenge (Table 3-2). Comparing studies, which used averages of 31% versus 41% of calories from fat, indicate that the incremental increase in plasma cholesterol levels per 100 mg dietary cholesterol fed were 2·2 ± 0·4 ($n = 21$) and 2·5 ± 0·3 ($n = 39$) mg/dl, respectively. The mean body weights, dietary cholesterol fed and baseline plasma cholesterol levels for these two groups were nearly identical as were the changes in plasma cholesterol levels. From these data it can be argued that the response to a dietary cholesterol challenge is unaffected by the quantity of dietary fat fed, within the range of 30–40%.

A commonly held belief is that the effects of dietary cholesterol on plasma cholesterol levels are maximal between intakes of zero to 500 mg/day with minimal changes in plasma levels occurring when dietary cholesterol is added to baseline intakes which exceed 500 mg (Grundy *et al.*, 1988). To test this theory the data in Table 3-1 were grouped according to initial dietary cholesterol intakes of less than 200 mg/day versus equal to or greater than 200 mg/day. As presented in Table 3-2, there was a small effect of initial dietary cholesterol intake on the incremental increase in plasma cholesterol per 100 mg dietary cholesterol fed. In the less than 200 mg/day baseline group plasma cholesterol increased 2·8 ± 0·3 ($n = 35$) mg/dl versus 1·8 ± 0·2 ($n = 33$) for the greater than 200 mg baseline group. The mean difference of 1 mg/dl per 100 mg dietary cholesterol fed suggests that the incremental increase may be greater when cholesterol intake is increased from a baseline of less than 200 mg/day, or else this difference may result from the decreased fractional absorption of cholesterol when intake exceeds 1500 mg/day (Quintao *et al.*, 1971). The data do not facilitate an analysis of this question since dietary cholesterol absorption values were not determined in the majority of the reported studies. Irrespective of the mechanisms involved, the data suggest that addition of dietary cholesterol to an already high dietary cholesterol intake has less of an effect than adding cholesterol to a low baseline consumption. However, in both cases the relative change in plasma cholesterol levels per 100 mg increment increase in dietary cholesterol is relatively small, i.e. 2–3 mg/dl.

A criticism of many dietary cholesterol feeding studies has been the use of study participants with low plasma cholesterol levels since there may be a difference in response to a dietary cholesterol challenge between normocholesterolemic and hypercholesterolemic study participants. Using the data in Table 3-1, one can test this concept using two groups of study subjects, i.e. those with baseline plasma cholesterol levels of less than 200 mg/dl versus those with levels of 200 or higher. As shown in Table 3-2 analysis of the data indicates that the incremental response to a dietary cholesterol challenge is equivalent for those in 48 studies where the mean plasma level was 173 mg/dl versus a mean level of 233 mg/dl for 20 studies. On average, dietary cholesterol intakes during the low and high periods and the changes in plasma cholesterol levels were identical for the two groups. These data would suggest that sensitivity to a dietary cholesterol challenge is the same for both normocholesterolemics and hypercholesterolemics as has been noted in some studies (McNamara *et al.*, 1987).

In summary, analysis of data from 68 studies with 1490 patients carried out over the past 27 years indicate that, on average, an increase in dietary cholesterol intake of 100 mg/day increases plasma cholesterol levels by 2·3 mg/dl, independent of the amount of dietary cholesterol fed, dietary fat quality or quantity, or the baseline plasma cholesterol level. It may be that increasing dietary cholesterol from a low initial baseline intake of less than 200 mg/day has a greater impact on plasma cholesterol levels than addition of cholesterol to an already cholesterol-rich diet. Whether this is a physiological response based on an increased sensitivity to dietary cholesterol or a decreased fractional absorption of the dietary cholesterol fed, or a response to a very high pharmacological dose of dietary cholesterol, cannot be determined. In either case, the incremental increase per 100 mg dietary cholesterol fed remains relatively small and would have an almost unmeasurable effect on plasma cholesterol levels.

What really is surprising about the data presented in Tables 3-1 and 3-2 is the consistency of the observations even with the variations in experimental design, diet compositions, amounts of cholesterol fed, and patient heterogeneity. The data provide a convincing argument that the effects of dietary cholesterol on plasma cholesterol levels are minimal at best, and that dietary cholesterol intake at almost any level does not play a major role in determining plasma cholesterol levels in the population as a whole.

(ii) Compensators versus non-compensators

The data presented above deal with average changes in plasma cholesterol levels of groups of patients; however, a consistent observation in almost all studies on the effects of dietary cholesterol on plasma cholesterol levels has been the heterogeneity of responses to the dietary cholesterol challenge. A number of studies have presented evidence indicating that within the population there exist two sub-groups, one sensitive to dietary cholesterol and one resistant to a hypercholesterolemic response (Nestel and Poyser, 1976; Maranhao and Quintao, 1983; Katan *et al.*, 1986; Beynen *et al.*, 1987; McNamara *et al.*, 1987). The metabolic basis for the hyporesponders (compensators) to dietary cholesterol appears to be the existence of precise feedback down regulation of endogenous cholesterol synthesis in response to an increased intake of dietary cholesterol. In contrast, hyperresponders (non-compensators) exhibit an increased plasma cholesterol level when challenged with dietary cholesterol due to an inability to effectively decrease endogenous cholesterol synthesis (Nestel and Poyser, 1976; Maranhao and Quintao, 1983; McNamara *et al.*, 1987).

In a study of 75 outpatients fed 250 versus 800 mg/day dietary cholesterol by McNamara *et al.* (1987), it was shown that 70% were compensators and had no change in plasma cholesterol levels and a 26% reduction in cholesterol synthesis ($P < 0{\cdot}001$) as measured by analysis of sterol synthesis in freshly isolated blood mononuclear leukocytes. In contrast, non-compensators represented 30% of the study group and had a mean 12% increase in plasma cholesterol levels ($P < 0{\cdot}001$) with a non-significant 12% decrease in sterol synthesis. This study also evaluated the effects of dietary fat quality on cholesterol absorption, endogenous sterol synthesis and the precision of the feedback control mechanisms and found that the type of dietary fat consumed did not influence any of these metabolic responses. The data indicate that a major determinant of the response to a dietary cholesterol challenge is the efficacy of the feedback control response and that the majority of individuals have effective compensatory mechanisms.

IV. BLOOD CHOLESTEROL LOWERING DIETS: EFFICACY AND SAFETY

A. Dietary Guidelines for the Public

There is little doubt that identifying and treating patients with plasma cholesterol levels in the high-risk range is an appropriate course of action in attempting to reduce the incidence of CVD in the population (Bilheimer, 1988). There does, however, remain some skepticism regarding the advisability of generalized dietary recommendations that all Americans should reduce their intake of dietary cholesterol as a modality to reduce their risk of CVD (Oliver, 1983; Samuel *et al.*, 1983; Ahrens, 1985; McNamara, 1987). The proposed approaches to CVD risk reduction are interventions as part of the public health approach, which treats the population as a whole irrespective of plasma cholesterol levels, and the clinical approach, which is to screen and treat the high risk hypercholesterolemic patients to reduce CVD risk in the individual. These approaches are not mutually exclusive and in many ways are complementary (Oliver, 1985, 1986; Sherwin and Lewis, 1988). While one may conclude that both approaches have value, the question of mechanisms and messages by which public health recommendations are given has much to do with potential efficacy of the public health approach. At the present time the over emphasis given to dietary cholesterol, the public's confusion regarding the relationship between dietary and plasma cholesterol, and the quantitative nature of the recommendations (does anyone really know what constitutes a diet with less than 100 mg dietary cholesterol per 1000 kilocalories?), negate much of the potential benefits of the public health approach. The recent National Cholesterol Education Program's public message emphasis to 'know your cholesterol number' addresses an important aspect of previous public health messages in that the high risk hypercholesterolemic individual, who changes his/her diet, and achieves an average plasma cholesterol reduction will have the benefit of medical care to try and reduce the plasma cholesterol level by other means.

B. Dietary Intervention Studies

A number of pharmacologic intervention trials to lower plasma cholesterol levels and CVD incidence have provided a basis for recommending that hypercholesterolemic individuals receive treatment (Lipid Research Clinics Program, 1984a, b; Canner *et al.*, 1986; Blankenhorn *et al.*, 1987; Frick *et al.*, 1987; Manninen *et al.*, 1988). However, there are no dietary intervention trials which have demonstrated a significant reduction in CVD mortality or morbidity, and there probably never will be such evidence. The total cost, patient numbers required and duration of such a study preclude initiation of such an ambitious clinical study. With this in mind, the question becomes whether it is reasonable to extrapolate from the positive drug trials and recommend dietary interventions for the public. Two major problems with the extrapolations are that most of the drug studies were carried out in hypercholesterolemic, high risk male populations and that the mechanisms of plasma cholesterol lowering by drug interventions differ substantially from mechanisms responsible for dietary effects. The problems associated with extrapolation of drug studies to dietary recommendations are numerous and the number of potentially erroneous assumptions involved necessitate that caution be used. What can be argued persuasively is that the hypercholesterolemic patient has the greatest potential to benefit from lowering an elevated plasma cholesterol level and that dietary intervention should be initiated and given a suitable trial prior to therapy with cholesterol lowering medication.

C. Risk–Benefit Considerations

Most advocates of generalized dietary recommendations to the public refute the possibility that the recommended changes will in any way have an associated risk. There are those who believe that some potential risks are associated with the proposed dietary changes (Reaven, 1986) and only future research can adequately address this very important question. From an overall nutritional balance point of view there are some serious questions, which need to be addressed in the context of the marketing, media and nutritional misinformation so prevalent today. When quantitative dietary recommendations are given to a public, which has little nutritional knowledge, there is a tendency for oversimplification towards a 'good food, bad food' approach to making dietary changes. Exclusion of animal products from the diet, because of a dietary cholesterol phobia, is neither the goal of the recommended dietary changes nor a dietary pattern which will provide the public with an optimal nutritional balance. Zero tolerance for cholesterol-containing 'bad foods' may have a pronounced effect on the nutritional balance for certain segments of the population. Young children and the elderly are two such groups, and therefore it is essential that the public be aware of the value of animal products in the diet as well as the question of any possible role in CVD risk. The public need will best be served when this balanced approach is taken by health promotion agencies and the mass media.

The second aspect of the risk–benefit consideration deals with the expected reduction to be gained from a population-wide decrease in dietary saturated fat and cholesterol intake. Using data from various epidemiological and intervention trials, Taylor *et al.* (1987) have formulated a model to quantitate the increase in life expectancy from life-long adherence to a 'prudent diet'. According to this model, a normotensive non-smoking 40 year old male with an average plasma cholesterol level, who adheres to the prudent diet for the rest of his life, would increase his life expectancy by an average of 0·3 months. One could predict, based on the evidence presented above, that dietary cholesterol plays a very minimal role in determining plasma cholesterol levels and that reduction of dietary cholesterol intake to less than 300 mg/day would have even a smaller effect on life expectancy. In light of these types of data one must question whether giving up animal products in the diet because they contain cholesterol is really worth the effort.

V. MEAT INTAKE AND BLOOD CHOLESTEROL LEVELS

Most of the cholesterol in the American diet comes from eggs, meat and dairy products, all of which are important sources of nutrients (Block *et al.*, 1985a) and have important roles to play in a balanced, nutritious diet. According to the results of the NHANES II survey, meat in the diet, in all forms and types, provides 34% of the cholesterol in our diet (Block *et al.*, 1985b). This would equal 153 mg of the average daily intake of 450 mg of cholesterol in the average American diet. At this level it may be that the cholesterol in meat products contribute between 3–4 mg/dl of our plasma cholesterol level or approximately 1·5–2% of the total. The rationale of labeling meat products as 'bad foods' based on their possible contribution to the plasma cholesterol level, when contrasted to the wide spectrum of important nutrients provided by this component of the American diet, would seem to be both unnecessary and unreasonable.

VI. SUMMARY AND CONCLUSIONS

The advice that all Americans reduce their dietary cholesterol intake from the current 450 mg/day to less than 300 mg/day needs to be evaluated in terms of our current knowledge of whole body cholesterol metabolism and the effect of dietary cholesterol on plasma cholesterol levels. Based on the analysis of the numerous cholesterol feeding studies described above, it would be predicted that a 150 mg/day reduction in dietary cholesterol intake would result in a decrease in the average plasma cholesterol level of 3–4 mg/dl, or slightly less than a 2% reduction. When considered in light of the fact that the entire population does not have plasma cholesterol levels above average risk and that only a small segment of the population is unable to compensate for an increase in dietary cholesterol, the effects of such a reduction in dietary cholesterol intake would be predicted to have a very small, if any, effect on CVD mortality or morbidity. Even if plasma cholesterol levels were to be reduced in some individuals by dietary cholesterol restriction there is no evidence for a reduction in overall mortality by reducing plasma cholesterol levels (Oliver, 1988).

To put this reduction in a different type of context let us consider the decrease in endogenous cholesterol input accomplished by having the population as a whole lose 5 kg of body weight. Sterol balance studies have shown that endogenous production of cholesterol increases 20 mg/day for every kg of excess body fat (Miettinen, 1971); therefore, losing 5 kg of body fat would reduce cholesterol production by 100 mg/day. In other words, reducing dietary cholesterol by 150 mg/day, of which 90 mg is absorbed into the body, actually results in a smaller reduction in cholesterol input than does losing 5 kg of fatty tissue. Considering the extent of obesity in the population, and the associated increased rate of cholesterol synthesis due to this obesity, it would seem that a greater number of individuals would benefit more from a little weight reduction than from reducing the intake of eggs, meats and dairy products, which provide a number of important and health maintaining nutrients. Recent studies have demonstrated that obesity is not only an independent risk factor for CVD but also is a contributing factor to other risk factors such as hypertension, glucose intolerance and a sedentary life style (Bjorntorp, 1988). Perhaps the public health approach needed should deal less with reducing dietary cholesterol intake and more on maintaining ideal body weight, eating a variety of foods, and moderate exercise, which would prove to be more effective in reducing CVD risk and would dispel the 'good food, bad food' demons that make every meal a life and death decision for many in the population.

VII. REFERENCES

ABBOTT, R. D., WILSON, P. W. F., KANNEL, W. B. and CASTELLI, W. P. (1988). High density lipoprotein cholesterol, total cholesterol screening, and myocardial infarction. The Framingham Study. *Arteriosclerosis* **8**, 207.

AHRENS, E. H., JR (1976). The management of hyperlipidemia: whether, rather than how. *Ann. Intern. Med.* **85**, 87.

AHRENS, E. H., JR (1985). The diet–heart question in 1985: Has it really been settled? *Lancet* **i**, 1085.

ANDERSON, J. T., GRANDE, F. and KEYS, A. (1976). Independence of the effects of cholesterol and degree of saturation of the fat in the diet on serum cholesterol in man. *Am. J. Clin. Nutr.* **29**, 1784.

APPLEBAUM-BOWDEN, D., HAFFNER, S. M., HARTSOOK, E., LUK, K. H., ALBERS, J. J. and HAZZARD, W. R. (1984). Down-regulation of the low-density lipoprotein receptor by dietary cholesterol. *Am. J. Clin. Nutr.* **39**, 360.

BEYNEN, A. C. and KATAN, M. B. (1985). Effect of egg yolk feeding on the concentration and composition of serum lipoproteins in man. *Atherosclerosis* **54**, 157.

BEYNEN, A. C., KATAN, M. B. and VAN ZUTPHEN, L. F. M. (1987). Hypo- and hyperresponders: individual differences in the response of serum cholesterol concentration to changes in diet. *Adv. Lipid Res.* **22**, 115.

BILHEIMER, D. W. (1988). Therapeutic control of hyperlipidemia in the prevention of coronary atherosclerosis: a review of results from recent clinical trials. *Am. J. Cardiol.* **62**, 1J.

BLANKENHORN, D. H., NESSIM, S. A., JOHNSON, R. L., SANMARCO, M. E., AZEN S. P. and CASHIN-HEMPHILL, L. (1987). Beneficial effects of combined colestipol–niacin therapy on coronary atherosclerosis and coronary venous bypass grafts. *JAMA* **257**, 3233.

BLOCK, G., DRESSER, C. M., HARTMAN, A. M. and CARROLL, M. D. (1985a). Nutrient sources in the American diet: quantitative data from the NHANES II survey. I. Vitamins and minerals. *Am. J. Epidemiol.* **122**, 13.

BLOCK, G., DRESSER, C. M., HARTMAN, A. M. and CARROLL, M. D. (1985b). Nutrient sources in the American diet: quantitative data from the NHANES II survey. II. Macronutrients and fats. *Am. J. Epidemiol.* **122**, 27.

BJORNTORP, P. (1988). The associations between obesity, adipose tissue distribution and disease. *Acta Med. Scand. Suppl.* **723**, 121.

BOWMAN, M. P., VAN DOREN, J., TAPER, L. J., THYE, F. W. and RITCHEY, S. J. (1987). Effect of dietary fat and cholesterol on plasma lipids and lipoprotein fractions in normolipidemic men. *J. Nutr.* **118**, 555.

BUZZARD, I. M., MCROBERTS, M. R., DRISCOLL, D. L. and BOWERING, J. (1982). Effects of dietary eggs and ascorbic acid on plasma lipid and lipoprotein cholesterol levels in healthy young men. *Am. J. Clin. Nutr.* **36**, 94.

CANNER, P. L., BERGER, K. G., WENGER, N. K., STAMLER, J., FRIEDMAN, L., PRINEAS, R. J. and FRIEDWALD, W. (1986). Fifteen year mortality in coronary drug project patients: long-term benefit with niacin. *J. Am. Coll. Cardiol.* **8**, 245.

CHENOWETH, W., ULLMANN, M., SIMPSON, R. and LEVEILLE, G. (1981). Influence of dietary cholesterol and fat on serum lipids in men. *J. Nutr.* **111**, 2069.

CONNOR, W. E., HODGES, R. E. and BLEILER, R. E. (1961a). The serum lipids in men receiving high cholesterol and cholesterol-free diets. *J. Clin. Invest.* **40**, 894.

CONNOR, W. E., HODGES, R. E. and BLEILER, R. E. (1961b). Effect of dietary cholesterol upon serum lipids in man. *J. Lab. Clin. Med.* **57**, 331.

EDINGTON, J., GEEKIE, M., CARTER, R., BENFIELD, L., FISHER, K., BALL, M. and MANN, J. (1987). Effect of dietary cholesterol on plasma cholesterol concentration in subjects following reduced fat, high fibre diet. *Brit. Med. J.* **294**, 333.

FLAIM, E., FERRERI, L. F., THYE, F. W., HILL, J. E. and RITCHEY, S. J. (1981). Plasma lipids and lipoprotein cholesterol concentrations in adult males consuming normal and high cholesterol diets under controlled conditions. *Am. J. Clin. Nutr.* **34**, 1103.

FLYNN, M. A., NOLPH, G. B., FLYNN, T. C., KAHRS, R. and KRAUSE, G. (1979). Effect of dietary egg on human serum cholesterol and triglycerides. *Am. J. Clin. Nutr.* **32**, 1051.

FLYNN, M. A., NOLPH, G. B., OSIO, Y., SUN, G. Y., LANNING, B., KRAUSE, G. and DALLY, J. C. (1986). Serum lipids and eggs. *J. Am. Dietetic Assoc.* **86**, 1541.

FRICK, M. H., ELO, O., HAAPA, K., HEINONEN, O. P., HEINSALMI, P., HELO, P., HUTTUNEN, J. K., KAITANIEMI, P., KOSKINEN, P., MANNINEN, V., MAENPAA, H., MALKONEN, M., MANTTARI, M., NOROLA, S., PASTERNACK, A., PIKKARAINEN, J., ROMO, M., SJOBLOM, T. and NIKKILA, E. A. (1987). Helsinki heart study: Primary-prevention trial with gemfibrozil in middle-aged men with dyslipidemia. Safety of treatment, changes in risk factors, and incidence of coronary disease. *N. Eng. J. Med.* **317**, 1237.

GILLUM, R. F., FOLSOM, A. R. and BLACKBURN, H. (1984). Decline in coronary heart disease mortality. Old questions and new facts. *Am. J. Med.* **76**, 1055.

GINSBERG, H., LE, N-A., MAYS, C., GIBSON, J. and BROWN, W. V. (1981). Lipoprotein metabolism in nonresponders to increased dietary cholesterol. *Arteriosclerosis* **1**, 463.

GORDON, T., CASTELLI, W. P., HJORTLAND, M. C., KANNEL, W. B. and DAWBER, T. R. (1977). High density lipoprotein as a protective factor against coronary heart disease. The Framingham Study, *Am. J. Med.* **62**, 707.

GRANDE, F., ANDERSON, J. T., CHLOUVERAKIS, C., PROJA, M. and KEYS, A. (1965). Effect of dietary cholesterol on man's serum lipids. *J. Nutr.* **87**, 52.

GRUNDY, S. M. (1979). Dietary fats and sterols. In *Nutrition, Lipids and Coronary Heart Disease* (R. I. Levy, B. M. Rifkind, B. H. Dennis and N. D. Ernst, Eds), p. 89. Raven Press, New York.

GRUNDY, S. M. (1983). Absorption and metabolism of dietary cholesterol. *Ann. Rev. Nutr.* **3**, 71.

GRUNDY, S. M., BARRETT-CONNOR, E., RUDEL, L. L., MIETTINEN, T. and SPECTOR, A. A. (1988). Workshop on the impact of dietary cholesterol on plasma lipoproteins and atherogenesis. *Arteriosclerosis* **8**, 95.

HAMSTEN, A. (1988). Apolipoproteins, dyslipoproteinaemia and premature coronary heart disease. *Acta Med. Scand.* **223**, 389.

HEGSTED, D. M. and AUSMAN, L. M. (1988). Diet, alcohol and coronary heart disease in men. *J. Nutr.* **118**, 1184.

HEGSTED, D. M. and NICOLOSI, R. J. (1987). Individual variation in serum cholesterol levels. *Proc. Natl Acad. Sci. USA* **84**, 6259.

HEGSTED, D. M., MCGANDY, R. B., MYERS, M. L. and STARE, F. J. (1965). Quantitative effects of dietary fat on serum cholesterol in man. *Am. J. Clin. Nutr.* **17**, 281.

HOPKINS, P. N. and WILLIAMS, R. R. (1981). A survey of 246 suggested coronary risk factors. *Atherosclerosis* **40**, 1.

KANNEL, W. B., CASTELLI, W. P. and GORDON, T. (1979). Cholesterol in the prediction of atherosclerotic disease. New perspectives based on the Framingham Study. *Ann. Intern. Med.* **90**, 85.

KATAN, M. B., BEYNEN, A. C., DE VRIES, J. H. M. and NOBELS, A. (1986). Existence of consistent hypo- and hyperresponders to dietary cholesterol in man. *Am. J. Epidemiol.* **123**, 221.

KEYS, A., ANDERSON, J. T. and GRANDE, F. (1965). Serum cholesterol response to changes in the diet. II. The effect of cholesterol in the diet. *Metabolism* **14**, 759.

Kummerow, F. A., Kim, Y., Pllard, J., Ilinov, P., Dorossiev, D. L. and Valek, J. (1977). The influence of egg consumption on the serum cholesterol level in human subjects. *Am. J. Clin. Nutr.* **30**, 664.

Lipid Research Clinics Program (1984a). The lipid research clinics coronary primary prevention trial results. I. Reduction in incidence of coronary heart disease. *JAMA* **251**, 351.

Lipid Research Clinics Program (1984b). The lipid research clinics coronary primary prevention trial results. II. The relationship of reduction in incidence of coronary heart disease to cholesterol lowering. *JAMA* **251**, 365.

Manninen, V., Elo, M. O., Frick, M. H., Haapa, K., Heinonen, O. P., Heinsalmi, P., Helo, P., Huttunen, J. K., Kaitaniemi, P., Koskinen, P., Maenpaa, H., Malkonen, M., Mantri, M., Norola, S., Pasternack, A., Pikkarainen, J., Romo, M., Sjoblom, T. and Nikkila, E. A. (1988). Lipid alterations and decline in the incidence of coronary heart disease in the Helsinki Heart Study. *JAMA* 260, 641.

Maranhao, R. C. and Quintao, E. C. R. (1983). Long term steroid metabolism balance studies in subjects on cholesterol-free and cholesterol-rich diets: comparison between normal and hypercholesterolemic individuals. *J. Lipid Res.* **24**, 167.

Martin, G. M. and Nestel, P. (1979). Changes in cholesterol metabolism with dietary cholesterol in children with familial hypercholesterolaemia. *Clin. Sci.* **56**, 377.

Mattson, F. H., Erickson, B. A. and Kligman, A. M. (1972). Effect of dietary cholesterol on serum cholesterol in man. *Am. J. Clin. Nutr.* **25**, 589.

McGill, H. C., Jr (1979). The relationship of dietary cholesterol to serum cholesterol concentration and to atherosclerosis in man. *Am. J. Clin. Nutr.* **32**, 2664.

McMurry, M. P., Connor, W. E., Lin, D. S., Cerquera, M. T. and Connor, S. L. (1985). The absorption of cholesterol and the sterol balance in the Tarahumara Indians of Mexico fed cholesterol-free and high cholesterol diets. *Am. J. Clin. Nutr.* **41**, 1289.

McNamara, D. J. (1987). Effects of fat-modified diets on cholesterol and lipoprotein metabolism. *Ann. Rev. Nutr.* **7**, 273.

McNamara, D. J., Kolb, R., Parker, T. S., Batwin, H., Samuel, P., Brown, C. D. and Ahrens, E. H., Jr (1987). Heterogeneity of cholesterol homeostasis in man: response to changes in dietary fat quality and cholesterol quantity. *J. Clin. Invest.* **79**, 1729.

Miettinen, T. A. (1971). Cholesterol production in obesity. *Circulation* **44**, 842.

Mistry, P., Miller, N. E., Laker, M., Hazzard, W. R. and Lewis, B. (1981). Individual variation in the effects of dietary cholesterol on plasma lipoproteins and cellular cholesterol homeostasis in man. *J. Clin. Invest.* **67**, 493.

Multiple Risk Factor Intervention Trial Group (1982). Multiple risk factor intervention trial. Risk factor changes and mortality results. *JAMA* **248**, 1465.

National Cholesterol Education Program Expert Panel (1988). Report on detection, evaluation, and treatment of high blood cholesterol in adults. *Arch. Intern. Med.* **148**, 36.

Nestel, P. J. and Poyser, A. (1976). Changes in cholesterol synthesis and excretion when cholesterol intake is increased. *Metabolism* **25**, 1591.

NESTEL, P. J. (1986). Fish oil attenuates the cholesterol induced rise in lipoprotein cholesterol. *Am. J. Clin. Nutr.* **43**, 752.

NESTEL, P. J. and BILLINGTON, T. (1983). Increased transport of intermediate density lipoproteins (IDL) with cholesterol loading. *Metabolism* **32**, 320.

NESTEL, P. J., HAVENSTEIN, N., HOMMA, Y., SCOTT, T. W. and COOK, L. J. (1975). Increased sterol excretion with polyunsaturated-fat high-cholesterol diets. *Metabolism* **24**, 189.

NESTEL, P., TADA, N., BILLINGTON, T., HUFF, M. and FIDGE, N. (1982). Changes in very low density lipoproteins with cholesterol loading. *Metabolism* **31**, 398.

O'BRIEN, B. C. and REISER, R. (1980). Human plasma lipid responses to red meat, poultry, fish and eggs. *Am. J. Clin. Nutr.* **33**, 2573.

OH, S. Y. and MONACO, P. A. (1985). Effect of dietary cholesterol and degree of fat unsaturation on plasma lipid levels, lipoprotein composition, and fecal steroid excretion in normal young men. *Am. J. Clin. Nutr.* **42**, 399.

OLIVER, M. F. (1983). The cholesterol–coronary question: why not a policy of selective intervention? *Internat. J. Cardiol.* **4**, 201.

OLIVER, M. F. (1985). Strategies for preventing and screening for coronary heart disease. *Br. Heart J.* **54**, 1.

OLIVER, M. F. (1986). Prevention of coronary heart disease—propaganda, promises, problems, and prospects. *Circulation* **73**, 1.

OLIVER, M. F. (1988). Reducing cholesterol does not reduce mortality. *JACC* **12**, 814.

PACKARD, C. J., MCKINNEY, L., CARR, K. and SHEPHERD, J. (1983). Cholesterol feeding increases low density lipoprotein synthesis. *J. Clin. Invest.* **72**, 45.

PORTER, M. W., YAMANAKA, W., CARLSON, S. D. and FLYNN, M. A. (1977). Effects of dietary egg serum cholesterol and triglyceride of human males. *Am. J. Clin. Nutr.* **30**, 490.

QUIG, D. W., THYE, F. W., RITCHEY, S. J., HERBERT, W. G., CLEVIDENCE, B. A., REYNOLDS, L. K. and SMITH, M. C. (1983). Effects of short-term aerobic conditioning and high cholesterol feeding on plasma total and lipoprotein cholesterol levels in sedentary young men. *Am. J. Clin. Nutr.* **38**, 825.

QUINTAO, E. C. R. and SPEROTTO, G. (1987). The role of dietary cholesterol in the regulation of human body cholesterol metabolism. *Adv. Lipid Res.* **22**, 173.

QUINTAO, E. C. R., GRUNDY, S. M. and AHRENS, E. H., JR (1971). An evaluation of four methods for measuring cholesterol absorption by the intestine in man. *J. Lipid Res.* **12**, 221.

QUINTAO, E. C. R., BRUMER, S. and STECHHAHN, K. (1977). Tissue storage and control of cholesterol metabolism in man on high cholesterol diets. *Atherosclerosis* **26**, 297.

REAVEN, G. M. (1986). Looking at the world through LDL-cholesterol colored glasses. *J. Nutr.* **116**, 1143.

ROBERTS, S. L., MCMURRY, M. P. and CONNOR, W. E. (1981). Does egg feeding (i.e. dietary cholesterol) affect plasma cholesterol levels in humans? The results of a double-blind study. *Am. J. Clin. Nutr.* **34**, 2092.

ROTTERDAM, E. P., KATAN, M. B. and KNUIMAN, J. T. (1987). Importance of time interval between repeated measurements of total or high density lipoprotein cholesterol when estimating an individual's baseline concentrations. *Clin. Chem.* **33**, 1913.

SACKS, F. M., SALAZAR, J., MILLER, L., FOSTER, J. M., SUTHERLAND, M., SAMONDS, K. W., ALBERS, J. J. and KASS, E. H. (1984). Ingestion of egg raises plasma low density lipoproteins in free-living subjects. *Lancet* **i**, 647.

SAMUEL, P., MCNAMARA, D. J. and SHAPIRO, J. (1983). The role of diet in the etiology and treatment of atherosclerosis. *Ann. Rev. Med.* **34**, 179.

SCHONFELD, G., PATSCH, W., RUDEL, L. L., NELSON, C., EPSTEIN, M. and OLSON, R. E. (1982). Effects of dietary cholesterol and fatty acids on plasma lipoproteins. *J. Clin. Invest.* **69**, 1072.

SHERWIN, R. and LEWIS, C. (1988). Why lower blood cholesterol in the whole population? *Prevent. Cardiol. Reports* **2**, 1.

SIMONS, L. A. (1986). Interrelations of lipids and lipoproteins with coronary artery disease mortality in 19 countries. *Am. J. Cardiol.* **57**, 5G.

SLATER, G., MEAD, J., DHOPESHWARKER, G., ROBINSON, S. and ALFIN-SLATER, R. B. (1976). Plasma cholesterol and triglycerides in men with added eggs in the diet. *Nutr. Rep. Int.* **14**, 249.

STAMLER, J., WENTWORTH, D. and NEATON, J. D. (1986). Is relationship between serum cholesterol and risk of premature death from coronary heart disease continuous and graded? Findings in 356 222 primary screenees of the Multiple Risk Factor Intervention Trial (MRFIT). *JAMA* **256**, 2823.

STEIN, E. A., SHAPERO, J., MCNERNEY, C., GLUECK, C. J., TRACY, T. and GARTSIDE, P. (1982). Changes in plasma lipid and lipoprotein fractions after alteration in dietary cholesterol, polyunsaturated, saturated, and total fat in free-living normal and hypercholesterolemic children. *Am. J. Clin. Nutr.* **35**, 1375.

TAYLOR, W. C., PASS, T. M., SHEPARD, D. S. and KOMAROFF, A. L. (1987). Cholesterol reduction and life expectancy. A model incorporating multiple risk factors. *Ann. Intern. Med.* **106**, 605.

TYROLER, H. A. (1987). Review of lipid-lowering clinical trials in relation to observational epidemiologic studies. *Circulation* **76**, 515.

WALLACE, R. B. and ANDERSON, R. A. (1987). Blood lipids, lipid-related measures, and the risk of atherosclerotic cardiovascular disease. *Epidemiol. Rev.* **9**, 95.

WHYTE, M., NESTEL, P. and MACGREGOR, A. (1977). Cholesterol metabolism in Papua New Guineans. *Europ. J. Clin. Invest.* **7**, 53.

ZANNI, E. E., ZANNIS, V. I., BLUM, C. B., HERBET, P. N. and BRESLOW, J. L. (1987). Effect of egg cholesterol and dietary fats on plasma lipids, lipoproteins, and apoproteins of normal women consuming natural diets. *J. Lipid Res.* **28**, 518.

4

Meat and Cancer

DAVID KRITCHEVSKY
The Wistar Institute of Anatomy and Biology, Philadelphia, Pennsylvania, USA

I. INTRODUCTION

There have been a number of epidemiological studies which have suggested a link between animal protein intake and predisposition to cancers at various sites. Lea (1967) examined data from 33 countries linking dietary patterns and mortality from a variety of cancers and found a correlation between animal protein and development of pancreatic cancer. Carroll and Khor (1975) plotted age-adjusted death rate from breast cancer in women against reported *per capita* consumption of animal protein and obtained a scatter diagram from which a straight line, significant relationship could be adduced. However, examination of the diagram reveals a number of unexplained inconsistencies. To cite a few, South Africa and New Zealand have virtually the same death rate (22–23/100 000) yet the animal protein intake in South Africa is about 29 g/day and that in New Zealand is about 76 g/day; animal protein intake in Finland, France, and Ireland is 57 g/day but the adjusted death rates in those countries (per 100 000) are 13 (Finland), 16 (France) and 22 (Ireland). Hungary, with about the same death rate as Finland, has an animal protein intake which is 44% lower (32 g/day). Among lesser developed nations we can compare Yugoslavia (death rate 8/100 000 and 22 g/day) with affluent Japan whose animal protein intake is 26 g/day and whose death rate is only 4/100 000.

II. EPIDEMIOLOGICAL STUDIES

Armstrong and Doll (1975) compared incidence rates for 27 cancers in 23 countries and mortality rates for 14 cancers in 32 countries and reported a positive correlation of meat intake with cancers of the pancreas, breast, colon, prostate and endometrium. One would be tempted to examine directly the correlation between colon cancer and meat intake in a population which largely abstains from meat (Seventh Day Adventists). Phillips (1975) did examine mortality rates in Seventh Day Adventists for cancer sites unrelated to drinking or smoking and found them considerably lower than those in the general American population. Cancer mortality rates for Seventh Day Adventist physicians and their counterparts who professed other religious preferences showed no differences, which could either be interpreted as backsliding in the first group or a health-message revelation in the second. Another religious group (Latter Day Saints or Mormons) who eat large amounts of meat also have significantly less colon cancer than the American average (Lyon *et al.*, 1976). Both Mormons and Seventh Day Adventists abstain from smoking, alcohol, tea and coffee.

Enstrom (1975) has shown that between 1940 and 1970 weekly beef consumption in the United States rose from 1·06 lb/*capita* to 2·25 lb/*capita* (a 112% increase) while cancer mortality (per 100 000) was virtually unchanged. He also reported that while there was a greater use of meat among more affluent Americans, risk of large bowel cancer showed no similar socioeconomic gradient. Graham *et al.* (1978) compared frequency of beef or meat eating with incidence of colon cancer in cases and controls and found no correlation (Table 4-1).

In a 1983 publication, Phillips *et al.* (1983) summarized epidemiological studies relating cancer risk to meat ingestion. In 11 case-control studies of colon cancer they found six which gave positive association, one which gave a negative association, and four which gave no association. Three studies of stomach cancer yielded no association, whereas one gave a

TABLE 4-1
BEEF INTAKE AND CANCER[a]

Frequency (times per week)	*Controls (632)* (%)	*Colon cancer cases (295)* (%)
0–1	8·7	10·8
2	17·4	15·4
3	25·0	30·2
4	22·5	20·0
5+	26·4	23·6

[a] After Graham *et al.* (1978).

positive association; a fifth study (Higginson, 1966) found a positive association with pork intake but a negative association with beef or lamb ingestion. Nomura *et al.* (1978) found no association between beef and lamb intakes and breast cancer in Hawaiian Japanese, whereas Lubin *et al.* (1981) found a positive correlation between beef and pork intake and breast cancer in Canada. Phillips *et al.* (1983) concluded:

> ...the available data does not provide convincing evidence that simply deleting meat from the typical American diet would substantially reduce cancer risk.

The National Academy of Sciences report on diet and cancer (Committee on Diet, Nutrition and Cancer, 1982) concluded the section on protein thus:

> Because of the relative paucity of data on protein compared to fat, and the strong correlation between intakes of fat and protein in the Western diet, the committee is unable to arrive at a firm conclusion about an independent effect of protein.

III. INFLUENCE OF SPECIFIC COMPONENTS OF MEAT

Meat provides three nutrients which might be involved in carcinogenesis—protein, cholesterol and fat, each of which is discussed below.

A. Protein

The specific influence of protein has been tested in experimental carcinogenesis. Tannenbaum and Silverstone (1949) fed mice diets in which the protein content ranged from 9–45% and found no general effects on benzpyrene (BP)-induced skin tumors. Shay *et al.* (1964) found that variation of dietary protein levels over reasonable ranges did not affect methylcholanthrene (MCA)-induced mammary tumors in rats. There was an increase in tumor incidence at protein levels of 64%, but this would be a rather unusual diet.

Visek *et al.* (1978) studied the effect of dietary protein levels on 1,2-dimethylhydrazine (DMH)-induced tumors in rats. Tumor incidence was not significantly different between rats fed 7·5, 15 or 22·5% casein, although larger tumors were observed in rats fed the two higher levels of protein. Walters and Roe (1964) observed that mice fed 25% casein exhibited the same incidence of 9,10-dibenzanthracene-induced tumors as did mice fed 15% casein but a lower multiplicity (tumors per tumor-bearing mouse). In another experiment, Clinton *et al.* (1977) fed female Sprague–Dawley rats 7·5, 15 or 45% casein for a month prior to administration of 7,12-dimethylbenz(a)anthracene (DMBA), and then placed them on a 15% protein diet after the carcinogen had been given. Palpable tumors appeared in the rats fed 7·5% protein much earlier than in the other two groups. At 24 weeks the incidence of palpable mammary tumors in the three groups was 78% in rats fed 7·5% protein, 40% in those fed 15% protein and 22% in those fed 45% protein.

It is difficult to compare effects of dietary factors in experimentally-induced tumors because rats and mice of different strains and gender are used; different carcinogens which require different pathways of activation and have different mechanisms of action are used; and the diets themselves are varied as is the accuracy of measurement of food intake. There are some early studies of dietary effects on spontaneous tumors in mice and rats but the questionable adequacy of the diets used renders interpretation hazardous. Tannenbaum and Silverstone (1949) also examined the incidence of spontaneous hepatomas in inbred mice fed diets containing 9–45% protein and found no significant effect on tumor latency or incidence. In another study, however, Silverstone and Tannenbaum (1951) found fewer tumors in mice fed 9% casein than in those fed 18 or 45% casein.

The author recognizes that this is a chapter in a book devoted to meat, but there are few cancer studies in which meat protein has been used. Casein is most often fed as a paradigm for animal protein and it was felt discussion of results obtained with casein were not out of place. In a study of DMH-induced colon cancer, Visek *et al.* (1978) compared raw beef, broiled beef and soy protein and concluded that the source of protein did not affect the results. Carroll (1975) compared the effects of casein and soy protein isolate on DMBA-induced mammary tumors and found no significant difference between the two sources of protein.

B. Cholesterol

The role of dietary cholesterol in carcinogenesis has rarely been tested. Cruse *et al.* (1978) reported that cholesterol was co-carcinogenic in rats when added to a defined liquid, but that experiment reflects very special dietary conditions.

Since cholesterol is a precursor of bile acids, which may act as co-carcinogens, some investigators have suggested that this metabolic pathway may tie dietary cholesterol into the cancer picture. High fat diets are associated with both hypercholesterolemia and cancer and this connection has also spurred interest into investigation of the role of cholesterol in carcinogenesis. Current data suggest that the connection between bile acids and colon cancer may be influenced by the concentration of fecal bile acids but not by their absolute amounts. Studies in Hong Kong (Crowther *et al.*, 1976) and Scandinavia (Jensen *et al.*, 1982) have shown that the concentration of bile acids in feces of groups prone to colon cancer is higher than in those at lower risk. New Yorkers and Finns excrete similar amounts of bile acid (275 mg) daily but the former group excrete about 11 mg/g of feces and the latter 4 mg/g (Reddy *et al.*, 1978). The incidence of colon cancer (per 100 000) is 7·9 in Finnish men and 24·6 in male New Yorkers. Hill (1975) showed that subjects ingesting low fat diets (less than 30 g/day) excreted 1·5–2·0 mg of bile acids per gram of feces, whereas controls eating 100–120 g of fat daily excreted 6·0–6·8 mg of bile acid per gram of feces.

There are data from some studies, including several coronary disease studies, suggesting a correlation between low levels of serum or plasma cholesterol and cancer mortality (Beaglehole *et al.*, 1980; Kark *et al.*, 1980; Garcia-Palmieri *et al.*, 1981; Kagan *et al.*, 1981; Kozararevic *et al.*, 1981; Peterson *et al.*, 1981; Williams *et al.*, 1981). Not all studies show this relationship, however (Dyer *et al.*, 1981). Rose and Shipley (1980) have suggested that the decline in cholesterol level may be a metabolic consequence of cancer. However, there are instances where the low levels of cholesterol precede the onset of cancer by a number of years. Lilienfeld (1981) does not think that the observed inverse correlations indicate a direct cause and effect relationship. McMichael *et al.* (1984) carried out an exhaustive review of the data and agreed that no cause and effect relationship could be easily adduced but suggested that further observation and analysis of data were warranted since in some studies there was no evidence of an undetected cancer or a pre-cancerous condition influencing cholesterol levels.

C. Fat

Epidemiological data suggest a strong relationship between diets high in fat and the incidence of certain tumors. What of the fat found in meat? Animal fat is described as a saturated fat, yet the line that divides saturated from unsaturated fats is never defined. Fats are high in saturated, monounsaturated or polyunsaturated fatty acids but virtually all dietary fats contain all three types of fatty acids. Beef tallow, for instance, contains about 42% oleic acid, a monounsaturated fatty acid, and 24 and 18% of the saturated fatty acids palmitic and stearic. Stearic acid has been shown not to be hypercholesterolemic for man (Bonanome and Grundy, 1988) and

TABLE 4-2

DIETARY FAT AND DMBA-INDUCED MAMMARY TUMORS IN RATS[a]

Fat[b] *(20% of diet)*	*Incidence (%)*	*Multiplicity*[c]	*Tumors per 30 rats*
Sunflower seed oil	96·6	4·8 ± 0·31	130
Soybean oil	100·0	4·0 ± 0·62	103
Corn oil	90·0	4·5 ± 0·75	110
Cottonseed oil	93·3	3·4 ± 0·46	127
Olive oil	86·6	4·5 ± 0·42	117
Lard	93·3	3·4 ± 0·47	97
Beef tallow	80·0	3·0 ± 0·49	72
Butter	86·6	3·3 ± 0·41	88
Coconut oil	96·6	2·5 ± 0·38	73

[a] After Carroll and Khor (1971).
[b] In order of descending iodine value.
[c] Tumors per tumor-bearing rat.

much less atherogenic than expected for rabbits (Kritchevsky and Tepper, 1965; Kritchevsky *et al.*, 1982). Discussion of the effects of individual fatty acids on blood cholesterol will be found in Chapter 2 and the relationship between dietary and blood cholesterol is reviewed extensively in Chapter 3.

Experimentally, Carroll and Khor (1971) fed DMBA-treated rats a number of fats as 20% of the diet. Rats fed more saturated fats exhibited lower tumor multiplicity (Table 4-2). Broitman *et al.* (1977) fed DMH-treated rats 20% coconut oil or 20% corn oil. The former group had 15% lower tumor incidence and 42% lower tumor multiplicity.

A study comparing colon cancer incidence in large and small cities in Denmark and Finland (Jensen *et al.*, 1982) has suggested saturated fat as a negative risk factor. A study of the relationship of dietary fat to mortality in the Honolulu Heart Program found that the percentage of calories as dietary saturated fatty acids is related inversely to cancer mortality (McGee *et al.*, 1985). Clearly this is an area of cancer epidemiology that requires more concentrated study.

IV. CALORIC INTAKE AND CANCER

The epidemiological data linking protein intake to cancer risk are almost always qualified by reference to the strong connection between protein and fat in the western diet, and it is often suggested that the protein data are innocent bystanders guilty only by association with fat. However, both the protein and the fat in our diet—level as well as quality—are a reflection of our affluence and consumption of a *luxus* diet. Berg (1975) suggested that many of the hormone-dependent cancers, such as mammary cancer, could be viewed as cancers of affluence. Affluence is reflected in excessive caloric ingestion and reduced calorie expenditure. Gregor *et al.* (1969) summarized the relationship between animal protein intake and rates of stomach and intestinal cancers in 28 countries. They found a direct correlation between increasing protein intake and increasing incidence of intestinal cancer and an inverse correlation between increasing protein intake and stomach cancer. In their comparative international study, Armstrong and Doll (1975) found gross national product (GNP) to be correlated directly with cancers of the colon, rectum, breast and kidney, and inversely with cancers

TABLE 4-3
GROSS NATIONAL PRODUCT AND COLON CANCER MORTALITY[a]

Country[b]	*Colon cancer*[c] (*1970*)	*GNP*[d] ($) (*1971*)
United Kingdom	22·7	2 430
Denmark	20·7	3 430
France	18·9	3 360
Sweden	18·8	4 240
New Zealand	17·9	2 470
USA	17·5	5 160
Norway	15·1	3 130
Italy	13·1	1 860
Portugal	10·1	730
Spain	8·8	1 100
Israel	8·2	2 190
Finland	7·5	2 550
Poland	4·8	1 350
Japan	3·9	2 130
Romania	3·8	740
Yugoslavia	3·4	730
Venezuela	1·9	1 060
Mexico	1·2	700
Egypt	0·6	220
Honduras	0·2	300

[a] After Kassira *et al.* (1976).
[b] From a total of 37.
[c] Mortality rate/100 000.
[d] *Per capita.*

of the stomach and liver. They also found inverse correlations between GNP and intake of cereals and pulses. Kassira *et al.* (1976) listed GNP for various countries and their colon cancer mortality rates and confirmed the inverse relationship shown by Armstrong and Doll (1975) (as shown in Table 4-3). Kassira *et al.* (1976) presented data from 37 countries. The seven most affluent countries (GNP > $3000) had an average GNP of $3810 ± 279 and average mortality of 18·3 ± 0·72: nine countries with GNP between $2000 and $3000 (average $2400 ± 333) had mortality of 13·7 ± 2·20; eight countries with GNP between $1000 and $2000 (average $1316 ± 92) had colon cancer mortality of 9·2 ± 2·19; and the 13 poorest countries (GNP = $559 ± 61) reported a mortality rate of 2·8 ± 0·86.

Could it be that the tumors of affluence are influenced less by specific dietary components than by total caloric intake? This question has been addressed experimentally for almost a century. Moreschi (1909) first demonstrated that underfeeding inhibited the growth of transplanted sarcomas in mice. A few years later Rous (1914) showed that fragments of tumors remaining after excision of the major tumor mass grew to new tumors in 83% of freely fed mice and only in 41% of underfed mice. In the 1940s Tannenbaum and Silverstone (1949) carried out numerous studies which showed that growth of both spontaneous and induced tumors was inhibited by underfeeding or caloric restriction. Underfeeding means simply feeding less of the same diet to one group of animals. Caloric restriction implies use of a diet which is replete in minerals and vitamins but may be low in a macronutrient, such as carbohydrate or fat. If animals subjected to caloric restriction continue to grow it is a sign that their diets are not severely limiting.

Lavik and Baumann (1943) tested the effects of fat and calories on MCA-induced skin tumors in mice and showed that tumor incidence on a high fat, low calorie diet was about half of that seen on a low fat, high calorie diet (Table 4-4).

Kritchevsky *et al.* (1984) studied the effects of 40% caloric restriction on the growth of DMBA-induced mammary tumors in rats. The calorie restricted diet contained about three times as much fat as did the *ad libitum* diet. When the fat was principally coconut oil (plus enough corn oil to insure against essential fatty acid deficiency), tumor incidence was 58% in the *ad libitum*-fed rats and 0% in the calorie restricted group. When the fat was corn oil (Klurfeld *et al.*, 1987), tumor incidence in the *ad libitum* and restricted groups was 80% and 20% respectively. These data suggest an effect for fat unsaturation even in a calorie restricted diet. It should be noted that the *ad libitum* diet contained 4% fat (0·11 g fat per kcal of diet). The

TABLE 4-4

EFFECT OF FAT AND CALORIES ON METHYLCHOLANTHRENE-INDUCED SKIN TUMORS IN MICE[a]

Regimen		*Tumor incidence (%)*
Fat	*Calories*	
Low	Low	0
Low	High	54
High	Low	28
High	High	66

[a] After Lavik and Baumann (1943). Carcinogen applied two times a week for 10 weeks; duration 6 months.

restricted diet, as fed contained 0·36 g fat per kcal. Caloric restriction by 40% reduced the incidence of DMH-induced colon tumors from 100% to 53% in rats fed corn oil (Klurfeld *et al.*, 1987), and from 85% to 35% in rats fed butter oil (Unpublished data). The data are summarized in Table 4-5.

In other studies (Kritchevsky and Klurfeld, 1987; Klurfeld *et al.*, 1989a) the influence of graded caloric restriction was tested in DMBA-treated rats.

TABLE 4-5

INFLUENCE OF 40% CALORIC RESTRICTION ON DMBA-INDUCED MAMMARY TUMORS AND DMH-INDUCED COLON TUMORS IN RATS

Regimen	*% fat*	*Incidence (%)*	*Multiplicity*
Mammary tumors[a]			
Ad libitum	4·0[b]	58	2·8 ± 0·5
Restricted	7·9	0	0
Ad libitum	4·0[c]	80	4·0 ± 0·5
Restricted	7·9	20	1·0 ± 0·0
Colon tumors[d]			
Ad libitum	4·0[e]	85	1·8 ± 0·3
Restricted	7·9	35	1·0 ± 0·0
Ad libitum	4·0[c]	100	3·5 ± 0·4
Restricted	7·9	53	2·1 ± 0·6

[a] Induced in female Sprague–Dawley rats.
[b] Coconut oil plus 1% corn oil.
[c] Corn oil.
[d] Induced in male F-344 rats.
[e] Butter oil plus 1% corn oil.

TABLE 4-6

DMBA-INDUCED MAMMARY TUMORS IN RATS SUBJECTED TO GRADED CALORIC RESTRICTION

Regimen	*Tumor incidence (%)*	*Multiplicity*
Ad libitum	60	4.7 ± 1.3
10% restricted	60	3.0 ± 0.8
20% restricted	40	2.8 ± 0.7
30% restricted	35	1.3 ± 0.3
40% restricted	5	1.0 ± 0
	$P < 0.005$	Not significant

The results are summarized in Table 4-6. It is evident that even 10% caloric restriction begins to influence tumorigenicity. Kritchevsky and Klurfeld (1987), and Klurfeld *et al.* (1989b) also examined the influence of caloric restriction (by 25%) in rats given DMBA and fed high levels of corn oil. Table 4-7 summarizes data which show that caloric restriction is effective in reducing tumor incidence even when large quantities of fat are present in the diet.

It is of interest that in some of the early studies showing protein effects on tumorigenicity the diets inhibited growth and the observed effects may well have been due to this factor rather than the gross effects of diet. White and Belkin (1944) showed that transplanted tumors grew poorly in mice fed a low nitrogen diet. Average weight changes (over 3 weeks) in 15 female mice fed the adequate and 16 female mice fed the low nitrogen diet were plus

TABLE 4-7

INFLUENCE OF FAT LEVEL AND 25% CALORIC RESTRICTION ON DMBA-INDUCED MAMMARY TUMORS IN RATS

Regimen	*Tumor incidence (%)*	*Multiplicity*	*Tumor weight (g)*
Ad libitum			
5% corn oil	65	1.9 ± 0.3	2.0 ± 0.7
15% corn oil	85	3.0 ± 0.6	2.3 ± 0.7
20% corn oil	80	4.1 ± 0.6	2.9 ± 0.5
Restricted			
20% corn oil	60	1.9 ± 0.4	0.8 ± 0.2
26.7% corn oil	30	1.5 ± 0.3	1.4 ± 1.0
	$P < 0.005$	$P < 0.0001$	$P < 0.0001$

TABLE 4-8

EFFECT OF EXERCISE AND CALORIC RESTRICTION ON DMH-INDUCED COLON TUMORS IN RATS

Experimental group	*Tumor incidence* (%)	*Multiplicity*
Ad libitum—sedentary	75	$2{\cdot}1 \pm 0{\cdot}4$
Ad libitum—exercised	36	$1{\cdot}3 \pm 0{\cdot}2$
25% restriction—sedentary	35	$1{\cdot}3 \pm 0{\cdot}2$
25% restriction—exercised	29	$1{\cdot}1 \pm 0{\cdot}1$
40% restriction—sedentary	21	$1{\cdot}2 \pm 0{\cdot}2$

$4{\cdot}05 \pm 0{\cdot}25$ and minus $3{\cdot}94 \pm 0{\cdot}29$ g, respectively. A diet low in cystine reduced the incidence of leukemia in mice, but restriction of lysine or tryptophan had no effect. All the amino acid-restricted diets were shown to inhibit growth of the mice (White *et al.*, 1946).

Another means of reducing calorie availability is by exercise. Comparison of the effects of caloric restriction and exercise on DMH-induced colon tumors in rats (Klurfeld *et al.*, 1988) shows exercise to be about as effective as 25% caloric restriction (Table 4-8). Over four decades ago, Potter (1945) suggested that exercise and reduced caloric intake might be effective in reducing the incidence of cancer.

V. SUMMARY

The accumulated evidence—epidemiological, case-control and experimental—do not support a connection between meat and colon cancer. Mormons and Seventh Day Adventists in the United States exhibit similar levels of colon cancer incidence despite large differences in meat intake. Between 1940 and 1970 meat consumption in the United States doubled while colon cancer mortality was unchanged.

If we examine effects of the principal components of meat we find little influence of dietary protein level in experimental colon carcinogenesis and none for cholesterol as well. The question of low levels of serum cholesterol and risk of cancer has been explained as a metabolic consequence of èxisting cancer. However, there are enough examples of hypo-cholesterolemia observed well before the onset of cancer to merit a deeper inquiry into this phenomenon.

The role of fat in promotion of carcinogenesis has received considerable attention. If we were to concentrate on beef tallow the data derived from animal studies suggest that it is less co-carcinogenic than fats which contain a greater proportion of unsaturated fatty acids. Some epidemiological studies in man suggest that saturated fat may be a negative risk factor for colon cancer (Jensen *et al.*, 1982).

The role of caloric flux (intake or expenditure) on carcinogenesis is being vigorously re-investigated. The findings indicate that intake of total calories, rather than their source, is the determinant of tumorigenicity. While meat is a common component of the diet of affluent populations, its contribution to cancer seems to be related only to its contribution to total caloric intake. There is no evidence of an independent link between meat consumption and cancer.

The data suggest that for a healthy life style we should adhere to the advice given in so many guidelines, namely, maintenance of ideal weight and ingestion of a variety of foods. This life style may not be glamorous, but we can live with it.

VI. ACKNOWLEDGEMENTS

This work was supported, in part, by a Research Career Award (HL-00734) from the National Institutes of Health and by funds from the Commonwealth of Pennsylvania.

VII. REFERENCES

ARMSTRONG, B. and DOLL, R. (1975). Environmental factors and cancer incidence and mortality in different countries with special reference to dietary practices. *Int. J. Cancer* **15**, 617.

BEAGLEHOLE, R., FOULKES, M. A., PRIOR, I. A. M. and EYLES, E. F. (1980). Cholesterol and mortality in New Zealand Maoris. *Brit. Med. J.* **280**, 285.

BERG, J. W. (1975). Can nutrition explain the pattern of international epidemiology of hormone-dependent cancers? *Cancer Res.* **35**, 3345.

BONANOME, A. and GRUNDY, S. M. (1988). Effect of dietary stearic acid on plasma cholesterol and lipoprotein levels. *New Engl. J. Med.* **318**, 1244.

BROITMAN, S. A., VITALE, J. J., VAVROUSEK-JAKUBA, E. and GOTTLIEB, L. S. (1977). Polyunsaturated fat, cholesterol and large bowel tumorigenesis. *Cancer* **40**, 2453.

CARROLL, K. K. (1975). Experimental evidence of dietary factors and hormone-dependent cancers. *Cancer Res.* **35**, 3374.

CARROLL, K. K. and KHOR, H. T. (1971). Effect of level and type of dietary fat on incidence of mammary tumors induced in female Sprague–Dawley rats by 7,12-dimethylbenz (a) anthracene. *Lipids* **6**, 415.

CARROLL, K. K. and KHOR, H. T. (1975). Dietary fat in relation to tumorigenesis. *Prog. Biochem. Pharmacol.* **10**, 308.

CLINTON, S. K., TRUEX, C. R. and VISEK, W. J. (1977). Dietary protein, arylhydrocarbon hydroxylase and chemical carcinogenesis. *J. Nutr.* **109**, 55.

COMMITTEE ON DIET, NUTRITION AND CANCER (1982). *Diet, Nutrition and Cancer.* National Academy Press, Washington, DC.

CROWTHER, J. S., DRASAR, B. S., HILL, M. J., MACLENNAN, R., MAGNIN, D., PECK, S. and TEAH-CHAN, C. H. (1976). Faecal steroids and bacteria and large bowel cancer in Hong Kong by socioeconomic group. *Brit. J. Cancer* **34**, 191.

CRUSE, J. P., LEWIN, M. R., FERULANO, G. P. and CLARK, C. G. (1978). Carcinogenic effects of dietary cholesterol in experimental colon cancer. *Nature* **276**, 822.

DYER, A. R., STAMLER, J., PAUL, O., SHEKELLE, R. B., SCHOENBERGER, J. A., BERKSON, D. M., LEPPER, M., COLLETTE, P., SHEKELLE, S and LINDBERG, H. A. (1981). Serum cholesterol and risk of death from cancer and other causes in three Chicago epidemiological studies. *J. Chronic Dis.* **34**, 249.

ENSTROM, J. E. (1975). Colorectal cancer and consumption of beef and fat. *Brit. J. Cancer* **32**, 432.

GARCIA-PALMIERI, M. R., SORLIE, P. D., COSTAS, R., JR and HAVLIK, R. J. (1981). An apparent inverse relationship between serum cholesterol and cancer mortality in Puerto Rico. *Am. J. Epidemiol.* **114**, 29.

GRAHAM, S., DAYAL, H., SWANSON, M., MITTELMAN, A. and WILKINSON, G. (1978). Diet in the epidemiology of cancer of the colon and rectum. *J. Natl. Cancer Inst.* **61**, 709.

GREGOR, O., TOMAN, P. and PRUSOVA, F. (1969). Gastrointestinal cancer and nutrition. *Gut* **10**, 1031.

HIGGINSON, J. (1966). Etiological factors in gastrointestinal cancer in man. *J. Natl Cancer Inst.* **37**, 527.

HILL, M. J. (1975). Metabolic epidemiology of dietary factors in large bowel cancer. *Cancer Res.* **35**, 3398.

JENSEN, D. M., MACLENNAN, R. and WAHRENDORF, J. (1982). Diet, bowel function, fecal characteristics and large bowel cancer in Denmark and Finland. *Nutr. Cancer* **4**, 5.

KAGAN, A., MCGEE, D. L., YANO, K., RHOADS, G. G. and NOMURA, A. (1981). Serum cholesterol and mortality in a Japanese-American population. *Am. J. Epidemiol.* **114**, 11.

KARK, J. D., SMITH, A. H. and HAMES, C. G. (1980). The relationship of serum cholesterol to the incidence of cancer in Evans County, Georgia. *J. Chronic Dis.* **33**, 311.

KASSIRA, E., PARENT, L. and VAHOUNY, G. (1976). Colon cancer: An epidemiological survey. *Am. J. Digestive Dis.* **21**, 205.

KLURFELD, D. M., WEBER, M. M. and KRITCHEVSKY, D. (1987). Inhibition of chemically induced mammary and colon tumor promotion by caloric restriction in rats fed increased dietary fat. *Cancer Res.* **47**, 2759.

KLURFELD, D. M., WELCH, C. B., EINHORN, E. and KRITCHEVSKY, D. (1988). Inhibition of colon tumor promotion by caloric restriction or exercise in rats. *FASEB J.* **2**, A433.

Klurfeld, D. M., Welch, C. B., Davis, M. J. and Kritchevsky, D. (1989a). Determination of degree of energy restriction necessary to reduce DMBA-induced mammary tumorigenesis in rats during the promotion phase. *J. Nutr.* **119**, 286.

Klurfeld, D. M., Welch, C. B., Lloyd, L. M. and Kritchevsky, D. (1989b). Inhibition of DMBA-induced mammary tumorigenesis by caloric restriction in rats fed high fat diets. *Int. J. Cancer* **43**, 922.

Kozararevic, D., McGee, D., Vojvodic, N., Gordon, T., Racic, Z., Zukel, W. and Dawber, T. (1981). Serum cholesterol and mortality. The Yugoslavia cardiovascular disease study. *Am. J. Epidemiol.* **114**, 21.

Kritchevsky, D. and Klurfeld, D. M. (1987). Caloric effects in experimental mammary tumorigenesis. *Am. J. Clin. Nutr.* **45**, 236.

Kritchevsky, D. and Tepper, S. A. (1965). Cholesterol vehicle in experimental atherosclerosis. VII. Influence of naturally occurring saturated fats. *Med. Pharmacol. Exp.* **12**, 315.

Kritchevsky, D., Tepper, S. A., Bises, G. and Klurfeld, D. M. (1982). Experimental atherosclerosis in rabbits fed cholesterol-free diets. 10. Cocoa butter and palm oil. *Atherosclerosis* **41**, 279.

Kritchevsky, D., Weber, M. M. and Klurfeld, D. M. (1984). Dietary fat versus caloric content in initiation and promotion of 7,12-dimethylbenz (a) anthracene-induced mammary tumorigenesis in rats. *Cancer Res.* **44**, 3174.

Lavik, P. S. and Baumann, C. A. (1943). Further studies on tumor-promoting action of fat. *Cancer Res.* **3**, 749.

Lea, A. J. (1967). Neoplasms and environmental factors. *Ann. R. Coll. Surg., Engl.* **41**, 432.

Lilienfeld, A. M. (1981). The humean fog: Cancer and cholesterol. *Am. J. Epidemiol.* **114**, 1.

Lubin, J. H., Burns, P. E., Blot, W. J., Ziegler, R. G., Lees, A. W. and Fraumeni, J. F. (1981). Dietary factors and breast cancer risk. *Int. J. Cancer* **28**, 685.

Lyon, J. L., Klauber, M. R., Gardner, J. W. and Smart, C. R. (1976). Cancer incidence in Mormons and non-Mormons in Utah, 1966–1970. *New Engl. J. Med.* **294**, 129.

McGee, D., Reed, D., Stemmerman, G., Rhoads, G., Yano, K. and Feinlieb, M. (1985). The relationship of dietary fat and cholesterol to mortality in 10 years: The Honolulu Heart Program. *Int. J. Epidemiol.* **114**, 97.

McMichael, A. J., Jensen, O. M., Parkin, B. M. and Zaridze, D. J. (1984). Dietary and endogenous cholesterol and human cancer. *Epidemiol. Rev.* **6**, 7192.

Moreschi, C. (1909). Beziehungen zwischen Ernahrung und Tumorwachstum. *Z. Immunitatsforsch* **2**, 651.

Nomura, A., Henderson, B. E. and Lee, J. (1978). Breast cancer and diet among the Japanese in Hawaii. *Am. J. Clin. Nutr.* **31**, 2020.

Peterson, B., Trell, E. and Sternby, N. H. (1981). Low cholesterol as risk factor for non-coronary death in middle-aged men. *J. Am. Med. Assoc.* **245**, 2056.

Phillips, R. L. (1975). Role of life-style and dietary habits in risk of cancer among Seventh Day Adventists. *Cancer Res.* **35**, 3513.

Phillips, R. L., Snowdon, D. A. and Brin, B. H. (1983). Cancer in vegetarians. In *Environmental Aspects of Cancer. The Role Macro and Micro Components of*

Foods (E. L. Wynder, G. A. Leveille, J. H. Weisburger and G. E. Livingston, (Eds), p. 53. Food and Nutrition Press, Inc., Westport, CT.

POTTER, V. R. (1945). The role of nutrition in cancer prevention. *Science* **101**, 105.

REDDY, B. S., HEDGES, A. R., LAAKSO, K and WYNDER, E. L. (1978). Metabolic epidemiology of large bowel cancer. *Cancer* **42**, 2832.

ROSE, G. and SHIPLEY, M. J. (1980). Plasma lipid and mortality: A source of error. *Lancet* **1**, 523.

ROUS, P. (1914). The influence of diet on transplanted and spontaneous mouse tumors. *J. Exp. Med.* **20**, 433.

SHAY, H., GRUENSTEIN, M. and SHIMKIN, M. B. (1964). Effects of casein, lactalbumin and ovalbumin on 3-methylcholanthrene induced mammary carcinoma in rats. *J. Natl Cancer Inst.* **33**, 243.

SILVERSTONE, H. and TANNENBAUM, A. (1951). Proportion of dietary protein and the formation of spontaneous hepatomas in the mouse. *Cancer Res.* **11**, 442.

TANNENBAUM, A. and SILVERSTONE, H. (1949). The genesis and growth of tumors. IV. Effects of varying the proportion of protein (casein) in the diet. *Cancer Res.* **9**, 162.

VISEK, W. J., CLINTON, S. K. and TRUEX, C. R. (1978), Nutrition and experimental carcinogenesis. *Cornell Vet.* **68**, 3.

WALTERS, M. A. and ROE, F. J. C. (1964). The effect of dietary casein on the induction of lung tumors by the injection of 9, 10-dimethyl-1,2- benzanthracene (DMBA) into newborn mice. *Brit. J. Cancer* **18**, 312.

WHITE, F. R. and BELKIN, M. (1944), Source of tumor proteins I. Effect of a low-nitrogen diet on the establishment and growth of a transplanted tumor. *J. Natl Cancer Inst.* **5**, 261.

WHITE, J., WHITE, F. R. and MIDER, G. B. (1946). Effects of diets deficient in certain amino acids on the induction of leukemia in dba mice. *J. Natl Cancer Inst.* **7**, 199.

WILLIAMS, R. R., SORLIE, P. D., FEINLIEB, M., MCNAMARA, P. M., KANNEL, W. B. and DAWBER, T. R. (1981). Cancer incidence by levels of cholesterol. *J. Am. Med. Assoc.* **245**, 247.

5

Toxic Compounds Produced During Cooking and Meat Processing

JOSEPH H. HOTCHKISS[a] AND ROBERT S. PARKER[b]
[a]*Institute of Food Science*, [b]*Division of Nutritional Sciences, Cornell University, Ithaca, New York, USA*

I. INTRODUCTION

Meats, like other complex foods, undergo substantial chemical changes during storage, processing, and cooking. These processes result in the formation of many compounds, only a few of which have been characterized. The majority of these non-intrinsic compounds may be of little significance or they may impart desirable characteristics such as flavor or increased microbiological stability to the meat. Some of the compounds produced may have undesirable biological properties when fed to laboratory animals at higher levels. They may, for example, produce tumors or cause circulatory system diseases.

The significance of potential toxicants found in processed and cooked meats, as well as in other foods, to human health is not understood. Acutely toxic contaminants derived from meats are usually avoided and, therefore, of less research interest. However, the long-term effects on human health of toxic compounds which, when fed to laboratory animals at high levels, are capable of causing chronic diseases, such as cancer and arteriosclerosis, are difficult to extrapolate in terms of the low levels to which humans are exposed.

This review will deal with chronic toxicants which are known to occur in meats as a result of storage, processing, and/or cooking. Each section will suggest methods by which the amount of toxicant formed can be reduced or minimized. It should be recognized that meats are not the only foods in which many of these same toxicants occur as a result of similar processes. In many cases, the process or cooking method is as great of a determinant of the type and amount of toxicant formed as is the nature of the food itself. Toxicants, such as drugs or other residues, toxic metals, environmental contaminants, package migrants or other adventitious additives, and direct additives are covered in other sections of this volume and will not be dealt with here. For more information on this topic see Chapter 6.

II. POLYCYCLIC AROMATIC HYDROCARBONS

It was discovered late in the 18th century that products of the pyrolysis of organic matter were capable of causing human cancer. However, it was not until the 1930s that polycyclic aromatic hydrocarbons (PAHs) were identified as causative agents (Cook *et al.*, 1932). Since then, considerable knowledge has been gained about not only the formation and carcinogenicity of PAHs but this research has led to an increased understanding of chemical carcinogenesis in general. Representative structures of PAHs which may be found in foods are given in Fig. 5-1. The most studied, and perhaps most commonly found, is benzo(a)pyrene (3,4-benzpyrene).

A. Structure and Formation

PAHs are annelated benzene (aromatic) rings and most are derivatives of the benzo(a)anthracene, which may or may not be substituted on one or more rings (Fig. 5-1). There have been at least 100 structurally distinct PAHs found in environmental and food samples. PAHs are pyrolysis products of organic matter and occur in the residue of smoke, tar, soot, coal, tobacco smoke, petroleum, or combustion effluent. They are formed from free radicals that are produced during pyrolysis of larger organic molecules. PAHs become contaminants in foods that have been cooked over open flames, treated with smoke condensate, or exposed to one of the above environmental sources. PAHs also form directly in foods which have themselves been partially pyrolyzed. In general, the water solubility of PAHs is quite low, being less than 100 μg/liter.

PAHs also are natural products of plant metabolism and some microorganisms are capable of *de novo* synthesis of low amounts (Knorr and Schenk, 1968). However, the major sources are derived from human activity. It is estimated (NAS–NRC, 1972) that 1 320 tons of PAHs are released into the atmosphere each year due to combustion processes. These combustion processes may result in the indirect contamination of some foods. However, smoking and open flame cooking processes are the major

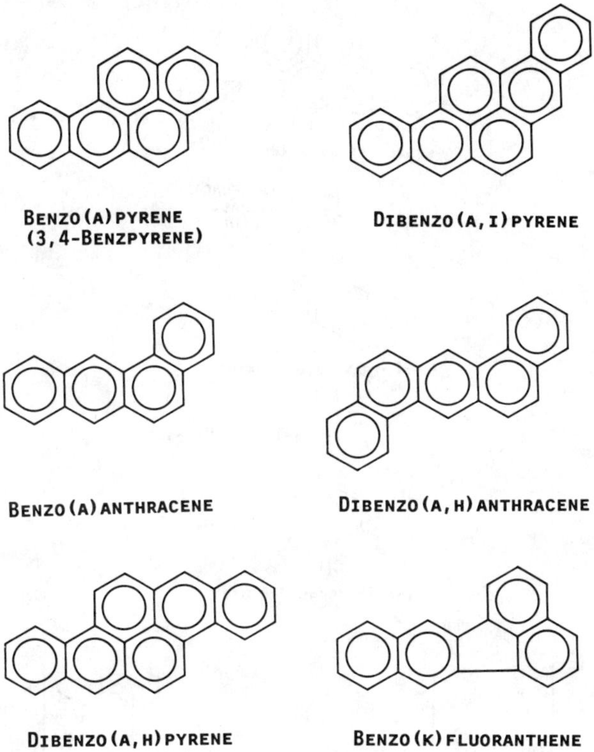

FIG. 5-1. Structures of some polynuclear aromatic hydrocarbons which can be found in foods.

factors that determine the PAH content of foods, with the most often contaminated products being smoked fish and meats.

B. Biological Activity

The biochemistry and metabolism of PAHs have been extensively studied over the last three decades, and in-depth overviews are available (Cook and Dennis, 1985). PAHs are not direct acting chemical carcinogens, but must first undergo a series of complex metabolic oxidations by the mixed function oxidase (P450) enzyme system (Selkirk, 1977). The first step in the activation is the formation of an epoxide by the P450 system, followed by hydrolysis to the diol which is further oxidized to a diol epoxide. The diol epoxide is thought to be the chemical species which binds to DNA and initiates the carcinogenic response (Yagi *et al.*, 1977). The location at which

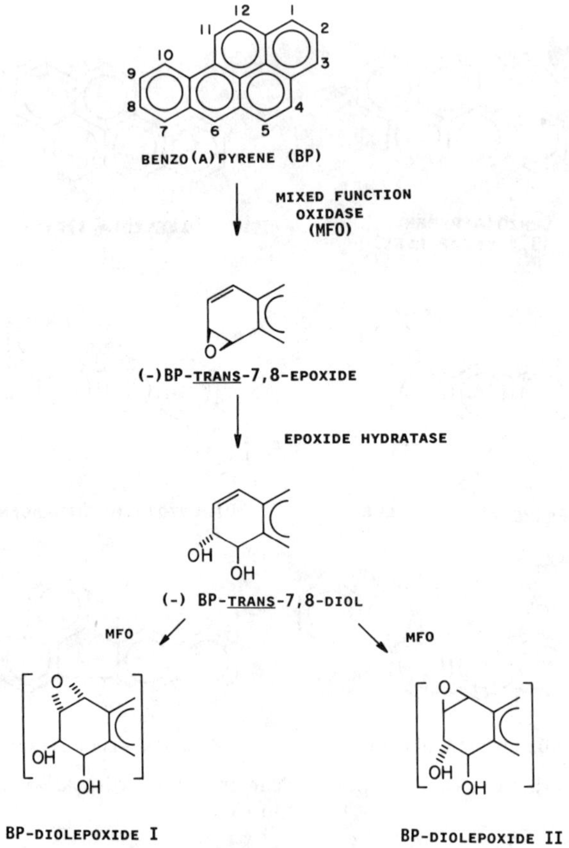

FIG. 5-2. Two step metabolic activation of benzo(a)pyrene by the microsomal mixed function oxidase enzyme system.

these epoxidations occur on the ring system is quite specific for carcinogenic activity, with the 7,8-diol-9,10 epoxide of benzo(a)pyrene being the most potent metabolite (Fig. 5-2).

C. PAHs in Foods

The first reports that foods contain carcinogenic PAHs were described more than 25 years ago. Benzo(a)pyrene was reported in roasted coffee (Kuratsune and Hueper, 1960), charred biscuits (Kuratsune, 1956), broiled meats (Lijinsky and Shubik, 1964), barbecued beef (Malanoski *et al.*, 1968), and broiled fish (Masuda *et al.*, 1966). Howard and Fazio (1980) have reviewed the occurrence of PAHs in smoked foods, fats and oils, plant materials, seafoods and water, liquid smokes, beverages, and the influence of cooking and heating on the PAH content. Detailed analytical methodology has recently been described by workers at the US Food and Drug Administration (Joe *et al.*, 1984; Fazio, 1987).

PAHs can enter meats and other foods by several routes. As pointed out above, charring or cooking by an open flame or exposed electrical element can result in the formation of PAHs. The compounds can be formed directly on the surface of the meat or can be transferred to the meat as melting fats drip onto the coals or element and are pyrolyzed to form PAHs, which then are volatilized and deposited on the surface of the food. Lijinsky and Ross (1967) showed that beef steaks cooked close to the coals contained considerably more PAHs than those cooked at greater distances. The fat content of the meat also affects the PAH content with a higher fat content causing more fat to drip onto the coals and, hence, causing more pyrolysis and an increase in PAH formation.

Cooking temperature is also an important factor in the PAH content of cooked meats as well as for other foods. Starches as well as fats will pyrolyze to form PAHs if sufficiently high temperatures are reached. Masuda *et al.* (1967) found that PAHs were not formed from starch at 300°C, but at 500–700°C as many as 19 different PAHs were detected. Davies and Wilmshurst (1960) showed that heating starch to 390°C formed only trace amounts of benzo(a)pyrene, while 650°C yielded 17 μg/kg. Normal temperatures for some cooking processes, such as broiling or charcoal broiling, are within these ranges.

PAHs can be transferred to foods through the use of liquid smoke in the cure-mix. Several workers have studied the PAH content of liquid smoke used in meat processing and found the levels of individual PAHs are 2–35 μg/liter, whereas the total is approximately 60 μg/liter (Lijinsky and Raha, 1965). The PAH content can be reduced by 90% by bubbling the smoke through cold water and filtering the resulting suspension.

Lo and Sandi (1978) have compiled much of the analytical data from the literature on the amounts of PAHs found in cooked foods. Perusal of these data shows that direct smoking, broiling and other high temperature processes and charring foods over an open flame or hot coals results in the highest concentrations (Table 5-1). The most extensive studies of PAHs in charcoal broiled meats were conducted by Lijinsky and Shubik (1964) and Lijinsky and Ross (1967). One or more PAHs were found in all samples including those cooked in commercial restaurants. The highest levels were found in T-bone steaks (up to 200 μg/kg total PAHs) that were cooked close

TABLE 5-1
PAH CONCENTRATION IN LABORATORY COOKED MEATS
(Adapted from Lijinsky and Ross, 1967)

Food	*Parts per billion*			
	BaA	*BaP*	*F*	*BaF*
Charcoal broiled				
Hamburger, fat,[a] hot[b]	2·7	2·6	13·3	—
Hamburger, fat,[a] cool[b]	—	—	6·4	—
Hamburger, lean,[a] hot[b]	—	—	0·3	—
Hamburger, lean,[a] cool[b]	—	—	1·3	—
Hamburger, no-drip pan	—	—	0·2	—
Hamburger (frozen), hot[b]	4·5	11·2	4·9	—
Pork chop, hot[b]	8·2	7·9	22·5	—
Chicken, hot[b]	3·2	3·7	1·1	—
Sirloin steak, hot[b]	10·3	11·1	12·6	4·3
T-bone steak, hot[b]	31·0	50·4	19·8	5·7
Flame broiled				
T-bone steak, hot[b]	3·9	4·4	19·0	—

[a] Fat = 21% fat, lean = 7% fat.
[b] Cool = 25 cm from heat source, hot = 7 cm from heat source.
PAH = polycyclic aromatic hydrocarbons.
BaA = benzo(a)anthracene.
BaP = benzo(a)pyrene.
F = fluorene.
BaF = benzo(a)fluorene.

to the coals. The source of the heat appeared to have some effect, flame broiling gave lower PAHs than charcoal broiling.

Smoked meats, cheese, ham, and fish also contain detectable amounts of PAHs but at levels that are at least an order of magnitude lower than charcoal broiled foods (Howard and Fazio, 1969). Malanoski *et al.* (1968) surveyed several smoked products including ham, barbecued beef, and sausages and found PAH levels of up to 13 μg/kg. Thorsteinsson (1969) found PAHs in Icelandic home smoked meats at levels greater than 2 000 μg/kg. Fretheim (1976) found PAH levels in Norwegian commercially smoked meats to be less than 1 μg/kg.

As with smoked meats, smoked fish can contain considerable amounts of PAHs. Masuda *et al.* (1966) and Masuda and Kuratsune (1971) have shown that Japanese smoked fish can contain more than 1 000 μg/kg of PAHs. Fish harvested from polluted environments can also contain PAHs in the hundreds of μg/kg range (Cahnmann and Kuratsune, 1957).

Other foods, in addition to smoked meats and fish, contain PAHs, but at much lower levels. Edible oils, including those of animal as well as plant sources, can have levels of a few μg/kg. Heating oils to frying temperatures may slightly elevate the levels (Lijinsky and Ross, 1967). On occasion, plant products have been shown to contain <1 μg/kg amounts of one or more PAHs. With the exception of roasted plant materials, such as coffee, the major sources of PAHs appear to be due to environmental pollution.

D. Reduction of PAHs in Meats

As indicated above, broiling over a direct flame source, especially charcoal, is the major source of PAHs in meats. Indirect cooking methods which separate the meat from the flame will greatly reduce PAHs. The second source is the smoking process. Meats which are treated with a liquid smoke have a much lower PAHs content, especially if the liquid smoke has been treated to remove the water insoluble fraction. Cooking foods at lower temperatures, regardless of the method used, in order to reduce surface charring will also further reduce PAHs.

III. *N*-NITROSO COMPOUNDS

A. Introduction

N-Nitroso compounds are, as a class, potent and versatile carcinogens and so are among the most studied of all chemical carcinogens. The occurrence of the *N*-nitroso group in a molecule gives a better than 90% chance that the compound will be capable of producing tumors in animals based on the over 300 compounds tested (Preussmann and Stewart, 1984).

N-Nitroso compounds can be divided into two general types based on their structure; nitrosamides (derivatives of amides and related compounds) and nitrosamines (derivatives of secondary amines; Fig. 5-3). Both classes are potent animal carcinogens but nitrosamides are environmentally unstable, while nitrosamines are quite stable, especially under conditions found in most foods. For this reason, nitrosamides have not been detected in foods while nitrosamines have been detected in the low μg/kg range in several foods including nitrite-cured meats, beer, dried products, and fish. The occurrence of *N*-nitroso compounds in foods has recently been reviewed in detail (Hotchkiss, 1987).

The suspicion that carcinogenic nitrosamines could be found in human foods stems from an incident in Norway in the early 1960s. Domestic animals were dying of liver necrosis after being fed nitrite-preserved fish

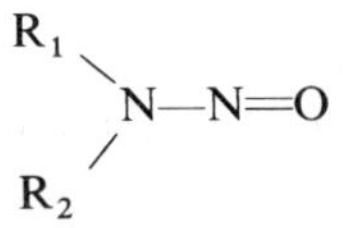

N-Nitrosamine

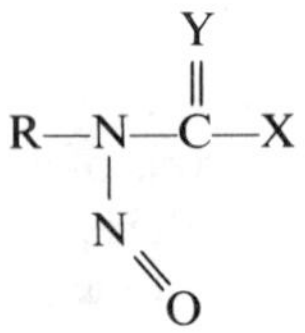

N-Nitrosamide*

*where:

Y	X	Compound
O	alkyl, aryl	*N*-Nitrosamide
O	NH_2, NHR, NR_2	*N*-Nitrosourea
O	RO	*N*-Nitrosocarbamate
NH	NH_2, NHR, NR_2	*N*-Nitrosoguanidine

FIG. 5-3. Generalized structures of *N*-nitrosamines and *N*-nitrosamides.

meal. *N*-Nitrosodimethylamine (NDMA) was shown to be the cause and it was thought that the toxicant was formed when the added nitrite reacted with the di- and trimethylamine in the meal (Ender *et al.*, 1964). Subsequent investigations confirmed these findings and it was suggested that human foods to which nitrite was added could be similarly affected (Ender *et al.*, 1967). This precipitated many investigations throughout the world in the 1960s but much of this early data is suspect due to inadequacies in the analytical methods (Hotchkiss, 1981).

Mass spectrometry was used in the early 1970s to confirm the presence of volatile (capable of analysis by gas chromatography) nitrosamines in nitrite-cured meats (Fazio *et al.*, 1971; Telling *et al.*, 1971; Crosby *et al.*, 1972; Sen, 1972). However, these procedures were laborious and time consuming. This led to a search for a selective detection technique so that larger numbers of foods could be analyzed. In 1974 the Thermal Energy Analyzer (TEA) was introduced (Fine *et al.*, 1975). The TEA enabled a single analyst to conduct several analyses per day. Because of this development, nearly every western food has been analyzed for volatile nitrosamines. The occurrence of non-volatile nitrosamines and nitrosamides has not been adequately addressed due to a lack of acceptable methodology for these compounds. The TEA has only recently been successfully interfaced with reverse-phase HPLC.

B. Chemistry of Formation of Nitrosamines

Nitrosamines form when a nitrosating agent reacts with a secondary, or under some circumstances, a tertiary amine. This can occur under a variety of conditions, the classical case being aqueous acid catalyzed nitrosation. In this case, nitrous acid (in equilibrium with nitrite and a proton) forms dinitrogentrioxide (N_2O_3) which nitrosates the unprotonated amine. The opposing pH requirements of unprotonated amine and nitrous acid formation means that this form of nitrosation occurs at an optimum pH. For dialkylamines pH 2·5–3·5 is optimum. Nitrosation can also occur at basic or neutral pH when oxides of nitrogen (NO_x) formed by combustion come in contact with amines. As is pointed out below, a third nitrosation mechanism, transnitrosation, may be responsible for the formation of nitrosamines in fried bacon and other cooked nitrite-cured meats. The chemistry of nitrosation has been reviewed by Ridd (1961) and updated by Challis (1981).

C. Function of Nitrite and Nitrate in Meats

Nitrite imparts three desirable properties to meats to which it is added. First, it fixes the red to pink color commonly associated with nitrite-cured meats. It accomplishes this by combining with the heme portion of myoglobin which after heat denaturation becomes relatively stable. Secondly, nitrite enhances the flavor (or retards its degradation) of cured meats. This appears to be accomplished more by inhibition of oxidation rather than by the direct formation of specific flavor compounds (Gray *et al.*, 1981). The third function is to inhibit toxin production by *Clostridium botulinum.* The mechanism by which this inhibition occurs is not understood but the extreme toxicity and lethality of the toxin produced by this anaerobic food-borne pathogen is well characterized. If nitrite were no longer permitted in meats many common products would either not be available or there would likely be an increase in botulism. While nitrite is a very reactive substance, nitrate is quite stable. Nitrate does not directly impart any specific properties to meats to which it is added but can serve as a reservoir for nitrite. A portion of the microorganisms that proliferate on stored meats contain nitrate reductase activity and as they grow they reduce the nitrate to nitrite. Thus, nitrate can indirectly inhibit toxin formation. However, the mechanism is not easily controlled and could result in an increased amount of nitrite and nitrosamine formation. The US Department of Agriculture allows nitrate addition only to meat products which are fermented and stored over extended periods, such as summer sausages and country-cured hams.

D. Nitrosamines in Fried Bacon

Fried bacon is the only nitrite-cured meat product in which the edible

TABLE 5-2
COMMERCIAL FRIED BACON RASHERS AND FRIED-OUT FAT[a]
(Taken from Hotchkiss, 1987)

Sample	*No. tested*	*NDMA*	*NPYR*	*NTHZ*
Edible	18	NR[b]	20·0 (4–75)	NR
Edible	17	NR	NR (5–63)	NR
Edible	12	3·4 (ND[c]–17·2)	9·3 (1·7–21·8)	NR
Fried-out fat	10	6·4 (2·6–11·9)	21·9 (15·1–24·0)	NR
Edible	NR	NR (0·1–5)	NR (1–20)	NR
Edible	21	NR	NR (3·4–11·8)	NR
Edible	7	NR	NR	21 (13–32)
Raw bacon	7	NR	NR	2·8 (ND–7·5)
Fried bacon	22	NR	NR	6·3 (ND–241)
Fried-out fat	6	NR	NR	1·0 (ND–2·5)
Edible	18	7 (ND–44)	21 (1–65)	NR
Fried-out fat	18	4 (ND–11)	27 (<1–75)	NR
Edible	39	4·0 (tr–23)	17 (ND–130)	8·9 (ND–30)
Fried-out fat	39	5·3 (ND–33)	32 (ND–120)	3·4 (ND–17)

[a] g/kg, average (range).
[b] Not reported.
[c] Not detected.
NDMA, *N*-nitrosodimethylamine; NPYR, *N*-nitrosopyrrolidine; NTHZ, *N*-nitrosothiazolidine.

portion consistently contains detectable amounts (roughly 1–20 μg/kg) of two or three volatile nitrosamines. Table 5-2 summarizes data from several recent reports of volatile nitrosamines in fried bacon and the fried-out fat. The amount of nitrosamines in fried bacon has declined over the last 10–15 years (Havery and Fazio, 1985) but some evidence suggests that the amount may have increased recently (Canas *et al.*, 1986; Vecchio *et al.*, 1986). The US Department of Agriculture regulates the amount of nitrosamine in fried bacon and initiates action if the level is 17 μg/kg or greater (Federal Register, 1978).

The major volatile nitrosamines found in fried bacon are *N*-nitrosopyrrolidine (NPYR), NDMA, and *N*-nitrosothiazolidine (NTHZ), in order of highest to lowest concentration (Hotchkiss and Vecchio, 1985). Considerable research has been directed at the occurrence of these nitrosamines in fried bacon and the topic reviewed by Gray (1976).

The amine precursor to NPYR has been shown to be predominately free proline but the mechanism through which it is formed is not known with certainty. *N*-Nitrosoproline (NPRO), or other nitrosamines, are not found in raw bacon which means that the process must be thermally induced. Two pathways are possible; proline may be first nitrosated to NPRO and then decarboxylated or proline could be first decarboxylated and the resulting pyrrolidine nitrosated. Kinetic data suggests that the former mechanism predominates under frying conditions (Bharucha *et al.*, 1979; Lee *et al.*, 1983). The precursor to NDMA has not been extensively researched, but Gray *et al.* (1978) have suggested that *N*-nitrososarcosine (NSAR) might be decarboxylated in a manner similar to NPRO.

The discovery of NTHZ in bacon and other foods was first reported in 1982 (Gray *et al.*, 1982; Kimoto and Fiddler, 1982). This nitrosamine occurs as a result of smoking (or adding liquid smoke) to nitrite-cured meats, fish, or other protein foods. Formaldehyde, or other aldehydes produced during smoke generation, can combine with cysteine to form thiazolidine carboxylic acid or alkyl homologs (Fig. 5-4). These thiol-containing amino

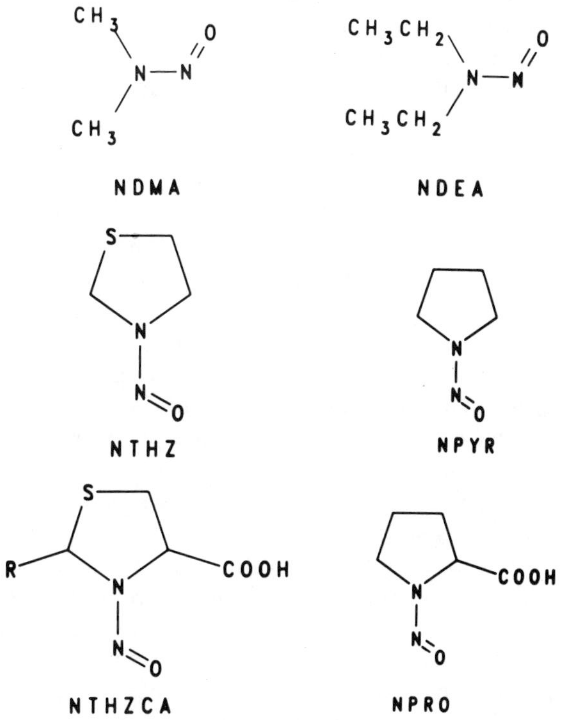

FIG. 5-4. Structures of some *N*-nitrosamines found in fried bacon and other cured meats. (NDMA, *N*-nitrosodimethylamine; NDEA, *N*-nitrosodiethylamine; NTHZ, *N*-nitrosothiazolidine; NPYR, *N*-nitrosopyrrolidine; NTHZCA, *N*-nitrosothiazolidine carboxylic acid; NPRO, *N*-nitrosoproline.)

acids can either be first nitrosated, then decarboxylated or first decarboxylated then nitrosated in a manner analogous to NPYR formation. Smoked nitrite-treated foods have been shown to contain *N*-nitrosothiazolidine carboxylic acid (NTHZCA) which upon thermal decarboxylation yields NTHZ. Recent reports have determined that NTHZ is not a carcinogen in the rat (Lijinsky *et al.*, 1988).

The concentration of nitrosamines found in bacon after frying depends on several factors including the method, time, and temperature of cooking, the amount of nitrite initially added, the presence of nitrosation inhibitors in the cure-mix, and the amount of free amine present in the bacon at the time of frying. The latter factor relates to the age of the bacon, with older more aged bacon having higher free amine/amino acid contents, thus favoring *N*-nitrosamine formation.

Cooking procedures are especially significant. Frying produces the greatest amounts of volatile nitrosamines. The nitrosamines are divided up between the edible portion, the fried-out fat and the vapor. Approximately 20% remains in the edible portion with the rest vaporizing with the water or remaining in the fried-out fat. The higher the frying temperature, the more nitrosamine formed. Lower temperature frying for longer periods of time results in less nitrosamine formation, even at the same degree of doneness, as frying at higher temperatures for shorter times. Other cooking methods such as broiling or baking result in less nitrosamine formation, whereas microwave cooking produces only trace amounts of volatile nitrosamines.

Bacon with a higher fat content and/or free amine content produces more nitrosamines during cooking. Nitrosamine formation in bacon has been shown to predominately occur in the fat phase. This and other evidence suggest that nitrosation may result from a radical mediated reaction (Bharucha *et al.*, 1979). This does not explain why uncooked bacon does not contain appreciable amounts of nitrosamine nor does it explain why the amount of nitrosamine formed increases as the nitrite content of bacon decreases during storage (Sen *et al.*, 1974). One explanation might be that nitrite reacts with components of the meat to form other compounds which are capable of nitrosation when heated during frying. Cassens *et al.* (1977) showed that nitrite does react with several meat components including lipids. We have investigated the nitrosation mechanism during bacon frying and have presented indirect evidence that nitrite reacts with unsaturated lipids during frying to form pseudonitrosites. These lipid–nitrite adducts release nitrosating oxides of nitrogen when heated to frying temperatures (Hotchkiss *et al.*, 1986; Ross *et al.*, 1987; Liu *et al.*, 1988). These compounds serve as a reservoir of nitrosating agents and decompose to produce oxides of nitrogen, which are capable of nitrosating proline or other amines when heated to frying temperatures.

Other composition factors such as the cure-mix makeup also affect nitrosamine formation. Chemical inhibitors of the nitrosation reaction are added to the cure-mix in order to reduce the formation of nitrosamines. USDA regulations require 500 mg/kg of ascorbic or erythorbic acids be added to the cure. These additives react with N_2O_3 to form nitric oxide (NO) which is not a nitrosating agent. The major drawback to ascorbic acid is its low solubility in the lipid phase which is the site of nitrosamine formation. Lipid soluble free radical scavengers, such as α-tocopherol, ethoxyquin (Coleman, 1978), acetals of ascorbic acid (Bharucha *et al.*, 1980), or *N*-alkyl anilines (Bharucha *et al.*, 1985; 1986), are more effective than ascorbate. A commercial product in which tocopherol is coated onto the salt used in the cure-mix has been introduced as a method of evenly dispersing the hydrophobic tocopherol in the mix (Gray *et al.*, 1982).

E. Nitrosamines in other Nitrite-Cured Meats

With the exception of fried bacon, the edible portions of most other nitrite-cured meats contain only very low or undetectable levels of volatile nitrosamines. Several possible explanations have been offered including a lack of precursors in other products (Fiddler *et al.*, 1974), differences in fat content that result in different temperature profiles (Scanlan, 1975), and loss of volatiles due to vaporization (Fazio *et al.*, 1973). Hotchkiss and Vecchio (1985) have studied the total (edible + fat + steam) formation of nitrosamines when nitrite-cured meats other than bacon are fried. These data clearly show that most nitrite-cured meats produce nitrosamines, up to 10 000 ng/portion in ham, when fried. However, the nitrosamines are nearly all carried away with the steam during frying. This points out the unusual nature of bacon. It is the only common cured meat which is cooked beyond the point at which the water is all vaporized. Cooking is stopped with other cured meats before all of the water is vaporized, hence, the nitrosamine content is very low in the edible portions.

F. Regulation of Nitrite in Meats

The US Department of Agriculture closely regulates the amount of nitrate and nitrite that can be added to meats (Table 4-3). Sodium or potassium salts of nitrite are required at levels of 120 or 148 mg/kg, respectively. Sodium ascorbate or erythorbate are also required at 550 mg/kg. The regulations were amended in 1986 to permit the lowering of sodium nitrite to 100 mg/kg with the demonstration of an acceptable quality control

TABLE 5-3
REGULATION OF NITRITE AND NITRATE IN FOODS
(Taken from Hotchkiss and Cassens, 1987)

Law/regulation	*Agency*	*Citation*	*Provision*
Federal Meat Inspection Act of 1906	USDA	21 USC[a] 601–605	Inspection of meat and meat products
Nitrate sanctioned in meats, 1908	USDA	USDA–BAI,[b] 25th Annual Report, p. 301	Use of nitrate (salt petre) detailed
Nitrite sanctioned in meats, 1925	USDA	USDA–BAI,[b] Order 211, Amendment 4	Meat curing regulations detailed
Food, Drug and Cosmetic Act of 1938, Food Additives Amendment 1958	FDA	21 USC[a] 301–392; 21 CFR[c] 172.160; 172.170; 172.175; 172.177	Regulates nitrate and nitrite in non-prior sanctioned uses (e.g. fish)
Nitrite and nitrate in bacon, 1978	USDA	43FR[d]:20992 (1978); 9 CFR[c] 318.7(b) (2)	Lowers nitrite, eliminates nitrate, requires ascorbate
Tocopherol addition to bacon	USDA	50FR[d]:27573 (1985); 9 CFR[c]318.7(c) (4)	Allows up to 500 ppm tocopherol in bacon
Nitrite levels in bacon	USDA	51FR[d]:21731 (1986) 9 CFR[c]318.7(b) (3), (4)	Allows 100 or 40 ppm sodium nitrite in some circumstances

[a] United States Code.
[b] United States Department of Agriculture, Bureau of Animal Industries.
[c] Code of Federal Regulations.
[d] Federal Register.

program, or the use of 40 mg/kg in combination with inoculation of a lactic acid culture (the Wisconsin Process). Nitrate is allowed only in certain dry-cured or fermented meat products.

G. Cured Meats as Compared to other Foods

Humans are exposed to nitrate, nitrite, and nitrosamines from a variety of food and non-food sources including occupational exposure, cosmetics, rubber products, and tobacco usage. It is important to understand the relative contribution of each source to overall exposure. In weighing each source, a Committee of the National Academy of Sciences (NAS–NRC, 1981) determined that the major source of exposure for US residents was cigarette smoke, which contributed approximately 100× as much nitrosamine as bacon consumption. Exposure resulting from beer consumption exceeded bacon by a factor of 2–6 and cosmetics exceeded bacon by a factor of 2–3. These data may not reflect current levels because there is evidence that the nitrosamine content of foods and other products is decreasing due to changes or alterations in processing. Bacon manufacturers, for example, have exercised increased control over the addition of nitrite to their products, which has, no doubt, decreased human exposure to nitrosamines from cured meats.

H. Control of Nitrosamines in Bacon and other Meats

As pointed out above, the occurrence of nitrosamines in cured meats results from actions of both the processor and the cook. The processor can reduce the ability of a given product to form nitrosamines by lowering and controlling the amount of nitrite added to the cure-mix, by the addition of nitrosation inhibitors to the mix, and by using fresher, unaged meats that have a lower fat content. The cook can reduce, or in the case of microwaving, nearly eliminate, the nitrosamine content of fried bacon by reducing the temperature and increasing the time of cooking.

IV. HETEROCYCLIC AMINES AND RELATED PYROLYSIS PRODUCTS

Sugimura and coworkers found in the 1970s that broiling fish resulted in the formation of potent bacterial mutagens that appeared at the charred surface of the cooked food as well as in the smoke condensate (Nagao *et al.*, 1977). The mutagenicity could not be accounted for by the polycyclic aromatic hydrocarbons present in the foods. Other work subsequently showed that the mutagenicity resulted from compounds formed during the pyrolysis of amino acids and proteins including glutamic acid, phenylalanine, ornithine, and soybean globulin (Sugimura and Sato, 1983a). Jaegerstad *et al.* (1984) and Grivas *et al.* (1985, 1986) have used model systems containing amino acids, creatinine, and sugars to show that heating these meat components under conditions similar to cooking results in the formation of mutagenic heterocyclic amines.

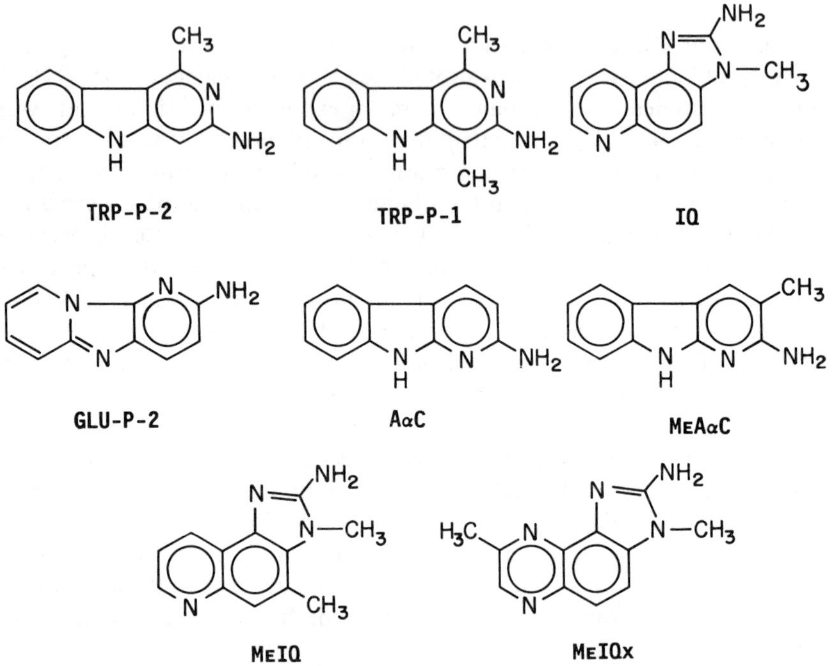

FIG. 5-5. Structures of some heterocyclic amines which are formed by heating proteins and amino acids.
Trp-P-2 = 3-Amino-1-methyl-5*H*-pyrido(4,3-*b*)indole.
Trp-P-1 = 3-Amino-1,4-dimethyl-5*H*-pyrido(4,3-*b*)indole.
IQ = 2-Amino-3-methylimidazo-(4,5-*f*)quinoline.
Glu-P-2 = 2-Aminodipyrido(1,2-*a*:3′,2′-*d*)imidazole.
AαC = 2-Amino-9*H*-pyrido(2,3-*b*)-indole.
MeAαC = 2-Amino-3-methyl-9*H*-pyrido(2,3-*b*)indole.
MeIQ = 2-Amino-3,4-dimethylimidazo(4,5-*f*)quinoline.
MeIQx = 2-Amino-3,8-dimethylimidazo(4,5-*f*)quinoxaline.

The structure of many of these compounds has been elucidated (Fig. 5-5). Heterocyclic amines can be divided into IQ types (derivatives of quinoline) and non-IQ types (Sugimura *et al.*, 1989). The structures of both classes are similar in that they are heterocyclic aromatic amine derivatives of either indole, α-carboline, quinoxaline, or quinoline. Some of the compounds are very potent bacterial mutagens. Subsequent work by a number of research groups has elucidated the structures of several heterocyclic compounds which are mutagens (Barnes *et al.*, 1983; Felton *et al.*, 1986a, b; Knize *et al.*, 1987).

A. Biological Activity

The complexity of foods is so great that it would not have been possible to test the biological activity of the many compounds formed during cooking of meats or other protein foods without a rapid screening technique. The Ames mutagenicity assay is a method of determining the ability of extracts from samples to cause genetic mutations in bacterial cultures (Ames *et al.*, 1973). Bacterial mutagenicity often, but not always, correlates with animal carcinogenicity. This procedure allows large numbers of complex and unpurified samples to be assayed for biological activity. Using this procedure, Sugimura *et al.* (1977) found that broiling sun-dried fish produced unknown potent mutagens. Later, Commoner *et al.* (1978) found an elevated background of mutagenicity in the Ames assay when beef extracts were used to culture the bacteria.

Further work has investigated the mechanism by which these mutagenic compounds are formed during the frying of hamburger. For example, Grivas and Jaegerstad (1984) have synthesized several related heterocyclic amines and determined their mutagenic activity. These data indicated a wide range of potencies and that the presence of the imidazole ring and the 2-amino group was required for high mutagenic activity.

The mutagenicity of various cooked meats and other foods has been tested and several specific compounds have been identified. Felton *et al.* (1986a, b) have shown that as many as 9 or 10 distinct mutagenic heterocyclic amines are formed when beef is fried at 300°C. Vuolo and Schuessler (1985) have reviewed the biological activity of protein pyrolyzates and the possible role that they may play in human cancer. These compounds require activation by mammalian mixed function oxidase enzymes (P450s) for mutagenic activity and are considerably more potent bacterial mutagens than aflatoxin B1 (Table 5-4; Sugimura and Sato, 1983b). MeIQ (Fig. 5-5) is capable of producing $>6{\cdot}6 \times 10^5$ revertants/μg in the TA98 strain of *Salmonella* commonly used in the Ames assay, while aflatoxin B1 produces 6×10^3 revertants/μg when tested in the same strain. Felton and Healy (1984) have shown that human liver microsomes have greater capacity to activate the mutagens formed when beef is fried than do uninduced rat or mouse microsomes. The authors speculated that human microsomes might be in an activated state as a result of exposure to these compounds through the diet.

At least eight of the mutagens, including MeIQ, have been tested for carcinogenicity in rodent systems. Tumors have been produced at a variety of sites in both mice and rats, with the liver being the most common location (Sugimura, 1985, 1986). The potency of these compounds is less

TABLE 5-4
MUTAGENICITIES OF SOME HETEROCYCLIC AMINES COMPARED TO AFLATOXIN B_1 ON *Salmonella typhimurium*
(Adapted from Sugimura *et al.*, 1989)

Compound	*Revertants/μg*	
	TA98	*TA100*
IQ	433 000	7 000
MeIQ	661 000	30 000
IQx	75 000	1 500
MeIQx	145 000	14 000
Trp-P-1	39 000	1 700
Trp-P-2	104 200	1 800
Glu-P-1	49 000	3 200
Glu-P-2	1 900	1 200
Phe-P-1	41	23
Orn-P-1	56 800	—
AαC	300	20
MeAαC	200	120
Aflatoxin B_1	6 000	28 000
Benzo(a)pyrene	320	660

IQ = 2-Amino-3-methylimidazo-(4,5-*f*)quinoline.
MeIQ = 2-Amino-3,4-dimethylimidazo(4,5-*f*)quinoline.
IQx = 2-Amino-3-methylimidazo-(4,5-*f*)quinoxaline.
MeIQx = 2-Amino-3,8-dimethylimidazo(4,5-*f*)quinoxaline.
Trp-P-1 = 3-Amino-1,4-dimethyl-5*H*-pyrido(4,3-*b*)indole.
Trp-P-2 = 3-Amino-1-methyl-5*H*-pyrido(4,3-*b*)indole.
Glu-P-1 = 2-Amino-6-methyldipyrido-(1,2-*a*:3′,2′-*d*)imidazole.
Glu-P-2 = 2-Aminodipyrido(1,2-*a*:3′,2′-*d*)imidazole.
Phe-P-1 = 2-Amino-5-phenylpyridine.
Orn-P-1 = 4-Amino-6-methyl-1*H*-2,5,10,10b-tetraazafluoranthene.
AαC = 2-Amino-9*H*-pyrido(2,3-*b*)-indole.
MeAαC = 2-Amino-3-methyl-9*H*-pyrido(2,3-*b*)indole.

than that expected on the basis of their mutagenicity (Miller and Miller, 1986).

B. Formation During Cooking

As pointed out above, the formation of these toxicants is not limited to one particular type of meat, but most, if not all, proteinaceous foods will similarly form mutagens upon pyrolysis. The basic chemical mechanism by which most of these compounds are formed was studied for decades before it was known that the result is the formation of mutagens. The overall reaction is thermally induced and is known as Maillard browning (Cheftel *et al.*, 1985). Jaegerstad *et al.* (1986) have reviewed the thermally induced Maillard browning reactions which result in the formation of mutagens in cooked foods.

Yoshida *et al.* (1986) found that several plant as well as animal proteins yielded amino-α-carboline upon pyrolysis. The yields from several grilled foods were also compared and while beef gave the greatest amount of α-carboline, smaller amounts were obtained from grilled vegetables.

It is also apparent that mutagens can be formed by a variety of cooking methods, with the most important determinant appearing to be the temperature to which the food is subjected (Pariza, 1982). For example, Pariza *et al.* (1979) found that mutagen formation was temperature dependent when hamburger patties were fried to an approximately equal doneness at temperatures of 143, 191, and 210°C. The lower temperature produced little mutagenesis while the highest temperature resulted in substantial mutagen formation. Others have pointed out that the mutagens are concentrated on the outer surface of the meat and that the greater the degree of charring the greater the degree of mutagenicity. Kasai *et al.* (1980, 1981) found that IQ and MeIQ were formed from dried fish under moderate broiling conditions, and that commercial beef extracts also contained IQ and MeIQx.

Much of the earlier work was done in model systems containing only amino acids or proteins heated to temperatures and for times that were higher and longer than might be encountered in normal cooking. An important question is whether or not these compounds are formed under widely used conventional cooking and commercial food processing conditions. Krone *et al.* (1986) and Krone and Iwaoka (1987) assayed for the formation of mutagens during commercial processing of foods. Several commercial processes which involved heating, including pasteurization, concentration, deep-fat frying, drying, and thermal processing were investigated. The greatest mutagenicity was produced when fish was thermally processed (i.e. canned) to commercial sterility (Krone and Iwaoka, 1984). The other processes resulted in little or no detectable mutagenicity. It should be noted that even the most mutagenic commercial processes were 2–15 times lower than fried or grilled protein foods.

Recent evidence suggests that several foods, including fried ground beef also contain compounds which are capable of modulating or reducing the carcinogenicity of heat-induced mutagens. For example, Ha *et al.* (1987) isolated and identified four isomeric derivatives of linoleic acid, each of which contained a conjugated double bond system. The development of skin tumors in mice was inhibited when the compounds were applied to the skin of the mouse prior to administration of a carcinogen. Previous work by this same group had shown that the semi-purified fraction isolated from fried ground beef could inhibit mutagenic activity, apparently by inhibiting the microsomal enzymes incorporated in the Ames assay (Pariza *et al.*, 1983).

C. Reducing the Formation of Heterocyclic Amines

Formation of this class of mutagens and carcinogens is thermally-induced. Therefore, the most appropriate way of reducing their formation is to cook foods at lower temperatures with less charring. Lower temperature processes, such as microwave cooking would, no doubt, result in less formation of mutagens. Indirect cooking processes which isolate foods from direct heat sources will also reduce mutagen formation. It may also be possible to include additives which can inhibit mutagen formation. However, Sugimura (1986) has pointed out that there is little if any evidence that heterocyclic amines pose a significant risk for human cancer.

V. LIPID OXIDATION PRODUCTS

Muscle and organ meats contain polyunsaturated fatty acids and cholesterol, both of which are susceptible to oxidation during heating and storage. While the process of fatty acid oxidation has been intensely scrutinized for several decades, the formation and occurrence of oxides of cholesterol has attracted attention only recently. The potential health risks of both classes of lipid oxidation products remain unclear and are topics of current research (Winston, 1981).

A. Fatty Acid Oxidation

Polyunsaturated fatty acids occur in meats primarily esterified to phospholipids in cellular membranes, although neutral lipids contain small amounts of these esters. However, in most muscle foods stored prior to heating, endogenous lipase activity will result in at least small quantities of free fatty acids, even during frozen storage. Polyunsaturated fatty acids contain methylene groups alpha to two double bonds, the hydrogen atoms of which are particularly susceptible to abstraction by metals, ultraviolet light, or other catalysts. The result is a carbon-centered free radical, which can react with molecular oxygen to yield fatty acid–peroxy radicals (FA—OO·) and hydroperoxides (FA—OOH). These hydroperoxides undergo homolytic decomposition to yield a variety of secondary products including aldehydes, esters, alcohols, ketones, and short chain carboxylic acids. Such compounds often have undesirable odors or flavors detectable by the human palate at very low concentrations, and thus can adversely impact the quality of foods.

While oxidation of polyunsaturated fatty acids can be catalyzed by oxidases in unheated muscle foods (Gardner, 1980; Hultin, 1980), non-enzymic oxidation (autoxidation) can pose problems in both heated and unheated foods. Autoxidation is accelerated by heat, and is influenced by the concentration of polyunsaturated fatty acids and prooxidant transition metals (e.g. heme and non-heme iron), oxygen tension, water activity, and added or endogenous antioxidants (Nawar, 1985). Meats are particularly susceptible to fatty acid oxidation due to their relatively high content of unsaturated membrane phospholipid species and of both heme and non-heme iron. Poultry lipids are more unsaturated than red meats, and lipid oxidation occurs most readily in turkey meat, followed by chicken, pork, beef, and mutton (Wilson *et al.*, 1976). The relative importance of heme versus non-heme iron is unclear, as both have been implicated as catalysts of fatty acid oxidation (Love, 1983; Chen *et al.*, 1984). Harel and Kanner (1985a) reported the occurrence of hydrogen peroxide in ground turkey muscle, and that the interaction of hydrogen peroxide with metmyoglobin or methemoglobin led to the formation of a reactive species capable of initiating lipid peroxidation (Harel and Kanner, 1985b; Kanner and Harel, 1985). Subsequently, Rhee *et al.* (1987) have identified significant roles for H_2O_2-activated myoglobin and non-heme iron in the initiation of lipid peroxidation of raw and cooked beef muscle lipids, as have Asghar *et al.* (1988) using raw beef and chicken dark muscle. Ang (1988) reported that fatty acid oxidation rate in broiler parts was positively correlated with phospholipid and non-heme iron content, but negatively correlated with neutral lipids, probably reflecting the generally less unsaturated nature of the latter.

B. Cholesterol Oxidation

Cholesterol in muscle meats occurs primarily as free cholesterol (DeVore, 1988) associated with cellular membranes. The mechanism of cholesterol oxidation in meats is unclear. Cholesterol oxidation products may form as the result of autoxidation or enzyme-catalyzed lipid peroxidation via the initial attack of triplet oxygen on the C-7 cholesteryl radical to yield a wide variety of stable and unstable products (Smith *et al.*, 1982; Smith, 1987). Cholesterol oxidation may also occur in conjunction with fatty acid oxidation, as the 7-ketocholesterol content and thiobarbituric acid (TBA) values were found to be highly correlated in fresh and cooked ground beef (DeVore, 1988). Microwaving did not increase the 7-ketocholesterol content of ground beef, but the concentration of this compound was increased by 10-fold in cooked patties stored four days relative to uncooked patties stored a similar length of time. The factors which contribute to the variable (and seemingly unpredictable) levels of oxidized cholesterol species in meat products have not been clarified, and additional investigation is warranted in this area. Time-dependent formation of 7-ketocholesterol and other oxidized cholesterol derivatives in heated beef tallow has been reported by Park and Addis (1986). For example, cooked lean bacon and raw hamburger contained levels of some cholesterol oxides ranging from trace levels to over 1000 mg/kg. Major oxidation products included 5-cholesten-3β, 19-diol, 5-cholesten-3β-01-22-one, the α- and β-epimers of 5-cholesten-3β,-7-diol and cholestan-3β,5α,6β-triol derivatives of cholesterol. Cholesterol oxides occur in highly variable concentrations in raw or processed meats. Park and Addis (1985) observed C-7 cholesterol oxides in raw processed organ meats (liver, brain) in concentrations up to 148 mg/kg, but could not detect these compounds in liver sausage, cooked hamburger, beef jerky or fried chicken. Similar variability, including undetectable levels in many meat products, has been reported by Higley *et al.* (1986).

C. Potential Adverse Health Effects of Lipid Peroxidation Products

In the past much of the research into lipid oxidation was primarily concerned with quality factors. However, recent evidence has raised the possibility that some of the products of oxidation are chronic toxicants in man and contribute to the aging process, cancer, and cardiovascular disease (Pearson *et al.*, 1983; Addis, 1986). Oxidation products of unsaturated fatty acids and cholesterol are absorbed by experimental animals and have been reported to elicit a variety of disorders, including hepatic dysfunction and aortic lesions. Cultured cell systems have also been utilized in the assessment of cytotoxicity and mutagenicity of these compounds. The fatty acid derivatives studied most intensely include hydroperoxides and malondialdehyde, although other secondary carbonyl products may also exhibit toxicity.

Intragastric administration of cholesterol autoxidation products has been reported to cause degeneration of aortic smooth muscle cells in rabbits (Peng and Taylor, 1983). Other reports of potential immunosuppression, carcinogenicity, and cytotoxicity of these products have prompted concern regarding their occurrence and consumption in human diets (Kandutsch, 1980; Sheppard and Shen, 1980). The finding of oxidized cholesterol species in atheromatous plaques has reinforced interest in the possible causal relationship between lipid oxidation and arteriosclerosis. However, it remains unclear whether such oxidation products are derived from the diet or are formed *in vivo.*

In general the levels of oxidized lipids in foods are below those required to elicit responses of acute toxicity. In addition, the low flavor and odor thresholds of many lipid oxidation products, particularly those derived from fatty acids, constitute one level of protection against short term exposure to large amounts of such products. The potential long term impact of ingestion of small quantities of these compounds on risk of chronic diseases such as cardiovascular disease and cancer remain undetermined.

VI. SUMMARY AND CONCLUSIONS

Perusal of the scientific literature leads to the inescapable conclusion that the normal storage, processing, and/or preparation of meats may result in the formation of trace amounts of compounds which can have undesirable biological effects. In nearly all cases, the untoward effects have only been demonstrated after considerable concentration from the meat products in which they occur. Much has been learned about the occurrence, amounts, precursors, mechanism of formation, and biological activity of these compounds. The critical missing knowledge concerns the relationship between low level exposure to these substances in meats and human disease. There are epidemiological data which suggest an association between meat consumption and certain chronic human diseases, but specific causal relationships have not been firmly established. The challenge for scientists is not to discover new trace toxicants in meats or other foods or their biochemistry, but rather to determine the significance, if any, of the toxicants we have already identified.

VII. REFERENCES

Addis, P. B. (1986). Occurrence of lipid oxidation products in foods. *Food Chem. Toxic.* **24**, 1021.

AMES, B. N., DURSTON, W. E., YAMASAKI, E. and LEE, F. D. (1973). Carcinogens are mutagens: Simple test system combining liver homogenates for activation and bacteria for detection. *Proc. Nat. Acad. Sci. USA* **70**, 2281.

ANG, C. Y. W. (1988). Comparison of broiler tissues for oxidative changes after cooking and refrigerated storage. *J. Food Sci.* **53**, 1072.

ASHGAR, A., GRAY, J. I., BUCKLEY, D. J., PEARSON, A. M. and BOOREN, A. M. (1988). Perspectives on warmed-over flavor. *Food Technol.* **42**(5), 102.

BARNES, W. S., MAHER, J. C. and WEISBURGER, J. H. (1983). High pressure liquid chromatographic method for the analysis of 2-amino-3-methylimidazo[4,5-*f*] quinoline, a mutagen formed during the cooking of food. *J. Agric. Food Chem.* **31**, 883.

BHARUCHA, K. R., CROSS, C. K. and RUBIN, L. J. (1979). Mechanism of *N*-nitrosopyrrolidine formation in bacon. *J. Agric. Food Chem.* **27**, 63.

BHARUCHA, K. R., CROSS, C. K. and RUBIN, L. J. (1980). Long-chain acetals of ascorbic and erythrobic acid as antinitrosamine agents for bacon. *J. Agric. Food Chem.* **28**, 1274.

BHARUCHA, K. R., CROSS, C. K. and RUBIN, L. J. (1985). Ethoxyquin, dihydroethoxyquin, and analogues as antinitrosamine agents for bacon. *J. Agric. Food Chem.* **33**, 834.

BHARUCHA, K. R., CROSS, C. K. and RUBIN, L. J. (1986). *p*-Alkoxyanilines as antinitrosamine agents for bacon. *J. Agric. Food Chem.* **34**, 814.

CAHNMANN, H. J. and KURATSUNE, M. (1957). Determination of polycyclic aromatic hydrocarbons in oysters collected in polluted water. *Anal. Chem.* **29**, 1312.

CANAS, B. J., HAVERY, D. C., JOE, F. L. and FAZIO, T. (1986). Current trends in levels of volatile *N*-nitrosamines in fried bacon and fried-out bacon fat. *J. Assoc. Offic. Anal. Chem.* **69**, 1020.

CASSENS, R. G., WOOLFORD, G., LEE, S. H. and GOUTEFONGEA, R. (1977). Fate of nitrite in meat. In *Proc. of 2nd Internat. Sympos. on Nitrite in Meat Products* (B. J. Tinbergen and B. Krol, Eds), p. 95. PUDOC, Wageningen, Holland.

CHALLIS, B. C. (1981). The chemistry of formation of *N*-nitroso compounds. In *Safety Evaluation of Nitrosatable Drugs and Chemicals* (G. G. Gibson and C. Ioannides, Eds) p. 16. Taylor & Francis Ltd, London.

CHEFTEL, J. C., CUZ, J.-L. and LORIENT, D. (1985). Amino acids, peptides, and proteins. In *Food Chemistry*, 2nd edn (O. R. Fennema, Ed.), p. 245. Marcel Dekker, Inc., New York and Basel.

CHEN, C. C., PEARSON, A. M., GRAY, J. I., FOOLADI, M. H. and KU, P. K. (1984). Some factors influencing the nonheme iron content of meat and its implications in oxidation. *J. Food Sci.* **49**, 581.

COLEMAN, M. H. (1978). A model system for the formation of *N*-nitrosopyrrolidine in grilled or fried bacon. *J. Food Technol.* **13**, 55.

COMMONER, B., VITHAYATHIL, A. J., DOLORA, P., NAIR, S., MADYASTHA, P. and CUCA, G. C. (1978). Formation of mutagens in beef and beef extract during cooking. *Science* **201**, 913.

COOK, J. W., HEIGER, I., KENNAWAY, E. L. and MAYNEORD, W. V. (1932). The production of cancer by pure hydrocarbons. Part I. *Proc. Roy. Soc. B.* **III**, 455.

COOK, M. and DENNIS, J. J. (Eds) (1985). *7th Internat. Sympos. on Polynuclear Aromatic Hydrocarbons: Mechanisms, Methods and Metabolism.* Battelle Press, Columbus, OH.

Crosby, N. T., Forman, J. K., Palframan, J. F. and Sawyer, R. (1972). Estimation of steam-volatile nitrosamines in foods at the μg/kg level. *Nature* **238**, 342.

Davies, W. and Wilmshurst, J. R. (1960). Carcinogens formed in the heating of foodstuffs. Formation of 3,4-benzopyrene from starch at 370–390°C. *Brit. J. Cancer* **14**, 295.

DeVore, V. R. (1988). TBA values and 7-ketocholesterol in refrigerated raw and cooked ground beef. *J. Food Sci.* **53**, 1058.

Ender, F., Harve, G., Helgebostad, A., Koppang, N., Madsen, R. and Ceh, L. (1964). Isolation and identification of a hepatotoxic factor in herring meal produced from sodium nitrite preserved herring. *Naturwissenschaften* **51**, 637.

Ender, F., Harve, G. N., Madsen, R., Ceh, L. and Helgebostad, A. (1967). Studies on conditions under which *N*-nitrosodimethylamine is formed in herring meal produced from nitrite-preserved herring. *Z. Tierphysiol. Tierernaehr. Futtermittelkd.* **22**, 181.

Fazio, T. (Ed.) (1987). Polynuclear aromatic hydrocarbons. In *Food Additives Analytical Manual*, Volume II, p. 205. Association of Official Analytical Chemists, Arlington, VA.

Fazio, T., White, R. H. and Howard, J. W. (1971). Analysis of nitrite- and/or nitrate-processed meats for *N*-nitrosodimethylamine. *J. Assoc. Offic. Anal. Chem.* **54**, 1157.

Fazio, T., White, R. H., Dusold, L. R. and Howard, J. W. (1973). Nitrosopyrrolidine in cooked bacon. *J. Assoc. Offic. Anal. Chem.* **56**, 919.

Federal Register (1978). Nitrite and nitrate in bacon. 43 FR 20992 (1978); 9 CFR 318·7(b) (2).

Felton, J. S. and Healy, S. K. (1984). Activation of mutagens in cooked ground beef by human-liver microsomes. *Mutat. Res.* **140**, 61.

Felton, J. S., Knize, M. G., Shen, N. H., Andresen, B. D., Bjeldanes, L. F. and Hatch, F. T. (1986a) Identification of the mutagens in cooked beef. *Environ. Health Perspect.* **67**, 17.

Felton, J. S., Knize, M. G., Wood, C., Wuebbles, B. J., Healy, S. K., Stuermer, D. H., Bjeldanes, L. F., Kimble, B. J. and Hatch, F. T. (1986b). Isolation and characterization of new mutagens from fried ground beef. *Carcinogenesis* **5**, 95.

Fiddler, W., Pensabene, J. W., Fagan, J. C., Thorne, E. J., Piotrowski, E. G. and Wasserman, A. E. (1974). The role of lean and adipose tissue in the formation of nitrosopyrrolidine in fried bacon. *J. Food Sci.* **39**, 1070.

Fine, D. H., Rufeh, F., Lieb, D. and Rounbehler, D. P. (1975). Description of the thermal energy analyzer (TEA) for trace determination of volatile and nonvolatile *N*-nitroso compounds. *Anal. Chem.* **47**, 1188.

Fretheim, K. (1976). Carcinogenic polycyclic aromatic hydrocarbons in Norwegian smoked meat. *J. Agric. Food Chem.* **24**, 976.

Gardner, N. W. (1980). Lipid enzymes: Lipases, lipoxygenases, and 'hydroperoxidases'. In *Autoxidation in Food and Biological Systems* (M. G. Simic and M. Karel, Eds), p. 447. Plenum Press, New York.

Gray, J. I. (1976). *N*-Nitrosamine precursors in bacon. A Review. *J. Milk Food Technol.* **39**, 686.

Gray, J. I., Collins, M. E. and MacDonald, B. (1978). Precursors of dimethylnitrosamine in fried bacon. *J. Food Protect.* **41**, 31.

GRAY, J. I., MACDONALD, B., PEARSON, A. M. and MORTON, I. D. (1981). Role of nitrite in cured meat flavor: A review. *J. Food Protect.* **44**, 302.

GRAY, J. I., REDDY, S. K., PRICE, J. F., MANDAGERE, A. and WILKENS, W. F. (1982). Inhibition of *N*-nitrosamines in bacon. *Food Technol.* **36**, 39.

GRIVAS, S. and JAEGERSTAD, M. (1984). Mutagenicity of some synthetic quinoline and quinoxalines related to IQ, MeIQ or $MeIQ_x$ in Ames test. *Mutat. Res.* **137**, 29.

GRIVAS, S., NYHAMMAR, T., OLSSON, K. and JAEGERSTAD, M. (1985). Formation of a new mutagenic $DiMeIQ_x$ (imidazoquinoxalinamine) compound in a model system by heating creatinine, alanine and fructose. *Mutat. Res.* **151** 177.

GRIVAS, S., NYHAMMAR, T., OLSSON, K. and JAEGERSTAD, M. (1986). Isolation and identification of the food mutagens IQ and $MeIQ_x$ from a heated model system of creatinine, glycine and fructose. *Food Chem.* **20**, 127.

HA, Y. L., GRIMM, N. K. and PARIZA, M. W. (1987). Anticarcinogens from fried ground beef: Heat-altered derivatives of linoleic acid. *Carcinogenesis* **8**, 181.

HAREL, S. and KANNER, J. (1985a). Hydrogen peroxide generation in ground muscle tissues. *J. Agric. Food Chem.* **33**, 1186.

HAREL, S. and KANNER, J. (1985b). Muscle membranal lipid peroxidation initiated by H_2O_2-activated metmyoglobin. *J. Agric. Food. Chem.* **33**, 1188.

HAVERY, D. C. and FAZIO, T. (1985). Human exposure to nitrosamines from foods. *Food Technol.* **39**(1), 80.

HIGLEY, N. A., TAYLOR, S. L., HERIAN, A. M. and LEE, K. (1986). Cholesterol oxides in processed meats. *Meat Sci.* **16**, 175.

HOTCHKISS, J. H. (1981). Analytical methods for *N*-nitrosamines in foods. *J. Assoc. Offic. Anal. Chem.* **64**, 1037.

HOTCHKISS, J. H. (1987). A review of current literature on *N*-nitroso compounds in foods. *Adv. Food Res.* **31**, 54.

HOTCHKISS, J. H. and CASSENS, R. G. (1987). Nitrate, nitrite, and nitroso compounds in foods. *Food Technol.* **41**(4), 127.

HOTCHKISS, J. H. and VECCHIO, A. J. (1985). Nitrosamines in fried-out bacon fat and its use as a cooking oil. *Food Technol.* **39**(1), 67.

HOTCHKISS, J. H., VECCHIO, A. J. and ROSS, H. D. (1986). *N*-nitrosamine formation in fried-out bacon fat: Evidence for nitrosation by lipid bound nitrite. *J. Agric. Food Chem.* **33**, 5.

HOWARD, J. W. and FAZIO, T. (1969). A review of polycyclic aromatic hydrocarbons in foods. *J. Agric. Food Chem.* **17**, 527.

HOWARD, J. W. and FAZIO, T. (1980). Review of polynuclear aromatic hydrocarbons in foods. *J. Assoc. Offic. Anal. Chem.* **63**, 1077.

HULTIN, H. O. (1980). Enzyme-catalyzed lipid oxidation in muscle microsomes. In *Autoxidation in Food and Biological Systems* (M. G. Simic and M. Karel, Eds), p. 505. Plenum Press, New York.

JAEGERSTAD, M., OLSSON, K., GRIVAS, S., NEGISHI, C., WAKABAYASHI, K., TSUDA, M., SATO, S. and SUGIMURA, T. (1984). Formation of 2-amino-3,8-dimethylimidazo-[4,5,*f*]quinoxaline in model system by heating creatinine, glycine and glucose. *Mutat. Res.* **126**, 239.

JAEGERSTAD, M., GRIVAS, S and OLSSON, K. (1986). Formation of food mutagens via Maillard reactions. *Prog. Clin. Biol. Res.* **206**, 155.

JOE, F. L., SALEMME, J. and FAZIO, T. (1984). Liquid chromatographic determination of trace residues of polynuclear aromatic hydrocarbons in smoked foods. *J. Assoc. Offic. Anal. Chem.* **67**, 1076.

KANDUTSCH, A. A. (1980). Biological effects of some products of cholesterol autoxidation. In *Autoxidation in Food and Biological Systems* (M. G. Simic and M. Karel, Eds), p. 589. Plenum Press, New York.

KANNER, J. and HAREL, S. (1985). Initiation of membranal lipid peroxidation by activated metmyoglobin and methemoglobin. *Arch. Biochem. Biophys.* **237**, 314.

KASAI, H., YAMAIZUMI, Z., WAKABAYASHI, K., NAGAO, M., SUGIMURA, T., YOKOYAMA, S., MIYAZAWA, T. and NISHIMURA, S. (1980). Structure and chemical synthesis of Me-IQ, a potent mutagen isolated from broiled fish. *Chem. Lett.* **1980**, 1391.

KASAI, H., NAGAO, M., SUGIMURA, T. and NISHIMURA, S. (1981). Structure of a potent mutagen isolated from fried beef. *Chem. Lett.* **1981**, 485.

KIMOTO, W. I. and FIDDLER, W. (1982). Confirmatory method for *N*-nitrosodimethylamine and *N*-nitrosopyrrolidine in food by multiple ion analysis with gas chromatography–low resolution mass spectrometry before and after ultraviolet photolysis. *J. Assoc. Offic. Anal. Chem.* **65**, 1162.

KNIZE, M. G., HAPPE, J. A., HEALY, S. K. and FELTON, J. S. (1987). Identification of the mutagenic quinoxaline isomers from fried ground beef. *Mutat. Res.* **178**, 25.

KNORR, M. and SCHENK, D. (1968). About the question of the synthesis of PA by bacteria. *Arch. Hyg.* **152**, 282.

KRONE, C. A. and IWAOKA, W. T. (1984). Occurrence of mutagens in canned foods. *Mutat. Res.* **141**, 131.

KRONE, C. A. and IWAOKA, W. T. (1987). Commercial food processing operations and mutagen formation. *J. Food Protect.* **50**, 167.

KRONE, C. A., YEH, S. M. J. and IWAOKA, W. T. (1986). Mutagen formation during commercial processing of foods. *Environ. Health Perspect.* **67**, 75.

KURATSUNE, M. (1956). Benzo(a)pyrene content of certain pyrogenic materials. *J. Natl Cancer Inst.* **16**, 1485.

KURATSUNE, M. and HUEPER, W. C. (1960). Polycyclic aromatic hydrocarbons in roasted coffee. *J. Natl Cancer Inst.* **24**, 463.

LEE, M. L., GRAY, J. I., PEARSON, A. M. and KAKUDA, Y. (1983). Formation of *N*-nitrosopyrrolidine in fried bacon: Model system studies. *J. Food Sci.* **48**, 817.

LIJINSKY, W. and RAHA, C. R. (1965). The detection of polycyclic aromatic hydrocarbons in liquid smoke and some foods. *Toxicol. Applied Pharmacol.* **7**, 337.

LIJINSKY, W. and ROSS, A. E. (1967). Production of carcinogenic polynuclear hydrocarbons in the cooking of food. *Food Cosmet. Toxicol.* **5**, 343.

LIJINSKY, W. and SHUBIK, P. (1964). Benzo(a)pyrene and other polynuclear hydrocarbons in charcoal-broiled meat. *Science* **145**, 53.

LIJINSKY, W., KOVATCH, R. M., KEEFER, L. K., SAAVEDRA, J. E., HANSEN, T. J., MILLER, A. J. and FIDDLER, W. (1988). Carcinogenesis in rats by cyclic *N*-nitrosamines containing sulfur. *Food Chem. Toxic.* **26**, 3.

LIU, R.-H., CONBOY, J. J. and HOTCHKISS, J. H. (1988). Nitrosation by nitro-nitroso derivatives of olefins: A potential mechanism for the formation of nitrosamines in fried bacon. *J. Agric. Food Chem.* **36**, 984.

LO, M.-T. and SANDI, E. (1978). Polycyclic aromatic hydrocarbons (Polynuclear) in foods. *Residue Rev.* **69**, 35.

LOVE, J. D. (1983). The role of heme iron in the oxidation of lipids in red meats. *Food Technol.* **37**(7), 117.

MALANOSKI, A. E., GREENFIELD, E. L., BARNES, C. J., WORTHINGTON, J. M. and JOE, F. L. (1968). Survey of polycyclic aromatic hydrocarbons in smoked foods. *J. Assoc. Offic. Anal. Chem.* **51**, 114.

MASUDA, Y. and KURATSUNE, M. (1971). Polycyclic aromatic hydrocarbons in smoked fish, 'Katsuobushi'. *Gann* **62**, 27.

MASUDA, Y., MORI, K. and KURATSUNE, M. (1966). Polycyclic aromatic hydrocarbons in common Japanese foods. I. Broiled fish, roasted barley, shoyu, and caramel. *Gann* **57**, 133.

MASUDA, Y., MORI, K. and KURATSUNE, M. (1967). Polycyclic aromatic hydrocarbons formed by pyrrolysis of carbohydrates, amino acids, and fatty acids. *Gann* **58**, 69.

MILLER, E. C. and MILLER, J. A. (1986). Carcinogens and mutagens that may occur in foods. *Cancer* **58**, 1795.

NAGAO, M., HONDA, M., SEINO, Y., YAHAGI, T. and SUGIMURA, T. (1977). Mutagenicities of smoke condensates and the charred surface of fish and meat. *Cancer Lett.* **2**, 221.

NAS–NRC (1972). *Particulate Polycyclic Organic Matter: Biological Effects of Atmospheric Pollutants.* National Research Council, Washington, DC.

NAS–NRC (1981). *The Health Effects of Nitrate, Nitrite, and* N-*Nitroso Compounds.* National Academy Press, Washington, DC.

NAWAR, W. F. (1985). Lipids. In *Food Chemistry* (O. R. Fennema, Ed.), p. 139. Marcel Dekker, Inc., New York.

PARIZA, M. W. (1982). Mutagens in heated foods. *Food Technol.* **36**(3), 53.

PARIZA, M. W., ASHOOR, S. H., CHU, F. S. and LUND, D. B. (1979). Effects of temperature and time of mutagen formation in pan-fried hamburger. *Cancer Lett.* **7**, 63.

PARIZA, M. W., LORETZ, L. J., STORKSON, J. M. and HOLLAND, N. C. (1983). Mutagens and modulator of mutagenesis in fried ground beef. *Cancer Res.* (*Suppl.*) **43**, 2444s.

PARK, S. W. and ADDIS, P. B. (1985). HPLC determination of C-7 oxidized cholesterol derivatives in foods. *J. Food Sci.* **50**, 1437.

PARK, S. W. and ADDIS, P. B. (1986). Identification and quantitative estimation of oxidized cholesterol derivatives in heated tallow. *J. Agric. Food Chem.* **34**, 653.

PEARSON, A. M., GRAY, J. I., WOLZAK, A. M. and HORENSTEIN, N. A. (1983). Safety implications of oxidized lipids in muscle foods. *Food Technol.* **37**(7), 121.

PENG, S. K. and TAYLOR, C. B. (1983). Atherogenic effect of oxidized cholesterol. In *Dietary Fats and Health* (E. G. Perkins and W. J. Visek, Eds), p. 919. American Oil Chemists' Society, Champaign, IL.

PREUSSMANN, R. and STEWART, B. W. (1984). *N*-Nitroso carcinogens in the environment. In *Chemical Carcinogens*, 2nd ed. (C. E. Searle, Ed.), p. 829. American Chemical Society, Washington, DC.

RHEE, K. S., ZIPRIN, Y. A. and ORDONEZ, G. (1987). Catalysis of lipid oxidation in raw and cooked beef by metmyoglobin–H_2O_2, non-heme iron, and enzyme systems. *J. Agric. Food Chem.* **35**, 1013.

Ridd, J. H. (1961). Nitrosation, diazotisation and deamination. *Quart. Rev. Chem. Soc. London* **15**, 418.

Ross, H. D., Henion, J., Babish, J. G. and Hotchkiss, J. H. (1987). Nitrosating agents from the reaction between methyl oleate and dinitrogen trioxide: Identification and mutagenicity. *Food Chem.* **23**, 207.

Scanlan, R. A. (1975). *N*-Nitrosamines in foods. *CRC Crit. Rev. Food Technol.* **5**, 357.

Selkirk, J. K. (1977). Benzo(a)pyrene carcinogenesis: A biochemical selection mechanism. *J. Toxicol. Environ. Health* **2**, 1245.

Sen, N. P. (1972). The evidence for the presence of dimethylnitrosamine in meat products. *Food Cosmet. Toxicol.* **10**, 219.

Sen, N. P., Donaldson, B., Charbonneau, C. and Miles, W. F. (1974). Effect of additives on the formation of nitrosamines in meat curing mixtures containing spices and nitrites. *J. Agric. Food Chem.* **22**, 1125.

Sheppard, A. J. and Shen, C-S. J. (1980). Activities of FDA's division of nutrition regarding cholesterol oxides. In *Autoxidation in Food and Biological Systems* (M. G. Simic and M. Karel, Eds), p. 133. Plenum Press, New York.

Smith, L. L. (1987). Cholesterol autoxidation 1981–1986. *Chem. Phys. Lipids* **44**, 87.

Smith, L. L., Teng, J. I., Liu, Y. Y., Seitz, P. K. and McGehee, M. F. (1982). Lipid peroxidations of cholesterol. In *Lipid Peroxides in Biology and Medicine* (K. Yagi, Ed.), p. 89. Academic Press, New York.

Sugimura, T. (1985). Carcinogenicity of mutagenic heterocyclic amines formed during the cooking process. *Mutat. Res.* **150**, 33.

Sugimura, T. (1986). Past, present, and future of mutagens in cooked foods. *Environ. Health Perspect.* **67**, 5.

Sugimura, T. and Sato, S. (1983a). Mutagens–carcinogens in foods. *Cancer Res. (Suppl.)* **43**, 2415s.

Sugimura, T. and Sato, S. (1983b). Bacterial mutagenicity of natural materials, pyrolysis products and additives in foodstuffs and their association with genotoxic effects in mammals. In *Developments in the Science and Practice of Toxicology* (A. W. Hayes, R. C. Schnell and T. S. Miya, Eds), p. 115. Elsevier, Amsterdam.

Sugimura, T., Nagao, M., Kawachi, T., Honda, M., Yahagi, T., Seino, Y., Sato, S., Matsukura, N., Matsushima, T., Shirai, A., Sawamura, M. and Matsumoto, H. (1977). Mutagen–carcinogens in food, with special reference to highly mutagenic pyrolytic products in broiled foods. In *Origins of Human Cancer. Book C.* (H. H. Hiatt, J. D. Watson and A. Winsten, Eds), p. 1561. Cold Springs Harbor Laboratory, Cold Springs Harbor, NY.

Sugimura, T., Wakabayashi, K., Nagao, M. and Ohgaki, H. (1989). Heterocyclic amines in cooked food. In *Food Toxicology: A Perspective on Relative Risks* (R. A. Scanlan and S. L. Taylor, Eds), Marcel Dekker, Inc., New York, p. 31.

Telling, G. M., Bryce, T. A. and Althorpe, J. (1971). Use of vacuum distillation and gas chromatography–mass spectrometry for determining low levels of volatile nitrosamines in meat products. *J. Agric. Food Chem.* **19**, 937.

Thorsteinsson, T. (1969). Polycyclic hydrocarbons in commercially and home-smoked food in Iceland. *Cancer* **23**, 455.

Vecchio, A. J., Hotchkiss, J. H. and Bisogni, C. A. (1986). Ingestion of *N*-nitrosamines from fried bacon: A consumer survey. *J. Food Sci.* **51**, 754.

VUOLO, L. L. and SCHUESSLER, G. U. (1985). Review: Putative mutagens and carcinogens in foods: VI. Protein pyrolysate products. *Environ. Mutagen* **7**, 577.

WILSON, B. R., PEARSON, A. M. and SHORLAND, F. B. (1976). Effect of total lipids and phospholipids on warmed-over flavor in red and white muscle from several species as measured by TBA analysis. *J. Agric. Food Chem.* **24**, 7.

WINSTON, M. (1981). Diet and coronary heart disease. *Contemp. Nutr.* **6**, 1.

YAGI, H., THAKKER, D. R., HERNANDEZ, O., KOREEDA, M. and JERINA, D. M. (1977). Synthesis and reactions of the highly mutagenic 7,8-diol 9,10-epoxides of the carcinogen benzo(a)pyrene. *J. Am. Chem. Soc.* **99**, 1604.

YOSHIDA, D., MATSUMOTO, T., OKAMOTO, H., MIZUSAKI, S., KUSHI, A. and FUKUHARA, Y. (1986). Formation of mutagens by heating foods and model systems. *Environ. Health Perspect.* **67**, 55.

6

Residues

Michael M. Pullen
Department of Large Animal Clinical Sciences, College of Veterinary Medicine, University of Minnesota, St. Paul, Minnesota, USA

I. INTRODUCTION

Since Rachel Carson (1962) published the book *Silent Spring*, consumers have been increasingly concerned about chemicals both in their environment and food supply. To the extent that the raw material for US meat and poultry is exposed to chemicals during livestock husbandry and through contact with the air, water and soil, the food supply provides a complex pathway for contamination by many different compounds (National Research Council, 1985).

Residues in food may present a hidden but serious threat to public health. Because residues generally cannot be seen, smelled or tasted, they are difficult to detect. The monitoring of raw meat and poultry for drug and chemical residues is necessary to ascertain that approved compounds are not being misused and are not presenting a danger to consumers. Residues in meat and poultry tissue can result from a variety of sources: animal drugs given to promote growth and treat or prevent disease, pesticides, feed, and other agricultural or industrial chemicals. Residues from drugs and medicated feeds often result when the drug is used too near the time of slaughter and the withdrawal period is not observed. Drug residues can also result from accidental mixing of medicated and non-medicated feeds at the feed mill, during transport, or on farm facilities.

Pesticides may be applied to animals to control insects or internal parasites, but most animal exposure results from the application of pesticides to buildings, crops used for feed, grazing areas, or feed storage areas. Livestock might ingest traces of pesticides from these sources and store them in their tissues in amounts higher than are legally permitted. Industrial chemicals used in equipment, such as polychlorinated biphenyls (PCBs), can also result in residues. If animals consume feeds or breathe air contaminated with certain chemicals, the substances may be stored in their tissues and then appear as residues at slaughter (Food Safety and Inspection Service, 1984).

The American consumer continues to regard both intentional and unintentional food additives as a major food safety concern (McBean, 1988). For example, Food Marketing Institute (FMI) surveys (1988) reveal that since 1984 residues, including pesticides and herbicides, lead the list of potential hazards in the perception of shoppers who consider them to be a serious hazard. In the FMI (1988) survey, 95% of all shoppers considered residues to be a serious hazard or something of a hazard. Fully three-fourths (75%) considered them to be a serious hazard. Over the past years, the proportions of shoppers who view 'antibiotics and hormones in poultry and livestock' as serious hazards has remained relatively constant at 61% (Food Marketing Institute, 1988).

The responsibility for assuring the safety of meat and poultry as it relates to residues falls on three federal governmental agencies: (1) US Food and Drug Administration (FDA); (2) USDA, Food Safety and Inspection Service (FSIS); and (3) US Environmental Protection Agency (EPA) (Food Safety and Inspection Service, 1984).

II. FEDERAL REGULATORY RESPONSIBILITY—RESIDUES IN MEAT AND POULTRY

The National Residue Program (NRP) began in 1967. The original concern was the effect of environmental contamination, primarily from pesticides, on animals utilized for food. Today, the program includes analyses for over 100 drugs and chemical residues. The regulation of illegal residues is a cooperative effort of FSIS, FDA and EPA. These three federal agencies act under provision of the Food, Drug and Cosmetic Act; the Federal Insecticide, Fungicide and Rodenticide Act; and the Toxic Substance Control Act. FDA is responsible for testing the safety of animal drugs and EPA tests for the safety of pesticides and toxic substances. Both FDA and EPA can prohibit the use of any substance that presents a danger to human health.

FDA and EPA prescribe the conditions under which approved drugs and chemicals may be used. They also establish the maximum allowable limits in meat and poultry. They determine levels considered safe in food consumed by humans by considering each chemical's potential for producing harmful effects, the maximum amount of food containing the residue that a person would be likely to consume, how the body metabolizes the substance, and interactions between the residue and other chemicals that may be ingested.

Raw meat and poultry containing residues above the action tolerance levels is considered adulterated and in violation of federal inspection laws (Food Safety and Inspection Service, 1984). USDA's Food Safety and Inspection Service (FSIS) conducts inspection in meat and poultry plants to assure the safety and wholesomeness of the meat and poultry food supply. As part of that responsibility FSIS continually monitors the incidence and levels of chemical or drug residues in meat and poultry slaughtered for human consumption.

As an added safeguard any new compound used in the production of food animals must serve a useful purpose. This means that any chemical or drug used in the production of animals or poultry must meet several criteria (Spaulding, 1975; Byrnes, 1988):

(1) they must be effective at the proposed dosage level for the proposed use;
(2) the drug or chemical must not create a residue in the edible tissue of the animal or bird that is at a level which is judged harmful to the consumer;
(3) the use of the drug or agricultural compound must serve a useful purpose in the production of the feed crop, animal or bird;
(4) an analytical detection method must be available which is capable of detecting the substance at or below the tolerance level; and
(5) the chemical and drug compounds must be used in a manner that would not contaminate their environment or the food supply.

FDA further requires animal drug manufacturers to demonstrate that each new animal drug is safe and effective before it is approved for marketing. Manufacturers also must develop a reliable assay method for detecting drug residues in slaughtered animals. These analytical methods are reviewed by FDA and FSIS before the drug is approved. FDA also establishes tolerance levels for residues of the drug in animal tissues. The tolerances include a built-in safety factor to assure that the drug will have no harmful effects on consumers of the food (Byrnes, 1988).

III. COMPOUND EVALUATION PROCEDURES

There are more than 300 pesticides approved for use in the United States, with varying potential for their occurrence as residues in meat and poultry. There are many others that may also occur as a result of environmental contamination or in imported foods from significant use in other countries. The number of potential residues from animal drugs and biologics is equally impressive, again with the foreign use of compounds adding to the total number of residues that may occur in meat and poultry. The potent biological activity of many of these compounds raises concern regarding the potential hazard to human health associated with the ingestion of meat and poultry containing residues from pesticides, drugs or other chemicals (Food Safety and Inspection Service, 1988).

It is neither feasible nor necessary to monitor for all chemical residues that could contaminate meat and poultry. However, in deciding where available resources and monitoring efforts should be assigned, it is imperative that FSIS can assess relative concerns for those residues most likely to have the greatest impact on public health. To assist the agency in the effective management of its resources and residue program activities, a compound evaluation system (CES) was developed, which is described by the Food Safety and Inspection Service (1988).

A FSIS compound evaluation system must satisfy certain basic

TABLE 6-1
CRITERIA FOR HAZARD CLASSIFICATION A, COMPOUND EVALUATION SYSTEM, FSIS

Category A—high health hazard potential
- —Acute toxicity is high in experimental animals: oral LD_{50} is 25 milligrams per kilogram of body weight (mg/kg bw), or less.
- —Severe or life-threatening hyperallergenic insults such as anaphylactic shock have been observed.
- —The compound is mutagenic or a confirmed carcinogen in at least two species.
- —Adverse reproductive effects, or teratogenic, have been demonstrated in both rodent and non-rodent species.
- —Irreversible damage to vital functions, such as the hematopoietic system, the immune system, or the hepatic or renal systems, has been observed.
- —Permanent, debilitating effects, known to drastically reduce the quality of life, e.g. neurologic/neuromuscular insults resulting in retardation or motor dysfunction, have been associated with the compound.
- —Major metabolites are of equal or greater toxicity and are known to have extended tissue residency times.

From: Food Safety and Inspection Service (1988).

requirements: (1) it must provide a well-defined and systemic approach for evaluating available data; (2) it must be a manageable and a dynamic system that can accommodate new information and permit rapid reassessment of the potential effect on public health of a given compound; and (3) it should be sufficiently flexible in the use of scientific judgement to allow definitive decisions to be made even with gaps in desired information (Food Safety and Inspection Service, 1988).

After consideration, FSIS (Food Safety and Inspection Service, 1988) developed a two-tiered, hierarchical compound evaluation system. A potential impact on public health is expressed as a function of two major elements in this system: (1) hazard (adverse effects that may be produced by a given compound), and (2) exposure (residue concentration: factors affecting concentration, such as use patterns, withdrawal times, duration of or frequency of consumption of product containing residues of concern). FSIS utilizing the two-tiered, hierarchical compound evaluation system, ranks a hazard in one of five categories:

A—Designation assigned to compounds for which experimental or clinical evidence demonstrates a *high health hazard* potential, based on acute or chronic toxicity data.

B—Designation assigned to compounds for which experimental or clinical evidence demonstrates a *moderate health hazard* potential, based on acute or chronic toxicity data.

C—Designation assigned to compounds for which experimental or clinical evidence demonstrates a *low health hazard* potential, based on acute or chronic toxicity data.

D—Designation assigned to compounds for which experimental or clinical evidence demonstrates a *negligible health hazard* potential.

Z—Designation assigned to compounds for which there is insufficient information available to conduct an adequate toxicological or pharmacologic evaluation.

Criteria for the different categories (A–D) are provided in Tables 6-1–6-4.

The second element of the FSIS two-tiered CES is human exposure to residues of pesticides, animal drugs, or other contaminants in meat and poultry. Human exposures to a compound are ranked in the following four categories:

Category 1—Designates a substance with a *high probability of exposure* of humans to a toxic concentration from meat or poultry, based on known conditions of use/misuse, metabolic patterns in animals or plants, environmental factors or historical presence.

Category 2—Designates a substance with a *moderate probability of exposure* of humans to a toxic concentration from meat or known conditions of use/misuse, metabolic patterns in animals or plants, environmental factors, or historical presence.

Category 3—Designates a substance with a *low probability of exposure* of humans to a toxic concentration from meat or poultry, based on known conditions of use/misuse. Metabolic patterns in animals or plants, environmental factors, or historical presence are considered under this category.

Category 4—Designates a substance with insufficient information available to estimate the *probability of exposure* of humans to a toxic concentration from meat or poultry.

After a pesticide, animal drug, or environmental contaminant has been evaluated according to hazard and exposure potential, the compound is assigned a dual ranking (Hazard vertical, Exposure horizontal). Compounds of greatest concern are designated A-1 (high health hazard potential; high likelihood of residue occurrence), while those compounds of least significance are designated D-4 (negligible health hazard potential; negligible likelihood of residue occurrence) (Food Safety and Inspection

TABLE 6-2
CRITERIA FOR HAZARD CLASSIFICATION B, COMPOUND EVALUATION SYSTEM, FSIS

Category B—moderate health hazard
- —Acute toxicity is moderate in experimental animals, e.g. oral LD_{50} is 25–250 mg/kg bw.
- —Severe but non-life-threatening hyperallergenic effects have been reported.
- —The compound is considered to be weakly mutagenic with evidence of carcinogenicity being invited to a single species, strain, or sex within that species.
- —The compound has caused or is suspected of causing reproductive disturbances without being directly teratogenic; confirmation in a second, non-rodent species has not been demonstrated.
- —Damage to vital functions may be serious but reversible, with no permanent debilitating effects.
- —The metabolism of the compound is well defined; metabolites are no more toxic than the parent compound and are not irreversibly bound in the tissues.

From: Food Safety and Inspection Service (1988).

TABLE 6-3

CRITERIA FOR HAZARD CLASSIFICATION C, COMPOUND EVALUATION SYSTEM, FSIS

Category C—low health hazard

—Acute toxicity is low in experimental animals, e.g. oral LD_{50} is 250–1 000 mg/kg bw

—Limited to mild hyperallergenic reactions.

—May be classified as weakly mutagenic, but with no evidence of carcinogenicity based on chronic studies in rodent and non-rodent species.

—Study results show no form of disturbance to the reproductive process in either sex, nor have any teratogenic insults been reported in the species tested.

—Damage to vital functions may be noted but is of a transient nature with no permanent impairment.

—Absorption of the compound from the gastrointestinal tract is limited.

—Metabolism is rapid, the major metabolites are less toxic than the parent compound, and there is no tissue accumulation.

From: Food Safety and Inspection Service (1988).

TABLE 6-4

CRITERIA FOR HAZARD CLASSIFICATION D, COMPOUND EVALUATION SYSTEM, FSIS

Category D—negligible health hazard

—Acute or chronic toxicity is slight in experimental animals, e.g. oral LD_{50} is greater than 1 000 mg/kg bw.

—Test results are negative for mutagenicity, carcinogenicity, reproductive toxicity and teratogenicity.

—No damage to vital functions has been reported: slight, transient alterations in specific enzyme systems may occur.

—The compound is not absorbed from the gastrointestinal tract or, if absorbed, metabolizes rapidly to non-toxic metabolites with complete elimination.

From: Food Safety and Inspection Service (1988).

Service, 1988). Of the 76 compounds ranked under the Compound Evaluation System two were designated A-1: furazolidone as well as heptachlor and heptachlor epoxide. Those classified as D-4 were hexazinone, methoxychlor and zinc (Food Safety and Inspection Service, 1987).

IV. NATIONAL RESIDUE PROGRAM, FSIS

The National Residue Program, FSIS, USDA which began in 1967 has five major components: (1) monitoring; (2) surveillance; (3) exploratory; (4) new

Quick Tests and (5) Residue Avoidance Program (Dubbert, 1984; Food Safety and Inspection Service, 1984, 1987; Byrnes, 1988).

A. Monitoring

To protect consumers from adulterated meat and poultry products, USDA regularly monitors tissue samples from slaughtered animals for residues of antibiotics, hormones, pesticides, and others. USDA's residue program is divided into the Monitoring and Surveillance Phases. The program includes analyses for over 100 drug and chemical residues (Food Safety and Inspection Service, 1984). In the *Monitoring Phase*, animals slaughtered at federally inspected establishments are sampled at random. In 1985, 24 000 animals were sampled in the monitoring phase, providing a statistically valid national drug residue picture. Each tissue sample collected is analyzed for one or more drugs (Food Safety and Inspection Service, 1984; Byrnes, 1988). Information gathered in the monitoring program is reviewed by FDA or EPA for use in making on-the-farm inspections to determine if chemicals were misused. A flagrant violation of the law or repeated misuse may result in criminal prosecution of producers (Food Safety and Inspection Service, 1984).

The number of samples tested in the monitoring phase is designed to ensure, at the 95% confidence level, that the chemical will be detected in at least one sample if it occurs in 1% or more of the population of animals being observed during a given year (National Research Council, 1985). The objective statistical sampling covers approximately 0·002% of swine, 0·005% of cattle and calves, 0·001% of sheep and 0·000 02% of chickens and 0·0004% of turkeys slaughtered annually under federal and state inspection (Beran, 1987).

In 1986 FSIS inspected 121 million red meat animals and almost 5 billion birds and supervised production of 67 billion pounds of processed meat and 60 billion pounds of processed poultry. Also in 1986, violative residues of chlorinated hydrocarbons were detected in 0·5% of swine tested, 0·1% of cattle and calves tested, and in 0·5% of sheep tested but in none of the chickens or turkeys tested. Organophosphate residues were not detected in any species. Antibiotic residues were reported in 1·2% of animals and 0·5% of poultry tested, and sulfonamide residues in 2·5% of animals and 1·6% of poultry tested (Beran, 1987).

The 1985 NAS Committee questioned the current residue testing strategy of FSIS to detect with 95% confidence whether or not a problem exists in 1% of the animal population. The committee considered this sampling plan inadequate to prevent consumer exposure to residues.

Because millions of animals are slaughtered annually, the chance of any animal being sampled in the United States is minuscule. Furthermore, because of the increasing number and variety of contaminating residues that may constitute possible health hazards, especially to susceptible subgroups in the population, and because the overall contamination rate of less than 1% may be considerably higher for certain food sources or consumer groups, the 1985 NAS Committee questioned whether the sampling plan was adequate (National Research Council, 1985).

B. Surveillance

The *Surveillance Phase* is designed to investigate and control the movement of potentially adulterated products. The sampling is biased and is directed at particular carcasses or products in response to information from monitoring or other sources or from observations during antemortem or postmortem inspection indicating that adulterating levels of residue may be present (Food Safety and Inspection Service, 1987). The animals are tested because they belong to producers who were recent violators or because the plant inspector observes marks of drug injection that suggests the animal may contain illegal residues. Animals suspected of being sick or diseased may also be sampled in the *Surveillance Phase* (Byrnes, 1988). Inplant testing procedures may be performed by the inspector, or samples may be submitted to a FSIS laboratory for analysis. Depending upon the weight of evidence that led to the testing, product may be retained until test results indicate appropriate disposition. Laboratory testing of surveillance samples is completed as rapidly as possible and takes precedence over monitoring samples (Food Safety and Inspection Service, 1987).

When an illegal drug residue is found, FDA can conduct a follow-up investigation and USDA can detain future shipments of meat/poultry from the affected producer while the tissue samples are analyzed. The FDA on-site investigation is aimed at determining the cause of the residue and identifying those responsible. In conjunction with FDA's investigation, USDA can require that subsequent shipments be free of illegal residues before carcasses and parts are approved for food (Food Safety and Inspection Service, 1984, 1987; National Research Council, 1985; Byrnes, 1988).

Imported meat is also re-inspected and tested for residues at the port of entry. Countries exporting meat to the United States must have a residue program comparable to that in the US (Food Safety and Inspection Service, 1984). Residue testing of imported products is an assurance check by USDA that the foreign country's residue control program is effective and that its products meet the same standards applied to meat/poultry products produced in the United States. Under the surveillance program, when a violation is found in the monitoring program, subsequent shipments from the same foreign establishment are retained at the port of entry under the surveillance program. All shipments of product from that country are placed on an increased monitoring schedule until a history of compliance is re-established. The rationale for sample collection for residues analysis is the same in both the domestic and foreign programs. The compounds selected for residue testing in imported products were chosen to closely parallel the domestic residue program to the extent possible (Food Safety and Inspection Service, 1987).

C. Exploratory Testing

In *Exploratory Testing*, random or non-random samples are taken to study chemicals in meat and poultry for which safe limits have not been established. The information derived from these tests is used to define the frequency, distribution and levels of occurrence of chemicals. The exploratory program also involves studies to help develop new methods for evaluating existing programs. Exploratory test results are not used to take regulatory action or to trigger follow-up surveillance testing since the study design is not suitable for this purpose (National Research Council, 1985; Food Safety and Inspection Service, 1987).

D. Residue Avoidance Program

In 1983, the *Residue Avoidance Program* was inaugurated. It was implemented due to growing concerns about the problem of drug and chemical residues in the meat/poultry supply. The testing of every animal for every possible drug or chemical that may be in the food supply was neither practical nor cost effective. Therefore, the importance of prevention as a successful means of dealing with residue problems was recognized. The *Residue Avoidance Program* aids the livestock producer in identifying points in their production systems where contamination could occur. The prevention of residues at all stages of production—from birth of an animal to its slaughter and processing—would achieve the residue avoidance goal. This approach is beneficial to both the food industry and consumers.

Approximately 1·5 million dollars was awarded by FSIS to land-grant universities for 35 projects addressing residue prevention. The projects encompassed a wide range of activities, including residue information programs for livestock producers; an animal medication survey to determine current animal drug-use practices and sources for both drugs and drug-use information; a residue avoidance training program using a microcomputer/television interface as a teaching technique; and a field test designed to reduce the incidence of drug residues in marketed dairy animals. Education of the livestock producer in residue avoidance is a critical element in residue prevention (Dubbert, 1984; Food Safety and Inspection Service, 1984; National Research Council, 1985).

E. New Quick Tests for Residues

FSIS is developing *Quick Tests* that speed residue analysis. USDA inspectors are utilizing a 'swab test on premises' (STOP) that detects antibiotic residues in animal tissues within 24 hours—as compared to 1–2 weeks for laboratory testing. The STOP test quickly informs an inspector whether antibiotics are present before a carcass leaves the slaughtering establishment. The test is performed by inserting cotton swabs into liver or kidney tissue and placing the swabs on a microbiologic plate coated with agar gel. The plate is then incubated at 26–29°C overnight. When antibiotics are present, bacterial growth is inhibited around the swab tips, indicating the need for further analysis before the carcass can leave the plant. If the carcass is free of antibiotics, bacteria grow uniformly right up to the swab tips, and the inspector can approve the carcass. Eight antibiotics commonly used in animal rearing were utilized in developing the screening procedure: chlortetracycline, oxytetracycline, tetracycline, erythromycin, neomycin, penicillin, streptomycin and tylosin (Johnston *et al.*, 1981). The test is approved for use on all species of meat and poultry.

USDA has adapted STOP for use on the farm with live animals. The 'live animal swab test' (LAST) involves testing animal urine and requires only cotton swabs, a test plate and an incubator. Farmers or their veterinarians are able to test live animals and determine whether there is a violation before the animals are marketed (Dubbert, 1984; Food Safety and Inspection Service, 1984). The two microbiological procedures (LAST and STOP) were evaluated to detect antibiotic residues in dairy cows at slaughter. The STOP test was used to detect antibiotic residues in kidney and muscle tissue and the LAST procedure was used to detect residues in urine of all dairy cows. Kidney samples from 3% of the cull dairy cows were positive for antibiotics. Confirmation by standard reference procedures and a subsequent investigation of antibiotic residues in urine from 317 cows and heifers with known antibiotics treatment histories suggested that a high percentage of false-positive readings occurred on urine. In addition, 23% of urine samples were difficult to interpret in that *Bacillus subtilis* growth surrounding swabs dipped in urine were reduced. The authors concluded that while dairy producer response was generally favorable for an on-farm screening test for antibiotic residue detection in cows going to slaughter, interpretation problems, difficulty in collecting urine samples, and concerns over both the complexity and sensitivity made it unlikely that the widespread of acceptance of the LAST for use on dairy farms would be forthcoming (Tritschler *et al.*, 1987).

More recently FSIS has introduced the Sulfa on Site (SOS) test for the detection of sulfamethazine. The SOS test is a thin layer chromatography test designed to screen swine serum, urine or feed for sulfamethazine and possibly other sulfonamides. The SOS test is designed for use in slaughtering plants as well as on the farm. The visually observed test which can be completed within two hours relies upon two standards to interpret the test. A high standard of 1·3 ppm and a low standard 0·4 ppm for sulfamethazine is utilized. Studies indicate that when the swine urine contains greater than 0·4 ppm sulfamethazine, the liver and other internal organs contain greater than 0·1 ppm violative levels of sulfamethazine. When the urine contains greater than 1·3 ppm sulfamethazine, the liver, other organs and muscle will contain greater than 0·1 ppm sulfamethazine. With the SOS test it is now possible to establish some type of farm-based pre-sulfamethazine slaughter testing program and/or some means to assume that swine presented for slaughter are not adulterated. Such plans, if established, would need to be individually approved, monitored and verified by FSIS (1987) as described by McKean (1987) and by Randecker *et al.* (1987).

Enzyme-linked Immunosorbent Assay (ELISA) is used to detect and measure antigens or antibodies. Several procedural variations of this technology have been used for the last decade. ELISA is an emerging technology in view of the added diagnostic specificity and potential applications available when monoclonal antibodies are used in the process. The antibodies produced by this technology are homogeneous and monospecific. The hybridoma–monoclonal antibody technique can also yield a specific antibody directed against a single antigen even when a mixture of antigens is injected into the mouse. The combination of ELISA and monoclonal antibodies should result in rapid and accurate tests for use both in the slaughtering establishment and on the farm. These screening tests will enable FSIS to evaluate more animals for residues at slaughter (National Research Council, 1985).

The NAS Committee (National Research Council, 1985) in its 1985 report identified essential features in an optimal program for monitoring chemical residues in meat and poultry as follows:

(1) The primary focus of the program should be prevention.
(2) There should be a clear, precisely stated quantitative limit (tolerance) for each chemical to be regulated under the program, and the tolerances as a whole should be consistent and adequately measurable in FSIS laboratories.
(3) Priorities should be determined in an open process by using specific, stated guidelines determined largely by consideration of public health.
(4) Sampling methods are critical to prevention.
(5) Formal risk assessment should play an explicit, prominent role in each of the features mentioned: setting of tolerances, focus on prevention and hazard characterization, priorities and sample design.
(6) Technical aspects of the testing program should be adequate to support the functions discussed above.
(7) The inspection service, including those who select the samples and those who collect them, must be trained and educated for their roles.
(8) Although prevention should be emphasized, the testing program as a whole should have close links to regulatory enforcement; each should have a substantial impact on the other.
(9) Information systems should be an integral part of the program.
(10) The program should be developed and operated in a fully open manner, with peer review, continuing and systematic use of advisory committees, public hearings encouraging public participation, and substantial efforts to improve public understanding.
(11) The program must be flexible enough to recognize and respond to changes in this rapidly changing field with minimum restrictions.

V. RISK ASSESSMENT/MANAGEMENT

Risk assessment as it relates to public health is an emerging discipline that has its origins in the investigation of chemicals as potential carcinogens. It is used to investigate a much broader range of health risks and has been defined as the qualitative or quantitative estimation of the likelihood of adverse effects from exposure to a specified health hazard or from the absence of beneficial influences (USDHHS, 1986; Hathaway *et al.*, 1988). In completing a risk assessment four analytical steps are required (USDHHS, 1986; National Research Council, 1987; Russell and Gruber, 1987; Hathaway *et al.*, 1988):

(1) *Hazard identification*—qualitative indication that a condition/substance may adversely affect human health.
(2) *Hazard characterization*—qualitative and quantitative evaluation of the nature of the adverse effects, including their expression as functions of the amount of exposure per dose. In toxicology, hazard characterization ideally represents a dose/response relationship between a specified statistical distribution of exposures and the probability of one or another set of health effects (USDHHS, 1986).
(3) *Exposure characterization*—qualitative and quantitative evaluation of the degree of human exposure likely to occur before or after application of controls.
(4) *Risk characterization*—integration of the aforementioned factors into a scientific determination of the degree of risk as a basis for policy consideration.

The 1985 NAS committee concluded that although significant strides have been made in protecting the public against exposure to hazardous chemicals in meat and poultry, the fundamental design of FSIS's residue monitoring program needs to be improved to ensure maximum protection. In particular, the committee questioned the adequacy of sampling size and procedures, the basis for and the establishment of tolerance levels for chemicals, and the basis for setting priorities for testing chemicals (National Research Council, 1985). The National Residue Program sampling plan was determined inadequate to provide maximum protection to consumers, there is no free communication with experts outside the agency, and has no formal risk assessment and risk management program. The committee believes that a program based on rational public health objectives and risk assessment should contain many of the characteristics previously identified and ensure that no one person would consistently be exposed to levels of chemicals in excess of established tolerance levels.

The 1985 NAS committee also concluded that the establishment of reasonable, measurable objectives for the nation's meat and poultry inspection program is imperative. To that end, the committee recommended the adoption of quantitative health risk assessment which it believed would aid FSIS in improving its program and achieving specific objectives. Quantitative health risk assessment has been discussed in connection with toxic substances, yet its roots go much deeper than that, into areas as diverse as transportation, national security policy, and business decision making (National Research Council, 1980, 1983). Although specific elements of this analytical tool may have to be adjusted for the meat and poultry inspection process, the concept is universal. Its application in food inspection and regulation is already much discussed in relation to the Federal Food, Drug and Cosmetic Act. The courts, including the Supreme Court, have indicated their willingness to accept the notion of quantitative health risk assessment in the context of indirect food additives (National Research Council, 1985).

Formal risk assessment is the key to capturing, organizing and interpreting the evidence that can be brought to bear on the optimum use of inspection resources. It will identify problems in a clear and organized way; produce the best possible estimate of the likelihood that a risk exists, and if so, its size; and make clear the kinds and degrees of uncertainty attached to that estimate. This information can then be translated into a detailed strategy to protect human health, including the development of specific regulations and instructions to inspection staff (National Research Council, 1987).

VI. RESIDUES ACTIVITY

Since the end of World War II, there has been revolutionary developments in synthetic organic chemistry. As of Spring 1985, the US Environmental Protection Agency (EPA) had a list of 60 000 marketed chemicals, and new compounds can be expected to be added at the current rate of 1200 each year (McCormick, 1985; National Research Council, 1985; Biehl and Buck, 1987). In 1976, the National Institute of Environmental Health Sciences noted that 'the chemical entities comprising those constituents of foods that are pertinent to food safety encompass a wide spectrum of substances that are introduced into foods through a number of routes. Such substances can be categorized into two groups: (1) those present as naturally occurring components or contaminants; and (2) those added by man in the course of food manufacture or preparation (US Department of Health, Education and Welfare, 1976; National Research Council, 1985)'. As it relates to the management of chemical hazards in both meat and poultry, two recent NAS reports fully address this area (National Research Council, 1985, 1987). Recent FSIS/FDA activities have concentrated on antimicrobial agents and environmental contaminants.

A. Antibiotic and Sulfa Residues

In 1985 only 1% of the animals sampled contained violative residues. In contrast, the annual residue rate of 1·9% was found 10 years previously

(Byrnes, 1988). More recently, USDA has been concerned about the continuing occurrence of antibiotic and sulfa residues at concentrations above the tolerances established by FDA for hogs, young calves and cull dairy cows. In 1987, 4% of swine sampled and tested had violative sulfa residues and 1·8% of all cows sampled and tested had violative antibiotic residues. A voluntary certification program and extensive cooperative education efforts by USDA and the industry were successful in lowering the violation rate in young calves from 5% to the 1987 rate of 1·7% (Federal Register, 1987). A special program was also developed toward violative sulfamethazine residues in swine.

Violative levels of residues occurred in calves because they were medicated on the farm and then slaughtered before the drugs had cleared the animal's system. The calf antibiotic and sulfonamide test (CAST) developed at FSIS is used at slaughtering establishments to determine whether calves up to three weeks of age contain violative residues. The CAST was designed to detect violative levels of antibiotics and sulfonamides in bob veal calf kidney tissues. The CAST is a microbiologic assay similar to, but more sensitive than STOP and LAST. If a clear zone ≥ 18 mm develops around the head of the test swab, the result is considered positive for antibiotics or sulfonamides at the violative level; if there is no zone of inhibition or if the zone is <18 mm, the result is considered negative. The CAST has been limited by FSIS to testing bob veal calves (Engel, 1988).

Under the CAST regulatory program begun in 1984; producers and dealers can certify that their calves do not contain violative levels of residues, in which case the healthy-appearing, certified calves can be processed without delay. In contrast, each lot of non-certified calves is held overnight until a statistically-based number of calves are tested and passed. All calves showing signs of disease or treatment or that are from previously-identified violative sources must be tested. The CAST program has been very successful in reducing violations from a high of 5·5% of calves tested during the summer of 1984, to about 1·7% during 1987.

Recent changes in treatment and marketing practices resulted in FSIS modifying the original CAST program. Originally, sulfonamides accounted for a large share of violations; however, other antibiotics, some which could not be identified by present methods, began to appear. The modified CAST program requires that a number of healthy-appearing calves be tested on a percentage of the estimated day's slaughter. Initially, the rate of testing in all establishments will be 5% for certified calves and 10% for non-certified, but the rate can increase or decrease at each establishment according to its compliance history (Miller, 1987).

Since 1978 sulfonamide residues in meat, especially sulfamethazine residues in pork, have been of special concern due to the prevalence of residues and the toxicity of the drugs. Hypersensitive reactions in sensitized human patients cause blood and kidney damage. Birth defects, particularly cleft palate and bone abnormalities, have occurred when rats were experimentally fed sulfonamides during gestation, but have not been clinically observed when women have been treated with these drugs during pregnancy. Although violative levels of sulfa residues in swine were reduced to 4·6% in 1986, FDA expressed an immediate goal of reducing sulfamethazine residues in swine to less than 1%. The National Pork Producers' Council recommended the adoption of a control program which included: (1) support of swine identification; (2) encouragement of FDA enforcement of avoiding use of soluble powdered sulfonamides; (3) encouragement of both industry and producers to test feed, ingredients and swine; and (4) conducting of industry-wide education (Beran, 1987). In 1988 several events occurred that increased the sulfamethazine reduction effort in swine. FDA reported that dosing of mice with sulfamethazine at various levels over 24 months resulted in low toxicity and adenoma in the thyroid gland at a low incidence. Japan tested some imported US pork and found sulfa residues in muscle. Pork in shipment was placed on hold and Japan threatened to discontinue purchase of US pork. The National Pork Producers' Council asked pork producers to discontinue using sulfa drugs for an indefinite period until FDA completed a review of new studies (Meyerholz, 1988a). FSIS in May 1988 began testing slaughtered hogs (6 per plant) in the 100 largest hog slaughtering establishments utilizing the SOS test (Anon., 1988). As of September 1988, SOS plant testing shows a violative rate of 0·6% (239 of 42 446 samples) (Meyerholz, 1988b). This decline in the prevalence of sulfamethazine residues in swine is due to the cooperative efforts of many groups.

A recent study by Moats (1988) states that ordinary cooking procedures for meat do not inactivate residues of even the most heat-sensitive antibiotics, such as penicillin and tetracyclines. The more severe heating process of canning will inactivate some of the more heat-sensitive compounds, but others such as neomycin and possibly streptomycin, survive canning. Prolonged cooking of tough cuts of meat with moist heat might also inactivate heat-sensitive antibiotics. This study emphasizes the importance of eliminating violative levels of antibiotic residues at the livestock production stage.

D. Environmental/Accidental/Chemical Contaminations

Periodically, FDA, FSIS and EPA are involved in the investigation and control of sporadic, isolated contamination incidents in food animals. These often involve the halogenated hydrocarbons. For example, in 1970 a heat exchanger in a fish meal plant developed a leak and the PCBs that were used as the heat exchange fluid leaked into the product. The contaminated fish meal was subsequently used in poultry feeds in a wide area of the Southwestern US. A similar situation occurred in the Western United States when a transformer developed a leak and PCBs contaminated wastes that were converted to rendered products. Again, the contaminated rendered products were used in poultry feeds. Another unanticipated source of residues was the use of PCBs (Aroclor 1254) in a silo sealant. Six plants in the Mid West and Mid South US manufactured these silos from about 1940 until about 1960. PCBs from the sealant diffused into silage and produced violative residues in a number of dairy herds (Fries, 1984).

The largest and most costly livestock contamination incident in history occurred in Michigan in 1973 when a fire retardant, polybrominated biphenyls (PBBs), was accidentally incorporated into animal feeds. Approximately 30 000 cattle, 6000 swine, 15 000 sheep and 1·5 million chickens were destroyed along with more than 50 000 pounds of dairy products and 5 million eggs (Biehl and Buck, 1987).

Heptachlor contamination of all dairy cattle on the island of Oahu, Hawaii also is an example of unanticipated consequences of what was thought to be an acceptable method of using the compound. Pineapple green-chop containing heptachlor was fed to dairy cattle. In addition to the direct loss of the violative products, there was an indirect loss by a 20% reduction in consumption of dairy products in Hawaii up to a year later. More recently in Arkansas, residues were found in dairy cattle fed heptachlor-contaminated stillage from gasohol production. Although various sources of contamination exist, generally at least 80% of all residues in food animals are estimated to occur through the feed (Fries, 1984; Biehl and Buck, 1987). In the 1970s, as a result of several major residue contamination problems there were major economic losses in the poultry industry. As a consequence, in 1976 a cooperative residue program was developed under which FSIS entered into a voluntary agreement with a poultry establishment. The purpose of voluntary agreements between FSIS and poultry establishments is to ensure that poultry slaughtered do not contain drugs, pesticides or other chemicals that would yield adulterated poultry products. An extension of the successful poultry residue prevention program applicable to all food animals is the newly proposed FSIS verified production control program as outlined by Engel (1988). This program has the following advantages for both the livestock producer and consumer:

(1) Consumers would be offered both red meat and poultry products that are produced under a program intended to produce products from livestock and poultry raised, slaughtered and handled under conditions ensuring that products are free of a violative level of residues.
(2) Those who wish to take economic advantage of the program would be allowed to label their products as produced under verified production control.

In May 1987 Verified Production Control (VPC) agreements were in force with 11 companies involving 47 slaughtering establishments. They represent a combined kill of seven billion pounds per year. By commodity, the agreements cover about 45% of young turkeys, about 30% of young chickens and about 3% of feed cattle (Miller, 1987).

After the Chernobyl USSR accident, FSIS developed a plan to assess the accident's impact on domestically produced and imported meat and poultry. In the absence of any international guidelines, FSIS followed the October 1982 FDA guidelines for the accidental radioactive contamination of human food and animal feed. The protective action guides took into consideration the type of contamination that might occur after such an event, the half-lives of resulting radioactive substances, and the biological pathways by which humans would be exposed to radioactive substances.

One month after the Chernobyl accident, FSIS was monitoring meat and poultry products imported from 14 European countries. By using the available information concerning the nature of the accident, five radionuclides were measured: cesium-134, cesium-137, strontium-89, strontium-90 and iodine-131. As of June 1987, FSIS had analyzed approximately 3100 samples of imported meat and poultry from 14 European countries.

FSIS established a total cesium (cesium-134 plus cesium-137) response level of 75 000 pico Curies per kilogram (pCi/kg) or 2775 Becquerels per kilogram (Bq/kg), and 1500 pCi/kg (56 Bq/kg) of iodine-131 for meat and poultry. Only Romania had values greater than 5000 pCi/kg (185 Bq/kg) with the highest reading being 21 460 pCi/kg (794 Bq/kg) (Engel *et al.*, 1988).

The Food Animal Residue Avoidance Databank (FARAD) is a computer-based system to provide veterinarians and livestock producers with practical information on drugs, pesticides and environmental contaminants that have the greatest potential for persisting in animal tissues at the time of slaughter. Funding for the program has been provided by the USDA through the Agricultural Extension Service and FSIS. A large percentage of calls to FARAD pertain to drugs used at greater-than-recommended dosages, in unapproved species or administered by unapproved routes. The telephone numbers for this information system are: East and Southeastern United States (904) 392-4085; Central United States (217) 333-3611 and Western United States (916) 752-7507 (Sundlof, 1988).

VII. SUMMARY

The concern of the United States consumer relative to residues in their food, including meat and poultry, is real and has been verified in numerous consumer surveys. It is also extremely important to weigh the benefits of chemical usage versus the potential contamination of our environment and food supply. Also, the actual risk of toxic injury after exposure to various chemicals needs to be fully examined. Through continued research many of these complex questions may be answered, enabling regulatory personnel to use sound scientific judgement coupled with an understanding of risk assessments to prevent the chemical contamination of our food supply. Two NAS reports clearly define the optimal meat–poultry inspection program for residue control. Recommendations of the National Academy of Sciences to FSIS for residue control can be summarized in four points: (1) prevention, (2) examination of an adequate number of samples, (3) use of risk assessment and (4) testing capacity.

VIII. REFERENCES

ANONYMOUS (1988). *Sulfamethazine Residues—FSIS Increases Testing*. Vet. Med. News from Washington. Government Relations Division, Am. Vet. Med. Assoc., Washington, DC, Vol. 12, No. 6 (March 15, 1988), 2 pp.

BERAN, G. W. (1987). Use of drugs in animals, an epidemiologic perspective. In *Proc.—Animal Drug Use, Dollars and Sense*, p. 3. Herndon, VA.

BIEHL, M. L and BUCK, W. B. (1987). Chemical contaminants: Their metabolism and their residues. *J. Food Prot.* **50**, 1058.

BYRNES, S. (1988). Drug residues in meat. *FDA Veterin.* **3**(4), 4.

CARSON, R. (1962). *Silent Spring*. Houghton Mifflin, Boston, Massachusetts.

DUBBERT, W. H. (1984). The new look of meat and poultry inspection. *J. Am. Vet. Med. Assoc.* **184**, 266.

ENGEL, R. E. (1988). Quality assurance through residue screening. *J. Am. Vet. Med. Assoc.* **192**, 268.

ENGEL, R. E., RANDECKER, V. W. and FRANKS, W. J. (1988). Lessons learned from Chernobyl: Public Health Aspects. *J. Assoc. Food and Drug Officials* **52**, 15.

FEDERAL REGISTER (1988). p. 18 572.

FOOD MARKETING INSTITUTE (1988). *Trends—Consumer Attitudes and the Supermarket.* 1988 update. Research Dept, FMI, Washington, DC.

FOOD SAFETY AND INSPECTION SERVICE (1984). The National Residue Program. FSIS Facts. FSIS-18, USDA, FSIS, Washington, DC. Food Safety and Inspection Service (1987). *Compound Evaluation and Analytical Capability National Residue Program Plan.* USDA, FSIS, Science Program, Washington, DC.

FOOD SAFETY AND INSPECTION SERVICE (1988). The compound evaluation system. The Residue and Planning Division. Science Program, Washington, DC.

FRIES, G. F. (1984). Accidental Toxicants: PCB, PBB, TCDD and other halogenated hydrocarbons. In *Animal Origin Residues*, Proc. Cont. Ed. Seminar, Am. Acad. Veter. Prev. Med., Rockville, MD.

FSIS (1987). *Performing the Sulfa on Site Test: A Self-Instructional Guide.* USDA, FSIS, Technical Services, Program Training Division, Denton, TX.

HATHAWAY, S. C., PULLEN, M. M. and MCKENZIE, A. I. (1988). A model for risk assessment of organoleptic postmortem inspection procedures for meat and poultry. *J. Am. Vet. Med. Assoc.* **192**, 960.

JOHNSTON, R. W., REAMER, R. H., HARRIS, E. W., FUGATE, H. G. and SCHWAAB, B. (1981). A new screening method for the detection of antibiotic residues in meat and poultry tissues. *J. Food Prot.* **44**, 828.

MCBEAN, L. D. (1988). A perspective on food safety concerns. *Dairy and Food Sanitation* **8**, 112.

MCCORMICK, D. (1985). One bug's meat. *Biotechnol.* **3**, 429.

MCKEAN, J. D. (1987). A veterinary approach to residue testing. *Large Anim. Veterin.* September/October 1987, 38.

MEYERHOLZ, G. W. (1988a). *Summary—Sulfamethazine in Swine. Events and Action Plan for Sulfamethazine.* USDA Extension Service, Washington, DC.

MEYERHOLZ, G. W. (1988b). Food Safety Summary. USDA Extension Service, Washington, DC.

MILLER, W. R. (1987). Violative drug residues. In *Proc.—Animal Drug Use, Dollars and Sense*, p. 67. Herndon, VA.

MOATS, W. A. (1988). Inactivation of antibiotics by heating in foods and other substrates—A review. *J. Food Prot.* **51**, 491.

NATIONAL RESEARCH COUNCIL (1980). Problems of Risk Estimation. *Drinking Water and Health, Vol. 3, 25.* Subcommittee on Risk Assessment, Safe Drinking Water Committee. Board on Toxicology and Environmental Health Hazards, Assembly of Life Sciences. National Academy Press, Washington, DC.

NATIONAL RESEARCH COUNCIL (1983). *Risk Assessment in the Federal Government: Managing the Process.* Committee on the Institutional Means for Assessment of Risks to Public Health, Commission on Life Sciences. National Academy Press, Washington, DC.

NATIONAL RESEARCH COUNCIL (1985). *Meat and Poultry Inspection: The Scientific Basis of the Nation's Program.* National Academy Press, Washington, DC.
NATIONAL RESEARCH COUNCIL (1987). *Poultry Inspection: The Basis for a Risk-Assessment Approach.* National Academy Press, Washington, DC.
RANDECKER, V. R., REAGAN, J. A., ENGEL, R. E., SODERBERG, D. L. and MCNEAL, J. E. (1987). Serum and urine as predictors of sulfamethazine levels in swine muscle, liver and kidney. *J. Food Prot.* **50**, 115.
RUSSELL, M. and GRUBER, M. (1987). Risk assessment in environmental policy-making. *Science* **236**, 286.
SPAULDING, J. (1975). Toxic Residues. In *Meat Hygiene*, 4th edn (J. A. Libby, Ed.), p. 470. Lea and Febiger, Philadelphia.
SUNDLOF, S. (1988). FARAD strives to reduce incidence of food-borne illness through practitioner awareness. *J. Am. Vet. Med. Assoc.* **192**, 1026.
TRITSCHLER, II, J. P., DUBY, R. T., OLIVER, S. P. and PRANGE, R. W. (1987). Microbiological screening tests to detect antibiotic residues in cull dairy cows. *J. Food Prot.* **50**, 97.
US DEPARTMENT OF HEALTH, EDUCATION AND WELFARE (1976). *Human Health and the Environment: Some Research Needs, Report of the Second Task Force for Research Planning in Environmental Health Science.* Public Health Service, National Institute of Environmental Health Sciences, National Institutes of Health, US Dept, of Health, Education and Welfare, Bethesda, MD.
USDHHS (1986). *Determining Risks to Health: Federal Policy and Practice.* Auburn House, Dover, MA.

7

Pathogenic Bacteria in Meat and Meat Products

E. A. ZOTTOLA AND L. B. SMITH

Department of Food Science and Nutrition, University of Minnesota, St. Paul, Minnesota, USA

I. MEAT AS A SOURCE OF FOODBORNE DISEASE

Foodborne illnesses implicating meat and meat products as the vehicles of transmission for pathogenic microorganisms have been well documented in the literature. Fresh meat and poultry are ideal sources of nutrients for proliferation and growth of both spoilage and pathogenic bacteria.

The microbial flora of raw red meats and poultry consists of mesophilic bacteria from the animal, the soil, the environment and water. Bacteria are also present as a contaminant from equipment surfaces and handling during processing (Empey and Scott, 1939; Barnes, 1976; Ingram and Roberts, 1976; Roberts, 1980). Mesophilic bacteria (10^2–10^4 bacteria/in^2) which originate from the alimentary tract and external surfaces of the animal make up a good portion of the surface flora of freshly slaughtered carcasses. The slaughtering area is normally heated in the winter months and ambient temperatures are prevalent during the summer, thus contributing to the proliferation of mesophilic bacteria. Although psychrotrophic microorganisms, which originate from the soil and water, are often present in smaller numbers (10^1/in^2), it is the presence of mesophilic bacteria that are important since they indicate the degree of sanitation during the slaughtering process.

A bactericidal step is not included in the slaughtering process, consequently a diverse microflora consisting of *Escherichia coli*, coliforms, enterococci, *Clostridium perfringens*, *Staphylococcus aureus* and *Salmonella* may be present on fresh meat. The levels and frequency of bacteria will fluctuate depending on the season of the year, the source of the animals, the mode of transport, the holding area and processing conditions. With the exception of *Salmonella*, many of them will be present at low levels, i.e. 10^1–10^2. The incidence of salmonellae, as reported by a summary of US and Canadian surveys for the period 1943–77 showed 1·9% in ground beef, 0·5% in other fresh beef, 15–16% in fresh pork and 0·5% in cooked meats (Tompkin, 1983). Fresh poultry has a higher incidence of salmonellae than red meats (Surkiewicz *et al.*, 1973; Pivnick, 1978; Green *et al.*, 1982; Tompkin, 1983). Cooking reduces the numbers of bacteria initially present on raw meat, yet the persistence of sporeformers and possibly some thermoduric microorganisms, i.e. lactobacilli, micrococci and enterococci, may occur. Subsequent refrigeration is conducive to the growth of psychrotrophic bacteria. These microorganisms are often present as post-processing contaminants and are responsible for spoilage and are frequently a measure of shelf-life stability.

II. PATHOGENIC BACTERIA ASSOCIATED WITH MEAT

A. *Salmonella* species

Salmonella are commonly present on raw meat and poultry and are therefore a part of normal flora. Incidence and numbers vary with: (1) species of the animal, (2) preslaughter holding conditions, and (3) processing conditions. The consumer and producer cannot depend on current technology to assure salmonellae-free meat and poultry since processing into retail cuts does not include a treatment that would be destructive to salmonellae.

(i) Characteristics

Salmonella sp. are motile, do not produce urease, do not liquefy gelatin, do not utilize sodium malonite and growth is inhibited in medium containing potassium cyanide. Decarboxylation of lysine, arginine and ornithine is observed and acid is produced in Jordan's tartrate medium. Dulcitol is fermented while sucrose, salicin, raffinose and lactose are not. Some strains will utilize inositol. Some nonmotile strains such as *S. gallinarum* and *S. pullorum* are found as well as some lactose- and sucrose-fermenting salmonellae. Serological analysis and identification of isolates based on the Kauffman–White scheme (Kauffman, 1966) of the O (somatic) and H (flagellar) antigens have been valuable in epidemiological investigations and are the basis for the CDC *Salmonella* surveillance program.

Host-preference grouping includes those species including *S. typhi*, *S.*

paratyphi, types A, B and C, and *S. sendai*, which are adapted to man. Only type B *S. paratyphi* has a known secondary host such as infections of dogs, fowl and swine. Characteristics of human-adapted serotypes include: (a) small disease-producing dosage, (b) incubation time of 10–20 or more days, (c) invasion of the bloodstream by the organism causing enteric fever, and (d) they often produce permanent carriers. Most often the infection is the result of consumption of contaminated food and water while person-to-person contact is less often the mode of transmission. Animal-adapted serotypes include *S. pullorum* (poultry), *S. abortus equi* (horses), *S. abortus ovis* (sheep) and *S. choleraesuis* and *S. typhisuis* (pigs). However human illness from all of these serotypes has been known to occur. The characteristics of the disease produced by a third group, which infects both man and animals, include: (a) gastroenteritis rather than enteric fever, (b) the bloodstream is not invaded and infection is localized in intestine, (c) a 48-h incubation time, which is considerably shorter than the animal-adapted infection, and (d) a shorter duration than that which causes enteric fever. The infection, however, if experienced by the very young, the aged or the debilitated patient can result in serious problems.

(ii) Epidemiology

Epidemiological records (Hobbs, 1974) have shown that meat and poultry are vehicles of transmission for outbreaks of salmonellosis. Factors which impact on salmonellosis in humans include not only animal-to-man linkage but also pinpoint mishandling during slaughtering and post-processing contamination. Poor manufacturing and sanitation processes are responsible for the perpetuation of salmonellae contamination of red meats and poultry.

(iii) Human salmonellosis

Most cases of human salmonellosis are due to the non-host-adapted group of salmonellae via the consumption of meat and poultry. Food poisoning symptoms include an incubation period ranging from 8–72 h but usually in the 24–48 h range, abdominal cramps, vomiting, diarrhea, headache and general malaise. A rise in temperature to 38–39°C may be experienced. Duration of the infection often is 2–5 days and it is during this time that the organism may be isolated from the feces. Both clinical symptoms and isolation of *Salmonella* from the feces should be included in the diagnosis. A summary of the estimates of infective doses was published by Silliker (1980) which indicated that relatively low numbers of salmonellae ranging from 60–15 000 were responsible for foodborne illness outbreaks. However interpretation of data must be tempered with caution since MPN procedures used in analysis may give highly variable results (Bryan *et al.*, 1979). It is postulated, however, that the minimum infectious dose responsible for salmonellosis may be low but the age and health of the host as well as the implicated food must also be considered as influencing factors of host-susceptibility to salmonellosis.

(iv) Growth, survival, destruction

The optimum temperature for growth of *Salmonella* is 35–37°C, but substrate, pH, water activity and competitive microbes may influence the effects. Mackey *et al.* (1980) summarized growth temperatures of salmonellae in various foods some of which are shown in Table 7-1.

(v) pH

The pH for *Salmonella* growth varies in fermented meats and poultry. Deibel *et al.* (1961) reported a pH from 4·6–5·3 in summer sausage from nine different suppliers. In dry salami (8 samples/all from different suppliers) the pH varied from 5·1–5·4, while Lebanon bologna had pH values of 4·6–4·7 (3 samples). Other researchers (Smith and Palumbo, 1973) reported pH from 4·6–4·9 in the same type of product. Smoking for 4 days at 35°C may account for the greater acidity of this product. A slow ripening process, such as that used in a dry sausage including Hungarian salami, contributes to pH levels of 5·9–6·2, and in some instances to 6·5 (Takaćs *et al.*, 1963). The American Meat Institute (1982) published voluntary guidelines for the

TABLE 7-1
GROWTH TEMPERATURES OF SALMONELLAE IN VARIOUS MEAT PRODUCTS

Food	*Temperature (°C)*		*Reference*
	Growth	*No growth*	
Beef and pork	—	4·4–10	Gomutputra and Fabian (1953)
Chicken à la king	6·7	5·6	Angelotti *et al.* (1961)
Ground pork	10	4·0	Alford and Palumbo (1969)
Ground pork	—	7·0	Sulzbacher (1952)
Ground beef	12·5	7·0	Goepfert and Kim (1975)
Ground beef	—	5·0	Tiwari and Maxcy (1972)
Ground beef (vacuum packed)	12	5·0	Davidson and Witty (1977)
Sterile beef	8	7·0	Shaw and Nicol (1969)
Bacon	16	5·0	Farrell and Upton (1978)

manufacture of semidry and dry sausage and prescribed a minimum pH of 5·3 for both products.

The results of a study by Goepfert and Chung (1970a) showed that over a 14-day period at 30°C *Salmonella typhimurium* multiplied in a sausage emulsion although a starter culture was absent. Using *Pediococcus* as a starter culture, a decline in population was observed during fermentation. No change was observed when nitrite was omitted from the formulation. When glucose was also omitted from the emulsion, only a small reduction of viable salmonellae was observed. However, when sodium chloride was excluded, salmonellae grew during the first 12 h of fermentation and then died as the pH dropped to 4·3 over the 24-h test period. It was concluded that a combination of sodium chloride and acidity was responsible for the death of salmonellae during the fermentation process.

In other studies on the survival of *S. dublin* and *S. typhimurium* during Lebanon bologna production, Smith *et al.* (1975) showed *S. dublin* populations declined 3–4 $\log_{10}$ cycles during a 4-day fermentation at 35°C but the *S. typhimurium* declined to undetectable levels. *S. pullorum* populations were reduced 4·5–5·3 $\log_{10}$ cycles and *S. senftenberg* by 1·5–2·0 $\log_{10}$ cycles during processing of dry fermented turkey sausage (Baran and Stevenson, 1975), with a final reported pH of 5·3. The greater survival of salmonellae in turkey in this study may have been due to a shorter fermentation time (12 h) than that reported by other researchers (Chung and Goepfert, 1970; Smith *et al.*, 1975).

(vi) a_w

Christian and Scott (1953) reported a minimum a_w of 0·941 for growth of three *Salmonella* species. This study also showed that maximum growth rates were obtained at a_w of 0·995 for 15 *Salmonella* strains. When a_w values were decreased below the optimum, the growth rates declined markedly and the length of lag time was increased. A concentration of 9% sodium chloride is equivalent to an a_w of 0·94.

Red meat and poultry have an a_w near the optimum for growth of salmonellae. The a_w is reduced in cured meats due to the salt and this results in an increased lag time and a reduction in growth rate. Nevertheless the growth of salmonellae in these products is influenced by the interaction of a_w, pH, the competitive microbes and the temperature of incubation. Lactic acid bacteria, the prevalent microbes isolated from cooked cured meats which have been vacuum packed and refrigerated, tend to suppress the growth of salmonellae. In the presence of a lactic acid bacteria starter culture salmonellae died rapidly during a 24-h fermentation at 30°C

(Chung and Goepfert, 1970). If salt was excluded from the emulsion formulation, however, *S. typhimurium* multiplied at 30–37°C during a 12-h incubation, which reinforces the influence of a_w. Interactions between brine, pH and competing microorganisms may inhibit growth of salmonellae, but some may survive for a period of time. Marazza and Crespi (1973) reported survival of salmonellae for two months at room temperature in a naturally contaminated salami with a brine content of 23%. It has also been reported by Takaćs and Simonfly (1970) that if the initial concentration of salmonellae was more than 20 000/g, viable salmonellae could be isolated from dried sausages up to the time of human consumption.

(vii) Packaging/gaseous atmosphere

Marriott *et al.* (1977) have reported that more than one-half of North American red meat is vacuum packaged in gas-impermeable films, while according to Wolfe (1980), a great number of carcasses and boned fresh meat are shipped in modified atmospheres, which contain elevated levels of CO_2 with varying concentrations of nitrogen and oxygen. These conditions inhibit Gram-negative psychrotrophs which are responsible for spoilage of fresh meat under aerobic conditions. The use of vacuum packaging itself creates a modified atmosphere due to the metabolism of meat enzymes that results in CO_2 accumulation within the package. Ledward *et al.* (1971) and Taylor (1971) reported that CO_2 levels of 10–20% are observed within 4 h of vacuum packaging, achieving a maximum level of 30% CO_2. Inhibition of salmonellae in ground meat stored at 10°C in a 60% CO_2 atmosphere was reported by Silliker and Wolfe (1980), but growth was observed on storage in air. At 20°C, however, samples stored in air and the CO_2 atmosphere showed increased numbers of salmonellae. Beef steaks stored at 10°C in oxygen-permeable film showed increased numbers of *S. typhimurium* but when packaged under vacuum or in oxygen barrier packaging films containing a mixture of 60:40 CO_2:O_2 the numbers of salmonellae were low.

(viii) Heat destruction

The heat sensitivity of salmonellae is well documented in the literature (Genigeorgis and Riemann, 1979) and temperatures of pasteurization and cooking are deemed to be adequate to kill salmonellae especially in high moisture products. As the a_w decreases, the heat resistance of salmonellae is increased. This interaction was shown by Goodfellow and Brown (1978) who reported that for the same period of time and at the same temperature a 7 $\log_{10}$ reduction of salmonellae in the interior of a beef roast occurred but the surface inoculum was not destroyed. They reported *D* values of 51–62 min at 51·6°C, 3·8–4·2 min at 57·2°C, and 0·6–0·7 min at 62·7°C for salmonellae in ground beef.

Although many perishable raw, cured and processed meats do not undergo a heat treatment during the manufacturing process they have not been considered a source of salmonellosis. Improper handling of these products can result in outbreaks, however, thorough cooking and the presence of salt in many of these meats reduce the possibility of a salmonellosis hazard.

A temperature of 137°F (58·3°C) is specified for raw pork in the United States in order to destroy trichinae. This is considered within the lower temperature range which is lethal to salmonellae. The destruction of trichinae, not salmonellae, is the primary purpose in heat processing of semidry sausages. To effect destruction of salmonellae in this product, consideration must be given to the interaction between not only the heat treatment but the pH, the a_w, and the competitive microbes present during fermentation. Some other pork products, which are considered ready-to-eat such as Italian and Polish sausages, are packaged commercially and distributed to the consumer under frozen or refrigerated storage conditions. The heat processing of these products must meet the minimal heat treatment standards for the destruction of trichinae which will also destroy salmonellae. Although there is the possibility of post-heat-processing contamination, the normal cooking temperatures before consumption generally would rule out a salmonellosis hazard.

Poultry and uncured cooked meats such as ground beef, sliced beef and chicken are used in food service establishments as well as in frozen entrées packaged for the individual consumer. Salmonellae contamination after cooking is possible but these products are not often involved as the vehicles in outbreaks of salmonellosis. Since these products usually receive a before-consumption cooking process, the *Salmonella* organisms are destroyed.

Precooked rare roast beef has been implicated in several outbreaks of human salmonellosis in recent years (Centers for Disease Control, 1981a,b). Consequently a regulation was issued by the USDA requiring a minimum internal processing temperature of 145°F (62·7°C) for all cooked beef and beef roasts (Angelotti, 1977), however, 'rare' roast beef could not be produced under this temperature constraint. At the request of the meat industry an equivalent longer time/lower temperature process was developed for USDA by Goodfellow and Brown (1978) which was based on the thermal destruction of salmonellae at temperatures ranging from 51·6–62·7°C. The USDA subsequently issued regulations permitting processing of roast beef based on the data generated by Goodfellow and Brown (1978). This process produced beef roast with the characteristic 'rare' roast beef red color and yet ensured the destruction of 10^6 *Salmonella* inoculated into the center of the roasts. Despite the initiation of these regulations, precooked roast beef has been implicated in salmonellosis outbreaks (Centers for Disease Control, 1981a,b). These outbreaks have occurred as the result of post cooking cross-contamination (R. W. Johnston, personal communication).

Several causes of cross-contamination have been cited including failure to separate raw and cooked product, rebagging of a heat processed product and, of course, an inadequate heat process or failure to comply with the required heat process regulations. Commercially prepared cooked 'roast beef' which is fabricated from meat trimmings and resembles sliced cooked roast beef usually receives a heat treatment during the production process that is adequate to kill most vegetative microorganisms.

Salmonellosis outbreaks have also been attributed to turkey rolls that were inadequately heat processed or were contaminated during post-processing. A USDA requirement now in effect specifying a minimum internal temperature of 160°F (71°C) for poultry rolls has been effective in controlling salmonellosis outbreaks implicating these products (R. W. Johnston, personal communication). Boneless turkey breasts and other cooked uncured poultry products which are marketed for retail and food service use must be cooked to an internal temperature of 160°F (Bailey, 1974) and, according to R. W. Johnston (personal communication), have not presented significant *Salmonella* problems.

Cooked cured meat products that are treated with salt and nitrite and receive a heat treatment include such products as bologna, frankfurters (domestic sausage), ham, bacon, corned beef, pepper and pimento loaf (luncheon meats). Certain of these meat products are considered ready-to-eat while others, such as smoked ham and frankfurters, are cooked before consumption to improve flavor and texture. Still other products, such as bacon that does not receive a heat treatment adequate to destroy trichinae or *Salmonella*, must be cooked before eating.

Heat processes used for cooked cured meat production is product-dependent. Bacon requires a final internal temperature between 120–130°F (49–54·5°C) to 'fix' the cured color. That along with the thorough cooking temperature of bacon by the consumer before consumption eliminates the *Salmonella* hazard. Smoked hams are heat processed to a temperature of

137°F (58·3°C) to assure destruction of trichinae, which may also eliminate salmonellae. However, this product is not considered a ready-to-eat item and requires additional cooking by the consumer. On the other hand, fully cooked hams must attain a minimum internal temperature of 158°F (70°C) which should pose no problem with respect to survival of salmonellae. Domestic sausages and luncheon meats that contain pork must be processed to a minimum internal temperature of 137°F (58·3°C) to destroy trichinae, but are usually processed to much higher temperatures to enhance shelf-life. Minimum heat processes for products such as those discussed have been published by Bailey (1974).

Cured and smoked poultry products, e.g. poultry frankfurters, must be heated to a minimum internal temperature of 155°F (68·3°C) which eliminates the presence of salmonellae. However, adequate as the heat process is, post-processing contamination may occur. If favorable conditions such as temperature exist, growth of salmonellae in these cured products is possible (Goepfert and Chung, 1970b; Davidson and Webb, 1973). These products have not, however, been important vehicles for salmonellosis.

The International Commission on Microbiological Specifications for Foods (1980) includes information for production of dried meats that may be dried in hot air tunnels at temperatures greater than 50°C, which is inhibitory to the growth of relevant microorganisms. Microbial growth is also inhibited by the low temperatures utilized in freeze drying of cooked or uncooked meats. Predrying cooking temperatures are sufficient to destroy salmonellae but the freeze drying of uncooked meats will not eliminate such contamination. Post-processing contamination of a dried product with salmonellae is a possibility and should the contaminated dried meat be rehydrated and if temperatures are conducive to *Salmonella* growth, the hazard is increased.

(ix) Control

Control of this bacteria is a problem both nationally and internationally. At the present time no microbiological criteria exists for eliminating *Salmonella* in red meats and poultry since the incidence is considered inherent in these products. It was established by Hobbs (1974) that epidemiologically meat and poultry are responsible for most outbreaks of salmonellosis. This is true on a world-wide basis. Between 1966 and 1975 CDC attributed 40% of the outbreaks of salmonellosis to meat and poultry and in a study by Gangarosa (1978) it was shown that 56% of the outbreaks were due to these foods.

B. Hemorrhagic *Escherichia coli* 0157:H7

Gastrointestinal symptoms due to infection by *E. coli* 0157:H7 are watery, bloody diarrhea, abdominal cramps, with a low grade fever either being present or absent. Transmission is via the fecal/oral route and the reservoir is presumed to be cattle resulting in contamination of meat during processing.

(i) Outbreaks

Several outbreaks attributed to this organism have been reported by CDC (Blaser and Reller, 1981) and also by the Canada Disease Weekly Report (1988). In Ontario, 31 of 353 persons in a home for aged were stricken. The suspected vehicle was hamburger; however, frozen samples of the meat did not test positive for *E. coli* 0157:H7. In 1982 an outbreak of hemorrhagic colitis due to the consumption of hamburger was reported by the Centers for Disease Control. Riley *et al.* (1983) reported 26 cases in White City, Oregon and 21 cases in Traverse City, Michigan. A total of 47 cases were involved with 33 persons being hospitalized. Suspicion was linked to the temperature of the grill which was 330°F when it should have been 350°F. Miscellaneous cases numbered 29 in 11 states—25% from a specific fast food restaurant and the balance at a variety of restaurants from hamburgers ingested by consumers. In 1982, there was a total of 107 cases of hemorrhagic colitis: 26 in Oregon, 21 in Michigan, 29 at miscellaneous locations and 31 in Canada.

(ii) Sources

Sources of *E. coli* 0157:H7 in meat were reported by Doyle and Schoeni (1987), to include the following: 6/164 ground beef = 3·7%; 4/263 poultry = 1·5%; 4/264 pork = 1·5%; and 4/205 lamb = 2·0%. This would indicate that *E. coli* contamination was associated not only with beef but with other animal sources.

A Calgary report indicated that 5/17 beef or 31% of beef samples and 1/14 pork or 7·1% of pork samples were contaminated. Doyle and Schoeni (1987) reported that the types of meat involved were ground beef, pork chops, pork loin, pork hock, ground pork, chicken leg, turkey drumstick, lamb riblet, lamb loin chop, lamb shoulder blade chops and lamb leg. *D* values as reported by Doyle and Schoeni (1984) from ground beef with 17–20% fat content are shown in Table 7-2. Doyle and Schoeni (1987) predicted that at 147°F *E. coli* 0157:H7 would be inactivated. They reported that 0157:H7 was first isolated in 1875 in California and it produces an exotoxin (cytolytic toxin) and lethality is determined by the

TABLE 7-2

COMPARISON OF *D* VALUES OF *E. COLI* 0157:H7 AND SALMONELLAE IN GROUND BEEF

Organism	*Temp. (°C)*	*D value (min)*	*Reference*
E. coli 0157:H7	54·4	39·8	Doyle and Schoeni (1984)
E. coli 0157:H7	57·2	4·5	
E. coli 0157:H7	58·9	1·16	
E. coli 0157:H7	60	0·75	
E. coli 0157:H7	62·8	0·4	
E. coli 0157:H7	64·3	0·16	
Salmonellae	51·6	51–62	Goodfellow and Brown (1978)
Salmonellae	57·2	3·8–4·2	
Salmonellae	62·7	0·6–0·7	

mouse test. A review by Kornacki and Marth (1982) stated any strain of *E. coli* that has the potential to cause diarrheal illness may be defined as EEC (enteropathogenic *E. coli.*). EPEC refers to serogroups of *E. coli* associated with outbreaks of diarrhea in infants and small children. FEEC defines facultatively enteropathogenic *E. coli* which are non-EPEC serogroups associated with sporadic diarrhea and often are found in normal intestinal flora. ETEC includes strains which produce ST (heat stable enterotoxin), LT (heat labile enterotoxin) and some which produce both ST and LT. Large numbers (10^6–10^9) when ingested are the cause of gastrointestinal illness resulting in diarrhea and are an indication of poor sanitation. LT or ST enterotoxin production by *E. coli*, are dependent on constituents of growth medium, pH of media, incubation time, age of culture, agitation and aeration of culture. The presence of antibiotics also influences LT production. Optimal pH of the medium for LT was 8·5, which more than doubled when the pH of specific medium was 7·5. At pH 9, growth diminished. In 1978 an outbreak in September in Oregon at a camp affecting 35 people was attributed to beef obtained from a foodservice establishment and was due to improper holding and cooking temperatures and contaminated equipment (Centers for Disease Control, 1981a,b).

Hall *et al.* (1967) examined samples of 490 food specimens from market foods, including cubed beef steak, pork liver, frozen gravy and sliced beef. *E. coli* serotype 026:B6 (two strains) were isolated from raw cubed beef and pork liver, and it was postulated that when the items were cooked, the organisms (410/g) would probably have been killed. However, the organisms isolated from gravy and sliced beef were from a prepared dish and the increase in numbers was attributed to possible mishandling.

Enrichment in lauryl sulfate tryptose broth (LST) was required to isolate the strain. Several reports of contaminated animals in the Philippines were reported by Escheverria *et al.* (1978). Reis *et al.* (1980) surveyed hamburger, sausage and a food consisting of bovine meat and wheat. His results indicated that 5% of the bovine/wheat samples, 7·5% of the hamburger and 10% of the sausage samples produced LT isolates. Sack *et al.* (1972) reported 8% of 240 isolates of *E. coli* found in soft cheeses, hamburger, crab meat and summer sausage produced LT.

Martin (1986) reported the isolation of *E. coli* 0157:H7 from dairy cattle to be associated with two cases of hamolytic uremic syndrome and stated that the reservoir of this bacteria was unknown, although epidemiological studies have demonstrated an association between infection by *E. coli* 0157:H7 and consumption of undercooked ground beef and raw milk. Because dairy cattle are a general source of both milk and meat for hamburgers, it was suspected that they might also be a reservoir for *E. coli* 0157:H7. Fecal specimens from animals on two farms were screened and *E. coli* 0157:H7 was isolated from healthy heifers from both herds supporting the reservoir theory (Riley *et al.*, 1983; O'Leary *et al.*, 1986; Ryan *et al.*, 1986). Anon. (1987b) published a report stating that Utah State officials were analyzing samples of ground beef, poultry, cheese and butter to determine the source of hemorrhagic *E. coli* 0157:H7, which apparently caused several cases of HUS (hemolytic uremic syndrome) in two state institutions for the mentally retarded. Two deaths were reported. The processed meat had been received from a state prison processing plant and the original source of beef had not been determined. The chicken eaten was not federally inspected.

A report in the 1984 Annual Report of the Food Research Institute (FRI) at the University of Wisconsin-Madison stated that vero cell toxin (VT) produced by *E. coli* was indistinguishable by Ouchterlony immunodiffusion from shiga toxin, a cytotoxin produced by Shigella dysenteriae I (Anon., 1984). A further report by MacDonald (1985) reported on an outbreak of *E. coli* 0157:H7 diarrheal illness in a Nebraska nursing home in which 17 of 19 residents were diagnosed with definite cases, but only 28 of 67 well residents had eaten hamburger (34 of 101 nursing home residents developed diarrheal illness). *E. coli* 0157:H7 was isolated from stool specimens from 4 of 11 definite cases, 1 of 3 probable cases and an asymptomatic resident who had eaten hamburger, but not from 6 well controls who did not eat hamburger. Results demonstrate that hamburger was the vehicle of transmission, with beef cattle probably serving as the animal reservoir for the pathogen.

Survival and growth characteristics of *E. coli* 0157:H7 which were published by Doyle and Schoeni (1984, 1987) show that one strain heated in ground beef was more heat sensitive than salmonellae, and the same strain survived in ground beef patties at −20°C with little change in numbers. Rapid growth occurred in tryptic soy broth (TSB) within the temperature range of 30–42°C; but growth was poor in range of 44–45·5°C which are standard methods for detecting *E. coli* in foods. Five strains of *E. coli* 0157:H7 were negative in the MUG assay.

C. *Listeria monocytogenes*

(i) Characteristics

L. monocytogenes are Gram-positive short rods, are not acid fast, do not form capsules and spores, and are motile by a few peritrichous flagella when cultured at 20–25°C. They are aerobic and facultative anaerobes. Their colonies appear bluish-gray under normal illumination but have a characteristic blue-green sheen produced by obliquely transmitted light. They are catalase positive and oxidase negative, but may give a negative catalase reaction if cultured on media containing low concentrations of meat and yeast extract. This organism produces cytochromes, and the fermentative metabolism of glucose results in production of L(+) lactic acid. They produce acid but no gas from other sugars. They are methyl red positive and Voges–Proskauer positive and exogenous citrate is not utilized. Organic growth factors are required. They do not produce indole. They hydrolyze esculin and sodium hippurate, but do not hydrolyze urea, gelatin, casein and milk. They produce soluble hemolysin in liquid culture (Sneath, 1986).

L. monocytogenes is sensitive to antibiotics *in vitro*, including ampicillin, carbenicillin, cephaloridine, chloramphenicol, erythromycin, furazolidone, neomycin, novobiocin, oleandomycion, ticarcillin, and azlocillin. Listeria is less sensitive to chlortetracyline, oxytetracycline, tetracycline, gentamycin, kanamycin, nitrofurantoin, penicillin G, streptomycin, methicillin, colistin sulfate, nalidixic acid, polymyxin B and sulfonamides (Sneath, 1986).

(ii) Sources

These organisms are widely distributed in nature, and the environment. They are isolated from soil, vegetation and feces of humans and animals, with poultry often being contaminated. Kwantes and Isaac (1971) reported that 57% (20 of 35 samples) of market poultry contained these organisms and later found 33% or 17 of 51 samples to be contaminated (Kwantes and Isaac, 1974). Gitter (1976) reported 10 of 68 swabs of frozen 'oven-ready' poultry samples from 26 shops or supermarkets showed contamination.

(iii) From meat and meat products

Gudkova *et al.* (1958) isolated *L. monocytogenes* from viscera of pigs on a farm at which several persons with mononucleosis due to *L. monocytogenes* had ingested pork. In a survey by Kampelmacher and Van Noorle Janssen (1969), 10–30% of workers in egg processing plants and slaughter houses were found to harbor these microorganisms. The carrier state is brief and is usually without diarrhea (Bojsen-Moller, 1972). *Listeria* has also been isolated from pasteurized milk and fried eggs with congealed whites and soft yolks.

(iv) Growth characteristics

Listeria grows well at refrigeration temperatures of 4–6°C. Petran and Zottola (1989) have reported growth temperatures of a minimum at 4·0°C, optimum of 37°C and maximum at 45°C for *L. monocytogenes* Scott A. Research in progress (Smith and Zottola, unpublished data) indicates that these organisms are heat resistant in meat emulsions and autoclaved ground beef. Gouet *et al.* (1978) reported that *L. monocytogenes* multiplied in ground beef, especially in the presence of pseudomonads, but that lactobacilli inhibited their growth.

(v) pH

Listeria grows best at slightly alkaline pH, range (5·5–9·6) according to Sneath (1986). Petran and Zottola (1989) have reported the following pH values: a minimum at 4·7, optimum at 7·0 and maximum at 9·2 for *L. monocytogenes* Scott A.

(vi) a_w

Listeria can grow in a complex media containing 10% NaCl. Some strains can tolerate 16–20% NaCl and are viable after one year in 16% NaCl at pH 6·0 (Seeliger *et al.*, 1982). A minimum a_w of 0·92 has been reported by Petran and Zottola (1989) for *L. monocytogenes* Scott A. All strains grow well in 10 and 40% bile agar and MacConkey's agar.

(vii) Other

Cold enrichment is used to facilitate isolation from foods. Several modified and new media are now being used to enhance growth and aid in isolation.

(McBride and Girard, 1960; Welshimer, 1968; Wilkins *et al.*, 1972; Martin *et al.*, 1984; Doyle and Schoeni, 1984, 1987; Anon., 1987a). A review of methods and media used to enumerate *L. monocytogenes* has been recently published by Cassiday and Brackett (1989).

(viii) Control mechanisms
Meat and poultry are frequently contaminated with *L. monocytogenes*, which can multiply at refrigeration temperatures. Heat resistance in meat products is presently unknown. Several research projects are in progress to determine *D* values for several strains of *L. monocytogenes*. Preliminary data suggests that *L. monocytogenes* is more heat resistant in meat than *Salmonella*. The necessity of proper hygiene and sanitization procedures in handling, processing, and packaging of meat products is emphasized.

D. *Yersinia enterocolitica*

(i) Characteristics
Y. enterocolitica are Gram-negative straight rods to coccobacilli. They are nonmotile at 37°C, but motile with peritrichous flagella when grown below 30°C. They do not produce capsules. This organism is facultatively anaerobic, oxidase negative and catalase positive. Nitrate is reduced to nitrite; glucose and other carbohydrates are fermented with acid production. Little or no gas production occurs (Krieg, 1984).

(ii) Sources
Animals, especially swine, are important reservoirs of *Yersinia*. They are often recovered from cecal or fecal material, tongues, mesenteric lymph nodes, and the throats of pigs. They have been isolated from cattle, sheep, chickens and rodents (Swaminathan *et al.*, 1982).

Leistner *et al.* (1975) reported contamination of beef samples in West Germany at a 10·8% level. According to Inoue and Kurose (1975), *Yersinia* was isolated from 15 of 61 samples in Japan. In the USA *Yersinia*-like organisms were isolated from 10 of 98 surface-swab samples of vacuum packaged beef and also from lambs (Hanna *et al.*, 1976). Johnson *et al.* (1982) reported that *Yersinia* was isolated from 66 of 150 vacuum packages of beef knuckles but it was only isolated from 4 of 150 samples of unpackaged hanging beef knuckles.

Leistner *et al.* (1975) also reported that 10 of 29 samples of pork from retail German markets contained the organism. In Belgium, Wauters and Janssens (1976) reported contaminated pork tongues, while in Japan

Asakawa *et al.* (1979) reported recovery of serotypes from fecal samples and from chopping blocks. In Canada, Schiemann (1980) reported contamination of 49% of 128 samples of raw pork and 7% of 169 samples of processed pork products from retail stores.

Poultry is also a reservoir of *Yersinia*. In Germany, *Yersinia* was isolated from 35 of 121 samples from chicken (Leistner *et al.*, 1975) and in Japan, 16 of 40 samples were contaminated (Inoue and Nagao, 1976). Other reports showed that *Yersinia* was isolated in 3 of 75 samples of turkey meat in the US (Guthertz *et al.*, 1976), while Norberg (1981) reported contamination of 24·5% of 82 samples from frozen chickens in retail stores in Sweden. Other reports indicated that 73 of 108 poultry carcasses from various processing plants and retail outlets were contaminated. Milk has also been reported as a source of *Yersinia* contamination (Lee *et al.*, 1981; Swaminathan *et al.*, 1982; Bryan, 1983).

(iii) Yersiniosis

The enteritis form of yersiniosis is manifested by abdominal pain, fever, diarrhea, nausea and vomiting and cannot be distinguished from salmonellosis, shigellosis and *E. coli* diarrhea without cultural or serological tests.

(iv) Outbreaks

Some of the identified vehicles of yersiniosis have been raw milk, pasteurized chocolate milk, pasteurized milk, tofu, and water (Bryan, 1983). Epidemiological association has been made between illness and meat ingestion, but laboratory confirmation is lacking.

(v) Growth factors

Temperatures for growth of *Yersinia* have been reported to be between 1–44°C (Sutherland and Varnam, 1977). Nilehn (1969) has reported that most strains could not grow above 43°C on raw beef; however, Hanna *et al.* (1979) reported growth to occur at 0°C. *Yersinia* grew in round steaks at 1–5°C when wrapped in polyvinyl chloride or in vacuum packages. Larger numbers of bacteria were found in the oxygen-permeable film than in vacuum packages. Hanna *et al.* (1979) also reported increased growth of *Yersinia enterocolitica* in either raw or cooked beef and pork when stored at 7°C for 10 days and even greater increases occurred when held at 25°C for 24 h. Freezing had an adverse effect on *Yersinia* in meat.

Hanna *et al.* (1977) showed a reduction of counts on roast beef stored at −23°C for 28 days. In ground beef, numbers declined 83% in 30 days when stored at $-20°C$ and the survivors were sublethally injured (El-Zawahry and Rowley, 1979). Ham stored at $-10°C$ for 7 days showed a $2 \log_{10}$ decrease (Asakawa *et al.*, 1979). A slight decrease in population was reported for chicken stored at $-18°C$ for 90 days (Leistner *et al.*, 1975).

(vi) Thermal treatment

Francis *et al.* (1980) reported a $D_{62·8}$ value in sterile whole milk ranging from 0·7–17 seconds. In roast beef, a population of 10^6 *Yersinia enterolitica* decreased to nondetectable levels when heated to 60–62°C (Hanna *et al.*, 1977).

(vii) pH

The pH range for *Yersinia enterocolitis* has been reported as 4·4–9·0 with an optimum of 7–8 (Hanna *et al.*, 1979; Kendall and Gilbert, 1980; Stern *et al.*, 1980). Some strains were inhibited in BHI (Brain Heart Infusion) with a concentration of 5–7% NaCl (Stern *et al.*, 1980).

(viii) Control and prevention

The sources of contamination are from the intestinal and oral cavities, hides, feathers and processing equipment of raw meat and poultry. Cooking of meat and poultry to an internal temperature of 60°C or above will destroy *Yersinia* unless the level of contamination is very high. Precautions to prevent cross contamination from raw to cooked products are essential. Prevention of growth of other pathogenic organisms by less than 7°C storage does not prevent growth of *Yersinia enterocolitica*, although the lag period is extended.

E. *Campylobacter jejuni*

(i) Characteristics

Campylobacter jejuni are Gram-negative tightly coiled spirals, and rapidly form coccoid bodies when exposed to air. They are motile with corkscrew-like motion by means of single polar flagellum at one or both ends of the cell. They require oxygen concentrations between 3–15% and carbon dioxide concentrations of 3–5%. These organisms are microaerophilic, methyl red and Voges–Proskauer negative. No lipase activity occurs. They are oxidase positive, and reduce nitrate. No pigment is produced (Kreig, 1984).

(ii) Sources

Campylobacter jejuni is found in the reproductive organs, intestinal tract and oral cavity of man and animals. They have been isolated from swine, cattle, sheep, rabbits, and goats, cecal contents of chickens, ducks, turkeys and wild birds. This microorganism is the cause of abortion in cattle and sheep, hepatitis in fowl and scours in swine and calves (Smibert, 1978; Blaser and Reller, 1981; Doyle, 1981).

(iii) Food sources

Campylobacter jejuni was isolated from 94% of 50 chicken carcass rinses collected from a poultry processing plant (Smeltzer, 1981). Simmons and Gibbs (1979) reported 72% (36 of 50 samples) contamination and the organisms were isolated from chickens both at the start and end of processing and were present in 24 (48%) after refrigerated delivery at simulated time of sale. Smith and Muldoon (1974) reported isolation of 2·1% of 140 rinses from necks and whole dressed broilers purchased at local outlets. In Ontario 62% of 100 whole market chickens purchased at the rate of 1 per week over a 5-week period from 20 different stores were positive for *C. jejuni* (Park *et al.*, 1981). Norberg (1981) isolated the organism from 22% of 82 samples of frozen chickens. They were also isolated from peritoneal cavities of chilled chicken carcasses and from liver which had been chilled (36% of counts $>10^3$ cfu/g).

Christopher *et al.* (1982) isolated the organism in small numbers from turkey gizzards. Hartog and deBoer (1981) showed wide cross-contamination in slaughterhouse equipment, with cooling water having 3×10^3 cfu/ml and air near scalding tanks and in evisceration areas resulting in populations of 5–6 cfu/m^3. There are numerous reports of contamination of carcasses and cuts of meat, but few of contamination at the retail source. Death of these organisms in the process from slaughtering to the retail source was probably due to their oxygen sensitivity.

(iv) *Campylobacter* enterocolitis

Campylobacter enterocolitis is a zoonosis. Infection is acquired orally and the infective dose can be small, with as few as 500 organisms causing illness (Robinson, 1981). The incubation period is 7–11 days. The infection results in a watery and sometimes cellular exudate (blood or pus). Other symptoms can be diarrhea, and severe abdominal pain. Illness may be preceded by malaise and fever. Aches of head, back and limbs as well as sweating and rigor may occur. Abdominal pain can be confused with appendicitis (Butzler and Skirrow, 1979).

(v) Growth factors

Campylobacter do not multiply well in or on food products. A lag phase of 2 days in cooked meat medium (CMM) at 37°C was reported and it took 2 days to increase from an initial population of 10^5 to 10^8. Temperature requirements for growth have been published by Doyle and Roman (1981). The organisms multiplied in Brucella broth at pH 6·9 at temperatures from 32–45°C. Populations declined at 47°C and at 25, 27 and 30°C. The most rapid generation time of 1·24–1·34 h occurred at 42–45°C while a slow generation time of 5·88–11·1 h at 32°C was observed. In Campylobacter Agar (pH 5·7–5·9), the maximum growth temperature was between 43–45°C, and the minimum was between 34–36°C. The populations increased from 10^4 to 10^9 in 6 h in sterile meat (pH 6·4) while stored at 37°C according to Gill and Harris (1982). These researchers concluded that *C. jejuni* could not grow on normal pH 5·0–5·5 meat, but could grow on high pH, dark, firm, dry meat only at temperatures around 40°C. They also stated that the organisms can multiply within the pH range of 4·9–9·5, but the most rapid growth occurs between pH 6 and 8. Doyle and Roman (1981) stated that in Brucella broth adjusted to pH 4·0 or less, incubated at 42°C, a 5 log decrease was observed within 4 h, and at pH 4·5, a 3 log decrease occurred within 8 h. Slight growth was observed at pH 5. In the same broth at 25°C (pH 3·5 or less), a 5 log decrease was observed in 4·5 h; at pH 4·0 a 24 h decrease and at pH 4·5 and 5·0 the decrease was 48 h.

(vi) Survival at storage temperatures

Svedhem *et al.* (1981) stated that a culture grown microaerobically at 42°C survived on chicken for 2 days, and minced meat at 4°C for 1 week and at −20°C for 3 months. Hanninen (1981) reported survival in ground beef liver was not affected at 4°C for 6 days but populations decreased when stored at −20°C for 12 weeks. Survival was 24 days at 4°C when packaged in air or CO_2 (Blankenship and Cravens, 1982). A more rapid decline on raw chicken in an air atmosphere than in CO_2 (4 log decrease) was reported by Stern and Kotula (1982), who also reported a 3 order of magnitude decline after 3 days at −15°C in ground beef, but it remained constant thereafter. The organism is not resistant to high temperatures. Svedhem *et al.* (1981) reported that none of 13 strains survived 60°C at greater than 30 min and 55°C for 60 min. Oven temperatures of 190 and 218°C resulted in a decrease to less than 30 cells/g after the internal temperature reached 70°C. Meat balls (100 g) decreased from 10^7 cfu/g to nondetectable in less than 10 min after the internal temperature reached 60°C (Stern and Kotula, 1982). D and z values in peptone broth, chicken, sterile skim milk, peptone–yeast extract broth at temperatures from 49–70°C have been published by Bryan (1986).

(vii) Control and prevention

It is difficult to prevent infection of animals, but fecal matter should be avoided on carcasses. Spray washing is helpful, but contaminated carcasses are the source of organisms on equipment surfaces and hands of workers. End of day, between shift cleanup and disinfection will help to eliminate the spread of contamination, but subsequent processing of newly contaminated carcasses can present new problems. Due to surface contamination and further grinding and incorporation of contamination into ground, rolled and fabricated meat, cooking to 60–70°C for few minutes may eliminate *Campylobacter* on the surface, but the geometric centers of ground, rolled, fabricated meat must also reach this temperature. Temperatures of 50–60°C can be effective if used for a longer time. Cooked foods should be held at or above these temperatures.

(viii) Routine practices

Separate equipment should be used to process raw and cooked meat and poultry. Use of separate utensils for each area, waxed paper and disposable gloves help to prevent cross-contamination. Do not hold meat products at room temperature, as organisms will not multiply below 30°C. Care should be taken to store cooked foods in small shallow containers under refrigerated conditions since foods stored in large containers remain warm at reduced redox potentials for several hours and multiplication of organisms can occur.

III. SUMMARY

This chapter reviews information about salmonellae and the more recently publicized pathogenic bacteria inherent in meat and meat products. These pathogens, which are transmitted by direct contact or by ingestion of meat, meat products and poultry, are of considerable concern because they constitute a severe health hazard to the consumer. Increased regulatory control practices of food service establishments such as those in place in food processing plants, including inspection and enforcement, can be instrumental in preventing foodborne illnesses. Control of pathogens is possible through improved food handling practices, but more importantly through education of food processors, food handlers, and consumers.

Education of the consumer concerning good sanitary procedures must be emphasized in food service establishments and in school health awareness programs. The information presented here concerns several of the 'emerging' pathogens: hemorrhagic *E. coli* 0157:H7, *Listeria monocytogenes*, *Campylobacter jejuni*, and *Yersinia enterocolitica*. Discussion about sources, outbreaks, growth and survival factors, pH, a_w, D values and control measures, where applicable, is included. With increased research in physiology, media formulations, the development of rapid methods for detection, and technological advances in instrumentation, these pathogens and the foodborne illnesses which they cause, may in the future be more easily identified and controlled in meat and meat products.

IV. REFERENCES

ALFORD, J. A. and PALUMBO, S. A. (1969). Interaction of salt, pH and temperature on the growth and survival of salmonellae in ground pork. *Appl. Microbiol.* **17**, 528.

AMERICAN MEAT INSTITUTE (1982). *Good manufacturing practices. I. Voluntary guidelines for the production of dry fermented sausage. II. Voluntary guidelines for the production of semi-dry fermented sausage.* American Meat Institute, Washington, DC.

ANGELOTTI, R. (1977). Cooking requirements for cooked roast beef. *Fed. Reg.* **42**(17), 44 217.

ANGELOTTI, R., FOTER, M. J. and LEWIS, K. H. (1961). Time–temperature effects on salmonellae and staphylococci in foods. I. Behavior in refrigerated foods. *Am. J. Publ. Health* **51**, 76.

ANON. (1984). *Hemorrhagic Colitis and Hemolytic Uremic Syndrome.* Food Research Institute Annual Report for 1984, p. 253. University of Wisconsin-Madison.

ANON. (1987a). *Product Information Sheet.* BBL Microbiology Systems. Cockeysville, MD.

ANON. (1987b). Utah investigating deaths of children from hemorrhagic *E. coli. Food Chemical News* July 27, 41.

ASAKAWA, Y., AKAHANE, S., SHIZAWA, K. and HONMA, T. (1979). Investigation of source and route of *Yersinia enterocolitica* infection. *Contrib. Microbial. Immunol.* **5**, 115.

BAILEY, J. W. (1974). *Encyclopedia of Labeling Meat and Poultry Products.* Meat Plant Mag., St. Louis, MO.

BARAN, W. L. and STEVENSON, K. E. (1975). Survival of selected pathogens during processing of a fermented turkey sausage. *J. Food Sci.* **40**, 618.

BARNES, E. M. (1976). Microbiological problems of poultry at refrigeration temperatures—A review. *J. Sci. Food Agric.* **27**, 777.

BLANKENSHIP, L. C. and CRAVENS, S. E. (1982). *Campylobacter jejuni* survival in chicken meat as a function of temperature. *Appl. Environ. Microbiol.* **44**, 88.

Blaser, M. J. and Reller, L. B. (1981). *Campylobacter* enteritis. *New Engl. J. Med.* **305**, 1444.

Bojsen-Moller, J. (1972). Human listeriosis. Diagnostic, epidemiological, and clinical studies. *Acta Pathol. Microbiol. Scand.* Suppl. **B229**, 1.

Bryan, F. L. (1983). Epidemiology of milk-borne diseases. *J. Food Prot.* **46**, 637.

Bryan, F. L. (1986). Miscellaneous pathogenic bacteria in meat and poultry products. In *Advances in Meat Research*, Vol. 2 (A. M. Pearson and T. R. Dutson, Eds), p. 254. AVI Publishing Company, Inc., Westport, Connecticut.

Bryan, F. L., Fanelli, M. J. and Riemann, H. (1979). *Salmonella* infections. In *Food Borne Infections and Intoxications* (H. Riemann and F. L. Bryan, Eds), p. 73. Academic Press, New York.

Butzler, J. P. and Skirrow, M. B. (1979). *Campylobacter* enteritis. *Clin. Gastroenterol.* **8**, 737.

Canada Disease Weekly Report (1988). Outbreak of gastroenteritis in a home for the aged—Ontario. *J. Food Prot.* **51**, 753.

Cassiday, P. K. and Brackett, R. E. (1989). Methods and media to isolate and enumerate *Listeria monocytogenes.* A review. *J. Food Prot.* **52**, 207.

Centers For Disease Control (1981a). Multistate outbreak of salmonellosis caused by precooked roast beef. *Morbidity Mortality Weekly Rpt.* **30**, 391.

Centers For Disease Control (1981b). Multiple outbreaks of salmonellosis associated with precooked roast beef—Pennsylvania, New York, Vermont. *Morbidity Mortality Weekly Rpt* **30**, 569.

Christian, J. H. B. and Scott, W. J. (1953). Water relations of salmonellae at 30°C. *Austral. J. Biol. Sci.* **6**, 565.

Christopher, F. M., Smith, G. C. and Vanderzant, C. (1982). Examination of poultry giblets, raw milk and meat for *Campylobacter fetus* subsp. *jejuni*. *J. Food Prot.* **45**, 260.

Chung, K. C. and Goepfert, J. M. (1970). Growth of *Salmonella* at low pH. *J. Food Sci.* **35**, 326.

Davidson, C. M. and Webb, G. (1973). The behavior of salmonellae in vacuum-packaged cooked cured meat products. *Canad. Inst. Food Sci. Technol. J.* **6**, 41.

Davidson, C. M. and Witty, J. K. (1977). Fate of salmonellae in vacuum-packaged ground meat during storage and subsequent cooking. *Canad. Inst. Food Sci. Technol. J.* **10**, 223.

Deibel, R. H., Niven, C. F., Jr and Wilson, G. D. (1961). Microbiology of meat curing. III. Some microbiological and related technological aspects in the manufacture of fermented sausages. *Appl. Microbiol.* **9**, 156.

Doyle, M. P. (1981). *Campylobacter fetus* subsp. *jejuni*. An old pathogen of new concern. *J. Food Prot.* **44**, 450.

Doyle, M. P. and Roman, D. J. (1981). Growth and survival of *Campylobacter fetus* subsp. *jejuni* as a function of temperature and pH. *J. Food Prot.* **44**, 596.

Doyle, M. P. and Schoeni, J. L. (1984). Survival and growth characteristics of *Escherichia coli* associated with hemorrhagic colitis. *Appl. Environ. Microbiol.* **48**, 855.

Doyle, M. P. and Schoeni, J. L. (1987). Isolation of *Escherichia coli* 0157:H7 from retail fresh meats and poultry. *Appl. Environ. Microbiol.* **53**, 2394.

El-Zawahry, Y. A. and Rowley, D. B. (1979). Radiation resistance and injury of *Yersinia enterocolitica*. *Egypt. J. Vet Sci.* **9**, 1.

EMPEY, W. A. and SCOTT, W. J. (1939). Investigations on chilled beef. I. Microbial contamination acquired in the meatworks. *Bull. No. 126. Counc. Sci. Ind. Res.*, Melbourne, Australia.

ESCHEVERRIA, P., ULYANGCO, C. V., HO, M. J., VERHAERT, L., KOMALARINI, S., ØRSKOV, F. and ØRSKOV, I. (1978). Search for heat-labile enterotoxigenic *Escherichia coli* in humans, livestock, food and water in a community in the Philippines. *J. Infect. Dis.* **138**, 87.

FARRELL, G. M. and UPTON, M. E. (1978). The effect of low temperature on the growth and survival of *Staphylococcus aureus* and *Salmonella typhimurium* when inoculated on to bacon. *J. Food Technol* **13**, 15.

FRANCIS, D. W., SPAULDING, P. L and LOVETT, J. (1980). Enterotoxin production and thermal resistance of *Yersinia enterocolitica* in milk. *Appl. Environ. Microbiol.* **40**, 174.

GANGAROSA, E. J. (1978). *History and Surveillance Programs for Salmonellosis*. Proc. Natl Salmonellosis Sem., Washington, DC.

GENIGEORGIS, C. and RIEMANN, H. (1979). Food processing and hygiene. In *Food Borne Infections and Intoxications* (H. Riemann and F. L. Bryan, Eds), p. 621. Academic Press. New York.

GILL, C. O. and HARRIS, L. M. (1982). Survival and growth of *Campylobacter fetus* subsp. *jejuni* on meat and cooked food. *Appl. Environ. Microbiol.* **44**, 259.

GITTER, M (1976). *Listeria monocytogenes* in 'oven-ready' poultry. *Vet Rec.* **99**, 336.

GOEPFERT, J. M. and CHUNG, K. C. (1970a). Behavior of *Salmonella* in sliced luncheon meat. *Appl. Microbiol.* **19**, 190.

GOEPFERT, J. M. and CHUNG, K. C. (1970b). Behavior of *Salmonella* during the manufacture and storage of a fermented sausage product. *J. Milk Food Technol.* **33**, 185.

GOEPFERT, J. M. and KIM, H. U. (1975). Behavior of selected food-borne pathogens in raw ground beef. *J. Milk Food Technol.* **38**, 449.

GOMUTPUTRA, C. and FABIAN, F. W. (1953). Acids and chloramphenicol as sanitizing agents for meat contaminated with food poisoning organisms. *J. Milk Food Technol.* **16**, 220.

GOODFELLOW, S. J. and BROWN, W. L. (1978). Fate of *Salmonella* inoculated into beef for cooking. *J. Food Prot.* **41**, 598.

GOUET, P. H., LABADIE, J. and SERRATORE, C. (1978). Development of *Listeria monocytogenes* in monoxenic and polyxenic beef mixtures. *Zentrabl. Bakteriol. Hyg. I.* Abt. Orig. **B166**, 87.

GREEN, S. S., MORAN, A. B., JOHNSTON, R. W., UHLER, P. and CHU, J. (1982). The incidence of *Salmonella* species and serotypes in young whole chicken carcasses compared with 1967. *Poultry Sci.* **61**, 288.

GUDKOVA, E. I., MORONOVA, K. A., KUSMINSKII, A. S. and GEINE, G. O. (1958). A second outbreak of listeriotic angina in a single populated locality. *J. Mikrobiol. Epidemiol. Immunobiol.* **29**, 1373.

GUTHERTZ, L. S., FRUIN, J. T., SPICER, D. and FOWLER, J. L. (1976). Microbiology of fresh comminuted turkey meat. *J. Milk Food Technol.* **39**, 823.

HALL, E. H., BROWN, D. F. and LEWIS, R. H. (1967). Examination of market foods for coliform organisms. *Appl. Microbiol.* **15**, 1062.

HANNA, M. O., ZINK, D. L., CARPENTER, Z. L. and VANDERZANT, C. (1976). *Yersinia enterocolitica*-like organisms from vacuum packaged beef and lamb. *J. Food Sci.* **41**, 1254.

HANNA, M. O., STEWART, J. C., CARPENTER, Z. L. and VANDERZANT, C. (1977). Effect of heating, freezing and pH on *Yersinia enterocolitica*-like organisms from meat. *J. Food Prot.* **40**, 689.

HANNA, M. O., STEWART, J. C., CARPENTER, Z. L., ZINK, D. L. and VANDERZANT, C. (1979). Isolation and characteristics of *Yersinia enterocolitica*-like bacteria from meats. *Contrib. Microbiol. Immunol.* **5**, 234.

HANNINEN, M. L. (1981). Survival of *Campylobacter jejuni/coli* in ground refrigerated and in ground frozen beef liver and in frozen broiler carcasses. *Acta. Vet. Scand.* **22**, 566.

HARTOG, B. J. and DE BOER, E. (1981). *Campylobacter jejuni* in poultry products from retail outlets and in poultry slaughter houses. In *Campylobacter, Epidemiology, Pathogenesis and Biochemistry* (D. G. Newell, Ed.), p. 270. MTP Press, Lancaster, Pennsylvania.

HOBBS, B. C. (1974). *Food Poisoning and Food Hygiene*. Edward Arnold Ltd, London.

INGRAM, M. and ROBERTS, T. A. (1976). The microbiology of the red meat carcass and the slaughterhouse. *Roy. Soc. Health J.* **96**, 270.

INOUE, M. and KUROSE, M. (1975). Isolation of *Yersinia enterocolitica* from cows intestinal contents and beef meat. *Japan J. Vet. Sci.* **37**, 91.

INOUE, M. and NAGAO, H. (1976). Isolation of *Yersinia enterocolitica* from bovine cecal contents, commercial meat and meatshops. *J. Japan Vet. Med. Assoc.* **29**, 612.

INTERNATIONAL COMMISSION ON MICROBIOLOGICAL SPECIFICATIONS FOR FOODS (1980). *Meats and Meat Products. Microbial Ecology of Foods. Vol. 2, Food Commodities*, p. 378. Academic Press, New York.

JOHNSON, R. W., HARRIS, M. E., MORAN, A. C., KRUMM, G. W. and LEE, W. H. (1982). A comparative study of the microbiology of commercial vacuum-packaged and hanging beef. *J. Food Prot.* **45**, 223.

KAMPELMACHER, E. H. and VAN NOORLE JANSSEN, L. M. (1969). *Zentrakbl. Bakteriol. Parasitenk, Infektionskr. Hyg.* Abt 1: Orig. **A211**, 353.

KAUFFMAN, F. (1966). *The Bacteriology of Enterobacteriaceae*. Einar Munksgard, Copenhagen, Denmark (Williams & Wilkins, Baltimore, MD).

KENDALL, M. and GILBERT, R. J. (1980). Survival and growth of *Y. enterocolitica* in broth media and in food. In *Microbial Growth and Survival in Extremes of Environment* (G. W. Gould and J. E. L. Corry, Eds), p. 215. Soc. Appl. Bacterial. Tech. Ser No. 15, Academic Press, London.

KORNACKI, J. L. and MARTH, E. H. (1982). Foodborne illness caused by *Escherichia*: A review *J. Food Prot.* **45**, 1051.

KRIEG, N. R. (ED.). (1984). *Bergey's Manual of Systematic Bacteriology*, Vol. 1, Williams & Wilkins, Baltimore, MD.

KWANTES, W. and ISAAC, M. (1971). Listeriosis. *Brit. Med. J.* **2**, 296.

KWANTES, E. and ISAAC, M. (1974). *Listeria* infection in West Glamorgan. In *Problems of Listeriosis. Proc. 6th Intern. Symp. on Listeriosis* (M. Woodbine, Ed.), p. 112. Leicester University Press, Leicester, UK.

LEDWARD, D. A., NICOL, D. J. and SHAW, M. K. (1971). Microbiological and color changes during aging of beef. *Food Technol. Austral.* **23**, 30.

LEE, W. H., VANDERZANT, C. and STERN, N. (1981). The occurrence of *Yersinia enterocolitica* in foods. In Yersinia enterocolitica (E. J. Bottone, Ed), p. 161. CRC Press, Boca Raton, FL.

LEISTNER, L., HECHELMANN, H., KASHIWAZAKI, M. and ALBERTZ, R. (1975). Nachweis von *Yersinia enterocolitica* in Faeces und Fleisch von Schwein, Rindern, und Geflugel, *Fleischwirtschaft* **55**, 1599.

MACDONALD, K. (1985). *Outbreak of* Escherichia coli *0157:H7 diarrheal illness in a nursing home, Nebraska.* Abst. Food Research Institute Ann. Spring Mtg, May 22, 1985, Madison, WI.

MACKEY, B. M., ROBERTS, T. A., MANSFIELD, J. and FARKAS, G. (1980). Growth of *Salmonella* on chilled meat. *J. Hyg. Cambridge* **85**, 115.

MARAZZA, V. and CRESPI, A., (1973). Osservazioni sulla sopravoivenza di *Salmonella cholerasuis* in insaccati naturalmente inquinati. *Atti. Soc. Ital. Sci. Vet.* **17**, 537.

MARRIOTT, N. G., SMITH, G. C., HOKE, K. E., CARPENTER, Z. L. and WEST, R. L. (1977). Long-distance transoceanic shipments of fresh beef. *J. Food Sci.* **42**, 316.

MARTIN, M. L. (1986). Isolation of *Escherichia coli* 0157:H7 from dairy cattle associated with two cases of Haemolytic uraemic syndrome. *Lancet*, Nov. 1, 1986. 1043.

MARTIN, R. S., SUMARAH, R. K. and MACDONALD, M. A. (1984). A synthetic based medium for the isolation of *Listeria monocytogenes. Clin. Investig. Med.* **7**(4), 233.

MCBRIDE, M. E. and GIRARD, K. F. (1960). A selective medium for the isolation of *Listeria monocytogenes* from mixed bacterial populations. *J. Lab. Clin. Med.* **55**(2), 153.

NILEHN, B. (1969). *Studies on* Yersinia enterocolitica *with Special Reference to Bacterial Diagnosis and Occurrence in Human Acute Enteric Disease*, Munksguard, Copenhagen.

NORBERG, P. (1981). Enteropathogenic bacteria in frozen chicken. *Appl. Environ. Microbiol.* **42**, 32.

O'LEARY, M. J., MACDONALD, K. L., WELLS, J. G., KOBAYASHI, J. M. and BLAKE, P. A. (1986). *Escherichia coli* 0157:H7 intestinal infections. Seattle. *Abst. 35th Annual EIS conference*, Atlanta, GA.

PARK, C. E., STANKCIEWICZ, Z. K., LOVETT, J. and HUNT, J. (1981). Incidence of *Campylobacter jejuni* in fresh eviscerated whole market chickens. *Canad. J. Microbiol.* **27**, 841.

PETRAN, R. L. and ZOTTOLA, E. A. (1989). A study of factors affecting growth and recovery of *Listeria monocytogenes* Scott A. *J. Food Sci.* **54**, 458.

PIVNICK, H. (1978). Canadian microbiological standards for foods. *Food Technol.* **32**, 50.

REIS, M. H. L., VASCONCELOS, J. C. and TRABULSI, L. R. (1980). Prevalence of enterotoxigenic *Escherichia coli* in some processed raw food from animal origin. *Appl. Environ. Microbiol.* **39**, 270.

RILEY, L. W., REMIS, R. S., HELGERSON, S. D., MCGEE, H. B., WELLS, J. G., DAVIS, B. R., HEBERT, R. J., OLCOTT, E. S., JOHNSON, L. M., HARGRETT, N. T., BLAKE, P. A. and COHEN, M. L. (1983). Hemorrhagic colitis associated with a rare *Escherichia coli* serotype. *New Engl. J. Med.* **308**, 681.

ROBERTS, T. A. (1980). Contamination of meat. The effects of slaughter practices on the bacteriology of the red meat carcass. *Roy. Soc. Health J.* **100**, 3.

ROBINSON, D. A. (1981). Infective dose of *Campylobacter jejuni* in milk. *Brit. Med. J.* **1**, 1584.

RYAN, C. A., TAUXE, R. V., HOSEK, G. W., WELLS, J. G., STOESZ, P. A., MCFADDEN, H. W., JR, SMITH, P. W., WRIGHT, G. F. and BLAKE, P. A. (1986). *Escherichia coli* 0157:H7 diarrhea in a nursing home: clinical, epidemiological, and pathological findings. *J. Infect. Dis.* **154**, 631.

SACK, R. B., SACK, D. A., MEHLMAN, J., ØRSKOV, F. and ØRSKOV, I. (1977). Enterotoxigenic *Escherichia coli* isolated from food. *J. Infect. Dis.* **135**, 313.

SCHIEMANN, D. A. (1980). Isolation of toxigenic *Yersinia enterocolitica* from retail pork products. *J. Food Prot.*, **43**, 360.

SEELIGER, H. P. R., SCHRETTENBRUNNER, A., PONGRATZ, G. and HOF, H. (1982). Zur Sonderstellung stark hamolysierender Stamme der Gattung Listeria. Special position of strongly haemolytic strains of the genus Listeria. *Zentralbl. Bakteriol. Parasitenkd. Infektionskr. Hyg.* I. Abt. Orig. **A252**, 176.

SHAW, M. K. and NICOL, D. J. (1969). Effect of the gaseous environment on the growth on meat of some food poisoning and food spoilage organisms. *Proc. 15th Europ. Mtg. Meat Res. Workers.* p. 226.

SILLIKER, J. H. (1980). Status of *Salmonella*—ten years later. *J. Food Prot.* **43**, 307.

SILLIKER, J. H. and WOLFE, S. K. (1980). Microbiological safety considerations in controlled atmosphere storage of meats. *J. Food Technol.* **34**, 59.

SIMMONS, N. A. and GIBBS, F. L. (1979). *Campylobacter* spp. in oven-ready poultry. *J. Infect. Dis.* **1**, 159.

SMELTZER, T. I. (1981). Isolation of *Campylobacter jejuni* from poultry carcasses. *Austral. Vet. J.* **57**, 511.

SMIBERT, R. M. (1978). The genus *Campylobacter. Ann. Rev. Microbiol.* **32**, 637.

SMITH, J. L. and PALUMBO, S. A. (1973). Microbiology of Lebanon bologna. *Appl. Microbiol.* **26**, 489.

SMITH, J. L., PALUMBO, S. A., KISSINGER, J. C. and HUTANEN, C. N. (1975). Survival of *Salmonella dublin* and *Salmonella typhimurium* in Lebanon bologna. *J. Milk Food Technol.* **38**, 150.

SMITH, M. V. and MULDOON, P. J. (1974). *Campylobacter fetus* subspecies *jejuni* (*Vibrio fetus*) from commercially processed poultry. *Appl. Microbiol.* **27**, 995.

SNEATH, P. H. A., (Ed.). (1986). *Bergey's Manual of Systematic Bacteriology*, Vol. 2. Williams & Wilkins, Baltimore, MD.

STERN, N. J. and KOTULA, A. W. (1982). Survival of *Campylobacter jejuni* inoculated into ground beef. *Appl. Environ. Microbiol.* **44**, 1150.

STERN, N. J., PIERSON, M. D. and KOTULA, A. W. (1980). Effects of pH and sodium chloride on *Yersinia enterocolitica* at room and refrigerator temperatures. *J. Food Sci.* **45**, 64.

SULZBACHER, W. L. (1952). Effect of freezing and thawing on the growth rate of bacteria in ground meat. *Food Technol.* **6**, 341.

SURKIEWICZ, B. F., HARRIS, M. E. and JOHNSTON, R. W. (1973). Bacteriological survey of frozen meat and gravy produced at establishments under federal inspection. *Appl. Microbiol.* **26**, 574.

Sutherland, J. P. and Varnam, A. H. (1977). Methods of isolation of potential importance of *Yersinia enterocolitica* in foods stored at low temperatures. *J. Appl. Bacteriol.* **43**, xiii (Abstr.).

Svedhem, A., Kaijser, B. and Sjogren, E. (1981). The occurrence of *Campylobacter jejuni* in fresh food and survival under different conditions. *J. Hyg.* **87**, 421.

Swaminathan, B., Harmon, M. C. and Mehlman, I. J. (1982). A review: *Yersinia enterocolitica. J. Appl. Bacteriol.* **52**, 151.

Takaćs, J. and Simonfly, Z. (1970). Das Salmonellen—Problem bei Dauerwursten. *Fleischwirtschaft* **50**, 1200.

Takaćs, J., Jirkovsky, M. and Hegyi, Z. (1963). Studies on the microbiological and biochemical changes involved in the ripening process of Hungarian salami. *Acta Vet. Hung.* **13**, 119.

Taylor, A. A. (1971). The gaseous environment of packaged fresh meat. *Proc. 17th Europ. Meat Res. Workers*, p. 662.

Tiwari, N. P. and Maxcy, R. B. (1972). Comparative growth of salmonellae, coliforms and other members of the microflora of raw and radurized ground beef. *J. Milk Food Technol.* **35**, 445.

Tompkin, R. B. (1983). Indicator organisms in meat and poultry products. *Food Technol.* **37**(6), 107.

Wauters, G. and Janssens, M. (1976). Carriage of *Yersinia enterocolitica* by slaughtering pigs. II. Search for *Yersinia enterocolitica* in pig tongues. *Med. Mal. Infect.* **6**, 517.

Welshimer, H. J. (1968). Isolation of *Listeria monocytogenes* from vegetation. *J. Bacteriol.* **95**, 300.

Wilkins, P. O., Bourgeois, R. and Murray, R. G. E. (1972). Psychrotrophic properties of *Listeria monocytogenes. Can. J. Microbiol.* **18**, 543.

Wolfe, S. K. (1980). Use of CO and CO_2 enriched atmospheres for meat, fish and produce. *Food Technol.* **34**(3), 55.

8

Iron

Bonnie Worthington-Roberts[a] and Elaine R. Monsen[b]

[a]*Nutritional Sciences/Epidemiology,* [b]*Nutritional Sciences/Medicine, University of Washington, Seattle, Washington, USA*

I. INTRODUCTION

While iron is found in only trace amounts in the human organism (National Research Council, 1979), it is the fourth most abundant element in the earth's crust. It can exist in a number of oxidation states but only the ferric form, Fe^{+3}, and the ferrous form, Fe^{+2}, are stable in an aqueous environment and thus are the only states that occur naturally in food. However, elemental iron, Fe^0, is also consumed since it is a common food fortificant with satisfactory bioavailability (Lee and Clydesdale, 1979). *It has long been known that iron is required for survival of the human organism. It is of interest, given its relative abundance, that iron deficiency is the most common specific nutrient deficiency observed around the world today.*

II. DISTRIBUTION AND FUNCTION OF BODY IRON

Most of the body iron is protein-bound, either as porphyrin or heme compounds in hemoglobin or myoglobin or as non-heme complexes such as transferrin, ferritin and hemosiderin (Morris, 1987). Less than 1% of total body iron is found in hemoprotein and flavoprotein enzymes and free iron is present in very small amounts. Needless-to-say, survival depends on the maintenance of sufficient body iron to support oxygen transport functions and an array of enzyme reactions (either as a component of the enzyme or a cofactor in the reaction). Ideally, iron is also stored for use as needed to maintain normal physiologic processes.

A. Iron in the Blood

Iron found in the hemoglobin complex represents 60–70% of total body iron in the normal adult human. Hemoglobin is made up of the protein globin and four ferroprotoporphyrin or 'heme' moieties. This structure stabilizes iron in the ferrous state and allows it to be reversibly bonded to oxygen, permitting hemoglobin to function as an oxygen carrier. The biosynthesis of heme and its attachment to globin takes place in the latter stages of red cell development in the bone marrow. Iron is carried to the bone marrow in the ferric form as transferrin, reduced to the ferrous form, and detached from transferrin, thus facilitating its transfer to protoporphyrin (Rimington, 1959). This process occurs continuously so it not surprising that more than 70% of plasma iron goes to the bone marrow (Bothwell *et al.*, 1979). While diet is the source of some plasma iron, the majority (some 20–24 mg daily) is liberated from the destruction of hemoglobin; this breakdown of the heme moiety and release of iron to the plasma is performed in the reticuloendothelial (RE) cells of the liver, spleen and bone marrow. The RE System, or monocyte:macrophage system, rapidly returns iron to the circulation ($t_{1/2}$, 34 minutes) or transfers it to a slowly exchanging pool of storage iron within the RE cell ($t_{1/2}$ for release to plasma, 7 days) (Fillet *et al.*, 1974). Each day in adult humans, 25–40 mg of iron are transported in the plasma, even though only 3–4 mg are present in the whole plasma volume at any one time (Morris, 1987).

Iron is incorporated into hemoglobin within the reticulocyte after its extraction from the carrier molecule, transferrin. Transferrin molecules first bind to cell membrane receptor sites (Jandl and Katz, 1963) and then move into the reticulocyte via endocytosis (Appleton *et al.*, 1971). Iron subsequently moves to membranous components of the cell for transport through the cytoplasm to the mitochondria. It is here that most of the iron is incorporated into hemoglobin (Sano *et al.*, 1959).

Normal blood hemoglobin levels in adult humans range from 13–17 g/dl (130–170 g/liter). Variations are related to age, sex, nutrition, pregnancy, lactation, altitude and disease. As far as nutrition is concerned, level of dietary iron is obviously important. However, anemia may also be caused by deficiencies of other nutrients, specifically folic acid, vitamin B_{12}, copper and protein.

Not only is iron found in blood as hemoglobin in the erythrocytes, it is also present as transferrin in the plasma. The amount of iron present in this form is only 1/1000 of that found in hemoglobin. Transferrin is a glycoprotein with two binding sites, each capable of binding one atom of ferric iron (Ehrenberg and Laurell, 1955). Transferrin is the principal carrier of iron in the blood and therefore plays a key role in iron metabolism. In addition, it also participates in the defense mechanisms of the body (Bullen *et al.*, 1972). Under normal circumstances, only 30–40% of the transferrin is saturated with iron; the remainder of the iron-binding potential is referred to as the latent iron-binding capacity.

Characteristic values for serum iron, total iron binding capacity (TIBC) and percentage transferrin saturation in humans are defined in Table 8-1. The range of values which are seen in human serum iron reflects the fact that it is a pool into which iron enters, leaves and is returned at varying rates. In iron deficiency, for example, low serum iron levels result from low intake, depletion of iron stores and reduced hemoglobin destruction accompanying anemia. The high serum iron characteristic of pernicious anemia can be associated with a block in hemoglobin synthesis in the presence of adequate iron stores. The high serum iron and percent transferrin saturation in hemachromatosis can be related to the excessive absorption and deposition of iron in the body (Morris, 1987).

Small quantities of iron are also present in the blood in the form of ferritin, a compound which can be isolated from erythrocytes, serum and leukocytes. The levels of ferritin in the serum vary with the iron status of the individual as well as with certain disease states. (The iron present in this form represents only 0·2–0·4% of the total serum iron normally present in the adult.) The serum ferritin assay has been shown to be a useful tool in the

TABLE 8-1

SERUM IRON, TOTAL IRON-BINDING CAPACITY (TIBC) AND PERCENT TRANSFERRIN SATURATION[a]

Condition	*Serum iron*[b] (*μg/dl*)	*TIBC*[b] (*μg/dl*)	*Mean transferrin saturation* (%)
Human adults			
Normal male	127 (67–191)	333 (253–416)	33
Normal female	113 (63–202)	329 (250–416)	37
Iron deficiency anemia	32 (0–78)	428 (204–705)	7
Late pregnancy	94 (22–185)	532 (373–712)	18
Hemochromatosis	250 (191–290)	263 (205–330)	96
Infections	47 (30–72)	260 (182–270)	20

[a] Data from Cartwright and Wintrobe (1949).
[b] Range given in parentheses.

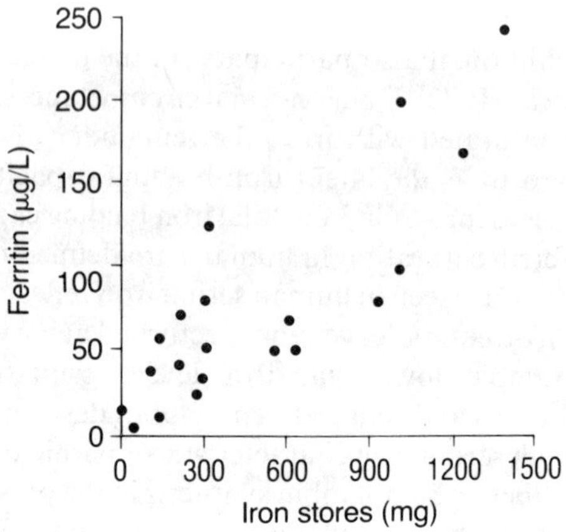

FIG. 8-1. Iron stores measured by phlebotomy and serum ferritin concentration. Data from Walters *et al.* (1973).

evaluation of iron status in humans as shown in Fig. 8-1 (Walters *et al.*, 1973). In the presence of certain pathologic conditions, however, serum ferritin values are known to rise, which is true for liver disease (Lipschitz *et al.*, 1974) as well as leukemia (Worwood *et al.*, 1974).

When hemolysis occurs within the vascular system, free hemoglobin is released into the plasma. Several proteins (hemopexin and haptoglobin) serve to return free heme or hemoglobin to the liver for breakdown and conservation of the iron; hemopexin binds heme and haptoglobin binds hemoglobin. In circumstances where intravascular hemolysis is significant, these proteins may be heavily utilized such that their levels (in free form) in the serum may drop. A test of free haptoglobin in the serum, for example, may provide evidence of existent hemolytic activity (Morris, 1987).

B. Storage Iron

Iron is a nutrient which the body can effectively store for use at a later time if dietary provisions are low. The predominant forms of storage iron are ferritin and hemosiderin, both of which are large iron–protein compounds that are distributed widely in body tissues, with the highest concentrations being found in the liver, spleen and bone marrow. A major difference between ferritin and hemosiderin is that the former is soluble in water and the latter is not. Ferritin contains up to 20% iron while hemosiderin may contain as much as 35% iron. In normal individuals, ferritin accounts for about 60% of the storage iron, whereas in conditions of iron overload, the proportion attributable to hemosiderin increases.

Under normal circumstances, iron is readily deposited in the liver and spleen and in roughly the same amounts as ferritin and hemosiderin. Research has shown that iron is utilized equally well from these two compounds for the demands of erythropoiesis and placental iron transfer to the fetus. The main factor affecting the relative distribution of iron between ferritin and hemosiderin is the total storage iron concentration. Morgan and Walters (1963) concluded that when total storage iron in the liver and spleen is below 500 μg/g of tissue, more iron is stored as ferritin than as hemosiderin. At storage levels above 1000 μg/g, more is stored as hemosiderin. In diseases, such as hemochromatosis, in which very high levels of iron are found in the tissues, most of the iron is present as hemosiderin (Morgan and Walters, 1963).

The average woman during her reproductive years will have iron stores of approximately 300 mg. Average iron intake reported in NHANES II for women 12–50 years of age is 11 mg/day (NCHS, 1983). To meet her average needs, a woman would need to absorb 13% of the ingested 11 mg. If menstrual losses were above average, absorption would need to increase and could reach 25% of ingested iron (Table 8-2).

TABLE 8-2

CHARACTERISTICS OF THEORETICAL SUBJECTS AT SELECTED LEVELS OF IRON STORES AND ESTIMATED OBLIGATORY IRON ABSORPTION TO MAINTAIN OR ACHIEVE STATED IRON STORES

Iron stores	
100 mg	*Iron deficient*
	Absorption up to maximum (25%)
	Anemia may develop
300 mg	*Average iron stores for 12–50 year old woman*
	11 mg iron average daily intake
	1·4 mg iron absorbed/day required for balance
	13% absorption of 11 mg intake allows 1·4 mg absorbed
	5% of 12–50 year old women require
	> 2·4 mg iron absorbed/day for balance
	22% absorption of 11 mg intake needed to absorb 2·4 mg iron
1 000 mg	*Average iron stores of adult man*
	17 mg iron average daily intake
	1·0 mg iron absorbed per day for balance
	to achieve 1000 mg store, additional absorption of 0·06 mg/day suffices
	6% absorption of 17 mg intake is needed

The average adult man consumes 17 mg iron/day (NCHS, 1983) and has iron stores approximating 1000 mg. If 6% of ingested iron were absorbed, an adult man could maintain iron balance plus store 0·06 mg iron/day; this modest retention would allow 1000 mg iron stores to be built up over 45 years (Table 8-2).

The level of body iron stores can be assessed by histochemical examination of aspirated samples of bone marrow. Use of both staining and chemical methods of evaluation allows for the detection of both the unstainable ferritin as well as the stainable hemosiderin (Shoden and Sturgeon, 1960). Since bone marrow aspiration is a rather invasive procedure, iron stores are often estimated indirectly. Several methods have been used for this purpose (Table 8-3) but the one traditionally considered most useful is serum ferritin. Since 1972, there have been a number of investigations of the serum ferritin assay as a method for evaluating iron stores. While some overlap between adequate and deficient groups is seen as well as some interlaboratory variation, its value in estimating iron stores is now appreciated (White, 1980).

In recent years, an assay for determination of the zinc protoporphyrin heme ratio has become available for assessing the presence or absence of marginal iron deficiency (Labbe *et al.*, 1987). This measure is useful since it has been shown that as the concentration of bone marrow iron decreases to a suboptimal level, zinc instead of iron is bound to protoporphyrin in the process of erythropoiesis. Iron depletion is thus associated with an increase in circulating zinc protoporphyrin, e.g. an increase from the usual level of 1 zinc protoporphyrin molecule per 30 000 heme molecules to 2 zinc protoporphyrin per 30 000 heme molecules. This was nicely shown in a 12-week study involving adult men placed on a metabolic ward and repeatedly subjected to blood draws (Rettmer *et al.*, 1985). The zinc protoporphyrin/heme ratio was determined with a customized hematofluometer (Rettmer *et al.*, 1987); measures of serum ferritin, serum iron and iron-binding capacity were also obtained. As illustrated in Fig. 8-2, the serum ferritin concentration in all subjects decreased from the beginning to the end of the experimental period, whereas, the zinc protoporphyrin/heme ratio uniformly increased. By contrast, the changes in percent transferrin saturation (not shown) were inconsistent. The hematocrit results were also inconsistent, but usually showed little change. The temporal relationship between changes in ferritin concentration and the zinc protoporphyrin/heme ratio were particularly significant, which clearly change in a concerted pattern, as shown in Fig. 8-3.

The fact that zinc protoporphyrin increases concomitantly with ferritin

TABLE 8-3

VALUES OBTAINED BY INDIRECT METHODS OF EVALUATION WITH NORMAL AND DEPLETED IRON STORES

Method, unit of measurement	*Iron stores*			*Comments*
	Normal		*Depleted*	
	Males	*Females*		
Desferrioxamine test (DFI), mg urinary Fe/24 h (500-mg i.m. test dose)	0·6–1·0	0·4–0·6	<0·4	Probably reflects liver parenchymal Fe; useful screening test for Fe overload
Serum ferritin, ng/ml (μg/liter)	*c.* 100	30–40	<5	Useful for detecting reduced iron stores
Sideroblast count, %	Both sexes 40–50		<10	Non-specific; affected by abnormalities of hemoglobin synthesis
Protoporphyrin, μg/dl RBC	50 (usually not >35)		>50	Non-specific; elevated in inflammation and infection
Serum Fe, μg/dl (μ mol/liter)	75–175 (13–31)		<60 (<11)	Non-specific; diurnal variation
Total iron-binding capacity (TIBC), μg/dl (μ mol/liter)	250–400 (45–72)		>400 (>72)	Correlates with direct methods better than does serum Fe
Transferrin saturation, %	18–50		<16	Diurnal variation; non-specific; low in inflammation and infection; best screening test for iron deficiency anemia
Iron absorption, % of 0·56-mg test dose, $^{59}Fe^{2+}$	28 (Range 6–46)		90 (Range 62–100)	Non-specific; most quantitative method for evaluating group

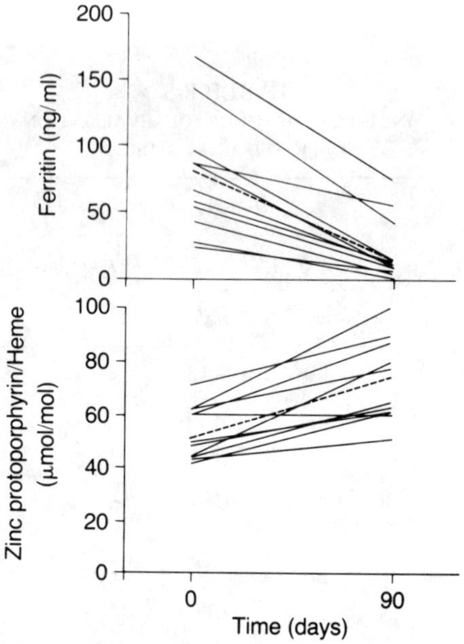

FIG. 8-2. The decrease in serum ferritin concentration and the increase in the whole blood zinc protoporphyrin/heme ratio in individual young men before and after becoming marginally iron deficient. From Labbe *et al.* (1987).

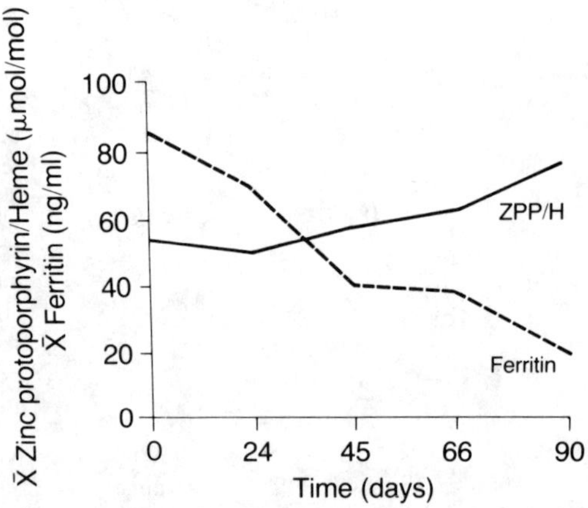

FIG. 8-3. The decrease in the serum ferritin concentration and the increase in the whole blood zinc protoporphyrin/heme (ZPP/H) ratio during the course of iron loss in young men. From Labbe *et al.* (1987).

decreases suggests that iron-deficient erythropoiesis should be considered an early rather than a late manifestation of iron deficiency. The very high sensitivity of the zinc protoporphyrin/heme ratio as an indicator of iron status is especially noteworthy. The test has been evaluated extensively in many subject groups; in each case, elevated zinc protoporphyrin levels have only been associated with iron-deficient erythropoiesis (Labbe *et al.*, 1987). Since the time and cost of determining the zinc protoporphyrin/heme ratio is substantially less than that of evaluating serum ferritin concentration, increasing use of this assessment tool is anticipated in the future.

C. Muscle Iron

The concentration of non-heme iron in the muscles is low but because of their large mass, the total amount is high. Research has shown that in human subjects with normal body iron stores, the total amount of non-heme iron in the muscles is at least equal to that in the liver (Torrance *et al.*, 1968). In individuals with iron overload the iron concentrations in muscles are raised, but to a much smaller extent than in the liver (Morris, 1987).

D. 'Functional Iron'

Most of the iron that is ultimately absorbed moves continuously through several metabolic circuits, the most important of which is:

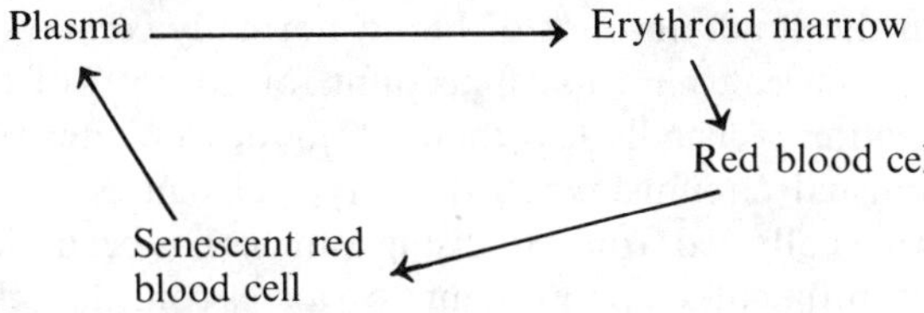

Other metabolic circuits also exist, including the cycles:

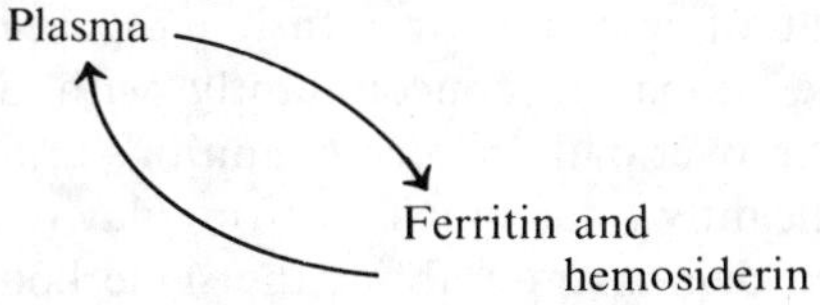

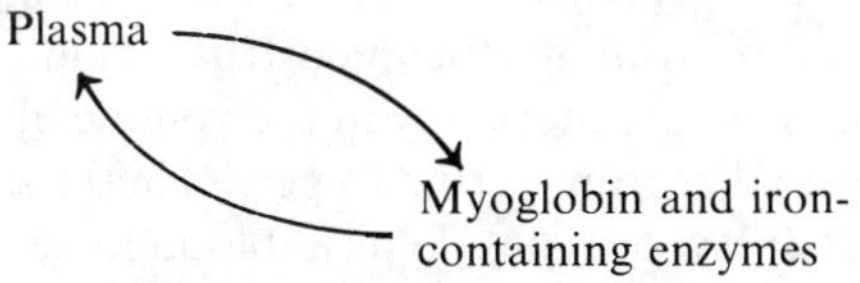

The iron transported via transferrin links the cycles and regulates the distribution of iron in the body.

The term 'functional iron' is often used to refer to the large proportion of body iron which is intimately associated with energy metabolism. Functional iron accounts for about 70% and 80% of the total in adult males and females, respectively. Hemoglobin contains about 80% of the functional iron. Most of the remaining 20% is present in myoglobin, which stores oxygen for energy metabolism in muscle cells. A very small proportion is found in iron–protein enzymes and in cofactors which play key roles in cellular energy metabolism. These include the cytochromes, catalase, and peroxidase, with an iron-containing nucleus, and non-heme enzymes such as certain of the iron-dependent flavoprotein dehydrogenases and oxidases (White, 1980).

III. USUAL BODY IRON LOSSES

Iron losses and body iron turnover have been evaluated in a number of populations of adult men using isotopic methods. Reports from different parts of the world indicate that normal adult men lose about 1 mg of iron/day. About three-fourths of the total body iron excretion occurs via the gastrointestinal tract and includes iron in the bile, in exfoliated mucosal cells, and in the small amount of blood normally escaping into the gut. Dermal losses (sweat, hair, nails) account for 20–25% of the total while urinary excretion is usually less than 100 μg/day (White, 1980).

Under unusual circumstances, these typical figures may change. For example, sweat collected from exercising athletes has been found to contain up to 1 mg iron/day in temperate climates; losses considerably greater than this might be anticipated in the tropics where the volume of sweat can be as much as 5 liters per day (Paulev *et al.*, 1983). Another example of an unusual situation is that of injection or infusion of chelating agents, such as desferrioxamine alone or concomitantly with ascorbic acid, in the treatment of iron overload. In such conditions urinary iron losses can be increased significantly to as much as 10 mg/day (Conte *et al.*, 1984).

While women demonstrate about the same body iron losses as men, maintenance of iron balance is more of a challenge due to the regular additional losses of iron in the menstrual blood, from menarche to menopause. Women vary markedly in the volume of menstrual blood loss but variation is smaller from period to period in the same woman (Morgan and Walters, 1963; Rybo, 1966). Typical blood losses range from 35–70 ml per period, a level containing 16–32 mg of iron (Johnston and McMillan, 1952). In a Scandinavian study of 12 young women over a 12-month period, the mean individual iron losses ranged from 4–26 mg per period and in adolescent girls ranged from 2–59 mg/period (Gregor and Buckley, 1977). Other investigators have reported higher losses with 60–80 ml of blood (27–37 mg iron) regarded as the upper limit or normal loss (Rybo, 1966). Most premenopausal women lose 0·5–0·8 mg/day of iron through menstruation when averaged over all days (not just days of menses), but some lose considerably more.

IV. DIETARY SOURCES OF IRON

A. Heme and Non-heme Iron

Iron in food may be classified as either heme or non-heme iron. Heme, as mentioned before, is the ferroprotoporphyrin component of hemoglobin, myoglobin and certain respiratory enzymes, such as the cytochromes. In human beings, heme is well absorbed; rates of absorption vary inversely with the quantity of iron stores and range from 15–35%. Non-heme iron is less well absorbed but since it is consumed in greater amounts, it makes an important contribution to maintenance of iron status. All the iron in plants—e.g. vegetables, fruits, grains, and nuts—and in non-cellular animal foods—e.g. eggs and dairy products—is non-heme. In addition, approximately half of the iron in meat, fish, and poultry is non-heme; the other half is heme iron. The absorption of non-heme iron ranges widely from 2–20% (Monsen, 1988a, b).

Meats represent a major source of dietary iron, much of which is found in the most absorbable form of heme iron. Non-meat sources of non-heme iron vary greatly in their iron content as a result of varietal differences and differences in the soil and climatic conditions under which the foods are grown or produced. The most concentrated sources of iron are the organ meats, egg yolk, dried legumes, cocoa, cane molasses and parsley; obviously one would have to eat a lot of parsley to obtain the amount of iron provided in one serving of liver. Other reasonable sources of iron include muscle meats, fish and poultry, nuts, green vegetables and whole-meal (or enriched) flour and bread. Boiling green vegetables (Sheets *et al.*, 1931) and milling of wheat (Czerniejewski *et al.*, 1964) lowers the iron content of the final product; similarly with cane sugars, refining reduces the concentration of iron (Hamilton and Minski, 1972–73).

B. Iron Fortification

Fortification of selected foods with stable iron compounds has had a significant impact on the level of potentially available dietary iron. Iron enrichment of white flour in the United States was started in 1945 with the intent of restoring the level of iron in white bread to that in whole-wheat bread. A proposal was made in 1974 to increase the iron fortification level of flour by about $2\frac{1}{2}$ times (Federal Register, 1971) but concerns related to efficacy and safety prevented this change. The safety aspects involved the potential increase in dietary iron intake and consequently more rapid development of iron overload by individuals with idiopathic hemochromatosis, Laennec's cirrhosis and iron-loading anemias (Crosby, 1970; Callender, 1973). Since that time, other foods have gained approval for iron fortification including infant formulas, infant cereals, and an array of breakfast cereals. The question of bioavailability (or absorbability) of the various iron fortificants has long been and still remains an issue of major concern (Pla and Fritz, 1970; Fomon, 1987).

Fortification of foods with bovine hemoglobin is currently under investigation in Chile (Stekel *et al.*, 1986). Initial studies show higher serum ferritin levels in females over 10 years of age who received daily 3–4 10-g cookies fortified with bovine hemoglobin compared to similar subjects receiving unfortified cookies.

As would be expected, total dietary iron intake varies with the total amount of food consumed as well as with the proportion of iron-rich and iron-poor foods selected. The degree of iron contamination may also be important in that processing, storing and cooking of foods and beverages may potentially contribute significant sources of this mineral. It has been estimated that in parts of the developing world, 13–47% of the total dietary iron might be surface contamination (Prabhavathi and Rao, 1981).

C. Contaminant Iron

The iron contributed by iron-containing cookware has long been of interest to food scientists and nutritionists. Recent efforts to reevaluate this issue provide clear evidence that the iron contribution of cookware may be significant (Table 8-4). Cooking time and pH of the food both affect the level of iron leaching; the number of occasions the pan has been used is also important since after numerous cooking episodes, less iron appears to be withdrawn from the container (Table 8-5). The mode of preparation is of keen import. Foods fried in iron pans appear to pick up no iron (Monsen and Cook, 1976); neither a ground beef patty nor an egg prepared in a

TABLE 8-4

COOKING TIME AND MEANS FOR pH, MOISTURE, AND IRON CONTENT OF 20 FOODS[a]

Food[b]	*Cooking order*	*pH (raw)*	*Cooking time (min)*	*Moisture content (%)*			*Iron content (mg/100 g)*		
				Raw	*Cooked in non-iron utensil*	*Cooked in iron utensil*	*Raw*	*Cooked in non-iron utensil*	*Cooked in iron utensil*
Applesauce, unsweetened	20	3·90	20·0	89·67	84·73	85·70[d]	0·35	0·28	7·38[d]
Spaghetti sauce	6	4·50	23·0	90·57	87·45	88·37[d]	0·61	0·69	5·77[d]
Chili with meat and beans	3	5·27	36·0	78·31	72·27	71·55	0·98	1·28	6·27[d]
Medium white sauce	12	6·48	12·0	71·00	70·35	70·21	0·22	0·18	3·30[d]
Scrambled egg	13	7·20	4·0	76·63	69·54	69·48	1·49	1·79	4·76[d]
Spaghetti sauce with meat	5	5·03	34·0	82·63	78·78	78·94	0·71	0·94	3·58[d]
Beef-vegetable stew	7	5·44	77·0	87·06	81·31	82·80[c]	0·66	0·81	3·40[d]
Fried egg	14	7·33	6·0	75·11	69·66	71·25[d]	1·92	1·84	3·48[d]
Spanish rice	10	4·61	27·0	67·56	68·52	68·62	0·87	0·83	2·25[d]
Rice, white	9	6·22	20·0	60·42	60·46	59·62	0·67	0·86	1·97[d]
Pan-broiled bacon	18	6·37	5·0	34·92	18·78	20·98	0·77	1·29	1·92[d]
Poached egg	15	7·58	5·0	75·95	77·60	77·46	1·87	1·71	2·32[d]
Fried chicken	2	6·15	17·5	66·83	52·10	52·18	0·88	1·37	1·89[d]
Pancakes	11	6·71	3·3	54·32	46·40	46·89[c]	0·63	0·81	1·31[d]
Stir-fried green beans	19	6·09	5·0	89·44	83·30	83·77	0·64	0·69	1·18[d]
Pan-broiled hamburger	1	5·77	9·0	58·89	59·22	56·75[c]	1·49	2·00	2·29[d]
Fried potatoes	16	5·94	3·0	80·87	59·07	58·45	0·42	0·59	0·80[d]
Fried corn tortillas	17	9·34	1·0	47·93	13·09	14·35[d]	0·86	1·14	1·23[c]
Pan-fried beef liver with onions	4	6·10	11·0	75·37	63·15	63·16	3·10	3·82	3·87
Baked cornbread	8	6·81	15·0	42·37	33·91	29·57[d]	0·67	0·83	0·86

[a] From Brittin and Nossaman (1986).
[b] Listed in descending order of increase in iron content of foods cooked in iron utensil over iron content of the same food cooked in non-iron utensil.
[c] Means for cooked in iron and cooked in non-iron utensils differ, $P < 0{\cdot}05$.
[d] Means for cooked in iron and cooked in non-iron utensils differ, $P < 0{\cdot}01$.

TABLE 8-5

MEAN IRON CONTENT OF THREE FOODS COOKED IN TWO IRON UTENSILS[a]

Food	*Iron content (mg/100 g) of foods cooked in:*	
	Iron skillet A[b]	*Iron skillet B*[c]
Spaghetti sauce	5·77	5·84
Scrambled egg	4·76	5·38
Apple sauce	7·38	16·36*

[a] From Brittin and Nossaman (1986).
[b] Skillet A—used daily for a week before the project.
[c] Skillet B—used 2–3 times prior to the study.
* $P < 0{\cdot}01$; other differences are non-significant at 0·05 level.

'seasoned' iron frying pan showed any increase in iron content compared to being cooked in a glass pan.

There has been some question about the bioavailability of iron derived from iron cookware. Efforts have been made to address this question, at least through work involving laboratory rats (Martinez and Vannucchi, 1986). Iron deficiency was produced in young Wistar rats over a period of five weeks; control rats received a complete diet throughout the experiment. After the period of iron depletion, the animals were subdivided into three groups: one continued to receive the basal diet, the second was fed a complete diet and the third received the basal diet cooked in an iron pot. After four weeks, the hematologic measures of the animals fed the diet cooked in the iron pot did not differ significantly from those of the animals fed the complete diet. Indirectly, this study suggests that the traditional habit of cooking food in iron pots may be effective in preventing or treating iron deficiency.

D. Iron Intake

Iron consumption in the United States today is about 14·6 and 10·2 mg/day for men and women, respectively, 15–64 years of age (Raper *et al.*, 1984). Over 50 years ago, daily iron intake was estimated to have been between 15 and 22 mg (Sherman, 1937). The basis for this change is believed to relate to multiple factors: (1) the food supply is not as frequently 'contaminated'; (2) more processed foods are produced; and (3) daily kcalorie intake has decreased. At the present time, available data suggest that healthy North Americans consume approximately 6–7 mg of iron per 1000 kcalories per day (McLennan *et al.*, 1973; Raper *et al.*, 1984) (Table 8-6). No matter what

TABLE 8-6
TOTAL AND AVAILABLE IRON INTAKE DENSITIES FOR 9 547 INDIVIDUALS IN THE 1977–78 NATIONWIDE FOOD CONSUMPTION SURVEY[a,b]

Sex and age (years)	*Total iron per 1 000 kcal (mg)*		*Available iron per 1 000 kcal (mg)*	
	Intake	*RDA*	*Intake*	*RDA*
Boys and girls				
1–2	6·9	12·5	0·4	1·3
3–5	6·6	7·7	0·5	0·8
6–8	6·4	4·8	0·5	0·5
Boys and men				
9–11	6·6	5·2	0·5	0·5
12–14	6·5	6·6	0·5	0·7
15–18	6·4	6·4	0·5	0·6
19–22	6·1	3·4	0·5	0·3
23–34	6·3	3·7	0·5	0·4
35–50	6·6	3·7	0·6	0·4
51–64	6·8	4·1	0·6	0·4
65–74	7·4	4·2	0·6	0·4
75 and over	7·1	4·9	0·5	0·5
Girls and women				
9–11	6·5	5·6	0·5	0·6
12–14	6·1	8·2	0·5	0·8
15–18	6·2	8·6	0·5	0·9
19–22	6·7	8·6	0·5	0·9
23–34	6·4	9·0	0·5	0·9
35–50	6·8	9·0	0·5	0·9
51–64	7·2	5·4	0·6	0·5
65–74	7·1	5·6	0·5	0·6
75 and over	7·6	6·3	0·5	0·6

[a] From Raper *et al.* (1984).
[b] Available iron was calculated using the original method developed by Monsen *et al.* (1978) and the refined model of Monsen and Balintfy (1982).

the composition of the diet, very little of the total food iron ultimately penetrates the mucosal barrier; factors affecting the absorptive process will be summarized later.

Improving the iron intake, especially of premenopausal women, has been a major goal in nutrition counseling and education programs for this population. A number of strategies have been developed and tested over the years; some have been far more successful than others. Hertzler and

TABLE 8-7

SERVING SIZES AND IRON POINTS OF FOODS IN THE IRON CHECK LIST[a]

Foods	*Quantity*	*Iron points*[b]	*Foods*	*Quantity*	*Iron points*[b]
Milk and milk products			Peach, dried	2 halves	3
Milk, skim, low-fat, whole	1 c	1	Prunes, dried	5	6
Milk chocolate	1 c	3	Raisins	2 tbsp	3
Cheese	1 oz	1			
Cottage cheese	$\frac{1}{2}$ c	1	*Breads and cereals*		
Custard	1 c	3	Biscuits	2–2 in	3
Pudding	1 c	3	Bread	1 slice	3
Yogurt	1 c	1	Cereal, cooked	$\frac{1}{2}$ c	3
			Cereal, ready-to-eat	1 oz	3
Fruits and vegetables			Cornbread	1 piece	3
Apple	$\frac{1}{2}$ c	1	Crackers	4	3
Asparagus	$\frac{1}{2}$ c	1	Macaroni	$\frac{1}{2}$ c	3
Banana	1 small	3	Muffin	1–3 in	3
Bean sprouts	$\frac{1}{2}$ c	1	Noodles	$\frac{1}{2}$ c	3
Beets	$\frac{1}{2}$ c	1	Rice	$\frac{1}{2}$ c	3
Broccoli	$\frac{1}{2}$ c	3	Roll	1 small	3
Brussels sprouts	$\frac{1}{2}$ c	3	Spaghetti	$\frac{1}{2}$ c	3
Cabbage	$\frac{1}{2}$ c	1	Tortilla chips	1 oz	3
Cantaloupe	$\frac{1}{2}$ c	3	Waffle	$4\frac{1}{2}$ in	3
Carrots	$\frac{1}{2}$ c	1	*High-calorie choices*		
Cauliflower	$\frac{1}{2}$ c	1	Chocolate cake	$\frac{1}{16}$ piece	3
Celery	$\frac{1}{2}$ c	1	Plain cake	$\frac{1}{16}$ piece	3
Corn	$\frac{1}{2}$ c	3	Coffee cake	$\frac{1}{16}$ piece	3
Cranberries	$\frac{1}{2}$ c	1	Fig bars	4	3
Grapefruit	$\frac{1}{2}$ c	1	Chocolate chip cookies	4	3

Grapes	$\frac{1}{2}$ c	1
Greens, cooked	$\frac{1}{2}$ c	6
Green beans	$\frac{1}{2}$ c	1
Lettuce	$\frac{1}{2}$ c	1
Lima beans	$\frac{1}{2}$ c	6
Lime	$\frac{1}{2}$ c	1
Okra	$\frac{1}{2}$ c	1
Onion	$\frac{1}{2}$ c	1
Orange	$\frac{1}{2}$ c	1
Parsley	$\frac{1}{2}$ c	1
Peach	$\frac{1}{2}$ c	1
Pear	$\frac{1}{2}$ c	1
Peas	$\frac{1}{2}$ c	6
Pineapple	$\frac{1}{2}$ c	1
Plums	$\frac{1}{2}$ c	1
Potato	1–$2\frac{1}{2}$ in	3
Pumpkin	$\frac{1}{2}$ c	3
Rhubarb	$\frac{1}{2}$ c	3
Squash, summer	$\frac{1}{2}$ c	1
Squash, winter	$\frac{1}{2}$ c	3
Strawberries	$\frac{1}{2}$ c	3
Sweet potato	1 small	3
Tomato	1 small	3
Watermelon	4 in × 8 in wedge	6
Apricots, dried	5 med. halves	3
Dates, dried	5	3
Doughnut	$3\frac{1}{2}$ in	3
Pie	$\frac{1}{7}$	3
Meat, fish, poultry		
Dry beans or dry peas, cooked	1 c	15
Beef	3 oz	9
Chicken	$\frac{1}{2}$ c	6
Clams	3 oz	15
Egg	1	3
Fish	3 oz	3
Lamb	2 oz	6
Liver	3 oz	24
Oysters	8	18
Pork	3 oz	9
Shrimp	3 oz	6
Tofu	$\frac{1}{4}$ block	6
Veal	3 oz	9
High-calorie choices		
Bacon	3 slices	3
Hot dog	2 oz	3
Braunschweiger	1 oz	3
Luncheon meat	1 oz	3
Sardines, in oil	3 oz	3
Tuna, in oil	3 oz	3
Peanut butter	4 tbsp	3
Peanuts	20 large	3

[a] From Hertzler and McAnge (1986).
[b] One iron point approximates 0·3 mg iron, or a range of 0·2–0·5 mg; 3 iron points approximate 0·9 mg iron.

TABLE 8-8
FREQUENCY DISTRIBUTION OF IRON POINTS BY FOOD GROUPS[a]

Food group	*Iron score*		*Subjects (no. = 89)*	
	Points	*mg*	*Frequency*	*%*
Milk	0	0	41	46·1
	1–5	≤0·9	37	41·6
	6–9	1·0–2·7	11	12·3
Fruit/vegetables	0	0	2	2·2
	1–5	≤0·9	4	4·5
	6–9	1·0–2·7	38	42·7
	10–21	3·0–6·3	39	43·8
	22–33	6·4–9·9	6	6·7
Bread/cereals	1–5	≤0·9	3	3·3
	6–9	1·0–2·7	21	23·6
	10–21	3·0–6·3	65	73·0
Meat/alternates	1–5	≤0·9	2	2·2
	6–9	1·0–2·7	18	20·2
	10–21	2·8–6·3	35	39·3
	22–60	6·4–18·0	34	37·2

[a] From Hertzler and McAnge (1986).

McAnge (1986) recently developed an iron checklist comprised of 93 foods to evaluate food choices in terms of iron concentration or frequency of use and to incorporate principles of iron nutriture. Foods were given points based on their iron content (Tables 8-7 and 8-8). The correlation between points scored on the iron checklist and the milligrams of iron calculated from the same 24-hour recall was 0·77. Results from the iron checklist indicated that almost half of the group (48%) had an iron intake below 75%

TABLE 8-9
FREQUENCY DISTRIBUTION OF IRON SCORES[a]

Iron score		*Subjects (no. = 89)*	
Points	*% 18 mg*	*No.*	*%*
18–30	≤50	4	4·5
31–47	51–75	39	43·8
48–60	76–100	30	33·7
60+	>100	16	18·0

[a] From Hertzler and McAnge (1986).

of 18 mg (Table 8-9). Helping women to use this tool may lead to improved iron intake over time.

V. IRON ABSORPTION

The term 'absorption' refers to the movement of iron from the gut, through mucosal cells and into the plasma. Uptake of iron by mucosal cells may exceed absorption, since some iron entering the cells may not be released into the plasma. Within the gut lumen, the amount of iron made available for uptake by the cells is influenced by both dietary components and digestive secretions (intraluminal factors). Uptake and absorption are further affected by mucosal and corporeal factors. Mucosal factors are those within the intestinal absorptive cells, while corporeal factors encompass those related to iron status and iron metabolism within the body (Conrad, 1970).

In humans, iron absorption takes place largely in the duodenum; iron from ferrous salts is generally absorbed to a greater extent than that from ferric salts but valency may not be critical since some ferric compounds are more bioavailable than some ferrous compounds (Fritz *et al.*, 1970). Effective absorption of iron from non-heme iron–protein compounds apparently requires that iron be released from conjugation, whereas the iron in heme compounds is absorbed as the heme moiety into the mucosal cells of the intestine without the necessity of release from its bound form (Hallberg and Slovell, 1967) as shown in Fig. 8-4.

A. Measurement of Iron Absorption

The availability of radioisotopes of iron have allowed for easier and more precise evaluation of iron absorption than was possible in years past. Absorption of iron from orally administered labeled compounds or biologically labeled foods can be determined from the amount of unabsorbed iron in the stools. In addition, methods of whole body counting of radioactivity have now become available for use in man. Both of these procedures are direct and quantitative. The former method is more subject to error and requires complete stool collections from one to two weeks. The latter is subject to little error and requires very little cooperation from the subject, although failure to record unusual blood loss will yield falsely low values for absorption.

Indirect measurement of iron absorption is possible by determining the amount of radioiron in the circulating red cell mass two weeks after oral

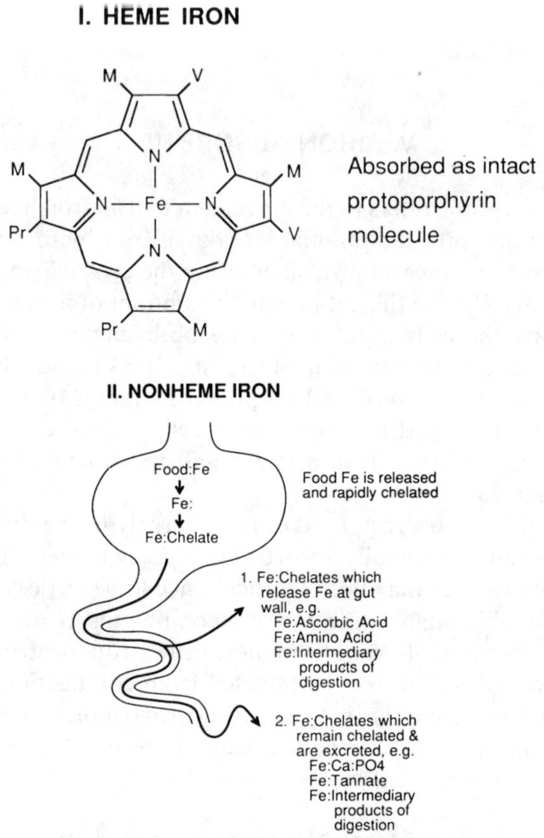

FIG. 8-4. Schematic diagram of the absorption of the two forms of food iron: heme and non-heme iron. From Monsen (1988b).

administration of a test dose. This is justified since most of the absorbed iron is rapidly incorporated into newly synthesized erythrocytes. Needless-to-say, falsely low results will be obtained when the rate of erythropoiesis or iron incorporation by erythrocytes is subnormal. A refinement of this procedure is a double isotope method in which one radioisotope of iron is administered orally and another intravenously. The amount of intravenously administered iron incorporated into red cells permits a correction of the estimated absorption of the orally given iron (accounting for the less than 100% incorporation of iron by red cells within the usual two-week period) as explained by White (1980).

B. Heme Iron Absorption

As mentioned previously, the heme portion of hemoglobin and myoglobin released by the action of proteases on the protein moieties is taken up without further change by mucosal cells. Heme is kept in solution by the products of protein degradation which help prevent the formation of insoluble heme polymers. Uptake of heme is little affected by chelating compounds which markedly influence the availability of inorganic iron. Once heme enters the intestinal mucosal cell, iron is removed from porphyrin and mixes with the inorganic iron which has entered the cell (Wheby *et al.*, 1970).

The effects of various culinary preparations on heme iron absorption from meat and on the denaturation of heme iron was recently examined in human volunteers (Martinez-Torres *et al.*, 1986). The iron absorption from heme in beef exposed to prolonged heating was markedly reduced, following the degree of denaturation of heme (Fig. 8-5). Inclusion of the overcooked meat within a vegetable-containing meal led to further (although modest) reduction in heme iron absorption (Table 8-10).

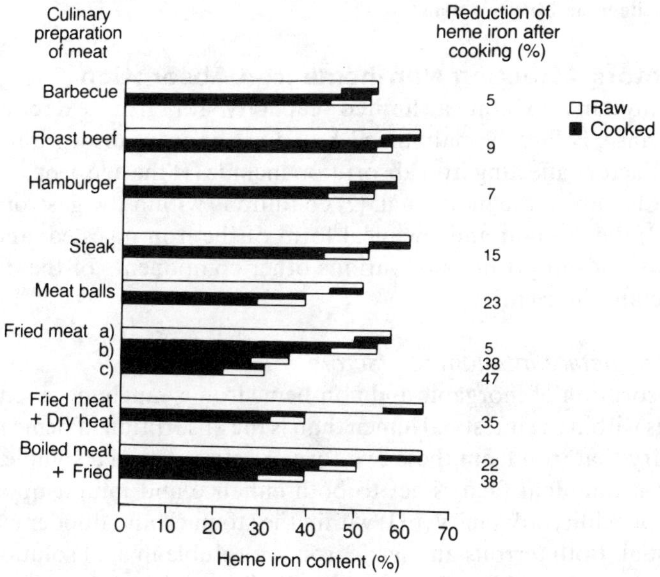

FIG. 8-5. Reduction of heme iron content in various kinds of meat culinary preparations: (a), (b) and (c) represent the reduction of heme in ground meat fried during 8, 18 and 30 minutes, respectively. The inset within each bar represents one standard deviation; $n = 4$ assays. From Martinez-Torres *et al.* (1986).

TABLE 8-10

IRON ABSORPTION FROM HEME IN COOKED BEEF (ALONE) AND FROM HEME IN COOKED BEEF IN A VEGETABLE-CONTAINING MEAL[a]

	Mean iron absorption (%)		
	From heme		*From reference dose (iron ascorbate)*
	Observed	*Expected*[b]	
Fried meat[c]	19·4	23·4	25·3[e]
Overcooked meat[d]	14·5	23·4	
Meal with fried meat[c]	26·7	25·2	31·8[e]
Meal with overcooked meat[d]	11·7	25·2	

[a] Data from Martinez-Torres *et al.* (1986).
[b] Expected iron absorption was determined using the formula $y = 14{\cdot}4 + 0{\cdot}31 \times x$, where y is the heme iron absorption and x is the reference dose absorption.
[c] The meat was fried for 10 minutes.
[d] The meat was fried for 10 minutes and kept hot in an oven at 350°F for 60 minutes.
[e] Composite mean from two trials.

C. Factors Affecting Non-heme Iron Absorption

Since humans exhibit a limited capacity for iron excretion, iron homeostasis is largely maintained by adjusting iron absorption to body needs. Factors affecting iron absorption include (1) the age, iron status and state of health of the individual; (2) conditions within the gastrointestinal tract; (3) the amount and chemical form of the iron ingested; and (4) the amounts and proportions of various other components of the diet, both organic and inorganic.

(i) Non-dietary intraluminal factors

The absorption of inorganic and non-heme iron is much more sensitive to changes within the intestinal lumen than is the absorption of heme iron. It is necessary that iron from these two former sources be in a soluble, ionized form. Intraluminal factors act to both enhance and inhibit uptake. The degree of acidity/alkalinity (pH) within the stomach and duodenum is very influential. Both ferrous and ferric iron are soluble in acid solution. Some ferrous iron remains in solution in the alkaline medium of the gut, but at a pH above 5, ferric iron forms insoluble complexes with hydroxyl ions. In the duodenum, ferric iron cannot remain in solution unless it forms soluble chelation compounds. Gastric hydrochloric acid helps to keep inorganic iron released from foods in solution, allowing more of it to be chelated (Krause, 1970).

Several iron-binding proteins have been isolated from gastric juice and it has been suggested that they may play a role in regulating iron absorption. Whether or not body iron status influences the concentration of these proteins in the gastric juice is the subject of some debate. Experts suggest that it appears unlikely that these gastric proteins play a significant role in modifying iron absorption (Turnbull, 1974).

The degree to which pancreatic secretions affect iron absorption is also uncertain. Higher than normal iron absorption has been observed in pathological conditions characterized by pancreatic insufficiency and in experimental animals following ligation of the pancreatic duct. However, other researchers have shown that iron absorption can be significantly reduced in hemachromatosis by addition of a pancreatic extract with the oral dose of iron. The full importance of pancreatic secretions in regulating iron absorption remains to be determined (White, 1980).

(ii) Corporeal and mucosal factors

The mechanism through which body iron status regulates the absorptive capacity of mucosal cells is still not completely understood. It is known, however, that body iron status or the amount of total body iron influences the process of iron absorption. Except in certain pathological conditions, iron absorption is directly related to the rate of erythropoiesis. The existence of a humoral factor for controlling iron absorption in response to body needs has been postulated but not proven (White, 1980).

Fletcher and Huehns (1968) proposed that iron absorption, in response to body iron needs, is regulated by the relative degree of saturation of the two iron-binding sites on the transferrin molecule. These researchers showed that these two binding sites are different and that the transferrin molecule demonstrates functional heterogeneity. If this idea is substantiated it means that transport iron cannot be considered a uniform pool; it also suggests a possible link between corporeal and mucosal factors.

A number of mucosal factors have been studied to determine their contribution to the regulation of iron uptake. Specific iron-receptor sites on brush-border membranes of mucosal cells have been identified by in-vitro studies (Greenberger *et al.*, 1969; Huebers *et al.*, 1971a, b). Some evidence was provided by these investigators for an effect of body iron status on brush-border binding capacity.

Studies conducted in animal models or in in-vitro systems have yielded interesting, but inconclusive findings. Radioiron, administered intravenously, has been shown to be incorporated into developing mucosal cells and the amount incorporated was related to body iron stores and inversely related to iron absorption (Conrad and Crosby, 1963; Conrad *et al.*, 1964; Weintraub *et al.*, 1965). Such findings suggest that total cellular iron plays a role in regulating absorption and that plasma iron serves as a 'messenger' to mucosal cells. However, research by other workers who have attempted to relate mucosal iron content to degree of iron absorption has yielded inconclusive results (Balcerzak and Greenberger, 1968).

The same can be said for investigations of the distribution of iron within mucosal cells, specifically the extent of its presence within mitochondria. While some evidence supports an association between lower mitochondrial iron concentration and iron deficiency (Richmond *et al.*, 1972), the opposite circumstance has not been observed in the iron-overloaded animal (Howard and Jacobs, 1972). Such findings suggest that the iron status of cellular mitochondria may play a role in the increased iron absorption associated with iron deficiency, but the decreased absorption of iron overload apparently cannot be explained by such a mechanism.

Finally, there is evidence for the existence of a transferrin-like, non-ferritin protein (or proteins) in the cytoplasm of mucosal cells, especially in those from iron-deficient animals (Huebers *et al.*, 1971a, b; Worwood and Jacobs, 1971; Worwood *et al.*, 1971). It has been suggested that such a protein (or proteins) may function as a carrier(s) to transfer iron across the cell, and that, since its concentration appeared to reflect body iron status, it may play a role in the regulation of iron absorption (Jacobs, 1973). One research team suggested that uptake of iron by mucosal cells might be controlled by a mucosal transport mechanism which was influenced by cellular iron status (Sheehan and Frenkel, 1972).

While an abundance of research has accumulated in this area, interpretation and comparison of results involving use of isolated mucosal cells (or subcellular fractions thereof) and of isolated segments of intestine have been complicated by differences in experimental techniques, by possible contamination of mucosal cell material with submucosal substances, and by the difficulty of duplicating in-vivo conditions in in-vitro experiments. There is in addition the obvious problem of applying to man the findings obtained with experimental animals.

(iii) Dietary factors: general

Using the radioisotopic methods referred to previously, absorption of non-heme iron has been found to be affected markedly by the dietary components that the non-heme iron comes in contact with in the gastrointestinal tract. Much of the research in this area has been conducted by Monsen and colleagues (Monsen, 1988a) who employed test meals providing 700 kcalories, 29 g protein, 68 g carbohydrate, 35 g fat, and 4·1 mg iron. The semi-synthetic meal was composed of egg albumin, dextrimaltose, and corn oil; the standard meal was composed of beef, potatoes, cornmeal, bread, margarine, ice milk, and peaches.

(iv) Dietary factors: enhancing

One of the more effective dietary factors that increases non-heme iron absorption is ascorbic acid. Adding ascorbic acid to the very low iron availability semi-synthetic meal enhanced non-heme iron absorption (Fig. 8-6). Above the 7·5 molar ratio of ascorbic acid:iron (i.e. 100 mg ascorbic acid:3 mg iron), the rate of increase was substantially more modest with larger additions of ascorbic acid. Addition of ascorbic acid to the higher bioavailable standard meal increased iron absorption (Cook and Monsen, 1977). However, the influence of ascorbic acid is greatest on low bioavailable meals, such as vegetarian meals.

The enhancing effect of ascorbic acid is seen only when it is consumed in the same meal (Cook and Monsen, 1977). Giving ascorbic acid 4 or 8 h

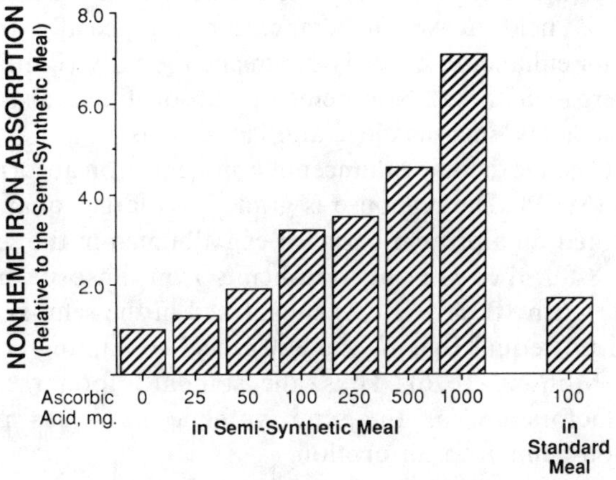

FIG. 8-6. Enhanced absorption of non-heme iron when ascorbic acid was added to a 700-kcal semi-synthetic meal fed to healthy adult men. Absorption of non-heme iron from the semi-synthetic meal with no addition of ascorbic acid was set at 1·0. The standard meal with ascorbic acid is compared with the standard meal with no ascorbic acid. From Cook and Monsen (1977).

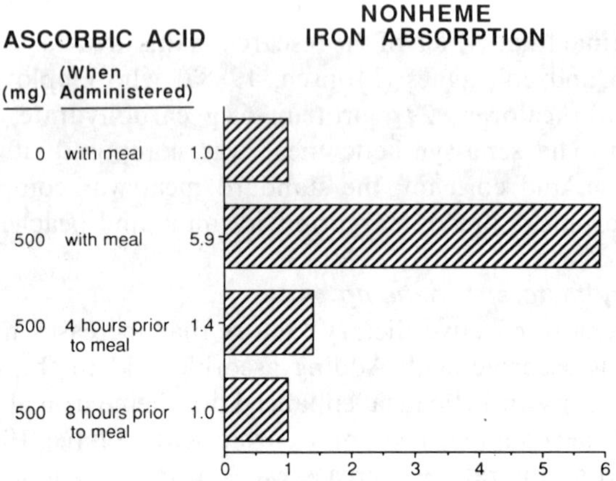

FIG. 8-7. The effect on non-heme iron absorption of administering ascorbic acid either with or prior to a 700-kcal meal presented to healthy adult men. Absorption of non-heme iron for the meal with no ascorbic acid was set at 1·0. From Cook and Monsen (1977).

before a test meal had no impact (Fig. 8-7). Ascorbic acid is a reducing agent and is capable of chelating iron. Thus, ascorbic acid can maintain iron as a soluble complex (Monsen, 1982). If ascorbic acid is oxidized, as occurs when food is held at warm temperatures, especially in non-acidic conditions, its enhancing effect is diminished greatly (Lynch and Cook, 1980; Hallberg *et al.*, 1982). Non-heme iron absorption is also enhanced by other organic acids, such as citric and lactic acids.

A second effective dietary enhancer of non-heme iron absorption is meat/fish/poultry (MFP). The response is graded. As larger quantities of beef were substituted on a protein basis for egg albumen in the semi-synthetic meal (Fig. 8-8), the rate of non-heme iron absorption increased. Nonetheless, when 100 g beef was substituted in the semi-synthetic meal, the rate did not equal that of the 100 g beef-containing standard meal (Cook and Monsen, 1976). Thus, the standard food meal has more enhancing factors and/or the semi-synthetic meal has more factors inhibiting non-heme iron absorption.

Substitutions of other animal proteins in both the semi-synthetic and standard meals showed that cellular proteins (i.e. liver, lamb, pork, chicken, and fish), had enhancing capabilities similar to those of beef (Fig. 8-9). However, non-cellular animal proteins (i.e. milk, cheese, and egg; Cook and Monsen, 1976), and the plant protein, soy, did not enhance non-heme iron

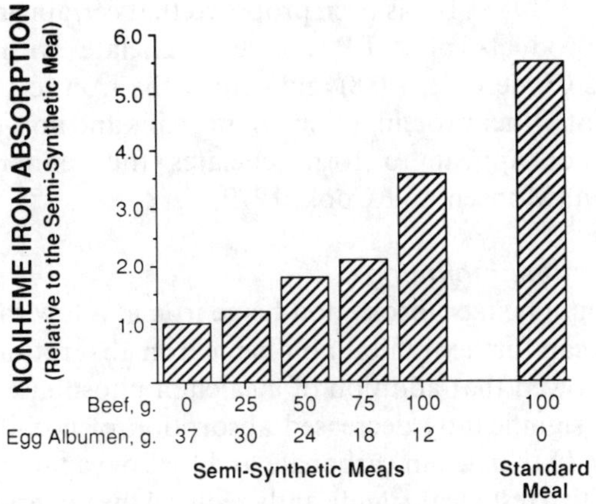

FIG. 8-8. Enhanced absorption of non-heme iron when increasing quantities of beef replaced egg albumen in 700-kcal meals presented to healthy adult women. The standard meal contained the same total protein and calories. Absorption of non-heme iron from the semi-synthetic meal (37 g egg albumen) was set at 1·0. From Cook and Monsen (1976).

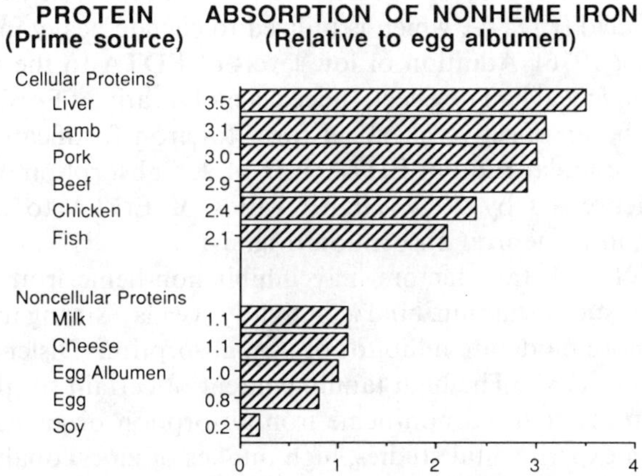

FIG. 8-9. Absorption of non-heme iron when an amount of protein equal to that in 25 g egg albumen or 100 g beef was presented in a 700-kcal meal to healthy adult subjects. Absorption of non-heme iron was set at 1·0 in the meal containing egg albumen. From Monsen (1988b).

absorption. In fact, soy inhibited absorption of non-heme iron (Cook *et al.*, 1981; Lynch *et al.*, 1985). It has been proposed that certain amino acids and intermediary products of MFP digestion chelate with soluble iron (Slatkavitz and Clydesdale, 1988) and deliver the iron to the gut mucosa (Monsen, 1988b). Other proteins (i.e. plant proteins and non-cellular animal proteins) do not appear to form chelates that enhance non-heme iron absorption (Monsen and Cook, 1979).

(v) Dietary factors: inhibiting

In general, human beings absorb non-heme iron at a low rate, and certain dietary factors can further inhibit non-heme iron absorption. Monsen and Cook (1976) showed that addition of a calcium phosphate salt to a semi-synthetic meal significantly decreased absorption of non-heme iron (Fig. 8-10). Similarly, both calcium carbonate and hydroxyapatite when given as supplements with a test meal, significantly reduced the retention of ^{59}Fe from the meal. The single addition of calcium as calcium chloride or phosphate as potassium phosphate had only a small effect on non-heme iron absorption (Monsen and Cook, 1976). The hypothesis proposed is that calcium phosphate and non-heme iron form an aggregate macromolecule that does not release iron. Phosphate alone, unless in very high levels, and calcium alone do not block non-heme iron absorption.

Another inhibitory compound is the food additive ethylene diamine tetra-acetic acid (EDTA), which is utilized to chelate heavy metals (Cook and Monsen, 1976). Addition of low levels of EDTA to the standard or semi-synthetic meal had no effect. Indeed, a molar ratio of Fe:EDTA of 1:1 appears to be an effective chemical form for iron fortification of food. However, at a molar ratio of EDTA:iron of 2:1, absorption of non-heme iron was depressed by 50%. Higher ratios of EDTA to iron further depressed non-heme iron absorption (Fig. 8-10).

Several other dietary factors may inhibit non-heme iron absorption. Polyphenols, such as tannin, bind iron tightly. Tea is a strong inhibitor and coffee is a more moderate inhibitor of iron absorption (Disler *et al.*, 1975; Gillooly *et al.*, 1983). The high tannin content of certain sorghum strains may explain the reduced non-heme iron absorption observed with their ingestion. In experimental studies, high intakes of zinc, cobalt, cadmium, copper, and manganese decrease iron absorption, which suggests common and competing absorption pathways. Another factor associated with poor iron bioavailability is pica, the eating of clay and earth. The greater the cation capacity of the clay, the greater the inhibition. Physical binding of iron by clay may explain the iron deficiency seen in geophagia.

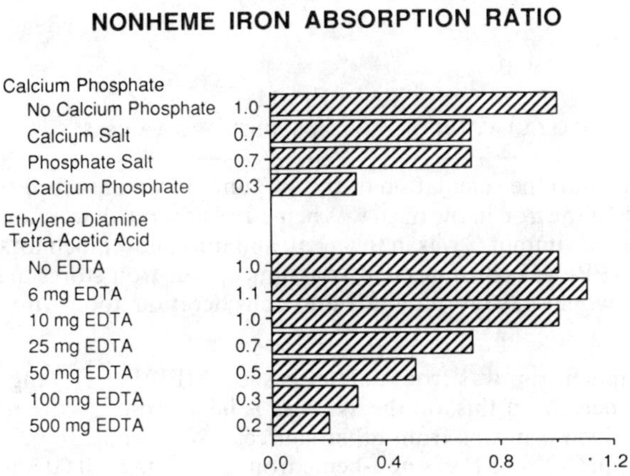

FIG. 8-10. Decreased absorption of non-heme iron in healthy adult men who were presented with 700-kcal semi-synthetic meals with the addition of calcium, phosphate, or EDTA. Absorption of non-heme iron was set at 1·0 in meals to which no calcium phosphate, or EDTA was added. From Monsen and Cook (1976), and Cook and Monsen (1976).

Wheat bran is associated with low iron bioavailability. It has been suggested that the phytate in bran binds with iron. Yet enzymatically dephytinized bran showed similar iron inhibition (Simpson *et al.*, 1981), while acid-washed dephytinized bran did not. Regardless, other foods with high phytate content, such as wheat germ and lentils, exhibit low iron bioavailability. The influence of soybeans on non-heme iron is also controversial. Although several experimental studies point to an inhibitory effect, no apparent differences were observed in long-term studies (Morris, 1987).

(vi) Dietary factors: accounting for them in estimating iron bioavailability in diets

Monsen *et al.* (1978) proposed a mathematical model to estimate iron bioavailability on the basis of composition of each eating occasion (Table 8-11). Use of this model provides a more precise estimate of bioavailability of dietary iron than the 10% absorption values used in setting the Recommended Daily Allowance. The Monsen *et al.* (1978) model is based on expected iron absorption in individuals with adequate iron stores: absorption in such individuals would be lower than that in iron-deficient individuals.

TABLE 8-11
CALCULATION OF IRON ABSORBED FROM MEALS[a]

Three factors go into the calculation of the amount of iron absorbed from a meal: first, how much of the iron in the meal was heme and how much was non-heme iron; second, how much vitamin C was in the meal; and third, how much total meat, fish, and poultry (MFP) was consumed. (It is assumed your iron stores are moderate; otherwise, you would have to take this into consideration, too.) Answer these six questions:

1. How much iron was from animal tissues (MFP)? ______ mg
2. Forty percent of this, on the average, is heme iron. ______ mg heme iron
3. How much iron was from other sources? ______ mg
4. This, plus 60% of (1), is non-heme iron. ______ mg + 0·60 × mg = ______ mg non-heme iron
5. How much vitamin C was in the meal? Less than 25 milligrams is low; 25–75 milligrams is medium; more than 75 milligrams is high
6. How much MFP was in the meal? Less than 1 ounce lean MFP is low; 1 to 3 ounces is medium; more than 3 ounces is high.

Now calculate:

You absorbed 23% of the heme iron (2), or ______ mg.

Now, take your best score from (5) and (6). If either vitamin C or MFP was high or if both were medium, the availability of your non-heme iron was high. If neither was high but one was medium, the availability of your non-heme iron was medium. If both were low, your non-heme iron had poor availability. You absorbed:

High availability: 8% of the non-heme iron.
Medium availability: 5%.
Poor availability: 3%.
Your total: ______ mg non-heme iron absorbed.

Add the two together:

______ mg heme iron absorbed
______ mg non-heme iron absorbed
Total = ______ mg iron absorbed

The RDA assumes you will absorb 10% of the iron you ingest. Thus, if you are a man of any age or a woman over 50 years old (RDA 10 milligrams), you need to absorb 1 milligram per day; if you are a woman 11–50 years old (RDA 18 milligrams), you need to absorb 1·8 milligrams. If you have higher menstrual losses than the average woman, you may still need more.

[a] After Monsen *et al.* (1978).

VI. IRON REQUIREMENTS

Sufficient iron needs to be consumed to replace losses and support growth during those periods of the life cycle when new tissue is being created. Acceptable data for average body iron losses are available. Requirements for growth can be calculated for increases in body size and hemoglobin mass. Since accumulation and maintenance of iron stores is a component of desirable iron status, enough iron must be consumed during growth and pregnancy to permit positive iron balance. Estimates of absorbed iron requirements for several age–sex categories are summarized in Table 8-12.

VII. RECOMMENDED IRON INTAKE

Translating physiological requirements for iron into dietary recommendations is hampered by individual differences in absorptive capacity as well as differing iron availability among foods and various combinations of foods. Further difficulty relates to the body's ability to increase iron absorption in the face of deficiency and reduce it in the face of excess. The estimates shown in column two of Table 8-12 assume an absorption of 10%. The Recommended Dietary Allowances (RDAs) for iron (column four of Table 8-12) also assume an overall average absorption of 10% (Food and Nutrition Board, 1980). Since the RDAs are meant to meet the needs of essentially all healthy, normal individuals, the RDAs for iron closely approximate the high values of ranges suggested by the American Medical Association committee in 1968 (column two of Table 8-12).

In 1970, the World Health Organization (WHO) also established recommendations for daily iron intake (Table 8-12). Recognizing the known differences in iron absorption from mixed diets containing varying amounts of animal foods, WHO recommended iron intakes for adult men of 9, 6, and 5 mg/day when diets contained, respectively, less than 10%, between 10 and 25% and over 25% of the kcalories from animal foods. The corresponding recommendations for menstruating women were 28, 19, and 14 mg (WHO, 1970, 1972). As it is now known that all animal food does not enhance iron absorption, it would be more precise to relate recommended iron intake to cellular animal protein, excluding non-cellular animal foods such as milk and eggs from the calculation.

Infants have been singled out by the American Academy of Pediatrics (1969) as needing special attention to the adequacy of dietary iron. A daily iron intake of 1 mg/kg per day (up to a maximum of 15 mg/day by the age of

TABLE 8-12

ESTIMATED IRON REQUIREMENTS AND RECOMMENDED DIETARY INTAKES[a] (From White, 1980)

	Am. Med. Assoc.		*Food Nutr. Bd*		*WHO*			
	Absorbed iron	*Dietary iron*	*Age*	*Dietary iron*	*Age*	*Animal foods providing*		
						<10% of cal.	*10–25% of cal.*	*>25% of cal.*
Infants	0·5–1·5	1·5/kg to max. of 15	0–6 months	10	0–4 months	[b]	[b]	[b]
			6–12 months	15	5–12 months	7	5	4
Children	0·4–1·0	4–10	1–3 years	15	1–12 years	10	7	5
			4–10 years	10				
Adolescents	1·0–2·0	10–20	11–18 years	18	13–16 years			
					Boys	18	12	9
					Girls	24	16	12
Adult males	0·5–1·0	5–10	19+ years	10	18+ years	9	6	5
Adult females								
Menst.	0·7–2·0	7–20	19–50 years	18	Menst.	28	19	14
Non-menst.	0·5–1·0	5–10	51+ years	10	Non-menst.	9	6	5
Pregnancy	2·0–4·8	20–48		18+[c]		[d]	[d]	[d]
Lactation				18				

[a] Compiled from American Medical Association (1968), Food and Nutrition Board (1974), and World Health Organization (1970, 1972). Values are expressed in mg iron/day.

[b] Breast feeding is assumed to be adequate.

[c] Use of supplements recommended to meet increased requirements.

[d] With adequate iron stores, recommendation same as for non-pregnant, menstruating females. Requirements of those without adequate stores cannot be met without supplementation.

three months) was recommended by this organization in 1969. Iron-fortified infant formulas and cereals are important dietary sources of iron for infants; however, the bioavailability of the type of iron added to infant diets is still under study. Breast milk is also an important source but its adequacy as the sole iron source beyond six months of age is questionable. Medicinal iron may be used when necessary to satisfy daily iron needs.

Both pregnancy and lactation increase iron requirements such that higher RDAs for these periods would seem justified. However, recognizing that the RDA for iron for non-pregnant, non-lactating premenopausal women (18 mg) is difficult to meet through diet alone, low-level iron supplementation, e.g. 30 mg, is recommended for pregnant and lactating women instead of augmentation in level of dietary iron. Typical prenatal iron supplements contain between 30 and 65 mg of iron/tablet.

With regard to the high RDA for iron in menstruating women, it is relevant to ask the question: What are the characteristics of a diet that provides 9 mg of iron/1000 kcalories (or 18 mg of iron/2000 kcalories). Farley *et al.* (1987) addressed this question by collection of food frequency information from 762 Utahns, aged 24–80 years. The diets were evaluated and divided into three categories according to iron per 1000 kcalories: category 1, 9·0 mg or more; category 2, 6·0–8·99 mg iron; and category 3, 5·99 mg or less iron. Twenty-seven percent of the women and 16% of the men reported consuming diets containing more than 9 mg iron/1000 kcalories. Individuals in the high iron density categories consumed greater proportions of their iron and energy from vegetable, fruit and cereal products; those in the low iron density category consumed more pastries, beverages, sweets and added fats. When fortified breakfast cereals were removed from the diets, only 14% of the women and 6% of the men consumed diets that provided at least 9 mg iron per 1000 kcalories. The authors calculated that women can meet the RDA for iron from their diets if they consume the recommended amount of energy distributed across food groups as follows: cereals 14–16%; vegetables, at least 11%; meat, fish, poultry, and eggs, 16–18%; fruits and juices, 13–18%; dairy, 15%; and beverages and other foods, 22–31%.

The extent to which iron needs can be met on vegetarian regimens has been questioned for several very obvious reasons. First, the lack of heme in the diet; second, the lack of meat proteins which increase the absorption of non-heme iron; and third, excessive use of foods such as bran cereals which are inhibitory to non-heme iron absorption (Hallberg *et al.*, 1987). The effects of long-term consumption of a vegetarian diet have been studied in Seventh Day Adventist women who have been vegetarians for 19 or more years by Anderson *et al.* (1981). In 56 women, 12·5 mg iron was consumed per day, 92% of which was from plant sources. Hemoglobin was satisfactory as was transferrin saturation. Unfortunately, serum ferritin was not evaluated.

In contrast, recent observations of vegetarians have shown them to have considerably lower ferritin levels than omnivores (Helman and Darnton-Hill, 1987). Unsupplemented omnivores had serum ferritin levels of 70 μg/liter while the vegetarians had 45 μg/liter. Thus the estimated iron stores were 36% lower for the vegetarians. It is interesting to note that approximately 22% of the vegetarians were taking vitamin or mineral supplements but few of these supplements contained iron.

A recent study compared 51 premenopausal women whose usual self-selected diets differed by the predominant protein source (Worthington-Roberts *et al.*, 1988), being classified as either red meat eaters (at least five times per week), fish/poultry eaters (with no more than one serving of red meat per week), or lacto-ovo vegetarians (with no red meat use and not more than one serving of fish/poultry per week). The data for hemoglobin

TABLE 8-13

IRON STATUS AND DIETARY PATTERNS OF PREMENOPAUSAL WOMEN[a]

	Predominant protein source		
	Red meat	*Fish/ poultry*	*Lacto-ovo vegetarian*
Subjects (*n*)	16	15	20
Age (years)	31	28	29
Menstrual cycle			
Interval (days)	29	30	29
Flow (days)	4·5	4·6	4·7
Diet intake/day			
Iron (mg)	13	12	12
Ascorbic acid (mg)	144	169	169
Kcalories	1 788	1 785	1 814
Protein (g)*	76	72	64
Carbohydrate (g)*	197	209	249
Fat (g)	78	70	64
Hemoglobin (g/d)*	14	13	13
Serum ferritin (μg/liter)*	30·5	15·6	19·1

*$P < 0·05$ difference between protein sources indicated by analysis of variance.
[a] From Worthington-Roberts *et al.* (1988).

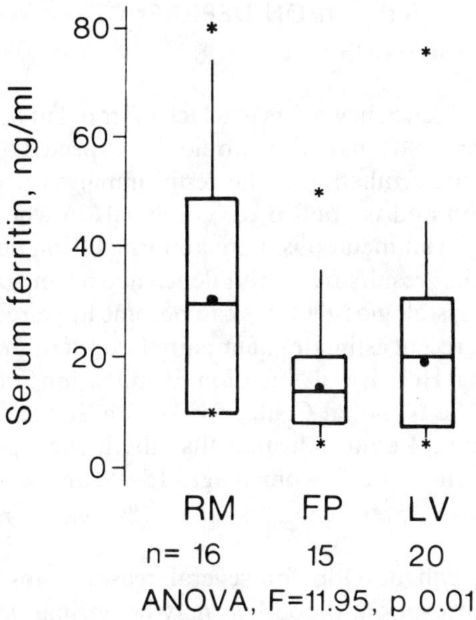

FIG. 8-11. Serum ferritin values in a group of premenopausal women whose diets were high (> 5 servings/week) in red meat (RM), high in fish/poultry (FP) or lacto-ovovegetarian (LV). Graphical display according to the method of Herbert and Waternaux (1983) and Worthington-Roberts *et al.* (1988).

and serum ferritin are shown in Table 8-13). No differences were seen in length of menses or menstrual cycle. Similar daily intakes of 1800 kcalories, 160 mg ascorbic acid, and 12 mg iron were recorded for the three groups. However, statistically different intakes of protein, carbohydrate and fat were reported: red meat eaters had the highest protein and fat and lowest carbohydrate intakes; the reverse was seen in the lacto-ovo vegetarians whose reported intakes were lowest in protein and fat and highest in carbohydrate. Iron status was adequate in all subjects, although serum ferritin was statistically higher in the red meat eaters (Fig. 8-11). Interestingly, the lowest serum ferritin levels were seen in the fish/poultry group. This suggests that long-term dietary patterns impact iron stores either through influences on absorption or metabolism of iron. While meat consumption is associated with higher iron stores, a well-designed and carefully-selected lacto-ovo vegetarian diet can support adequate hemoglobin levels and modest iron stores.

VIII. IRON DEFICIENCY

A. Definition

In this chapter, iron deficiency refers to a lack of iron that not only results in loss of iron stores, but that also would be expected to impair iron-dependent physiologic functions. The term 'impaired iron status' has a similar connotation and is applied to individuals in whom two or more laboratory tests of iron metabolism are abnormal. Iron deficiency anemia refers to anemia that results from iron deficiency or impaired iron status. Iron-dependent physiologic functions can become impaired before anemia develops. The best recent estimates of impaired iron status are derived from the second National Health and Nutrition Examination Survey (NHANES II) conducted by the National Center for Health Statistics between 1976 and 1980. Biochemical data indicated that the highest prevalences were seen among children ages 1–2, women ages 15–19, and women ages 20–44 (Fig. 8-12); the lowest prevalence, less than 1%, was in men between 15 and 64.

Iron deficiency can develop for several reasons—loss of blood and insufficient iron absorption. Blood loss may be normal (menstruation) or

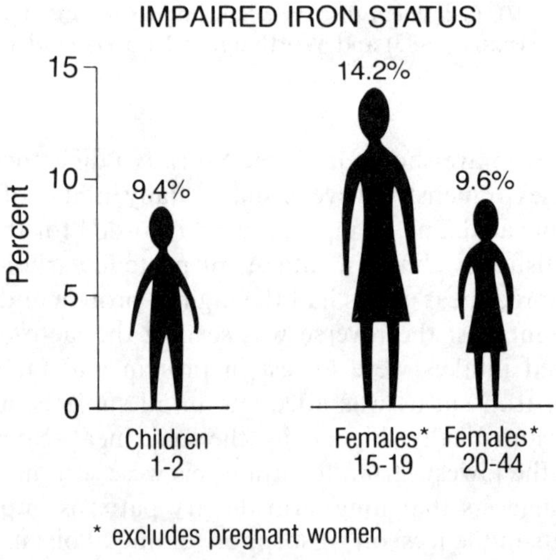

FIG. 8-12. Subgroups in the United States demonstrating the highest prevalence of impaired iron status. Data from the Second National Health and Nutrition Examination Survey (1976–1980).

pathological (due to bleeding lesions which require therapeutic intervention). Limited iron absorption may occasionally be the consequence of bleeding peptic ulcers, gastric surgery or ulcerative colitis. Usually, however, dietary composition limits either the quantity of dietary iron or its availability. Limited quantity and availability may be present simultaneously. In those parts of the world where iron deficiency is common, both dietary composition and blood loss (i.e. hookworm infestation) may adversely affect iron balance (Finch and Cook, 1984).

B. Diagnosis

Diagnosis of iron deficiency is best achieved by use of three laboratory tests. The first is plasma ferritin which, as mentioned previously, provides a reliable estimate of iron stores (provided inflammation has been excluded). In the normal adult, 1 μg of ferritin is roughly equivalent to 8 mg of storage iron; expressing ferritin stores on a per kg basis, this is equivalent to about 120 μg iron/kg body weight. The second measurement is transferrin saturation, which is a gauge of iron supply to tissues. When this value is less than 16%, normal erythropoiesis is impaired due to an inadequate iron supply. The third useful measure is zinc:protoporphyrin which increases when iron available to the developing red blood cells is deficient. The results of these three tests (along with the hemoglobin concentration) allow for the appropriate classification of the iron-deficient individual:

—those who are iron replete;
—those with depleted iron stores (decreased ferritin);
—those with iron deficiency but no anemia (decreased ferritin and transferrin saturation and increased zinc:protoporphyrin); and
—those with anemia (the indices of iron deficiency plus a decrease in hemoglobin).

In diagnosis of anemia and iron deficiency, age-related changes in laboratory values must be taken into account. Data from the Second National Health and Nutrition Examination Survey (NHANES II) allowed for the definition of some of the age-related changes in laboratory results which relate to iron nutrition (Yip *et al.*, 1984). The survey included a large number of subjects who were randomly selected in a manner that allowed extrapolation to the population of the United States as a whole. Analyses included hemoglobin, hematocrit, red blood cell count, red cell indices, iron, iron-binding capacity, transferrin saturation, and erythrocyte protoporphyrin. Computations of median values and 95% ranges by age and sex for each laboratory test were performed on 15 093 subjects between

TABLE 8-14

AGE-RELATED CHANGES IN BLOOD COUNTS BY AGE AND SEX: MEDIAN VALUES AND 95% RANGES (IN PARENTHESES) ARE SHOWN[a]

Sex	*Age* (*year*)	*n*	*Hb* (*g/dl*)	*Hct* (*%*)	*RBC* (10^{12}/*liter*)	*MCV* (*fl*)	*MCH* (*pg*)	*Mean corpuscular Hb concentration* (*μg/dl*)
Males and females								
	1–2	122	12·3 (10·7–13·8)	35·9 (32–40)	4·34 (3·8–4·8)	79 (67–88)	27·4 (22–30)	34·4 (32–38)
	3–5	587	12·5 (10·9–14·4)	36·3 (32–42)	4·34 (3·7–4·9)	81 (73–91)	28·1 (25–31)	34·5 (32–37)
	6–8	315	12·8 (11·0–14·3)	37·2 (33–41)	4·41 (3·8–4·9)	82 (74–92)	28·6 (25–31)	34·5 (32–37)
	9–11	430	13·2 (11·4–14·8)	38·4 (34–43)	4·51 (3·9–5·1)	84 (76–94)	28·7 (26–32)	34·5 (32–37)
Males								
	12–14	278	14·0 (12·0–16·0)	40·5 (35–45)	4·71 (4·1–5·2)	85 (77–94)	29·1 (26–32)	34·4 (32–37)
	15–17	371	14·8 (12·3–16·6)	43·0 (37–48)	4·92 (4·2–5·6)	87 (79–95)	29·9 (27–32)	34·4 (32–36)
	18–44	2 195	15·3 (13·2–17·3)	44·5 (39–49)	4·99 (4·3–5·7)	89 (80–99)	30·5 (27–34)	34·5 (32–37)
	45–64	1 433	15·2 (13·1–17·2)	44·3 (39–50)	4·91 (4·2–5·6)	90 (81–101)	30·9 (27–35)	34·3 (32–35)
	65–74	884	14·9 (12·6–17·4)	44·0 (37–51)	4·82 (3·8–5·8)	91 (81–103)	30·9 (27–34)	34·0 (31–35)
Females								
	12–14	299	13·4 (11·5–15·0)	39·0 (34–44)	4·47 (3·8–5·0)	86 (73–95)	29·4 (26–32)	34·1 (32–36)
	15–17	260	13·5 (11·7–15·3)	39·5 (34–44)	4·48 (3·9–5·1)	88 (78–98)	30·0 (26–34)	33·9 (32–36)
	18–44	1 999	13·5 (11·7–15·5)	40·0 (35–45)	4·42 (3·8–5·1)	90 (81–100)	30·6 (27–34)	33·9 (32–36)
	45–64	1 400	13·7 (11·7–16·0)	40·6 (35–47)	4·47 (3·8–5·3)	90 (81–101)	30·7 (27–34)	33·9 (31–36)
	65–74	974	13·8 (11·7–16·1)	40·8 (35–47)	4·50 (3·8–5·2)	90 (81–102)	30·6 (27–35)	33·9 (32–36)

[a] From Yip *et al.* (1984).

1 and 74 years of age who had complete laboratory data on venous blood (after excluding those subjects with an abnormality in one or more of three other laboratory tests). These age-related changes in laboratory measurements (Table 8-14) should be useful in identifying individuals with anemia and iron deficiency.

Just how applicable these reference standards are to blacks remains an unresolved question. Evidence to date indicates that blacks normally have a hemoglobin concentration that is about 0·5 g/dl (5 g/liter) below that of whites at all ages, except perhaps in the perinatal period. This difference does not appear to be due to iron deficiency, thalassemia trait, or differences in socioeconomic status.

C. Prevalence

The worldwide prevalence of iron deficiency is exceedingly high although marked differences are seen from one country to another, largely related to differences in socio-economic status (Fig. 8-13). Data from the World Health Organization indicate that the prevalence of iron deficiency in some developing countries is as high as 50% in adult menstruating women; over half of these women have frank anemia. The other extreme was seen in many developed countries where iron fortification programs exist and where many individuals voluntarily take iron supplements. Iron deficiency in menstruating women in these settings is as low as 10%. Throughout the world, iron deficiency in male populations is much less frequent (Finch and Cook, 1984).

Efforts have been initiated in the United States to monitor the prevalence of anemia. Using data from NHANES II (1976–1980), anemia (measured as

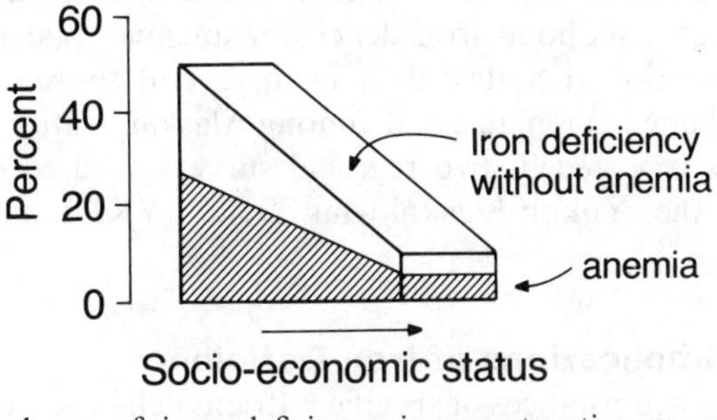

FIG. 8-13. Prevalence of iron deficiency in menstruating women, indicating diagrammatically the general relationship between prevalence socioeconomic status as one moves from disadvantaged (left) to privileged (right). Redrawn from Finch and Cook (1984).

TABLE 8-15

PREVALENCE OF IRON DEFICIENCY ANEMIA AMONG ALASKAN NATIVE CHILDREN—YUKON-KUSKOKWIM DELTA AND BRISTOL BAY REGIONS, ALASKA[a]

Age	*Anemia criteria*	*Yukon-Kuskokwim Delta*			*Bristol Bay*		
		Total no.	*Anemic*		*Total no.*	*Anemic*	
			No.	*(%)*		*No.*	*(%)*
6–11 Years	Hb < 11·5 g/dl	352	15	(4·3)	161	30	(18·6)
12–17 Years							
Female	Hb < 12·0 g/dl	243	35	(14·4)	76	18	(23·7)
Male	Hb < 12·5 g/dl	281	37	(13·2)	81	24	(29·6)
Total		876	87	(9·9)	318	72	(22·6)

[a] From Thiele *et al.* (1988).
Hb = hemoglobin.

those with hemoglobin values below the 95% reference range for age and sex) was highest in teenage girls (5·9%), young women (5·8%), infants (5·7%) and elderly men (4·4%) (Dallman *et al.*, 1984). Other data from the Pediatric Nutrition Surveillance System (CDC, 1986), which largely derives from WIC records, indicate that anemia in children declined from 7·8% in 1975 to 2·9% in 1985; prevalences among middle income children were even lower (Yip *et al.*, 1987a, b). Age-specific analysis using six-month age intervals demonstrated that the decline occurred among all age groups (CDC, 1986). In general, anemia prevalences were lower among children seen at follow-up visits than among children of the same age seen for initial visits, although both prevalences declined over the decade.

Even though childhood iron deficiency anemia appears to be on the decline in the United States, data from several sources show that the prevalence of anemia remains high among Alaskan Native children (CDC, 1988) as was reported in two regional surveys focused on school-aged children in the Yukon-Kuskokwim Delta (YKD) and Bristol Bay (Table 8-15).

D. Health Implications of Iron Deficiency

Unlike some circumstances of specific nutrient deficiency, overt symptoms of iron deficiency are generally inconspicuous. The potential deficit in oxygen transport is often prevented through compensatory mechanisms (i.e. increased cardiac volume) unless cardiopulmonary disease prevents this phenomenon. Under extremes of stress, however, these compensatory adjustments may not be sufficient to optimize oxygen delivery to body tissues. Work performance may then be affected (Gardner *et al.*, 1977). In fact, a number of studies of individuals engaged in hard physical labor suggest that productivity and therefore income are reduced in the presence of iron deficiency (Basta *et al.*, 1979; Edgerton *et al.*, 1979; Griesen, 1986).

Not only is oxygen transport hampered by limited supplies of iron but iron-dependent tissue enzyme activities are simultaneously depressed (Dallman, 1982). In the iron-deficient rat, it has been possible to demonstrate a marked decrease in work capacity unassociated with anemia (Finch *et al.*, 1976). The chief abnormality has been shown to be a decrease of iron-dependent mitochondrial oxidases (Finch *et al.*, 1976; Dallman, 1982; McKay *et al.*, 1983).

Iron deficiency (unassociated with anemia) has also been associated with an elevation in blood and urinary catecholamines, especially norepinephrine. In the rat, this leads to cardiac hypertrophy and it may also compensate for an impairment in temperature maintenance. In human subjects, metabolic requirements have been found to be higher for the iron-deficient individual when placed in a cold environment. Recent research in Pennsylvania and North Dakota suggest that non-anemic iron-deficient women demonstrate an impaired ability to maintain body temperature in the face of exposure to cold (Kirn, 1988). It has been proposed that the paucity of iron results in the lack of adequate stores of the thyroid hormones, which prevents the body from increasing cellular metabolism when necessary. The elevated norepinephrine levels indicate more intense activity by the sympathetic nervous system in an attempt to compensate.

Considerable evidence has accumulated during the last several decades for an association between iron deficiency and adverse effects on attention, intelligence test performance and school achievement (Pollitt *et al.*, 1986). Analysis of data derived from recent studies in which experimental design is judged to be satisfactory suggest that the effects of iron deficiency with and without anemia on the behavior of infants and children are the following:

(1) in comparison to infants without signs of iron deficiency, infants with iron deficiency (with and without anemia) tend to score lower on the Bayley Scale of Mental Development;
(2) there is no evidence for an association between iron deficiency and delayed motor development;
(3) iron repletion therapy implemented over a period of 7–10 days is likely to result in an improvement in the performance on the Bayley

Scale of Mental Development among infants with iron deficiency with or without associated anemia;

(4) there is yet no evidence available on the specific mental abilities and skills affected among iron-deficient infants that explains their comparatively low performance on the Bayley scale;

(5) in comparison with preschool children without iron deficiency, preschool children with iron deficiency with or without anemia are less likely to pay attention to relevant cues in problem solving situations;

(6) in populations where there is a high prevalence of protein–calorie malnutrition, iron-deficient infants and preschool children tend to be smaller and lighter than children without signs of iron deficiency;

(7) in these populations, the iron-deficient infants and preschool children are not likely to improve their performance in mental development scales and specific measures of cognitive function following iron repletion therapy;

(8) in these populations, preschool children with iron deficiency anemia are more likely to show selective deficits in attention and higher order cognitive functions.

The results of these studies are not conclusive but the behavioral abnormalities should not be taken lightly. It is possible that the brain's rapid rate of growth and differentiation during infancy might make it particularly vulnerable to nutrient deficiencies. But since the same adverse environmental factors that lead to iron deficiency could also be responsible for behavioral deficits, interpretation of much of this research is difficult. It must therefore be concluded at the present time that the long-term significance of these observations has yet to be determined.

The impact of iron deficiency on the immune response has been of much interest to researchers for at least several decades. Examination of the rather large body of research in this area indicates that abnormalities in cell-mediated immunity and ability of neutrophils to kill several types of bacteria are well established under experimental conditions in iron-deficient patients. It is still uncertain, however, whether these abnormalities result in an increased incidence and duration of infections. Well controlled clinical trials are required to satisfactorily address this question. In the meantime, experts anticipate that the substantial laboratory abnormalities in immune function in iron deficiency will eventually be shown to be associated with a decreased resistance to infection (Dallman, 1987).

IX. ADVANTAGES OF RED MEAT

There is no question about the potential value of lean meat in an individual's diet. In terms of iron, no other category of foods provides as high a level of bioavailable iron. This advantage is further augmented by the enhancing effect that meat appears to have on the absorption of non-heme iron from other foods. The merits of lean meat as a source of iron are particularly great for women of reproductive age; impaired iron status is common in this group, especially among those individuals who regularly consume well under 2000 kcalories daily. Lean meat provides a high level of total iron per serving (Fig. 8-14) as well as a high level of total iron per 100 kcalories (Fig. 8-15). While some non-meat sources of iron look favorable from an iron density standpoint (Table 8-16), the low iron bioavailability in most of these foods detracts markedly from their nutritional significance. Nonetheless, a well selected vegetarian diet can support iron nutriture adequately for most individuals.

TABLE 8-16
IRON CONTENT OF SELECTED NON-MEAT SOURCES OF IRON

Food	*Portion*	*Iron content (mg)*	*Kcalorie content*	*mg iron/100 kcal*
Oysters	$\frac{1}{2}$ cup	8·4	80	10·5
Spinach (cooked)	$\frac{1}{2}$ cup	3·2	20	15·7
Lima beans (cooked)	$\frac{1}{2}$ cup	3·0	130	2·3
Peaches (dried)	10 halves	5·3	311	1·7
Navy beans (cooked)	$\frac{1}{2}$ cup	2·6	112	2·3
Soybeans (cooked)	$\frac{1}{2}$ cup	2·5	117	2·1
Kidney beans (cooked)	$\frac{1}{2}$ cup	2·3	115	2·0
Sauerkraut (cooked)	$\frac{1}{2}$ cup	1·7	22	7·9
Prune juice	$\frac{1}{2}$ cup	1·0	90	1·7
Beet greens (cooked)	$\frac{1}{2}$ cup	1·4	20	6·9
Sardines (canned)	3 oz	2·6	175	1·5
Clam meat	3 oz	2·6	65	4·0

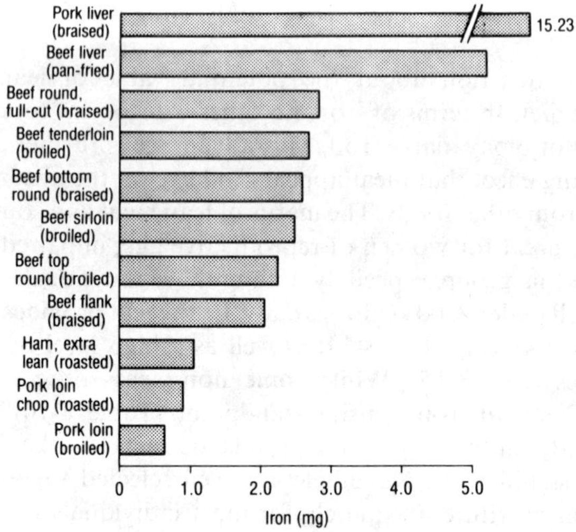

FIG. 8-14. Total iron content of 3 oz portions of selected meats. Data on total iron content from *Agriculture Handbook No. 8-10* (1983) and *No. 8-13* (1986), United States Department of Agriculture.

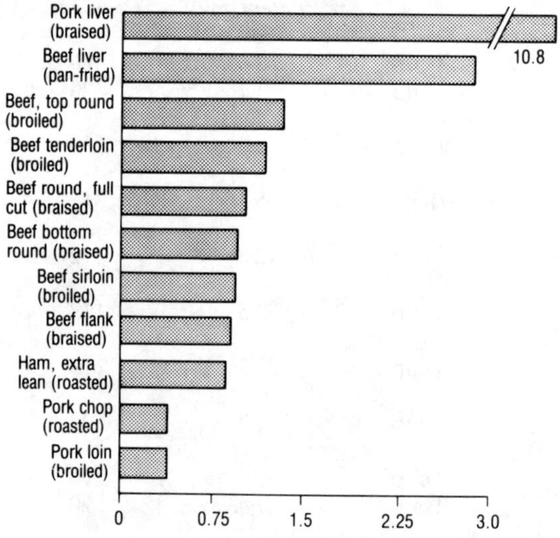

FIG. 8-15. Iron content of selected meats, expressed as mg per 100 kcalories. Calculated from data provided in *Agriculture Handbook No. 8-10* (1983) and *No. 8-13* (1986), United States Department of Agriculture.

Finally, it is now well recognized that diets including lean meat and lean meat products are effective in lowering plasma lipids in hyperlipidemic individuals. Watts and colleagues (1988) reported that free-living men with hyperlipidemia showed a significant reduction in total- and LDL-cholesterol when placed on moderately low-fat diets (27–35% fat) including lean meats. The authors conclude that a modified diet including a moderate amount of lean meat and meat products is compatible with a reduced lipoprotein mediated risk of atherosclerotic heart disease.

X. REFERENCES

AMERICAN ACADEMY OF PEDIATRICS, COMMITTEE ON NUTRITION (1969). Iron balance and requirements in infancy. *Pediatrics* **43**, 134.

AMERICAN MEDICAL ASSOCIATION, COMMITTEE ON IRON DEFICIENCY, COUNCIL ON FOODS AND NUTRITION (1968). Iron deficiency in the United States. *J. Am. Med. Assoc.* **203**, 61.

ANDERSON, B. M., GIBSON, R. S. and SABRY, J. H. (1981). The iron and zinc status of long-term vegetarian women. *Am. J. Clin. Nutr.* **34**, 1042.

APPLETON, T. C., MORGAN, E. H. and BAKER, E. (1971). *Proceedings International Symposium Erythropoieticum—1970* (T. Travnicek and J. Neuwert, Eds), p. 310. Univ. of Karlova, Prague.

BALCERZAK, S. P. and GREENBERGER, N. J. (1968). Iron content of isolated intestinal epithelial cells in relation to iron absorption. *Nature* **220**, 270.

BASTA, S. S., SOEKIRMAN, D., KARYADI, D. and SCRIMSHAW, N. S. (1979). Iron deficiency anemia and the productivity of adult males in Indonesia. *Am. J. Clin. Nutr.* **32**, 916.

BOTHWELL, T. H., CHARLTON, R. W., COOK, J. D. and FINCH, C. A. (1979). *Iron Metabolism in Man.* Blackwell Press, London.

BRITTIN, H. C. and NOSSAMAN, C. E. (1986). Iron content of food cooked in iron utensils. *J. Am. Diet. Assoc.* **86**, 897.

BULLEN, J. J., ROGERS, H. J. and GRIFFITHS, E. (1972). Iron binding proteins and infection. *Brit. J. Haematol.* **23**, 389.

CALLENDER, S. T. (1973). Fortification of food with iron—is it necessary or effective? In *Nutritional Problems in a Changing World* (D. Hollingsworth and M. Russell, Eds), p. 205. John Wiley and Sons, New York.

CARTWRIGHT, G. E. and WINTROBE, M. M. (1949). Chemical, clinical and immunological studies on the products of human plasma fractionation. XXXIX. The anemia of infection. Studies on the iron-binding capacity of serum. *J. Clin. Invest.* **28**, 86.

CENTERS FOR DISEASE CONTROL. MORBIDITY AND MORTALITY WEEKLY REPORT (1986). Declining anemia prevalence among children enrolled in public nutrition and health programs, selected states, 1975–1985. *J. Am. Med. Assoc.* **256**, 2165.

CENTERS FOR DISEASE CONTROL. MORBIDITY AND MORTALITY WEEKLY REPORT (1988). High prevalence of iron deficiency anemia among Alaskan Native children. *J. Am. Med. Assoc.* **259**, 2532.

CONRAD, M. E. (1970). Factors affecting iron absorption. In *Iron Deficiency* (L. Hallberg, H. G. Harweth and A. Vannotti, Eds), p. 87. Academic Press, New York.

CONRAD, M. E. and CROSBY, W. H. (1963). Intestinal mucosal mechanisms controlling iron absorption. *Blood* **22**, 406.

CONRAD, M. E., WEINTRAUB, L. R. and CROSBY, W. H. (1964). The role of the intestine in iron kinetics. *J. Clin. Invest.* **43**, 963.

CONTE, D., BRUNELLI, L., FERRARIO, L., MANDELLI, C., QUATRINI, M., VELIO, P. and BIANCHI, P. (1984). Effect of ascorbic acid on desferrioxamine-induced urinary excretion in idiopathic hemochromatosis. *Acta Haematol.* **72**, 117.

COOK, J. D. and MONSEN, E. R. (1976). Food iron absorption in human subjects: III. Comparison of the effects of animal protein on non-heme iron absorption. *Am. J. Clin. Nutr.* **29**, 859.

COOK, J. D. and MONSEN, E. R. (1977). Vitamin C, the common cold and iron absorption in man. *Am. J. Clin. Nutr.* **30**, 235.

COOK, J. D., MORCK, T. A. and LYNCH, S. R. (1981). The inhibitory effect of soy products on non-heme iron absorption in man. *Am. J. Clin. Nutr.* **34**, 2622.

CROSBY, W. J. (1970). Iron enrichment: One's food, another's poison. *Arch. Intern. Med.* **126**, 911.

CZERNIEJEWSKI, C. P., SHANK, C. W., BECHTEL, W. G. and BRADLEY, W. B. (1964). The minerals of wheat, flour and bread. *Cereal Chem.* **41**, 65.

DALLMAN, P. R. (1982). Manifestations of iron deficiency. In *Seminars in Hematology* (P. A. Miescher and E. R. Jaffe, Eds), **19**, 19.

DALLMAN, P. R. (1987). Iron deficiency and the immune response. *Am. J. Clin. Nutr.* **46**, 329.

DALLMAN, P. R., YIP, R. and JOHNSON, C. (1984). Prevalence and causes of anemia in the United States, 1976–1980. *Am. J. Clin. Nutr.* **39**, 437.

DAWSON-HUGHES, B., SELIGSON, F. H. and HUGHES, V. A. (1986). Effects of calcium carbonate and hydroxyapatite on zinc and iron retention in postmenopausal women. *Am. J. Clin. Nutr.* **44**, 83.

DISLER, P. B., LYNCH, S. R., CHARLTON, R. W., TORRANCE, J. D., BOTHWELL, T. H., WALKER, R. B. and MAYET, F. (1975). The effect of tea on iron absorption. *Gut* **16**, 193.

EDGERTON, V. R., GARDNER, G. W., OHIRA, Y., GUNAWARDENA, K. A. and SENEWIRATNE, B. (1979). Iron deficiency anaemia and its effect on worker productivity and activity patterns. *Brit. Med. J.* **2**, 1546.

EHRENBERG, A. and LAURELL, C.-B. (1955). Magnetic measurements on crystallized Fe-transferrin isolated from the blood plasma of swine. *Acta Chem. Scand.* **9**, 68.

FARLEY, M. A., SMITH, P. D., MAHONEY, A. W., WEST, D. W. and POST, J. R. (1987). Adult dietary characteristics affecting iron intake: A comparison based on iron density. *J. Am. Diet. Assoc.* **87**, 184.

FEDERAL REGISTER (1971). Wheat flour and related products and baked products. *Fed. Regist.* **36**, 23 074.

FILLET, G., COOK, J. D. and FINCH, C. A. (1974). Storage iron kinetics VII. A biologic model for reticuloendothelial iron transport. *J. Clin. Invest.* **53**, 1527.

FINCH, C. A. and COOK, J. D. (1984). Iron deficiency. *Am. J. Clin. Nutr.* **39**, 471.

FINCH, C. A., MILLER, L. R., INAMDAR, A. R., PERSON, R., SEILER, K. and MACKLER, B. (1976). Iron deficiency in the rat. Physiological and biochemical studies of muscle dysfunction. *J. Clin. Invest.* **58**, 447.

FLETCHER, J. and HUEHNS, E. R. (1968). Function of transferrin. *Nature (London)* **218**, 1211.

FOMON, S. J. (1987). Bioavailability of supplemental iron in commercially prepared dry infant cereals. *J. Ped.* **110**, 660.

FOOD AND NUTRITION BOARD, NATIONAL ACADEMY OF SCIENCES—NATIONAL RESEARCH COUNCIL (1980). *Recommended Dietary Allowances*, 9th edn. National Academy of Sciences, Washington, DC.

FRITZ, J. C., PLA, G. W., ROBERTS, T., BOEHNE, J. W. and HOVE, E. L. (1970). Biological availability in animals of iron from common dietary sources. *J. Agric. Food Chem.* **18**, 647.

GARDNER, G., EDGERTON, V., SENEWIRATNE, B., BARNARD, R. and OHIRA, Y. (1977). Physical work capacity and metabolic stress in subjects with iron deficiency anemia. *Am. J. Clin. Nutr.* **30**, 910.

GILLOOLY, M., BOTHWELL, T. H., TORRANCE, J. D., MACPHAIL, A. P., DERMAN, D. P., BEZWODA, W. R., MILLS, W. and CHARLTON, R. W. (1983). The effects of organic acids, phytates and polyphenols on the absorption of iron from vegetables. *Brit. J. Nutr.* **49**, 331.

GREENBERGER, N. J., BALCERZAK, S. P. and ACKERMAN, G. A. (1969). Iron uptake by isolated intestinal brush borders: Changes induced by alterations in iron stores. *J. Lab. Clin. Med.* **73**, 711.

GREGOR, J. L. and BUCKLEY, S. (1977). Menstrual loss of zinc, copper, magnesium and iron by adolescent girls. *Nutr. Rep. Intern.* **16**, 639.

GRIESEN, G. (1986). Mild anemia in African school children: Effect on running performance and an intervention. *Acta Paediatr. Scand.* **75**, 662.

HALLBERG, L. and SLOVELL, L. (1967). Absorption of hemoglobin iron in man. *Acta Med. Scand.* **181**, 335.

HALLBERG, L., ROSSANDER, L., PERSSON, H. and SVAHN, E. (1982). Deleterious effects of prolonged warming of meals on ascorbic acid content and iron absorption. *Am. J. Clin. Nutr.* **36**, 846.

HALLBERG, L., ROSSANDER, L. and SKANBERG, A. B. (1987). Phytates and the inhibitory effect of bran on iron absorption in man. *Am. J. Clin. Nutr.* **45**, 988.

HAMILTON, E. I. and MINSKI, M. J. (1972–73). Abundance of the chemical elements in man's diet and possible relations with environmental factors. *Sci. Total Environment* **1**, 375.

HELMAN, A. D. and DARNTON-HILL, I. (1987). Vitamin and iron status of new vegetarians. *Am. J. Clin. Nutr.* **45**, 785.

HERBERT, J. R. and WATERNAUX, C. (1983). Graphical display of growth data. *Am. J. Clin. Nutr.* **38**, 145.

HERTZLER, A. A. and MCANGE, T. R. (1986). Development of an iron checklist to guide food intake. *J. Am. Diet. Assoc.* **86**, 782.

HOWARD, J. and JACOBS, A. (1972). Iron transport by rat small intestine *in vitro*. *Brit. J. Haematol.* **23**, 595.

HUEBERS, H., HUEBERS, E., FORTH, W., LEOPOLD, G. and RUMMEL, W. (1971). Binding of iron and other metals in brush borders of jejunum and ileum of the rat in vitro. *Acta Pharmacol. Toxicol.* **29** (suppl. 4), 22 (abstract).

HUEBERS, H., HUEBERS, E., FORTH, W. and RUMMEL, W. (1971). Binding of iron to a non-ferritin protein in the mucosal cells of normal and iron-deficient rats during absorption. *Life Sci.* **10**(1), 1141.

JACOBS, A. (1973). The mechanism of iron absorption. In *Clinics in Hematology*, Vol. 2, No. 2, (S. T. Chandler, Ed.) p. 323. W. B. Saunders, Philadelphia.

JANDL, J. H. and KATZ, J. H. (1963). The plasma-to-cell cycle of transferrin. *J. Clin. Invest.* **42**, 314.

JOHNSTON, F. A. and MCMILLAN, T. J. (1952). Iron requirements of six young women. *J. Am. Diet. Assoc.* **28**, 633.

KIRN, T. F. (1988). Do low levels of iron affect body's ability to regulate temperature, experience cold? *J. Am. Med. Assoc.* **260**, 607

KRAUSE, U. (1970). Iron deficiency after gastrectomy. In *Iron Deficiency* (J. Hallberg, H. G. Harwerth and A. Vannotti, Eds), p. 505. Academic Press, New York.

LABBE, R. F., RETTMER, R. L., SHAH, A. G. and TURNLAND, J. R. (1987). Zinc protoporphyrin. Past, present and future. *Ann. NY Acad. Sci.* **514**, 7.

LEE, K. and CLYDESDALE, F. M. (1979). Iron sources used in food fortification and their exchanges due to food processing. *Crit. Rev. Food Sci. Nutr.* **11**, 117.

LIPSCHITZ, D. A., COOK, J. D. and FINCH, C. A. (1974). A clinical evaluation of serum ferritin as an index of iron stores. *New Engl. J. Med.* **290**, 1213.

LYNCH, S. R. and COOK, J. D. (1980). Interaction of vitamin C and iron. *Ann. NY Acad. Sci.* **355**, 32.

LYNCH, S. R., DASSENKO, S. A., MORCK, T. A., BEARD, J. L. and COOK, J. D. (1985). Soy protein products and heme iron absorption in humans. *Am. J. Clin. Nutr.* **41**, 13.

MARTINEZ, F. E. and VANNUCCHI, H. (1986). Bioavailability of iron added to the diet by cooking in an iron pot. *Nutr. Res.* **6**, 421.

MARTINEZ-TORRES, C., LEETS, I., TAYLOR, P., RAMIREZ, J., DEL VALLE CAMACHO, M. and LAYRISSE, M. (1986). Heme, ferritin and vegetable iron absorption in humans from meals denatured of heme iron during the cooking of beef. *J. Nutr.* **116**, 1720.

MCKAY, R. H., HIGUCHI, D. A., WINDER, W. W., FELL, R. D. and BROWN, E. B. (1983). Tissue effects of iron deficiency in the rat. *Biochim. Biophys. Acta* **757**, 352.

MCLENNAN, W. J., ANDREWS, G. R., MACLEOD, C. and CAIRD, F. I. (1973). Anemia in the elderly. *Quart. J. Med.* **42**, 1.

MONSEN, E. R. (1982). Ascorbic acid: An enhancing factor in iron absorption. In *Nutritional Bioavailability of Iron* (C. Kies, Ed.), ACS Symposium Series No. 203, p. 85. American Chemical Society, Washington, DC.

MONSEN, E. R. (1988a). Protein–iron interactions: Influences on absorption, metabolism and status. In *Nutrient Interactions* (C. E. Bodwell and J. W. Erdman, Eds), p. 149. Marcel Dekker, New York.

MONSEN, E. R. (1988b). Iron nutrition and absorption: Dietary factors which impact iron bioavailability. *J. Am. Diet. Assoc.* **88**, 786.

MONSEN, E. R. and BALINTFY, J. L. (1982). Calculating dietary iron bioavailability: Refinement and computerization. *J. Am. Diet. Assoc.* **80**, 307.

MONSEN, E. R. and COOK, J. D. (1976). Food iron absorption in human subjects. IV. The effects of calcium and phosphate salts on the absorption of non-heme iron. *Am. J. Clin. Nutr.* **29**, 1142.

MONSEN, E. R. and COOK, J. D. (1979). Food iron absorption in human subjects: V. Effects of the major dietary constituents of a semi-synthetic meal. *Am. J. Clin. Nutr.* **32**, 804.

MONSEN, E. R., KUHN, I. N. and FINCH, C. A. (1967). Iron status of menstruating women. *Am. J. Clin. Nutr.* **20**, 842.

MONSEN, E. R., HALLBERG, L., LAYRISSE, M., HEGSTED, D. M., COOK, J. D., MERTZ, W. and FINCH, C. A. (1978). Estimation of available dietary iron. *Am. J. Clin. Nutr.* **31**, 134.

MORGAN, E. H. and WALTERS, M. N. I. (1963). Iron storage in human disease: Fractionation of hepatic and splenic iron into ferritin and haemosiderin with histochemical correlations. *J. Clin. Pathol.* **16**, 101.

MORRIS, E. R. (1987). Iron. In *Trace Elements in Human and Animal Nutrition* (W. Mertz, Ed.), p. 79. Academic Press, San Diego.

NATIONAL CENTER FOR HEALTH STATISTICS (1983). *Dietary Intake Source Data: United States, 1976–1980.* Vital and Health Statistics Series 11, No. 231, DHHS Pub. No. (PHS) 83-1681, US Government Printing Office, Washington, DC.

NATIONAL RESEARCH COUNCIL (1979). *Iron.* University Park Press, Baltimore, MD.

PAULEV, P. E., JORDAL, R. and PEDERSEN, N. S. (1983). Dermal excretion of iron in intensely training athletes. *Clin. Chem. Acta* **127**, 19.

PLA, G. W. and FRITZ, J. C. (1970). Availability of iron. *J. Assoc. Offic. Anal. Chem.* **53**, 791.

POLLITT, E., SACO-POLLITT, C., LEIBEL, R. L. and VITERI, F. E. (1986). Iron deficiency and behavioral development in infants and preschool children. *Am. J. Clin. Nutr.* **43**, 555.

PRABHAVATHI, T. and RAO, B. S. N. (1981). Contaminant iron in foods and its bioavailability predicted by in vitro method. *Ind. J. Med. Res.* **74**, 37.

RAPER, N. R., ROSENTHAL, J. C. and WOTEKI, C. E. (1984). Estimates of available iron in diets of individuals 1 year old and older in the Nationwide Food Consumption Survey. *J. Am. Diet. Assoc.* **84**, 783.

RETTMER, R. L., FERNANDEZ-CANO, P., SAYERS, M. L., ASHWOOD, E. R. and LABBE, R. F. (1985). The zinc protoporphyrin/heme ratio in laboratory diagnosis. *Clin. Chem.* **31**, 1026.

RETTMER, R. L., GUNTER, E. W. and LABBE, R. F. (1987). Overcoming the limitations of hematofluorometry for assaying zinc protoporphyrin. *Ann. NY Acad. Sci.* **514**, 345.

RICHMOND, V. S., WORWOOD, M. and JACOBS, A. (1972). The iron content of intestinal epithelial cells and its subcellular distribution: Studies on normal, iron-overloaded and iron-deficient rats. *Brit. J. Haematol.* **23**, 605.

RIMINGTON, C. (1959). Biosynthesis of haemoglobin. *Brit. Med. Bull.* **15**, 19.

RYBO, G. (1966). Clinical and experimental studies on menstrual blood loss. *Acta Obstet. Gynecol. Scand.* **45** (suppl.), 1.

SANO, S., INOUE, S., TANABE, Y., SUMIYA, C. and KOIKE, S. (1959). Significance of mitochondria for porphyrin and heme biosynthesis. *Science* **129**, 275.

SHEEHAN, R. G. and FRENKEL, E. P. (1972). The control of iron absorption by the gastrointestinal mucosal cell. *J. Clin. Invest.* **51**, 224.

SHEETS, O., FRAZIER, E. and DICKENS, D. (1931). Conservation of iron in vegetables by methods of preparation and cooking. *Miss. Agric. Exp. Sta. Bull.* **291**, 291–7.

Sherman, H. C. (1937). *Chemistry of Food and Nutrition*, 5th edn, p. 323. MacMillan, New York.

Shoden, A. and Sturgeon, P. (1960). Hemosiderin. *Acta Haematol.* **23**, 376.

Simpson, K. M., Morris, E. R. and Cook, J. D. (1981). The inhibitory effect of bran on iron absorption in man. *Am. J. Clin. Nutr.* **34**, 1469.

Sisson, T. R. C. (1964). Iron therapy of infants: Quantitative aspects (abstract). *Fed. Proc.* **23**, 879.

Slatkavitz, C. A. and Clydesdale, F. M. (1988). Solubility of inorganic iron as affected by proteolytic digestion. *Am. J. Clin. Nutr.* **47**, 487.

Stekel, A., Monckeberg, F. and Beyda, V. (1986). *Combating Iron Deficiency in Chile: A Case Study*. International Nutritional Anemia Consultative Group (INACG), Sept., 1986.

Thiele, M., Geddes, M. E., Nobmann, E. and Peterson, K. (1988). High prevalence of iron deficiency anemia among Alaskan native children. *J. Amer. Med. Assoc.* **259**, 2532.

Torrance, J. D., Charlton, R. W., Schmaman, A., Lynch, S. R. and Bothwell, T. H. (1968). Storage iron in 'muscle'. *J. Clin. Path.* **21**, 495.

Turnbull, A. (1974). Iron absorption. In *Iron in Biochemistry and Medicine* (A. Jacobs and M. Worwood, Eds), p. 369. Academic Press, New York.

Walters, G. O., Miller, F. M. and Worwood, M. (1973). Serum ferritin concentration and iron stores in normal subjects. *J. Clin. Path.* **26**, 770.

Watts, G. F., Ahmed, W., Quiney, J., Houlston, R., Jackson, P., Iles, C. and Lewis, B. (1988). Effective lipid lowering diets including lean meat. *Brit. Med. J.* **296**, 235.

Weintraub, L. R., Conrad, M. E. and Crosby, W. H. (1965). Regulation of the intestinal absorption of iron by the rate of erythropoiesis. *Brit. J. Haematol.* **11**, 432.

Wheby, M. S., Suttle, G. E. and Ford, K. T. (1970). Intestinal absorption of hemoglobin iron. *Gastroenterology* **58**, 647.

White, H. S. (1980). Iron-hemoglobin. In *Nutrition and the Adult, Micronutrients* (R. B. Alfin-Slater and D. Kritchevsky, Eds), p. 287. Plenum Press, New York.

World Health Organization (1970). *Requirements of Ascorbic Acid, Vitamin D, Vitamin B_{12}, Folate, and Iron.* Report of a joint FAO/WHO Expert Group, WHO Tech. Rep. Ser. No. 452.

World Health Organization (1972). *Nutritional Anaemias.* Report of a WHO Group of Experts, WHO Tech. Rep. Ser. No. 503.

Worthington-Roberts, B., Breskin, M. W. and Monsen, E. R. (1988). Iron status of premenopausal women in a university community and its relationship to habitual dietary sources of protein. *Am. J. Clin. Nutr.* **47**, 275.

Worwood, M. and Jacobs, A., (1971). Absorption of ^{59}Fe in the rat: Iron-binding substances in the soluble fraction of intestinal mucosa. *Life Sci.* **10**(1), 1363.

Worwood, M., Edwards, A. and Jacobs, A. (1971). Non-ferritin iron compound in rat small intestinal mucosa during iron absorption. *Nature* (*London*) **229**, 409.

Worwood, M., Summers, M., Miller, F., Jacobs, A. and Whittaker, J. A. (1974). Ferritin in blood cells from normal subjects and patients with leukemia. *Brit. J. Haematol.* **28**, 27.

Yip, R., Johnson, C. and Dallman, P. R. (1984). Age-related changes in laboratory values used in the diagnosis of anemia and iron deficiency. *Am. J. Clin. Nutr.* **39**, 427.

YIP, R., BINKIN, N. J., FLESHOOD, L. and TROWBRIDGE, F. L. (1987a). Declining prevalence of anemia among low-income children in the United States. *J. Am. Med. Assoc.* **258**, 1619.

YIP, R., WALSH, K. M., GOLDFARB, M. G. and BINKIN, N. J. (1987b). Declining prevalence of anemia in childhood in a middle-class setting: A pediatric success story. *Pediatrics* **80**, 330.

9

Role of Zinc and the Contribution of Meat to Human Nutrition

H. H. SANDSTEAD, L. S. DARNELL AND J. C. WALLWORK
University of Texas Medical Branch,
Preventive Medicine and Community Health,
Galveston, Texas, USA

I. HISTORY OF ZINC AS A NUTRIENT

More than a century ago, zinc (Zn) was shown to be required for the growth of *Aspergillus niger* (Raulin, 1869). Sixty-five years later, Todd *et al.* (1934) induced Zn deficiency in rats. The importance of Zn for animal husbandry became evident when Tucker and Salmon (1955) recognized that porcine parakeratosis is caused by Zn deficiency. Evidence of conditioned Zn deficiency in humans with alcoholic cirrhosis was published by Vallee *et al.* in 1956. Primary human Zn deficiency seemed unlikely until Prasad *et al.* (1961) postulated that dwarfism and hypogonadism in Iranian adolescent village boys from Shiraz was caused by Zn deficiency. Their hypothesis was subsequently substantiated by metabolic studies and intervention trials (Prasad *et al.*, 1963a,b; Sandstead *et al.*, 1967; Halsted *et al.*, 1972).

Since the discovery of primary Zn deficiency in humans, many functions of Zn have been identified (Halsted *et al.*, 1974). These advances have occurred through clinical investigations of patients with primary and conditioned Zn deficiencies, the induction of experimental Zn deficiency in humans, and through research utilizing animal model systems. Advances in analytical chemistry, stable and radioisotopic technology and immunochemistry have made much of this progress possible. Results of some of this work are reviewed in this chapter.

A. Primary Deficiency

The Prasad–Halsted syndrome of growth stunting and hypogonadism in adolescents was characterized by Prasad and co-workers (Prasad *et al.*,

1963a,b; Sandstead *et al.*, 1967) working in Egypt, and Halsted *et al.* (1972) working in Iran. Similar patients were described from Turkey (Arcásoy *et al.*, 1978), the United States (Caggiano *et al.*, 1969) and China (Chao-ling *et al.*, 1959). The major putative cause of the Prasad–Halsted Syndrome is consumption of diets rich in unrefined cereals and low in sources of readily bioavailable Zn such as red meat, fish and poultry. Phytate from cereal brans, pulses and other plant sources inhibits Zn bioavailability through the formation of insoluble calcium–phytate–Zn complexes at alkaline pH (Mills, 1985). Conditioning factors, which also contribute to Zn deficiency in the Prasad–Halsted Syndrome, include parasitic infections that cause blood loss, geophagia, and recurrent bouts of diarrheal diseases and other infections.

Evidence of Zn deficiency among young children in the US was reported by Hambidge *et al.* (1972). They described improved growth and taste acuity in growth retarded infants and young children who were serendipitously found to have low concentrations of Zn in their hair, while plasma Zn levels were within the normal range. A retrospective dietary assessment suggested that selection of foods low in bioavailable Zn was the cause of the deficiency. More recently, Buzina *et al.* (1980) reported growth stunting associated with low Zn status among school children in Yugoslavia, and Xue-Cun *et al.* (1985) reported Zn-responsive growth stunting among Chinese preschool children. In the United States, Zn-responsive growth stunting of preschool children has been reported from Denver among Hispanic-Americans (Walravens *et al.*, 1983; Krebs *et al.*, 1984). Most recently, Gibson *et al.* (1989) reported Zn-responsive growth failure in young boys from southern Ontario. Low hair Zn and reduced taste acuity identified the boys that were responsive to Zn treatment.

Evidence of Zn deficiency associated with protein-energy malnutrition (PEM) was reported from Egypt in 1965 (Sandstead *et al.*, 1965). Subsequently, thymic hypoplasia and impaired delayed cutaneous hypersensitivity related to Zn deficiency was discovered in Jamaican infants with PEM (Golden *et al.*, 1977, 1978), and the beneficial effects of Zn on clinical outcome was described (Golden and Golden, 1981a,b). It seems evident from these reports that Zn deficiency is an important component of the PEM syndrome.

Zn deficiency also occurs in pregnancy (Jameson, 1976, 1982; Cherry *et al.*, 1981, 1989; Hunt *et al.*, 1984; Mukherjee *et al.*, 1984). Since Zn requirements increase during pregnancy (Sandstead, 1973), a probable cause of the observed deficiencies is a failure to select foods rich in bioavailable Zn. Among women who practice pica, retention of Zn may be impaired by the formation of insoluble complexes of Zn with components of the consumed material (Danford, 1982). Findings of Hambidge *et al.* (1975) in women with acrodermatitis enteropathica, an inborn error of Zn absorption, indicate that severe maternal Zn deficiency in humans can result in terata. Less severe deficiency may be associated with impaired fetal growth (Meadows *et al.*, 1981) and fetal distress syndrome (Mukherjee *et al.*, 1984; Cherry *et al.*, 1989). A variety of maternal complications may also occur (Jameson, 1976, 1982; Hunt *et al.*, 1984; Cherry *et al.*, 1981, 1989).

Another group that seems at significant risk of primary Zn deficiency is the elderly (Sandstead *et al.*, 1982; Bogden *et al.*, 1987, 1988). A survey of US elderly (Pilch and Senti, 1985) showed that 3·0% of the subjects had plasma levels of Zn that were below the normal range. Because plasma Zn is an insensitive index of Zn status (Solomons, 1979), humans display a remarkable tendency to maintain normal plasma Zn levels, and at the same time to display other biochemical and functional evidence of Zn deficiency (Hambidge *et al.*, 1972; Milne *et al.*, 1983, 1987; Lukaski *et al.*, 1984; Gibson *et al.*, 1989). It is, therefore, likely that this 3% is indicative of a substantially higher incidence of latent Zn deficiency.

B. Conditioned Deficiency

Conditioned Zn deficiency occurs when an underlying illness, behavior, or medication impairs absorption, utilization, or retention of Zn. Such conditions include malabsorption syndromes, liver and renal disease, anorexia nervosa, alcoholism, inborn errors of metabolism, cancer, chronic infections, parasitic diseases, acute catabolic states including major burns, certain medications, and pica (Sandstead, 1985).

A Zn deficiency syndrome occurs in infants with the autosomal recessive metabolic disorder acrodermatitis enteropathica (Hambidge *et al.*, 1978; Walravens *et al.*, 1978). Symptoms usually begin after weaning from breast milk. They include a vesicular dermatitis, hyperkeratosis over pressure points, angular stomatitis, perionychia, alopecia, diarrhea, apathy, irritability, failure to thrive, depressed immunity, infections, and death if untreated. This syndrome is very similar to the inborn error of Zn absorption of cattle known as lethal trait A46 or Adema disease (Weissmann and Flagstad, 1976). A second inborn error, which appears to increase the risk of Zn deficiency, is trisomy-21, otherwise known as Down's Anomaly, or Down's Syndrome (DS). Very low levels of plasma Zn have been reported in such patients (Halsted and Smith, 1970). A more recent study (Justice *et al.*, 1988) found that one third of DS subjects had low plasma Zn levels. Findings of Björksten *et al.* (1980) indicate that low Zn nutriture can substantially impair immune function of DS patients. Fabris *et al.* (1984) found low thymulin activity in plasma of DS patients. Deficits in activity of this Zn-requiring hormone might account, in part, for reduced cell mediated immunity in DS.

Congenital hemolytic anemias including sickle cell anemia and thalassemia may be complicated by Zn deficiency (Prasad *et al.*, 1965, 1975, 1981). Causes probably include increased losses of Zn from the body following hemolysis of red blood cells, and selection of diets low in bioavailable Zn. Manifestations of deficiency include growth retardation and delayed puberty in children, poor healing of leg ulcers and other injuries, and impaired immunity.

Increased losses of Zn in urine appear to be the major cause of Zn deficiency in alcoholics and cirrhotic patients (Vallee *et al.*, 1956; Sullivan and Burch, 1976). Other factors include selection of diets low in bioavailable Zn, and intestinal malabsorption syndromes that can seriously impair Zn nutriture (Solomons *et al.*, 1977). Manifestations are similar to those found in patients with hemolytic anemias and Zn deficiency. Patients with chronic renal failure may become Zn deficient. According to Mahajan *et al.* (1979, 1982), some of these patients develop clinical signs of Zn deficiency including impotence.

The striking effects of Zn nutriture on appetite have led to questions concerning the role of Zn in patients with anorexia nervosa. According to Bryce-Smith and Simpson (1984), and Safai-Kutti and Kutti (1984) some patients have displayed improved appetite subsequent to Zn supplementation.

Iatrogenic Zn deficiency caused by inadequate Zn in enteral or parenteral formulas can result in severe dermatitis, suppressed immunity and increased morbidity (Arakawa *et al.*, 1976; Kay *et al.*, 1976; Okada *et al.*, 1976; Pekarek *et al.*, 1979; Wolman *et al.*, 1979; McClain *et al.*, 1980).

Patients with severe catabolism experience massive losses of Zn in the urine. If inadequately repleted during refeeding, such patients can rapidly become Zn deficient. Such patients may display poor healing, and depressed immunity (Pories and Strain, 1974).

II. ZINC IN FOODS

Food selection and processing are critical factors affecting human Zn nutriture in that they determine both Zn content and bioavailability. Reports of the aforementioned Zn deficiency syndromes underscore the health significance of these factors.

Beef is the major dietary source of Zn in the US food supply (Welsh and Marston, 1982; USDA, 1986), the second most important source is pork (Pekkarinen, 1973). USDA (1986) data indicate that the shift in the US food supply over the past century has resulted in an increased consumption of meat and other animal products, with a concomitant decrease in foods of plant origin. Economics have an important effect on Zn nutriture. During the years between 1920 and 1940 Zn intakes declined in this country. Subsequently, as the economy improved, Zn intakes increased as a result of increasing meat consumption. The mean Zn intake of adults today is about 10·5 mg daily with a wide range within the population. Current data suggest that meat provides about half (50%) of the Zn in the US diet followed by dairy products (20%). Cereals and pulses provide most of the remaining Zn. Prior to 1950 proportions were: meat 35%, dairy 20%, and cereals 25%, a distribution with much less emphasis on meat, and similar to that of other western countries today (Lyon *et al.*, 1979; Milne *et al.*, 1980; Gibson and Scythes, 1982; USDA, 1986). In contrast to omnivorous diets, lacto-ovovegetarians receive the majority of Zn from cereal products (26%), beans and nuts (26%), and milk and eggs (18%) (Anderson *et al.*, 1981).

A. Ecological Influences on Food Zinc

Zn content of soil, season of the year, genotype of the plants, pH and other chemical factors in soil influence the levels of Zn in plants. In general, Zn is less available to plants from alkaline soil. Some plants grow and produce quite well on such soils, but contain less Zn than is required by grazing animals (Allaway, 1986). Livestock raised on confined areas where the availability of Zn from plants or directly from ingestion of soil is extremely low, may become Zn deficient. It should be noted however, that the Zn content of the muscle from grazing animals is generally not influenced by the Zn content of the plants or pastures on which they graze (Binnerts *et al.*, 1986). Animals actually constitute a safety advantage as an intermediate link in the food chain when soils are unbalanced or deficient. Some plants such as peas and other seed crops will accumulate Zn in their seeds from soils rich in available Zn. This process can be enhanced by the application of soil amendments that contain Zn. Such soil amendments are necessary for optimal performances of grazing animals in some regions of the US.

B. Bioavailability

Animal products contain considerable amounts of Zn, while lesser amounts are found in dried legumes, milk and grains (Table 9-1). Dietary components which are potential inhibitors of Zn bioavailability for either

TABLE 9-1

ZINC CONTENT OF COMMON HOUSEHOLD PORTIONS OF SELECTED FOODS

Food	*Portion*	*Zinc (mg)*	*Protein (g)*
Fish: flounder, tuna, salmon	3 oz	00·58	22·89
Oysters	3 oz	77·51	06·00
Crab	3 oz	06·48	16·46
Poultry, d-c meat	3 oz	02·20	22·08
Poultry, light	3 oz	00·87	25·34
Beef	3 oz	04·60	26·82
Pork	3 oz	04·40	26·72
Bologna	3 oz	01·70	13·02
Liver (chicken, beef, pork)	3 oz	04·90	23·48
Whole egg	1 large	00·70	06·07
Dried beans and lentils	½ cup	00·95	07·70
Milk	1 cup	00·93	08·03
Cheese, Cheddar	1 oz	00·88	07·05
Bread, white	1 sl	00·15	02·07
Bread, whole wheat	1 sl	00·47	02·69
Rice, white	½ cup	00·35	02·00
Rice, brown	½ cup	00·60	01·80
Cornmeal, cooked	½ cup	00·15	01·50
Oatmeal, cooked	½ cup	00·58	03·00
Bran flakes, 40%	1 oz	01·16	03·20
Corn flakes	1 oz	00·03	00·95

Source: United States Department of Agriculture. *Agricultural Handbooks* (1976–1988).

animal or vegetable Zn sources include phytate (inositol hexaphosphate), oxalate, lignin, certain hemicelluloses, Maillard browning products, ferrous salts, calcium, cadmium, copper, and calcium caseinate from cow's milk (Solomons *et al.*, 1979, 1983; Harzer and Kauer, 1982; Sandstead, 1982, 1985; Mills, 1985; Sandstead *et al.*, 1989a,b).

(i) Phytate complexes

Bioavailability is reduced by phytate and other binding ligands in foods of plant origin such as cereals and pulses. Refining of cereals reduces their phytate content, but also their Zn content because the Zn in cereal grains is primarily located in the bran. Inhibition of Zn retention by phytate was first shown in chicks (O'Dell and Savage, 1960). After the interaction of calcium–phytate and Zn was demonstrated in rats (Oberleas *et al.*, 1966), phytate was shown to impair Zn absorption of humans (Turnland *et al.*, 1984; Mills, 1985; Sandström *et al.*, 1987; Sandstead *et al.*, 1989a). Zn forms insoluble complexes with phytate at alkaline pH which are even more insoluble as a calcium–phytate–Zn complex (Mills, 1985). Studies in humans (Turnland *et al.*, 1984; Sandström *et al.*, 1987) showed that sodium phytate added to meals and cereal-based meals rich in phytate, impaired Zn absorption. Inhibition was found to be inversely proportional to the amount of phytate present in the meal.

(ii) Retention and absorption from cereals

Small additions of wheat bran (26 g daily) to low fiber, mixed diets were found to impair Zn retention of normal men in metabolic balance studies ($p < 0{\cdot}01$) (Sandstead, 1988; Sandstead *et al.*, 1989a). Sandström *et al.* (1987) reported an 8% absorption of ^{65}Zn by normal subjects fed oatmeal porridge containing 600 mmol of phytate with milk. In contrast, about 25% of the ^{65}Zn was absorbed from a meal of rye cereal with milk, containing 100 mmol of phytate. Absorption from meals of whole wheat and barley were intermediate between the oatmeal and rye. In addition, it was found by regression analyses of balance data that dietary Zn, nitrogen and the interaction of calcium and phytate were significant predictors of Zn retention ($R^2 = 0{\cdot}20$, $p < 0{\cdot}0001$) (Sandstead, 1988; Sandstead *et al.*, 1989a). These various studies, which demonstrate phytate and calcium–phytate interactions with Zn, clearly establish the importance of these phenomena for human nutrition.

Limited data suggest that products of non-enzymatic Maillard browning are potentially important inhibitors of Zn bioavailability. Findings of Lykken *et al.* (1986) showed that absorption of a ^{65}Zn tracer from corn flakes, which contain Mallard browning products, was significantly inferior to absorption from corn grits, which do not.

Solomons *et al.* (1979) found that tortillas, which are high in phytate, Maillard browning products, and lime ($CaCO_3$) significantly inhibited the increase in plasma Zn that normally occurs when humans are fed oysters, a rich source of bioavailable Zn. These findings showed that the above relationships may be of practical importance to populations of less developed countries who subsist on diets of poorly refined cereal grains and pulses.

Unfortunately, findings of Brune *et al.* (1989) show that humans do not adapt to high phytate diets even after many years of diets rich in phytate due to an inability to hydrolyze dietary phytate. On the other hand, findings of Sandström *et al.* (1989) suggest that the protein in legumes improves Zn absorption in spite of their high phytate content. The extent to which the enhancement of Zn absorption and retention by protein is counterbalanced by phytate–calcium complexes in free-living populations is not evident. Based on historical evidence linking high-phytate diets with primary Zn deficiency (Prasad *et al.*, 1963a,b; Sandstead *et al.*, 1967; Halsted *et al.*, 1972), humans who self-select diets rich in phytate must be considered at risk of Zn deficiency, particularly if the dietary calcium intakes are high as well.

(iii) Retention and absorption from milk

The absorption of Zn from cow's milk is generally less than from human milk (Sandström *et al.*, 1983). Findings of Pecoud *et al.* (1975) indicate that milk and cheese suppressed the rise in plasma Zn after an experimental meal. Observations of Harzer and Kauer (1982) indicate that the phosphopeptides of casein produced by tryptic digestion form insoluble complexes with Zn at alkaline pH. *In vitro*, calcium caused the casein phosphate–Zn complex to precipitate. Clinical experimental findings of Sandstead *et al.* (1989a) were consistent with these findings. They fed normal men diets that provided 15% of their energy intake from protein of which about 40% was from cow's milk products. Zn retention of the men was substantially less ($p < 0{\cdot}01$) on this diet than when they were fed diets that provided 8% of energy from protein. These findings and those of Pecoud *et al.* (1975) appear to conflict with those of Sandström *et al.* (1980) who reported that sodium caseinate did not impair absorption of ^{65}Zn. Natural milk proteins are rich in calcium, which according to Harzer and Kauer (1982) is a key factor in the precipitation of Zn–casein phosphopeptide complexes.

(iv) Dietary factors which enhance Zn absorption

Experiments indicate that histidine and glutamate, citrate, picolinate and ethylenediaminetetraacetic acid (EDTA) (Evans and Johnson, 1980; Oestreicher and Cousins, 1982; Seal and Heaton, 1983; Wapnir *et al.*, 1983) can facilitate Zn absorption under some conditions. Citrate, EDTA and glutamate are often used as antioxidants in processed meats, which might account for Solomons *et al.* (1979) finding that Zn absorption was greater from processed than unprocessed meats.

C. Toxicity

Zn has a fairly wide range between nutritional efficacy and toxicity (Hambidge *et al.*, 1986). Very high intakes from consumption of acidic drinks such as lemonade, which have been stored in galvanized containers, will result in acute poisoning. Symptoms include nausea, vomiting, abdominal pain, vertigo, headache and muscle incoordination.

A more subtle but potentially more important type of toxicity occurs when the Zn level in the intestinal contents is sufficient to interfere with intestinal absorption of other nutrients. This phenomenon was illustrated in patients treated with 150 mg Zn daily for sickle cell anemia. Copper deficiency, expressed through leukopenia and anemia occurred (Prasad *et al.*, 1978a). Copper absorption was impaired because the Zn induced the synthesis of metallothionein in the intestinal mucosal cells. Metallothionein has a higher binding affinity for copper than for Zn (Bremner, 1987). This phenomenon has been used successfully to inhibit intestinal absorption of copper in patients with Wilson's Disease (Brewer *et al.*, 1983). Inhibition of copper absorption by Zn might explain the decrease in HDL cholesterol observed in young men who were experimentally supplemented with about 150 mg Zn daily (Hooper *et al.*, 1980). Copper deficiency in experimental rats causes an increase in total plasma cholesterol and a relative decrease in HDL cholesterol (Allen and Klevay, 1980).

III. BIOCHEMISTRY AND PHYSIOLOGY OF ZINC

A. Zinc Metalloenzymes

In 1940, with the purification of carbonic anhydrase, the first Zn metalloenzyme was described (Keilin and Mann, 1940). To date, over 200 Zn metalloenzymes have been reported and are represented in all of the six categories of the International Nomenclature of Enzymes (Galdes and Vallee, 1983). Galdes and Vallee (1983) categorize several roles for Zn in metalloenzymes: catalytic, structural, regulatory or modulatory, and noncatalytic. Zn metalloenzymes are important components of several essential cell functions. The synthesis, repair and structural integrity of nucleic acids requires Zn (Burnet, 1981; Wu and Wu, 1983). The syntheses of proteins, including histones, also appear to need Zn (Mazus *et al.*, 1984; Wallwork and Duerre, 1985; Castro *et al.*, 1986; Duerre and Wallwork, 1986; Falchuk *et al.*, 1986; Hicks and Wallwork, 1987). Furthermore, interactions of Zn and lipid metabolism have been reported. The metabolism of cholesterol, fatty acids, phospholipids and triglyceride have all been reported to be influenced by Zn nutriture in experimental animals (Klevay, 1973; Patel *et al.*, 1975; Cornatzer *et al.*, 1984; Cunnane *et al.*, 1984; Koo and Lee, 1988). However, as Cunnane (1988) points out, it is difficult to correlate the activities of many Zn metalloenzymes to either altered tissue levels of Zn or to morphologic abnormalities that occur subsequent to Zn deficiency.

B. Zinc and the Genome

This subject was reviewed recently (Wallwork and Sandstead, 1990). Most of the common signs of Zn deficiency in experimental animals, e.g. growth depression, poor wound healing, depressed immune function, terata, and hypogonadism are probably mediated, at least in part, through impairment of nucleic acid synthesis and repair, suppressed expression of the genetic code, and depressed synthesis of proteins. Depressed levels of cellular Zn may also impair binding of Zn to apoenzymes, receptors, hormones, or other proteins (e.g. Zn finger proteins) so as to influence their tertiary structure, biological activity, or receptivity.

Adverse effects of severe Zn deficiency on the genome include reduced activity of Zn-dependent enzymes that mediate DNA replication, repair, transcription, and translation. Examples include terminal deoxyribonucleotidyl transferase, deoxythymidine kinase, nucleoside phosphorylase, elongation factor I, and a topoisomerase. In Zn-deficient rats incorporation of thymidine into liver nuclei and brain DNA is reduced (Sandstead and Rinaldi, 1969; Sandstead *et al.*, 1972); activity of liver DNA-dependent RNA polymerase is suppressed in weanling rats (Terhune and Sandstead, 1972); incorporation of uridine into RNA is decreased (Sandstead and Terhune, 1974); and polysomes are decreased on sucrose density profiles of liver and brain homogenates (Fosmire *et al.*, 1975, 1976). Protein synthesis is also decreased. Activity of amino acyl-tRNA synthetase in livers is low (Hicks and Wallwork, 1987) and amino acid utilization is reduced (Hsu *et al.*, 1969; Grey and Dreosti, 1972). This phenomenon decreases the synthesis of histones and non-histone chromosomal protein (Duerre *et al.*, 1977; Wallwork and Duerre, 1985) including histone H1° (Castro *et al.*, 1986). H1° histones are apparently responsible for the higher order coiling of nucleosome chains (Thoma *et al.*, 1979; Lennox, 1984), and in this capacity are believed to influence expression of the genetic code. Thus, it is evident that severe Zn deficiency impairs function of the genome at the levels of DNA, RNA, and of protein synthesis.

C. Zinc's Role in Nuclear Receptors for Steroids and other Compounds that Modulate DNA Function

Recently, a polypeptide receptor structure has been reported to be common to several steroid hormones (testosterone, estrogen, progesterone, corticosterone, aldosterone, and calcitonin) plus organic compounds with varied structures, e.g. 1,25-dihydroxy vitamin D_3 (biologically active form), retinoic acid, thyroxine, interleukin-2 and prolactin (Loosfelt *et al.*, 1986; Weinberger *et al.*, 1986; Arriza *et al.*, 1987; Hollenberg *et al.*, 1987; Green *et al.*, 1988; Minghetti and Norman, 1988). Of these compounds, the glucocorticoid receptor has been shown to contain two Zn ions in a region with 87 peptide residues with a configuration containing cysteine and histidine. This domain is involved in binding to DNA. The other two parts of this receptor that are involved in the transcriptional response and binding to the steroid hormone, are the amino-terminal and carboxy-terminal, respectively.

The amino-terminal and carboxy-terminal regions of the receptors for these various compounds can vary widely depending on their structure and function. The structure of the DNA-binding region is a highly conserved domain with many similar structural features in all the receptors to the compounds listed above. These domains are similar to that described in the transcription factor IIIA of *Xenopus laevulis*, which contains two Zn ions in the polypeptide chains with a structure described as Zn-finger proteins (Miller *et al.*, 1985; Klug and Rhodes, 1987). The configuration of these regions are essential for gene regulation and genetic circuitry.

D. Appetite Control

Depressed food intake is one of the first signs of Zn deficiency in experimental animals. Young growing rats fed diets low in Zn and high in protein display loss of appetite after 3–4 days. They subsequently feed in a cyclic manner with about 1–2 days of a low food intake, followed by 1–2 days of higher food consumption (Chesters and Quarterman, 1970). The mechanism of this phenomenon is unclear, but is believed to be related to changes in plasma Zn that are inverse to the feeding behavior (Wallwork *et al.*, 1981). Perhaps the changes in plasma Zn affect a nucleus in the hypothalamus that modulates appetite (O'Dell and Reeves, 1988).

E. Gustatory Function

The importance of Zn for taste function has been reviewed by Russell *et al.* (1983). Research of Henkin (Henkin and Bradley, 1970; Henkin *et al.*, 1975a, 1976) has shown a relationship between Zn status and taste and smell acuity in humans. The clearest association was found in subjects who were deprived of Zn experimentally and then repleted (Henkin *et al.*, 1975a). A double-blind intervention trial of Zn treatment of patients with dysgeusia however, was interpreted as negative, suggesting the presence of confounding factors in the population studied (Henkin *et al.*, 1976). In rats, Zn deficiency causes a reduction in the ability to taste sodium chloride (McConnell and Henkin, 1974) and sucrose, and increases tolerance for sour and bitter solutions (Catalanotto and Lacy, 1977). The mechanisms of these phenomena are unknown, as Catalanotto and Nanda (1977) found no relationship between taste function in rats and changes in the tongue epithelium to be induced by Zn deficiency.

It has been speculated that changes in saliva in some way influence taste. In rats, Zn deficiency caused no change in the Zn concentration of whole saliva (Everett and Apgar, 1979). However, in humans, Zn deprivation decreased the Zn content of whole saliva (Greger and Sickles, 1979; Freeland-Graves *et al.*, 1981). Henkin *et al.* (1975a) reported that parotid Zn concentrations were decreased in patients with impaired gustatory activity. They also found a Zn-containing protein with a molecular weight of 37 000 daltons in parotid saliva, which they termed 'gustin' because of its presumed role in taste function (Henkin *et al.*, 1975c).

Lack of understanding of the mechanisms whereby Zn nutriture influences taste has not precluded the clinical use of taste acuity as a functional indicator of Zn status (Hambidge *et al.*, 1972; Henkin *et al.*, 1975a; Gibson *et al.*, 1989). The relationship of this function to Zn status has been demonstrated through experimental depletion studies (Henkin *et al.*, 1975a) and studies of the relationship between growth retardation and Zn nutriture in children (Hambidge *et al.*, 1972; Gibson *et al.*, 1989). In these latter two studies, poor taste acuity was a feature of the syndrome.

F. Sexual Development

Zn deficiency has been shown to damage the germinal epithelium of the testis, reduce testosterone secretion, and suppress spermatogenesis in several species including humans (Millar *et al.*, 1958; Pitts *et al.*, 1966; Underwood and Somers, 1969; Diamond *et al.*, 1971; Abbasi *et al.*, 1980; Taneja and Nirmal, 1980; Mason *et al.*, 1982). Sperm contains a high concentration of Zn, and Zn deficiency causes malformed sperm (Dinsdale and Williams, 1980). Sperm tail components such as the dense fibers are rich in —SH groups which bind Zn (Wallace *et al.*, 1984). The high Zn content of seminal fluid is believed important for sperm integrity (Arver and Eliasson, 1982). Björndahl and Kvist (1982) postulated that Zn is essential for the head–tail detachment process that occurs when the egg is fertilized.

Evidence that Zn deficiency can cause hypogonadism in humans was first reported from Egypt (Prasad *et al.*, 1963b; Sandstead *et al.*, 1967), and Iran (Halsted *et al.*, 1972). Subsequent research has shown similar findings in

Zn-deficient patients with sickle cell disease (Prasad *et al.*, 1975; 1981; Abbassi *et al.*, 1976) and in experimentally Zn-deprived humans (Abbassi *et al.*, 1980). In rats, testosterone, dihydrotestosterone, androstenedione and growth hormone secretion were decreased by Zn deficiency, while synthesis and/or secretion of pituitary gonadotrophins (e.g. follicle stimulating hormone, luteinizing hormone, thyrotropin and prolactin) were increased (Lei *et al.*, 1976; Root *et al.*, 1979; Salem *et al.*, 1984). McClain *et al.* (1984) suggested that hypothalamic function of the Zn-deficient animals is intact, and that a depletion of Leydig cells is responsible for the hypogonadism associated with Zn deficiency.

Reversibility of testicular damage in Zn deficiency is dependent on the severity and timing of the deficiency. Mason *et al.* (1982) reported that testicular damage induced by severe short-term Zn deficiency in prepubertal male rats was reversed by Zn repletion, whereas severe Zn deprivation in postpubertal male rats caused permanent testicular damage. Studies in humans showed that suppressed testicular function, i.e. low sperm count and a low Leydig cell function, recovered slowly (over 6–10 months) in subjects who were Zn-deprived and then repleted (Abbassi *et al.*, 1980).

In some patients with alcoholism, sickle cell disease, and uremia, Zn treatment has improved sexual function (Abbassi *et al.*, 1976; Antoniou *et al.*, 1977; Levy *et al.*, 1981; Prasad *et al.*, 1981; Mahajan *et al.*, 1982). However, the findings are inconsistent among reports (Brook *et al.*, 1980; Goldiner *et al.*, 1983). Patient selection, compliance and length of treatment may contribute to these conflicting findings.

There have been few reports of Zn deprivation in immature females (Halsted *et al.* 1972). It was speculated that the delayed puberty, irregular menses, or amenorrhea in girls infected with hookworm in the southern US and Australia early in this century was caused by Zn deficiency (Sandstead *et al.*, 1967). Halsted *et al.* (1972) clearly showed that sexual development of girls required Zn, just as does sexual development of boys.

G. Gestation and Parturition

The induction of terata by Zn deficiency was first described in chickens by Blamberg *et al.* (1960). Subsequently, Hurley and Swenerton (1966) reported the teratogenic effect of Zn deficiency in rats. Their findings have been confirmed in rats and other species (Warkany and Petering, 1972; Palludan and Wegger, 1976; Apgar and Fitzgerald, 1985; Record *et al.*, 1987). Prolonged gestation and difficult parturition occur in Zn-deficient rats and pigs (Apgar, 1985).

Reports consistent with endemic Zn deficiency in Egypt and Iran (Prasad *et al.*, 1961, 1963a, b; Sandstead *et al.*, 1967) led to speculation that Zn deficiency was one of the causes of the high incidence of fetal abnormalities in the Middle East (Sever and Emmanuel, 1973). Subsequently, maternal Zn deficiency has been associated with spina bifida (Bergmann *et al.*, 1980), anencephaly (Hambidge *et al.*, 1975; Buamah *et al.*, 1984), and other abnormalities in pregnancy outcome such as prolonged pregnancy, low birth-weight, and fetal distress at birth (Jameson, 1976; Cherry *et al.*, 1981, 1989; Meadows *et al.*, 1981; Mukherjee *et al.*, 1984).

H. Brain Development and Function

Zn is essential for normal development of the brain. Zn deficiency in mice or rats causes anencephaly, microcephaly, hydrocephaly and other malformations of the brain (Hurley and Swenerton, 1966; Hurley and Shrader, 1972; Record *et al.*, 1987). Zn deficiency during intrauterine brain development has been associated with subsequent abnormalities in behavioral function in rats including increased aggression in response to shock (Halas *et al.*, 1975) and impaired avoidance of shock (Halas and Sandstead, 1975). Mild or severe maternal Zn deprivation throughout pregnancy and lactation in rats impairs subsequent working-memory in offspring (Halas *et al.*, 1983, 1986). In non-human primates, intrauterine Zn deprivation causes subsequent behavioral and learning deficits (Sandstead *et al.*, 1977; Strobel and Sandstead, 1984; Golub *et al.*, 1985). The hippocampal mossy fiber boutons are rich in Zn (Ibata and Otsuka, 1969). Zn deficiency has been reported to reduce the Zn content of the mossy fiber area of the hippocampus in the rat (Wensink *et al.*, 1987). A role for Zn in processes of neurotransmission has been suggested (Assaf and Chung, 1984; Howell *et al.*, 1984). Indeed, severe Zn deprivation in the rat causes increases in catecholamines in brain (Wallwork *et al.*, 1982). In humans, severe Zn deficiency can cause abnormal cerebellar function, and impair thought processes (Henkin *et al.*, 1975a).

I. Membrane Function

Findings of Bettger and O'Dell (1981), Cunnane (1988) and others suggest that Zn influences the structure and function of cell membranes. Its role in the activity of δ-6- and δ-5-desaturase enzymes, which convert linoleic acid to γ-linoleic acid and dihomo-γ-linolenic acid to arachidonic acid, has been put forth by Cunnane (1988) as evidence of this possible influence. Synthesis of phospholipids in microsomal membranes from liver, brain and spleen, has also been found to have been altered by Zn deficiency in rats (Cornatzer *et al.*, 1984).

J. Antioxidant Function

Findings of Sullivan *et al.* (1980), Bray *et al.* (1986) and Willson (1988) indicate that Zn deficiency results in an increased susceptibility of cells to peroxidation. Mechanisms of this phenomenon have not been established *in vivo* but *in vitro* findings by Thornalley and Vasak (1985) indicate that the level of metallothionein (MT) in cells is probably a crucial factor. They found that this cysteine-rich protein reacts avidly as its metal-thiolate clusters with free hydroxyl radicals (HO·). According to Sato *et al.* (1984) and Bremner *et al.* (1987) the synthesis of MT is proportional to the amount of Zn available to cells. Thornalley and Vasak (1985) also reported that reduced glutathione will restore the HO· scavaging capacity of MT. Their findings suggest that the activity of glutathione reductase is a critical factor in the detoxification of HO· by MT. It appears possible (but has been incompletely proven) that Zn nutriture influences the activity of glutathione reductase indirectly by mediating the phosphorylation of riboflavin to FMN (flavin mononucleotide, riboflavin-5′-phosphate), the precursor of FAD (flavin adenine dinucleotide) (McCormick, 1962). FAD is an essential co-factor for the activity of glutathione reductase.

K. Immune Development and Function

Zn is essential for the normal development and function of the immune system. Young adult male mice fed severely Zn-deficient diets for 28 days display atrophy of the thymus, lymphopenia and altered proportions of lymphocytes and polymorphonuclear neutrophils, depressed responses of T cells to mitogens, decrease cytolytic T cell responses and suppressed delayed cutaneous hypersensitivity to antigens (Fraker *et al.*, 1986). Children with acrodermatitis enteropathica and cattle with the lethal trait A46 display similar abnormalities of immune function (Weismann and Flagstad, 1976). In addition, one of the thymic hormones, thymulin, requires Zn for activity (Bach *et al.*, 1977). Zn complexes with apo-thymulin in the plasma to form active thymulin. Beach *et al.* (1982, 1983) found that gestational Zn deficiency suppressed subsequent formation of immunoglobulins by B-lymphocytes across two generations. Treatment of elderly persons with Zn was found to improve certain immune functions (Duchateau *et al.*, 1981). Findings of Bogden *et al.* (1987, 1988) suggest that impaired immunity of some elderly persons is related to low Zn nutriture. Björksten *et al.* (1980) found that Zn supplementation of 11 or 12 patients with Down's Anomaly, who also had low levels of plasma Zn, resulted in improvement of white cell chemotaxis, skin-test reactivity to antigens, and lymphocyte mitogen responses. Pekerak *et al.* (1979) showed that anergy and suppressed lymphocyte response to phytohemagglutinin were corrected by a Zn supplement in a man who had primary, iatrogenic Zn deficiency.

L. Skeletal Development

The essentiality of Zn for skeletal development has been reviewed by Wallwork and Sandstead (1990). Skeletal abnormalities occur in the fetuses of several species exposed to maternal Zn deprivation (Blamberg *et al.*, 1960; Hurley and Swenerton, 1966; Leek *et al.*, 1988). Zn deprivation decreases linear and radial bone growth, collagen synthesis, and biomechanical competence of bone and collagen (Suwarnasarn *et al.*, 1982). Adolescents with Zn deficiency may display delayed closure of epiphysis (Sandstead, 1972).

Zn in bone is relatively sequestered and insufficiently available to other organ systems to prevent clinical signs of Zn deficiency when dietary deprivation is severe. However, factors that increase the turnover of bone, such as increased parathyroid hormone activity, will cause bone Zn to be mobilized. Thus, Hurley and Tao (1972) found that diets low in calcium protected fetuses from the effects of severe maternal Zn deprivation.

M. Parakeratosis and Cancer of the Esophagus in Zinc Deficiency

The Zn-deficient epidermis, esophageal, and tongue epithelium display hyperplasia, hyperkeratosis and parakeratosis (Follis *et al.*, 1941; Tucker and Salmon, 1955; Legg and Sears, 1960; Barney *et al.*, 1968; Joseph *et al.*, 1981). While DNA synthesis and cell division are suppressed by Zn deficiency in most organs, the Zn-deficient oral and esophageal mucosa display increases in cell division, protein synthesis and enzyme activity. These increases occur even though Zn concentrations of these tissues are decreased about 50% by severe Zn deficiency in the rat (Gerson *et al.*, 1985).

The effects of Zn deficiency on the esophagus is believed to predispose this organ to cancer. Studies from China suggest that methylbenzylnitrosoamine (MBN) is particularly carcinogenic in Zn-deficient humans (Lin *et al.*, 1977; Van Rensberg, 1981). A possible explanation is the finding that Zn modulates the activity of certain cytochrome P450 enzymes which metabolize MBN. Barch and Iannaccone (1986) found that Zn is a noncompetitive inhibitor of this P450 reaction *in vivo*. Thus, in Zn deficiency, activity of the enzymes is increased as is the synthesis of carcinogenic species.

IV. ASSESSMENT OF ZINC STATUS

Zn status is a reflection of the Zn economy of the total body. As a general rule, a neutral or positive Zn balance is indicative of adequate Zn status. With Zn deprivation, homeostatic mechanisms reduce Zn losses. If deprivation continues for a sufficiently long period, homeostatic mechanisms break down and losses of Zn in urine and feces increase, resulting in a negative balance. Since mechanisms for maintenance of Zn homeostasis are so powerful, changes in blood-plasma and hair Zn tend to occur late in depletion. Decreases in the Zn content of urine and sweat occur much sooner in Zn-deprived individuals than for those on adequate Zn-containing diets (Solomons, 1979; Milne *et al.*, 1983; Lukaski *et al.*, 1984).

Plasma or serum Zn, a commonly used parameter of Zn nutriture in man and animals, is relatively simple to measure and, in well-controlled experiments of mild Zn deficiency, decreases after Zn deprivation has continued for a period of time. Generally, a decrease in plasma Zn is a rather late reflector of impaired Zn status. In addition, it is subject to a variety of influences which can cause confusion. Typically plasma Zn is increased by fasting, lowered by infection and stress, and decreased in pregnancy by physiologic mechanisms. Because albumin is its transport protein, plasma Zn will tend to decrease in hypoalbuminemia, although the binding sites for Zn on albumin are unsaturated (Solomons, 1979). Plasma Zn has a diurnal variation (Markowitz *et al.*, 1985). Erythrocyte Zn is also affected by Zn status, though more slowly. In experiments on humans, erythrocyte Zn reflected Zn status in men fed a Zn-deficient diet (Buerk *et al.*, 1973; Prasad *et al.*, 1978b). In addition, erythrocyte Zn was significantly decreased in adolescent Zn-deficient Egyptian boys (Prasad *et al.*, 1963b). In other clinical studies, erythrocyte Zn did not decrease in Zn-deprived young men (Baer and King, 1984).

Zn content of white blood cells has been used to assess Zn nutriture (Prasad *et al.*, 1978b; Keeling *et al.*, 1980; Jones *et al.*, 1981; Meadows *et al.*, 1981; Patrick *et al.*, 1982; Patrick and Dervish, 1984; Simmer and Thompson, 1985; Bogden *et al.*, 1987, 1988; Wells *et al.*, 1987). The Zn concentration of crude isolates of buffy coat of blood cells (polymorphonuclear neutrophils (PMNs) + mononucleated cells (MNCs) + platelets) has been used by some investigators as an indicator of Zn status. A potential problem with this method is that different cell types contain different levels of Zn, and various conditions alter the proportions of these cells from what is considered normal (Wallwork, 1987). The Zn concentration of polymorphonuclear neutrophils is perhaps a more reliable indicator of human Zn status (Prasad *et al.*, 1978b; Rabbani *et al.*, 1987). In contrast to humans, the Zn content of PMN and MNC were not indicative of Zn deficiency in severely Zn-deficient rats (Kramer, 1984; Milne *et al.*, 1985). Platelet Zn content has also been used as an indicator of Zn status (Bogden *et al.*, 1987, 1988). Further studies are needed to evaluate its usefulness. Other indices have been assessed as well, including skin Zn, fingernail Zn, salivary Zn, activities of certain serum enzymes that require Zn for activity, such as alkaline phosphatase, carbonic anhydrase, RNA-ase, taste and smell acuity and dark adaptation. All have limitations which are reviewed by Solomons (1979).

Recently, Bremner *et al.* (1987) proposed that plasma and/or cellular MT might be a useful indicator of Zn status. In rats, they found that MT levels were directly related to levels of tissue Zn (Bremner *et al.*, 1987). Findings of Grider *et al.* (1990) suggest that MT levels in erythrocytes reflect Zn nutriture of humans.

Prasad and Rabbani (1981), have proposed erythrocyte nucleoside phosphorylase activity as a useful index of Zn status. This enzyme is activated by Zn. Based on observations on humans, Prasad *et al.* (1988) have also suggested that the activity of thymulin in plasma is a useful indicator of Zn nutriture. Milne *et al.* (1987) have shown that the clearance of ethanol from the peripheral blood is reduced in mildly Zn-deprived humans. Application of this method to clinical situations has not been reported. Lukaski *et al.* (1984) have shown that release of Zn from muscle into blood in response to exercise is decreased in Zn deficiency, but application of this knowledge to clinical assessment has not been reported. Zn content of sweat is markedly reduced by Zn deficiency (Milne *et al.*, 1983). However, collection of total body sweat is difficult. It is unclear whether assay of sweat from specific regions of the skin is a useful method for Zn assessment.

V. ZINC REQUIREMENTS

Dietary Zn requirements are related to the bioavailability of food Zn, and to the level of anabolism and losses of Zn by excretion and other means.

Dietary factors affecting bioavailability have been noted previously. The influence of anabolism is related to the requirement of Zn for enzyme activity and protein synthesis. Increased anabolism increases the requirement for Zn. Losses of Zn from the body are mediated by homeostatic mechanisms of the intestine, kidkeys, and skin.

A. Infants

Healthy lactating mothers provide about 2·7 mg Zn/day in their milk during early lactation. Later, levels fall to about 0·9 mg/day (Hambidge *et al.*, 1986). Zn in human milk is highly bioavailable, presumably because of the relatively low casein content, and possibly because it is facilitated by other Zn-binding ligands (Evans and Johnson, 1980; Sandström *et al.*, 1983; Lönnerdal *et al.*, 1984). Because of the lower bioavailability of Zn from cow's milk, infant formulas are usually supplemented with levels of Zn that are substantially higher than levels in human milk. Provisional factorially estimated Zn requirements for infants up to one year of age are from 1·1–1·25 mg/day (WHO, 1973) (Table 9-3). The recommended daily allowance in the US for Zn is 3–5 mg/day for infants, which assumes 20% availability of Zn and 16% of calories as protein (FNB, 1980). According to Dauncey *et al.* (1977), preterm infants may display negative Zn balance for over 60 days when fed 0·6 mg of Zn/kg. Findings of Cavel and Widdowson (1964), showed that full-term infants were often in negative Zn balance at the end of the first week of life. Reasons for these negative balances are unclear. Feeding cow's milk or unenriched formulas can result in Zn deficiency in infants (Walravens and Hambidge, 1976). Zn absorption from infant soy formulas is lower than from cow's milk or human milk as a result of the formula's phytate content (Sandström *et al.*, 1983; Lönnerdal *et al.*, 1984).

B. Children

Dietary intakes of 7–8 mg of Zn appear to be adequate for young children if between 3·4 and 2·1 mg/day are absorbed (Scoular, 1939; Engle *et al.*, 1966). Increasing dietary protein intake will increase plasma Zn levels and Zn retention of children (Price *et al.*, 1970). The Recommended Daily Allowance in the US for Zn is 10 mg/day in children, assuming a 20% absorption from food and 16% of calories as protein (FNB, 1980). The USDA (1986) has reported that intakes of US children ages 1–3 are about 75% of the RDA. From Table 9-2, it appears that many populations of children receive potentially marginal dietary intakes of Zn, i.e. from 5–6·36 mg Zn/daily. Whether the children become Zn deficient or not will depend on the bioavailability of the dietary Zn.

TABLE 9-2

ZINC INTAKES IN DIETS OF CHILDREN, ADULTS AND VEGETARIANS

Age	*Sex*	*n*	*Zn intake mg/day*	*SD*	*Population*	*Reference*
1 month	M and F	35	1·90	0·20	Breast-fed, Canada	MacDonald *et al.* (1982)[a]
1 month	M and F	25	3·60	0·60	Bottle-fed, Canada	
6 months	M and F	16	2·70	0·50	Breast-fed, Canada	
6 months	M and F	23	4·60	0·70	Bottle-fed, Canada	
2–7 years	M and F	96	6·30	0·44	Middle income, USA	Hambidge *et al.* (1979)[b]
2–6 years	M and F	85	5·00	[m]	Low income, USA	Walravens *et al.* (1983)[c]
3–5 years	M and F	5	6·36	0·83	Norwegian children	Schlage and Wortberg (1972)[d]
10–13 years	M and F	6	10·16	1·42	Norwegian pre-teens	
14–16 years	F	15	12·00	5·00	High school, USA	White (1969)[e]
18–30 years	F	21	13·80	7·27	College women, USA	
14–64 years	M and F	22	8·60	0·52	Middle income, USA	Holden *et al.* (1979)[f]
30	F	100	10·10	3·30	Canadians, omnivorous	Gibson and Scythes (1982)[g]
Adult	F	5	6·40	1·69	Vegetarians, USA	King *et al.* (1981)[h]
Adult	M	5	20·30	8·80	Military, USA	Milne *et al.* (1980)[i]
81·7 years	M and F	21	5·53	[b]	Geriatric hospital	Thomas *et al.* (1988)[j]
85·5 years	M and F	24	8·90	2·53	Healthy elderly at home	Bunker *et al.* (1984)[k]
25–48 years	M and F	112	8·5	4·5	Vegetarians (Punjabi) Canada	Bindra *et al.* (1986)[l]

[a] 3-day records taken at home visits.
[b] 24-h recall and food checklist.
[c] 24-h recall and food checklist.
[d] 2-week food records.
[e] Weighed 24-h diets with duplicate food composite.
[f] 14-day food record and 132 diet composites.
[g] 3-day food records and 24 h food composite.
[h] 3-day food records.
[i] 6 days of duplicate chemical diet composites.
[j] Duplicate chemical diet composites.
[k] Duplicate chemical diet composites.
[l] 3-day weighed records and 30 1-day duplicate composites.
[m] Value not reported.

C. Adolescents

Because of accelerated growth, the Zn requirements of adolescents are relatively greater than those of children (Sandstead, 1985). Dietary requirements have been estimated at 12·3 mg/day before and 11·9 mg/day after menarche for girls, and 11 mg/day for boys.

D. Adults

Zn requirements are relatively decreased after growth is completed. In adults, requirements are related to metabolic mass. Balance studies on normal men who were consuming diets low in fiber and phytate, living in an air-conditioned environment, and having moderate exercise, indicated that about 7·8 mg of Zn in the diet was sufficient to maintain balance when the protein content of the diet approximated the RDA (Sandstead *et al.*, 1979). Holden *et al.* (1979) reported an average Zn content of self-selected diets of a small group of normal, middle-income men and women ($n = 22$) of 8·6 mg daily. The Zn content of vegetarian diets tends to be less than omnivorous diets (Table 9-2). The US Department of Agriculture (USDA, 1986) has reported that the Zn intake of women 19–50 years is about 60% of the RDA. Balance studies in adults suggest that the minimum requirement for dietary Zn from a low fiber, low phytate mixed diet is about 4·0–4·5 mg daily (Milne *et al.*, 1983; Lukaski *et al.*, 1984).

E. Pregnant Women

Zn requirements are increased during pregnancy (Table 9-3). The Recommended Daily Allowance for Zn in pregnancy adds 5 mg/day for pregnancy and 10 mg/day for lactation to the 15 mg recommended daily for non-pregnant adults (FNB, 1980).

F. Elderly

Dietary Zn requirements of elderly persons are likely to be relatively higher than those of younger persons. Capacity for intestinal absorption of Zn is apparently reduced in the elderly (Aamodt *et al.*, 1983; Bales *et al.*, 1986; Turnland *et al.*, 1986). Reported intakes of dietary Zn among groups of elderly are about 9 mg daily with a considerable range (Sandstead *et al.*, 1982). In general, one would expect elderly persons to consume less Zn than younger adults. Age-related reduced requirements for energy are associated with reduced appetite, and thus a tendency to have a decreased intake of micronutrients.

TABLE 9-3

FACTORIAL BASIS OF PROVISIONAL REQUIREMENTS OF DIETARY ZINC IN RELATION TO ESTIMATES OF ASSUMED LOSSES AND AVAILABILITY

Age	*Peak daily retention (mg)*	*Urinary excretion (mg)*	*Sweat excretion (mg)*	*Total required (mg)*	*Milligrams necessary in daily diet if content of available Zn is:*		
					10%	*20%*	*40%*
Infants:							
0–4 months	0·35	0·4	0·5	1·25	12·5	6·3	3·1
5–12 months	0·2	0·4	0·5	1·1	11·0	5·5	2·8
Males:							
1–10 years	0·2	0·4	1·0	1·6	16·0	8·0	4·0
11–17 years	0·8	0·5	1·5	2·8	28·0	14·0	7·0
18 years plus	0·2	0·5	1·5	2·2	22·0	11·0	5·5
Females:							
1–9 years	0·15	0·4	1·0	1·55	15·5	7·8	3·9
10–13 years	0·65	0·5	1·5	2·65	26·5	13·3	6·6
14–16 years	0·2	0·5	1·5	2·2	22·0	11·0	5·5
17 years plus	0·2	0·5	1·5	2·2	22·0	11·0	5·5
Pregnant women:							
0–20 weeks	0·55	0·5	1·5	2·55	25·5	12·8	6·4
20–30 weeks	0·9	0·5	1·5	2·9	29·0	14·5	7·3
30–40 weeks	1·0	0·5	1·5	3·0	30·0	15·0	7·5
Lactating women:	3·45	0·5	1·5	5·45	54·5	27·3	13·7

Explanation: The above estimates are based on the assumption that the fat-free tissue concentration of Zn in man is approximately 30 μg/g. This figure is equivalent to 2·0 g of Zn in the soft tissues of an adult male and 1·2 g in the soft tissues of an adult female, as determined from lean body mass. The Zn requirement at various ages was determined from the change in lean body mass with age. Bone Zn was not included in these calculations, as Zn in bone is relatively sequestered from the metabolically active pool of body Zn. The excretion of Zn in sweat is based on an assumed Zn content in sweat of 1 mg/liter. The estimated requirement for lactation is based on a Zn content in milk of 5 mg/liter and a daily milk secretion of 650 ml. The urinary excretions of Zn are based on levels reported.
Source: Adapted from WHO (1973).

VI. SUMMARY

The history of zinc (Zn) as a nutrient and its recognition as an essential element for human nutrition is described. Primary dietary deficiency of Zn as well as a number of conditioned Zn deficiencies, i.e. those secondary to underlying illnesses, are defined. Meat presently supplies approximately 50% of the total Zn intake in the average US diet, although shifts in the major Zn sources over the years have followed economic changes. The Zn content of plants can be affected by environmental conditions, so that livestock raised in confined areas with compromised Zn availability may become Zn deficient. However, the muscle content of Zn is generally not influenced by the Zn content of the plants or pastures on which they graze.

Animal products contain considerable amounts of Zn, while dried legumes, milk and grains contain lesser amounts. In comparison to meat products, the bioavailability of the Zn is reduced in foods of plant origin due to the inhibitory effects of phytate, oxalate, lignin, and certain hemicelluloses. Other factors, which can reduce Zn absorption, include Maillard browning products, ferrous salts, calcium, cadmium, copper and calcium caseinate from cow's milk. Dietary factors, which enhance absorption, include histidine, glutamate, citrate, picolinate and ethylenediaminetetraacetic acid (EDTA). Citrate, EDTA and glutamate are often used as antioxidants in processed meats, and may account for the increased Zn absorption from processed meats.

Toxicity from Zn intake is relatively rare. On the other hand, high dietary Zn can influence the metabolism of Cu causing symptoms of Cu deficiency. The biochemical role of Zn in metalloenzymes and consequently, the genome is discussed. The depressed activity of Zn metalloenzymes due to low Zn or the absence of Zn to bind to the finger proteins could affect many cellular systems. Zn deficiency is also thought to disturb cell metabolism by altering the membrane. Loss of appetite and changes in taste and smell function are early signs of Zn deficiency in man and animals, although the mechanism for this abnormality is unclear. Another early sign of Zn deficiency is depressed growth. Zn deficiency is thought to predispose to esophageal cancer. Zn is essential for normal sexual development and function. Behavioral and learning deficits have been observed in rats and non-human primates following intrauterine Zn deficiency. Immune development and function are also impaired in Zn-deficient animals and humans making them more susceptible to infection.

Some of the common methods used to assess Zn status including measurement of white cell Zn, sweat Zn, plasma metallothionein, erythrocyte nucleoside phosphorylase, plus several functional tests are discussed. Although some of these methods are promising, there is still not an ideal procedure to establish Zn status. Dietary Zn requirements are discussed for various subpopulations as a function of the bioavailability of food Zn, of the level of anabolism and of losses of Zn by excretion and other means.

VII. REFERENCES

AAMODT, R. L., RAMBLE, W. F. and HENKIN, R. I. (1983). Zinc absorption in humans: Effects of age, sex, and food. In *Nutritional Bioavailability of Zinc* (G. E. Inglett, Ed.) p. 61. Am. Chem. Society, Washington, DC.

ABBASI, A. A., PRASAD, A. S., ORTEGA, J., CONGCO, E. and OBERLEAS, D. (1976). Gonadal function abnormalities in sickle cell anemia: studies in adult male patients. *Ann. Intern. Med.* **85**, 601.

ABBASI, A. A., PRASAD, A. S., RABBANI, P. and DUMOUCHELLE, E. (1980). Experimental zinc deficiency in man. Effect on testicular function. *J. Lab. Clin. Med.* **96**, 544.

ALLAWAY, W. H. (1986). Soil–plant–animal and human interrelationships in trace element nutrition. In *Trace Elements in Human and Animal Nutrition*, Vol. 2, 5th Edn (W. Mertz, Ed.), p. 465. Academic Press, Inc.

ALLEN, K. G. D. and KLEVAY, L. M. (1980). Hyperlipoproteinia in rats due to copper deficiency. *Nutr. Rep. Intern.* **22**, 295.

ANDERSON, B. M., GIBSON, R. S. and SABRY, J. H. (1981). The iron and zinc status of long-term vegetarian women. *Am. J. Clin. Nutr.* **34**, 1042.

ANTONIOU, L. D., SHALHOUB, R. J., SUDHAKAR, T. and SMITH, J. C., JR (1977). Reversal of uraemic impotence by zinc. *Lancet* **2**, 895.

APGAR, J. (1985). Zinc and reproduction. *Ann. Rev. Nutr.* **5**, 43.

APGAR, J. and FITZGERALD, J. A. (1985). Effect on the ewe and lamb of low zinc intake throughout pregnancy. *J. Anim. Sci.* **60**, 1530.

ARAKAWA, T., TAMURA, T., IGARASHI, Y., SUZUKI, H. and SANDSTEAD, H. H. (1976). Zinc deficiency in two infants during total parenteral alimentation for diarrhea. *Am. J. Clin. Nutr.* **29**, 197.

ARCÁSOY, A., ÇAVDAR, A. O. and BABACAN, E. (1978). Decreased iron and zinc absorption in Turkish children with iron deficiency and geophagia. *Acta Haematol.* **60**, 76.

ARRIZA, J. L., WEINBERGER, C., CERELLI, G., GLASER, T. M., HANDELIN, B. L., HOUSMAN, D. E. and EVANS, R. M. (1987). Cloning of human mineralocorticoid receptor complementary DNA: Structural and functional kinship with the glucocorticoid receptor. *Science* **237**, 268.

ARVER, S. and ELIASSON, R. (1982). Zinc and zinc ligands in human seminal plasma. II. Contribution by ligands of different origin to the zinc binding properties of human seminal plasma. *Acta Physiol. Scand.* **115**, 217.

ASSAF, S. Y. and CHUNG, W-H. (1984). Release of endogenous Zn^{2+} from brain tissue during activity. *Nature* **308**, 734.

BACH, J.-F., DARDENNE, M., PLEAU, J.-M. and ROSA, J. (1977). Biochemical characterization of a serum thymic factor. *Nature* **266**, 55.

BAER, M. T. and KING, J. C. (1984). Tissue zinc levels and zinc excretion during experimental zinc depletion in young men. *Am. J. Clin. Nutr.* **39**, 556.

BALES, C. W., STEINMAN, L. C., FREELAND-GRAVES, J. H., STONE, J. M. and YOUNG, R. K. (1986). The effect of age on plasma zinc uptake and taste acuity. *Am. J. Clin. Nutr*, **44**, 664.

BARCH, D. H. and IANNACCONE, P. M. (1986). Role of zinc deficiency in carcinogenesis. In *Essential Nutrients in Carcinogenesis* (L. A. Porier, P. M. Newberne and M. W. Pariza, Eds) p. 517. Plenum Publ. Corp., New York.

BARNEY, G. H., ORGEBIN-CRIST, M. C. and MACAPINLAC, M. P. (1968). Genesis of esophageal parakeratosis and histological changes in the testes of the zinc-deficient rat and their reversal by zinc repletion. *J. Nutr.* **95**, 526.

BEACH, R. S., GERSHWIN, M. E. and HURLEY, L. S. (1982). Gestational zinc deprivation in mice: Persistence of immunodeficiency for three generations. *Science* **218**, 469.

BEACH, R. S., GERSHWIN, M. E. and HURLEY, L. S. (1983). Persistent immunological consequences of gestational zinc deprivation. *Am. J. Clin. Nutr.* **38**, 579.

BERGMANN, K. E., MAKOSCH, G. and TEWS, K. H. (1980). Abnormalities of hair zinc concentration in mothers of newborn infants with spina bifida. *Am. J. Clin. Nutr.* **33**, 2145.

BETTGER, W. J. and O'DELL, B. L. (1981). A critical role of zinc in the structure and function of biomembranes. *Life Sci.* **28**, 1425.

BINDRA, G. S., GIBSON, R. S. and THOMPSON. L. U. (1986). [Phytate][calcium]/[zinc] ratios in Asian immigrant lacto-ovo vegetarian diets and their relationship to zinc nutriture. *Nutr. Res.* **6**, 475.

BINNERTS, W. T., HERMSEN, S., VAN DER KAMP, M., LOYENS, L. and RUVEN, H. J. T. (1986). Radioactivity and food choice: Risk factors and their perception. *Voeding.* **47**, 337.

BJÖRKSTEN, B., BACK, K. H., GUSTAVSON, G., HALLMANS, B., HÄGGLÖF, B. and TARNVIK, A. (1980). Zinc and immune function in Down's syndrome. *Acta Paediatr. Scand.* **69**, 183.

BJÖRNDAHL, L. and KVIST, U. (1982). Importance of zinc for human sperm head–tail connection. *Acta Physiol. Scand.* **116**, 51.

BLAMBERG, D. L., BLACKWOOD, U. B., SUPPLEE, W. C. and COMBS, G. F. (1960). Effect of zinc deficiency on hatchability and embryonic development. *Proc. Soc. Exp. Biol. Med.*, **104**, 217.

BOGDEN, J. D., OLESKE, J. M., MUNVES, E. M., BRUENING, K. S., KEMP, F. W., HOLDING, K. J., DENNY, T. N. and LOURIA, D. B. (1987). Zinc and immunocompetence in the elderly: Baseline data on zinc nutriture and immunity in unsupplemented subjects. *Am. J. Clin. Nutr.* **46**, 101.

BOGDEN, J. D., OLESKE, J. M., LAVENHAR, M. A., MUNVES, E. M., KEMP, F. W., BRUENING, K. S., HOLDING, K. J., DENNY, T. N., GUARINO, M. A., KRIEGER, L. M. and HOLLAND, B. K. (1988). Zinc and immunocompetence in elderly people: Effects of zinc supplementation for 3 months. *Am. J. Clin. Nutr.* **48**, 655.

BRAY, T. M., KUBOW, S. and BETTGER, W. J. (1986). Effect of dietary zinc on endogenous free radical production in rat lung microsomes. *J. Nutr.* **116**, 1054.

BREMNER, I. (1987). The involvement of metallothionein in the hepatic metabolism of copper. *J. Nutr.* **117**, 19.

BREMNER, I., MORRISON, J. N., WOOD, A. M. and ARTHUR, J. R. (1987). Effects of changes in dietary zinc, copper and selenium supply and of endotoxin administration on metallothionein I concentrations in blood cells and urine in the rat. *J. Nutr.* **117**, 1595.

BREWER, G. J., HILL, G. M., PRASAD, A. S., COSSACK, Z. T. and RABBANI, P. (1983). Oral therapy for Wilson's disease. *Ann. Intern. Med.* **99**, 314.

BROOK, A. C., WARD, M. K., COOK, D. B., JOHNSTON, D. G., WATSON, M. J. and KERR, D. N. S. (1980). Absence of a therapeutic effect of zinc in the sexual dysfunction of hemodialyzed patients. *Lancet* **2**, 618.

BRYCE-SMITH, D. and SIMPSON, R. I. D. (1984). Case of anorexia nervosa responding to zinc sulphate. *Lancet* **2**, 350.

BRUNE, M., ROSSANDER, L. and HALLBERG, L. (1989). Iron absorption: No intestinal adaptation to a high-phytate diet. *Am. J. Clin. Nutr.* **49**, 542.

BUAMAH, P. K., RUSSELL, M., BATES, G., MILFORD, W. A. and SKILLEN, A. W. (1984). Maternal zinc status: A determination of central nervous system malformation. *Brit. J. Obstet. Gyn.* **91**, 788.

BUERK, C. A., CHANDY, M. G., PEARSON, E., MACAULY, A. and SOROFF, H. S. (1973). Zinc deficiency: Effect on healing and metabolism in man. *Surg. Forum* **24**, 101.

BUNKER, V. W., HINKS, L. J., LAWSON, M. S. and CLAYTON, B. E. (1984). Assessment of zinc and copper status of healthy elderly people using metabolic balance studies and measurement of leukocyte concentrations. *Am. J. Clin. Nutr.* **40**, 1096.

BURNET, F. M. (1981). A possible role of zinc in the pathway of dementia. *Lancet* **1**, 186.

BUZINA, R., JUSIC, M., SAPUNAR, J. and MILANOVIC, N. (1980). Zinc nutrition and taste acuity in school children with impaired growth. *Am. J. Clin. Nutr.* **33**, 2262.

CAGGIANO, J., SCHNITZLER, R., STRAUSS, W., BAKER, R. K., CARTER, A., JOSEPHSON, A. S. and WALLACH, S. (1969). Zinc deficiency in a patient with retarded growth, hypogonadism, hypogammaglobulinemia and chronic infection. *Am. J. Med. Sci.* **257**, 305.

CASTRO, C. E., ALVARES, O. F. and SEVALL, J. S. (1986). Zinc deficiency decreases histone H1° in rat liver. *Nutr. Rep. Intern.* **34**, 67.

CATALANOTTO, F. A. and LACY, P. (1977). Effect of a zinc-deficient diet upon fluid intake in the rat. *J. Nutr.* **107**, 436.

CATALANOTTO, F. A. and NANDA, R. (1977). The effects of feeding a zinc-deficient diet on taste acuity and tongue epithelium in rats. *J. Oral Pathol.* **6**, 211.

CAVEL, P. A. and WIDDOWSON, E. M. (1964). Intakes and excretions of iron, copper and zinc in the neonatal period. *Arch. Dis. Child.* **39**, 496.

CHAO-LING, C., SHIH-T'AO, C., KUOCH'EN, C., LAN-SHENG, Y., SHENG-CH'ING, L., CHIN-SEN, L., CH'ING-YUN, K., YU-FEN, L. and CHING-YA, H. (1959). Schistosomal hypophyseal dwarfism—Study of 72 cases. *Chinese Med. J.* **79**, 26.

CHERRY, F. F., BENNETT, E. A., BAZZANO, G. S., JOHNSON, L. K., FOSMIRE, G. J. and BATSON, H. K. (1981). Plasma zinc in hypertension/toxemia. *Am. J. Clin. Nutr.* **34**, 2367.

CHERRY, F. F., SANDSTEAD, H. H., ROJAS, P., JOHNSON, L. K., BATSON, H. K. and WANG, X. B. (1989). Adolescent pregnancy: Associations between body weight, zinc nutriture, and pregnancy outcome. *Am. J. Clin. Nutr.* **50**, 945.

CHESTERS, J. K. and QUARTERMAN, J. (1970). Effects of zinc deficiency on food intake and feeding patterns of rats. *Brit. J. Nutr.* **24**, 1061.

CORNATZER, W. E., HANING, J. A., WALLWORK, J. C. and SANDSTEAD, H. H. (1984). Effect of zinc deficiency on the biosynthesis of phosphatidylcholine in rat microsomes. *Biol. Trace Element Res.* **6**, 393.

CUNNANE, S. C. (Ed.) (1988). *Zinc: Clinical and Biochemical Significance.* CRC Press, Inc., Boca Raton, FL.

CUNNANE, S. C., HORROBIN, D. F. and MANKU, M. S. (1984). Essential fatty acids in tissue phospholipids and triglycerides of the zinc-deficient rat. *Proc. Soc. Exp. Biol. Med.* **177**, 441.

DANFORD, D. E. (1982). Pica and nutrition mineral. *Ann. Rev. Nutr.* **2**, 303.

DAUNCEY, M. J., SHAW, J. C. L. and URMAN, J. (1977). The absorption and retention of magnesium, zinc and copper by low birth weight infants fed pasteurized human breast milk. *Pediatr. Res.* **11**, 991.

DIAMOND, I., SWENERTON, H. and HURLEY, L. S. (1971). Testicular and esophageal lesions in zinc-deficient rats and their reversibility. *J. Nutr.* **101**, 77.

DINSDALE, D. and WILLIAMS, R. B. (1980). Ultrastructural changes in the sperm-tail of zinc-deficient rats. *J. Comp. Pathol.* **90**, 559.

DUCHATEAU, J., DELEPESSE, G., VRIJENS, R. and COLLET, H. (1981). Beneficial effects of oral zinc supplementation on the immune response of old people. *Am. J. Med.* **70**, 1001.

DUERRE, J. A. and WALLWORK, J. C. (1986). Methionine metabolism in isolated perfused livers from rats fed on zinc-deficient and restricted diets. *J. Nutr.* **56**, 395.

DUERRE, J. A., FORD, K. M. and SANDSTEAD, H. H. (1977). Effect of zinc deficiency on protein synthesis in brain and liver of suckling rats. *J. Nutr.* **107**, 1082.

ENGLE, R. W., MILLER, R. F. and PRICE, N. O. (1966). Metabolic patterns in preadolescent children. XIII. Zinc balance. In *Zinc Metabolism* (A. S. Prasad, Ed.), p. 326. Charles C. Thomas, Springfield, IL.

EVANS, G. W. and JOHNSON, P. E. (1980). Characterization and quantitation of a zinc binding ligand in human milk. *Pediatr. Res.* **14**, 847.

EVERETT, G. A. and APGAR, J. (1979). Effect of zinc status on salivary zinc concentrations in the rat. *J. Nutr.* **109**, 406.

FABRIS, N., MOOCHEGIANI, E., AMADIO, L., ZANNOTTI, M., LICASTRO, F. and FRANCHESCHI, C. (1984). Thymic hormone deficiency in normal aging and Down's Syndrome: Is there a primary failure of the thymus? *Lancet* **1**, 983.

FALCHUK, K. H., GORDON, P. R., STANKIEWICZ, A., HILT, K. L. and VALLEE, B. L. (1986). *Euglena gracilis* chromatin: Comparison of effects of zinc, iron, magnesium, or manganese deficiency and cold shock. *Biochem.* **25**, 5388.

FNB, FOOD AND NUTRITION BOARD, NATIONAL RESEARCH COUNCIL (1980). *Recommended Daily Dietary Allowances.* National Academy of Sciences.

FOLLIS, R. H., DAY, H. G. and MCCOLLUM, E. V. (1941). Histological studies of the tissues of rats fed a diet extremely low in zinc. *J. Nutr.* **22**, 223.

FOSMIRE, G. J., AL-UBAIDI, Y. Y. and SANDSTEAD, H. H. (1975). Some effects of postnatal zinc deficiency on developing rat brain. *Pediatr. Res.* **9**, 89.

FOSMIRE, G. J., FOSMIRE, M. A. and SANDSTEAD, H. H. (1976). Zinc deficiency in the weanling rat: Effects on liver composition and polysomal profiles. *J. Nutr.* **106**, 1152.

FRAKER, P. J., GERSHWIN, M. E., GOOD, R. A. and PRASAD, A. S. (1986). Interrelationships between zinc and immune function. *Fed. Proc.* **45**, 1474.

FREELAND-GRAVES, J. H., HENDRICKSON, P. J., EBANGIT, M. L. and SNOWDEN, J. Y. (1981). Salivary zinc as an index of zinc status: In women fed a low-zinc diet. *Am. J. Clin. Nutr.* **34**, 312.

GALDES, A. and VALLEE, B. L. (1983). Categories of zinc metalloenzymes. In *Metal Ions and Biologic Systems, Vol. 15, Zinc and its Role in Biology and Nutrition* (H. Siegel, Ed.), p. 1. Marcel Dekker, Inc. New York.

GERSON, S. J., MEYER, J. and GANDOR, D. (1985). Decreased zinc concentration does not lead to atrophy of rat oral epithelium. *J. Nutr.* **115**, 820.

GIBSON, R. S. and SCYTHES, C. A. (1982). Trace element intakes of women. *Brit. J. Nutr.* **48**, 241.

GIBSON, R. S., SMIT VANDERKOOY, P. D., MACDONALD, A. C., GOLDMAN, A., RYAN, B. A. and BERRY, M. (1989). A growth-limiting, mild zinc-deficiency syndrome in some Southern Ontario boys with low height percentiles. *Am. J. Clin. Nutr.* **49**, 1266.

GOLDEN, B. E. and GOLDEN, M. H. N. (1981a). Plasma zinc, rate of weight gain, and the energy cost of tissue deposition in children recovering from severe malnutrition on a cow's milk or soya protein based diet. *Am. J. Clin. Nutr.* **34**, 892.

GOLDEN, M. H. N. and GOLDEN, B. E. (1981b). Effect of zinc supplementation on the dietary intake, rate of weight gain, and energy deposition in children recovering from severe malnutrition. *Am. J. Clin. Nutr.* **34**, 900.

GOLDEN, M. H. N., JACKSON, A. A. and GOLDEN, B. E. (1977). Effect of zinc on thymus of recently malnourished children. *Lancet* **2**, 1057.

GOLDEN, M. H. N., GOLDEN, B. E., HARLAND, P. S. and JACKSON, A. A. (1978). Zinc and immunocompetence in protein-energy malnutrition. *Lancet* **2**, 1226.

GOLDINER, W. H., HAMILTON, B. P., HYMAN, P. D. and RUSSELL, R. M. (1983). Effect of the administration of zinc sulfate on hypogonadism and impotence in patients with chronic stable hepatic cirrhosis. *J. Am. Coll. Nutr.* **2**, 157.

GOLUB, M. S., GERSHWIN, M. E., HURLEY, L. A., HENDRICKX, A. G. and SAITO, W. Y. (1985). Studies of marginal zinc deprivation in Rhesus monkeys: Infant behavior. *Am. J. Clin. Nutr.* **42**, 1229.

GREEN, S., KUMAR, V., THEULAZ, I., WAHLI, W. and CHAMBON, P. (1988). The N-terminal DNA-binding 'zinc finger' of the oestrogen and the glucocorticoid receptors determines target gene specificity. *EMBO J.* **7**, 3037.

GREGER, J. L. and SICKLES, Y. S. (1979). Saliva zinc levels: Potential indicators of zinc status. *Am. J. Clin. Nutr.* **32**, 1859.

GREY, P. C. and DREOSTI, I. E. (1972). Deoxyribonucleic acid and protein metabolism in zinc-deficient rats. *J. Comp. Pathol.* **82**, 223.

GRIDER, A., BAILEY, L. B. and COUSINS, R. J. (1990). Erythrocyte metallothionein as an index of zinc status in humans. Proc. Nat. Acad. Sci. **87** (in press).

HALAS, E. S. and SANDSTEAD, H. H. (1975). Some effects of prenatal zinc deficiency on behavior of the adult rat. *Pediatr. Res.* **9**, 94.

HALAS, E. S., HANLON, M. J. and SANDSTEAD, H. H. (1975). Intrauterine nutrition and aggression. *Nature* **257**, 221.

HALAS, E. S., EBERHARDT, M. J., DIERS, M. A. and SANDSTEAD, H. H. (1983). Learning and memory impairment in adult rats due to severe zinc deficiency during lactation. *Physiol. Behav.* **30**, 371.

HALAS, E. S., HUNT, C. D. and EBERHARDT, M. J. (1986). Learning and memory disabilities in young adult rats from mildly zinc deficient dams. *Physiol. Behav.* **37**, 451.

HALSTED, J. A. and SMITH, J. C., JR (1970). Plasma zinc in health and disease. *Lancet* **1**, 322.

HALSTED, J. A., RONAGHY, H. A., ABADI, P., HAGHSHENASS, M., AMIRHAKENI, G. H., BARAKAT, R. M. and REINHOLD, J. C. (1972). Zinc deficiency in man: the Shiraz experiment. *Am. J. Med.* **53**, 277.

HALSTED, J. A., SMITH, J. C., JR and IRWIN, M. I. (1974). A conspectus of research on zinc requirements of man. *J. Nutr.* **104**, 345.

HAMBIDGE, K. M., HAMBIDGE, C., JACOBS, M. and BAUM, J. D. (1972). Low levels of zinc in hair, anorexia, poor growth, and hypogeusia in children. *Pediatr. Res.* **6**, 868.

HAMBIDGE, K. M., NELDNER, K. Y. H. and WALRAVENS, P. A. (1975). Zinc, acrodermatitis enteropathica and congenital malformations. *Lancet* **1**, 577.

HAMBIDGE, K. M., NELDNER, K. Y. H., WALRAVENS, P. A., WESTON, W. L., SILVERMAN, A., SABOL, J. L. and BROWN, R. M. (1978). Zinc and acrodermatitis enteropathica. In *Zinc and Copper in Clinical Medicine* (K. M. Hambidge and B. L. Nichols, Eds), p. 81. Spectrum, New York.

HAMBIDGE, K. M., CHAVEZ, M. N., BROWN, R. M. and WALRAVENS, P. A. (1979). Zinc nutritional status of young middle-income children and effects of consuming zinc-fortified breakfast cereal. *Am. J. Clin. Nutr.* **37**, 2532.

HAMBIDGE, K. M., CASEY, C. E. and KREBS, N. F. (1986). Zinc. In *Trace Elements in Human and Animal Nutrition* (W. Mertz, Ed), p. 1. Academic Press, Orlando, FL.

HARZER, G. and KAUER, H. (1982). Binding of zinc to casein. *Am. J. Clin. Nutr.* **35**, 981.

HENKIN, R. I. and BRADLEY, D. F. (1970). Hypogeusia corrected by Ni^{++} and Zn^{++}. *Life Sci.* **9**, 701.

HENKIN, R. I., PATTEN, B. M., RE, P. K. and BRONZERT, D. A. (1975a). A syndrome of acute zinc loss. Cerebellar dysfunction, mental changes, anorexia, and taste and smell dysfunction. *Arch. Neurol.* **32**, 745.

HENKIN, R. I., MUELLER, C. W. and WOLF, R. O. (1975b). Estimation of zinc concentration in parotid saliva by flameless atomic absorption spectrophotometry in normal subjects and in patients with idiopathic hypogeusia. *J. Lab. Clin. Med.* **86**, 175.

HENKIN, R. I., LIPPOLDT, R. E., BILSTAD, J. and EDELHOCH, H. (1975c). A zinc protein isolated from human parotid saliva. *Proc. Nat. Acad. Sci. USA* **72**, 488.

HENKIN, R. I., SCHECHTER, P. J., FRIEDWALD, W. T., DEMETS, D. L. and RAFF, M. (1976). A double blind study of the effects of zinc sulfate on taste and smell dysfunction. *Am. J. Med. Sci.* **272**, 285.

HICKS, S. E. and WALLWORK, J. C. (1987). Effect of dietary zinc deficiency on protein synthesis in cell-free systems isolated from rat liver. *J. Nutr.* **117**, 1234.

HOLDEN, J. M., WOLF, W. R. and MERTZ, W. (1979). Zinc and copper in self-selected diets. *J. Am. Diet. Assoc.* **75**, 23.

HOLLENBERG, S. M., GIGUERE, V., SEGUL, P. and EVANS, R. M. (1987). Colocalization of DNA-binding and transcriptional activation functions in the human glucocorticoid receptor. *Cell* **49**, 39.

HOOPER, P. L., VISCONTI, L., GARRY, P. E. and JOHNSON, G. E. (1980). Zinc lowers high density lipoprotein cholesterol levels. *J. Am. Med. Assoc.* **244**, 1960.

HOWELL, G. A., WELCH, M. G. and FREDERICKSON, C. J. (1984). Stimulation-induced uptake and release of zinc in hippocampal slices. *Nature* **308**, 736.

HSU, J. M., ANTHONY, W. L. and BUCHANAN, P. J. (1969). Zinc deficiency and incorporation of ^{14}C-labeled methionine into tissue proteins in rats. *J. Nutr.* **99**, 425.

HUNT, I. F., MURPHY, N. J., CLEAVER, A. E., FARAJI, B., SWENDSEID, M. E., COULSON, A. H., CLARK, V. A., BRONDY, B. J., CABALUM, M. D. and SMITH, J. C., JR (1984). Zinc supplementation during pregnancy: Effects on selected blood constituents and on program and outcome of pregnancy in low income women of Mexican descent. *Am. J. Clin. Nutr.* **40**, 508.

HURLEY, L. S. and SHRADER, R. E. (1972). Congenital malformations of the nervous system in zinc-deficient rats. In *Neurobiology of the Trace Metals Zinc and Copper* (C. C. Pfeiffer, Ed.), p. 51. Academic Press, New York.

HURLEY, L. S. and SWENERTON, H. (1966). Congenital malformations resulting from zinc deficiency in rats. *Proc. Soc. Exp. Biol. Med.* **123**, 692.

HURLEY, L. S. and TAO, S. H. (1972). Alleviation of teratogenic effects of zinc deficiency by simultaneous lack of calcium. *Am. J. Physiol.* **222**, 322.

IBATA, Y. and OTSUKA, N. (1969). Electron microscopic demonstration of zinc in hippocampal formation using Timm's sulfide silver technique. *J. Histochem. Cytochem.* **17**, 171.

JAMESON, S. (1976). Effects of zinc deficiency in human reproduction. *Acta Med. Scand.* **593**, 89 (Suppl).

JAMESON, S. (1982). Zinc status and pregnancy outcome in humans. In *Clinical Applications of Recent Advances in Zinc Metabolism* (A. S. Prasad, I. E. Dreosti and B. S. Hetzel, Eds), p. 39. Alan R. Liss, Inc., New York.

JONES, R. B., KEELING, P. W. N., HILTON, P. J. and THOMPSON, R. P. H. (1981). The relationship between leucocyte and muscle zinc in health and disease. *Clin. Sci.* **60**, 237.

JOSEPH, C. E., ASHRAFI, S. H. and WATERHOUSE, J. P. (1981). Structural changes in rabbit oral epithelium caused by zinc deficiency. *J. Nutr.* **111**, 53.

JUSTICE, P. M., KAMATH, S., LANGENBERG, P. W., SANDSTEAD, H. H., MILNE, D. B. and SMITH, G. F. (1988). Micronutrients status of children with Down Syndrome: A comparative study of the effects of vitamins with minerals or placebo. *Nutr. Res.* **8**, 1251.

KAY, E. F., TASMAN-JONES, C., PYBUS, J., WHITING, R. and BLACK, H. (1976). A syndrome of acute zinc deficiency during total parenteral alimentation in man. *Ann. Surg.* **183**, 331.

KEELING, P. W. N., JONES, R. B., HILTON, P. J. and THOMPSON, R. P. H. (1980). Reduced leucocyte zinc in liver disease. *Gut* **21**, 561.

KEILIN, D. and MANN, T. (1940). Carbonic anhydrase. Purification and nature of the enzyme. *Biochem. J.* **34**, 1163.

KING, J. C., STEIN, T. and DOYLE, M. (1981). Effect of vegetarianism on the zinc status of pregnant women. *Am. J. Clin. Nutr.* **3**, 1049.

KLEVAY, L. M. (1973). Hypercholesterolemia in rats produced by an increase in the ratio of zinc to copper ingested. *Am. J. Clin. Nutr.* **26**, 1060.

KLUG, A. and RHODES, D. (1987). 'Zinc fingers': a novel protein motif for nucleic acid recognition. *Trends Biolog. Sci.* **12**, 464.

KOO, S. I. and LEE, C. C. (1988). Compositional changes in plasma high-density lipoprotein particles in marginally zinc-deficient male rats. *Am. J. Clin. Nutr.* **47**, 120.

KRAMER, T. R. (1984). Reevaluation of zinc deficiency on concanavalin-A-induced rat spleen lymphocyte proliferation. *J. Nutr.* **114**, 953.

KREBS, N. F., HAMBIDGE, K. M. and WALRAVENS, P. A. (1984). Increased food intake of young children receiving a zinc supplement. *Am. J. Dis. Child.* **138**, 270.

LEEK, J. C., KEEN, C. L., VOGLER, J. B., GOLUB, M. S., HURLEY, L. S., HENDRICKX, A. G. and GERSHWIN, M. E. (1988). Long-term marginal zinc deprivation in rhesus monkeys. IV. Effects on skeletal growth and mineralization. *Am. J. Clin. Nutr.* **47**, 889.

LEGG, S. P. and SEARS, L. (1960). Zinc sulphate treatment of parakeratosis in cattle. *Nature* **186**, 1061.

LEI, K. Y., ABBASI, A. and PRASAD, A. S. (1976). Function of the pituitary–gonadal axis in zinc-deficient rats. *Am. J. Physiol.* **230**, 1730.

LENNOX, R. W. (1984). Differences in evolutionary stability among H1 subtypes. Implications for the role of H1 subtypes in chromatin. *J. Biol. Chem.* **259**, 669.

LEVY, C. M., KANAGASUNDARAM, N. and SMITH, F. (1981). Treatment of liver disease of the alcoholic: A composite approach. *Semin. Liver Dis.* **1**, 254.

LIN, H. J., CHAN, W. C., FONG, Y. Y. and NEWBERNE, P. M. (1977). Zinc levels in serum, hair and tumors from patients with esophageal cancer. *Nutr. Rep. Inter.* **15**, 635.

LÖNNERDAL, B., CEDERBLAD, Å., DAVIDSSON, L. and SANDSTRÖM, B. (1984). The effect of individual components of soy formula and cow's milk formula on zinc bioavailability. *Am. J. Clin. Nutr.* **40**, 1064.

LOOSFELT, H., ATGER, M., MISRAHI, M., GUIOCHON-MANTEL, A., MERIEL, C., LOGEAT, F., BENAROUS, R. and MILGROM, E. (1986). Cloning and sequence analysis of rabbit progesterone-receptor complementary DNA. *Proc. Nat. Acad. Sci. USA* **83**, 9045.

LUKASKI, H. C., BOLONCHUK, W. W., KLEVAY, L. M., MILNE, D. B. and SANDSTEAD, H. H. (1984). Changes in plasma zinc content after exercise in men fed a low-zinc diet. *Am. J. Physiol.* **247**, E88.

LYKKEN, G. I., MAHALKO, J., JOHNSON, P. E., MILNE, D., SANDSTEAD, H. H., DINTZIS, F. R. and INGLETT, G. E. (1986). Effects of browned and unbrowned corn products intrinsically labelled with ^{65}zinc on absorption of ^{65}zinc in humans. *J. Nutr.* **116**, 795.

LYON, T. D., SMITH, H. and SMITH, L. B. (1979). Zinc deficiency in the west of Scotland? *Brit. J. Nutr.* **42**, 413.

MACDONALD, L. D., GIBSON, R. S. and MILES, J. E. (1982). Changes in hair zinc and copper concentration of breast fed and bottle fed infants during the first six months. *Acta Paediatr.* **71**, 785.

MAHAJAN, S. K., PRASAD, A. S., RABBANI, P., BRIGGS, W. A. and MCDONALD, F. D. (1979). Zinc metabolism in uremia. *J. Lab. Clin. Med.* **94**, 693.

MAHAJAN, S. K., ABBASI, A. A., PRASAD, A. S., RABBANI, P., BRIGGS, W. A. and MCDONALD, F. D. (1982). Effect of oral zinc therapy on gonadal function in hemodialysis patients. *Ann. Intern. Med.* **97**, 357.

MARKOWITZ, M. E., ROSEN, J. F. and MIZRUCHI, M. (1985). Circadian variations in serum zinc (Zn) concentrations: Correlation with blood ionized calcium, serum total calcium and phosphate in humans. *Am. J. Clin. Nutr.* **41**, 689.

MASON, K. E., BURNS, W. A. and SMITH, J. C., JR (1982). Testicular damage associated with zinc deficiency in pre- and postpubertal rats: Response to zinc repletion. *J. Nutr.* **112**, 1019.

MAZUS, B., FALCHUK, K. H. and VALLEE, B. L. (1984). Histone formation, gene expression, and zinc deficiency in *Euglena gracilis*. *Biochem.* **23**, 42.

MCCLAIN, C. J., SOUTOR, C., STEELE, N., LEVINE, A. S. and SILVIS, S. E. (1980). Severe zinc deficiency presenting with acrodermatitis during hyperalimentation: Diagnosis, pathogenesis and treatment. *J. Clin. Gastroenterol*, **2**, 125.

MCCLAIN, C. J., SU, L.-C., GILBERT, H. and CAMERON, D. (1983). Zinc deficiency-Induced retinal dysfunction in Crohn's disease. *Dig. Dis. Sci.* **28**, 85.

McClain, C. J., Gavaler, J. S. and Van Thiel, D. H. (1984). Hypogonadism in the zinc-deficient rat: Localization of the functional abnormalities. *J. Lab. Clin. Med.* **104**, 1007.

McConnell, S. D. and Henkin, R. I. (1974). Altered preference for sodium chloride, anorexia and changes in plasma and urinary zinc in rats fed a zinc-deficient diet. *J. Nutr.* **104**, 1108.

McCormick, D. B. (1962). The intracellular localization, partial purification and properties of flavokinase from rat liver. *J. Biol. Chem.* **237**, 959.

Meadows, N. J., Smith, M. F., Keeling, P. W. N., Ruse, W., Day, J., Scopes, J. W., Thompson, R. P. H. and Bloxam, D. L. (1981). Zinc and small babies. *Lancet* **2**, 1137.

Millar, M. J., Fischer, M. I., Elcoate, P. V. and Mawson, C. A. (1958). The effects of dietary zinc deficiency on the reproductive system of male rats. *Canad. J. Biochem. Physiol.* **36**, 557.

Miller, J., McLachlan, A. D. and Klug, A. (1985). Repetitive zinc-binding domains in the protein transcription factor IIIA from Xenopus oocytes. *EMBO J.* **4**, 1609.

Mills, C. F. (1985). Dietary interactions involving the trace elements. *Ann. Rev. Nutr.* **5**, 173.

Milne, D. B., Schnakenberg, D. D., Johnson, H. L. and Kuhl, G. L. (1980). Trace element mineral intake of enlisted military personnel. *J. Am. Diet. Assoc.* **76**, 41.

Milne, D. B., Canfield, W. K., Malhalko, J. R. and Sandstead, H. H. (1983). Effect of dietary zinc on whole body surface loss of zinc: Impact on estimation of zinc retention by balance method. *Am. J. Clin. Nutr.* **38**, 181.

Milne, D. B., Ralston, N. V. C. and Wallwork, J. C. (1985). Zinc content of blood cellular components and lymph node and spleen lymphocytes in severely zinc deficient rats. *J. Nutr.* **115**, 1073.

Milne, D. B., Canfield, W. K., Gallagher, S. K., Hunt, J. R. and Klevay, L. M. (1987). Ethanol metabolism in postmenopausal women fed a diet marginal in zinc. *Am. J. Clin. Nutr.* **46**, 688.

Minghetti, P. P. and Norman, A. W. (1988). 1,25$(OH)_2$-Vitamin D_3 receptors: Gene regulation and genetic circuitry. *FASEB J.* **2**, 3043.

Mukherjee, M. D., Sandstead, H. H., Ratnaparkhi, M. V., Johnson, L. K., Milne, D. B. and Stelling, H. P. (1984). Maternal zinc, iron, folic acid, and protein nutriture and outcome of human pregnancy. *Am. J. Clin. Nutr.* **40**, 496.

Oberleas, D., Muhrer, M. E. and O'Dell, B. L. (1966). Dietary metal-complexing agents and zinc availability in the rat. *J. Nutr.* **90**, 56.

O'Dell, B. L. and Reeves, P. G. (1988). Zinc status and food intake. In *Zinc in Human Nutrition* (C. F. Mills, Ed.), p. 173. Springer-Verlag, London.

O'Dell, B. L. and Savage, J. E. (1960). Effect of phytic acid on zinc availability. *Proc. Soc. Exp. Biol. Med.* **103**, 304.

Oestreicher, P. and Cousins, R. J. (1982). Influence of intraluminal constituents on zinc absorption by isolated, vascularly perfused rat intestine. *J. Nutr.* **112**, 1978.

Okada, A., Takagi, Y., Itakura, T., Satani, M., Manabe, H., Iida, Y., Tanigaki, T., Iwasaki, M. and Kasahara, N. (1976). Skin lesions during intravenous hyperalimentation: Zinc deficiency. *Surgery* **80**, 629.

PALLUDAN, B. and WEGGER, I. (1976). Importance of zinc for foetal and post-natal development in swine. In *Nuclear Techniques in Animal Production and Health*, p. 191. International Atomic Energy Agency, Vienna, Austria.

PATEL, P. B., CHUNG, R. A. and LU, J. Y. (1975). Effect of zinc deficiency on serum and liver cholesterol in the female rat. *Nutr. Rep. Intern.* **12**, 205.

PATRICK, J. and DERVISH, C. (1984). Leukocyte zinc in the assessment of zinc status. *CRC Crit. Rev. Clin. Lab. Sci.* **20**, 95.

PATRICK, J., DERVISH, C. and GILLIESON, M. (1982). Zinc and small babies. *Lancet* **1**, 169.

PECOUD, A., DONZEL, P. and SCHELLING, J. L. (1975). Effect of foodstuffs on the absorption of zinc sulfate. *Clin. Pharmacol. Ther.* **17**, 469.

PEKAREK, R. S., SANDSTEAD, H. H., JACOB, R. A. and BARCOME, D. F. (1979). Abnormal cellular immune response during acquired zinc deficiency. *Am. J. Clin. Nutr.* **32**, 1466.

PEKKARINEN, M. (1973). World food consumption patterns. In *Man, Food, and Nutrition* (M. Rechcigl, Ed.) p. 16. CRC Press, Boca Raton, FL.

PILCH, S. M. and SENTI, F. R. (1985). Analysis of zinc data from the Second National Health and Nutrition Examination Survey (NHANES II). *J. Nutr.* **115**, 1393.

PITTS, W. J., MILLER, W. J., FOSGATE, O. T., MORTON, J. D. and CLIFTON, C. M. (1966). Effect of zinc deficiency and restricted feeding from two to five months of age on reproduction in Holstein bulls. *J. Dairy Sci.* **49**, 995.

PORIES, W. J. and STRAIN, W. H. (1974). Zinc sulfate therapy in surgical patients. In: *Clinical Applicants of Zinc Metabolism* (W. J. Pories, W. H. Strain, J. M. Hsu and R. L. Woosley, Ed.), p. 139. Charles C. Thomas, Springfield, IL.

PRASAD, A. S. and RABBANI, P. (1981). Nucleoside phosphorylase in zinc deficiency. *Trans. Assoc. Am. Physicians* **94**, 314.

PRASAD, A. S., HALSTED, J. A. and NADIMI, M. (1961). Syndrome of iron deficiency, anemia, hepatosplenomegaly, dwarfism, hypogonadism and geophagia. *Am. J. Med.* **31**, 532.

PRASAD, A. S., MIALE, A. J., FARID, Z., SANDSTEAD, H. H., SCHULERT, A. R. and DARBY, W. J. (1963a). Biochemical studies on dwarfism, hypogonadism and anemia. *Arch. Intern. Med.* **111**, 407.

PRASAD, A. S., MIALE, A., FARID, Z., SANDSTEAD, H. H. and SCHULERT, A. R. (1963b). Zinc metabolism in patients with the syndrome of iron deficiency anemia, hepatosplenomegaly, dwarfism, and hypogonadism. *J. Lab. Clin. Med.* **61**, 537.

PRASAD, A. S., DIWANY, M., GABR, M., SANDSTEAD, H. H., MOKTAR, N. and EL HEFNY, A. (1965). Biochemical studies in thalassemia. *Ann. Intern. Med.* **62**, 87.

PRASAD, A. S., SCHOOMAKER, E. B., ORTEGA, J., BREWER, G. J., OBERLEAS, D. and OELSCHLEGEL, F. J. J. (1975). Zinc deficiency in sickle cell disease. *Clin. Chem.* **21**, 582.

PRASAD, A. S., BREWER, G. J., SCHOOMAKER, E. B. and RABBANI, P. (1978a). Hypocupremia induced by zinc therapy in adults. *J. Am. Med. Assoc.* **240**, 2166.

PRASAD, A. S., RABBINI, P., ABBASSI, A., BOWERSOX, E. and SPIVEY FOX, M. R. (1978b). Experimental zinc deficiency in humans. *Ann. Intern. Med.* **89**, 483.

PRASAD, A. S., ABBASI, A. A., RABBANI, P. and DUMOUCHELLE, E. (1981). Effect of zinc supplementation on serum testosterone level in adult male sickle cell anemia subjects. *Am. J. Hematol.* **10**, 119.

PRASAD, A. S., MEFLAH, S., ABDALLAH, J., KAPLAN, J., BREWER, G. J., BACH, J. F. and DARDENNE, M. (1988). Serum thymulin in human zinc deficiency. *J. Clin. Invest.* **82**, 1202.

PRICE, N. O., BUNCE, G. E. and ENGEL, R. W. (1970). Copper, manganese and zinc balance in preadolescent girls. *Am. J. Clin. Nutr.* **23**, 258.

RABBANI, P. I., PRASAD, A. S., TSAI, R., HARLAND, B. F. and SPIVEY FOX, M. R. (1987). Dietary model for production of experimental zinc deficiency in man. *Am. J. Clin. Nutr.* **45**, 1514.

RAULIN, J. (1869). Études cliniques sur la vegetation. *Ann. Sci. Natl. Biol. Ser. 5* **11**, 93.

RECORD, I. R., DREOSTI, I. E. and TULDI, R. S. (1987). Growth and development of the zinc-deficient mouse embryo. *Nutr. Res.* **7**, 1209.

ROOT, A. W., DUCKETT, G., SWEETLAND, M. and REITER, E. O. (1979). Effects of zinc deficiency upon pituitary function in sexually mature and immature male rats. *J. Nutr.* **109**, 958.

RUSSELL, R. M., COX, M. E. and SOLOMONS, N. (1983). Zinc and the special senses. *Ann. Intern. Med.* **99**, 227.

SAFAI-KUTTI, S. and KUTTI, J. (1984). Zinc and anorexia nervosa. *Ann. Intern. Med.* **100**, 317.

SALEM, S. I., COWARD, W. A., LUNN, P. G. and HUDSON, G. J. (1984). Response of the reproductive system of male rats to protein and zinc deficiency during puberty. *Ann. Nutr. Metab.* **28**, 44.

SANDSTEAD, H. H. (1972). The zinc-deficiency syndrome. In *The State of Nutrition in the Arab Middle East* (V. N. Patwardhan and W. J. Darby, Eds), p. 122. Vanderbilt University Press, Nashville, TN.

SANDSTEAD, H. H. (1973). Zinc nutrition in the United States. *Am. J. Clin. Nutr.* **26**, 1251.

SANDSTEAD, H. H. (1982). Requirements and availability of dietary zinc for humans. In *Clinical and Public Health Significance of Trace Elements in the World Population* (A. S. Prasad, Ed.), p. 83. Alan R. Liss, Inc., NY.

SANDSTEAD, H. H. (1985). Requirement of zinc in human subjects. *J. Am. Coll. Nutr.* **4**, 73.

SANDSTEAD, H. H. (1988). Interactions that influence bioavailability of essential metals to humans. In *Metal Speciation: Theory, Analysis and Applications* (J. R. Kramer and H. E. Allen, Eds), p. 315. Lewis Publishers, Inc., Chelsea, Michigan.

SANDSTEAD, H. H. and RINALDI, R. A. (1969). Impairment of deoxyribonucleic acid synthesis by dietary zinc deficiency in the rat. *J. Cell. Physiol.* **73**, 81.

SANDSTEAD, H. H. and TERHUNE, M. W. (1974). Zinc deficiency: Effect on the activity of liver RNA polymerase, sucrose density gradients and *in vitro* uridine incorporation. In *Clinical Applications of Zinc Metabolism* (W. J. Pories, W. H. Strain, J. M. Hsu and R. L. Woosley, Eds), p. 9. Charles C. Thomas, Springfield, Il.

SANDSTEAD, H. H., SHURKRY, A. S. and PRASAD, A. S. (1965). Kwashiorkor in Egypt. I. Clinical and biochemical studies with special reference to plasma zinc and serum lactic dehydrogenase. *Am. J. Clin. Nutr.* **17**, 15.

SANDSTEAD, H. H., PRASAD, A. S. and SCHULERT, A. R. (1967). Human zinc deficiency, endocrine manifestations and response to treatment. *Am. J. Clin. Nutr.* **20**, 422.

Sandstead, H. H., Gillespie, D. D. and Brady, R. N. (1972). Zinc deficiency: Effect on brain of suckling rat. *Pediatr. Res.* **6**, 119.

Sandstead, H. H., Fosmire, G. J., Halas, E. S., Jacob, R. A., Strobel, D. A. and Marks, E. O. (1977). Zinc deficiency: Effects on brain and behavior of rats and Rhesus monkeys. *Teratology* **16**, 229.

Sandstead, H. H., Klevay, L. M., Jacob, R. A., Munoz, J. M., Logan, G. M., Jr, Reck, S. J., Dintzis, F. R., Inglett, G. E. and Shuey, W. C. (1979). Effects of dietary fiber and protein level on mineral element metabolism. In *Dietary Fibers: Chemistry and Nutrition* (G. E. Inglett and S. I. Falkehag, Eds), p. 147. Academic Press, New York.

Sandstead, H. H., Henriksen, L. K., Greger, J. L., Prasad, A. S. and Good, R. A. (1982). Zinc nutriture in the elderly in relation to taste acuity, immune response and wound healing. *Am. J. Clin. Nutr.* **36**, 1046.

Sandstead, H. H., Johnson, L., Jacob, R. A., Hunt, J., Hendriksen, L. K., Dintzis, F. R., Lykken, G. I., Johnson, P. E., Milne, D. B., Lukaski, H. C. and Klevay, L. M. (1989a). Bioavailability of zinc from human diets. In *Bioavailability of Micronutrients and its Human Consequences* (E. G. High and W. L. Stone, Eds), p. 23. Meharry Medical College, Nashville, TN.

Sandstead, H. H., Dintzis, F. R., Bogyo, T. P., Milne, D. B., Jacob, R. A. and Klevay, L. M. (1989b). Dietary factors that can impair calcium and zinc nutriture of the elderly. In *Nutrition and Aging* (D. M. Prinsley and H. H. Sandstead, Eds), p. 241. Alan R. Liss Inc. (In press).

Sandström, B., Arvidsson, B., Cederblad, Å. and Bjorn-Rasmussen, E. (1980). Zinc absorption from composite meals. I. The significance of wheat extraction rate, zinc, calcium, and protein content in meals based on bread. *Am. J. Clin. Nutr.* **33**, 739.

Sandström, B., Cederblad, Å and Lönnerdal, B. (1983). Zinc absorption from human milk, cow's milk, and infant formulas. *Am. J. Dis. Child.* **137**, 726.

Sandström, B., Almgren, A., Kivistö, B. and Cederblad, Å. (1987). Zinc absorption in humans from meals based on rye, barley, oatmeal, triticale and whole wheat. *J. Nutr.* **117**, 1898.

Sandström, B., Almgren, A., Kivistö, B. and Cederblad, Å. (1989). Effect of protein level and protein source on zinc absorption in humans. *J. Nutr.* **119**, 48.

Sato, M., Mehra, R. K. and Bremner, I. (1984). Measurement of plasma metallothionein-I in the assessment of the zinc status of zinc-deficient and stressed rats. *J. Nutr.* **114**, 1683.

Schlage, C. and Wortberg, B. (1972). Zinc in the diet of healthy preschool and school children. *Acta Paediatr. Scand.* **61**, 421.

Scoular, F. L. (1939). A quantitative study by means of spectrographic analysis of zinc in nutrition. *J. Nutr.* **17**, 103.

Seal, C. J. and Heaton, F. W. (1983). Chemical factors affecting the intestinal absorption of zinc *in vitro* and *in vivo*. *Brit. J. Nutr.* **50**, 317.

Sever, L. E. and Emanuel, I. (1973). Is there a connection between maternal zinc deficiency and congenital malformations of the central nervous system in man? *Teratology* **7**, 117.

Simmer, K. and Thompson, R. P. H. (1985). Maternal zinc and intrauterine growth retardation. *Clin. Sci.* **68**, 395.

Solomons, N. W. (1979). On the assessment of zinc and copper nutriture in man. *Am. J. Clin. Nutr.* **32**, 856.

SOLOMONS, N. W., ROSENBERG, I. H., SANDSTEAD, H. H. and VO-KHACTU, K. P. (1977). Zinc deficiency and Crohn's disease. *Digestion* **16**, 87.

SOLOMONS, N. W., JACOB, R. A., PINEDA, O. and VITERI, F. (1979). Studies on the bioavailability of zinc in man. II. Absorption of zinc from organic and inorganic sources. *J. Lab. Clin. Med.* **94**, 335.

SOLOMONS, N. W., PINEDA, O., VITERI, F. E. and SANDSTEAD, H. H. (1983). Studies on the bioavailability of zinc in humans: Mechanism of the intestinal interaction of non-heme iron and zinc. *J. Nutr.* **113**, 337.

STROBEL, D. A. and SANDSTEAD, H. H. (1984). Social and learning changes following prenatal or postnatal zinc deprivation in rhesus monkeys. In *Neurobiology of Zinc, Part B, Deficiency, Toxicity and Pathology* (C. J. Frederickson, G. A. Howell and E. J. Kasarskis, Eds), p. 121. Alan R. Liss, Inc., New York.

SULLIVAN, J. F. and BURCH, R. E. (1976). Potential role of zinc in liver disease. In *Trace Elements in Human Health and Disease* (A. S. Prasad and D. Oberleas, Eds), p. 67. Academic Press, New York.

SULLIVAN, J. F., JETTON, M. S., HAHN, H. J. K. and BURCH, R. E. (1980). Enhanced lipid peroxidation in liver microsomes of zinc-deficient rats. *Am. J. Clin. Nutr.* **33**, 51.

SUWARNASARN, A., WALLWORK, J. C., LYKKEN, G. I., LOW, F. N. and SANDSTEAD, H. H. (1982). Epiphyseal plate development in the zinc-deficient rat. *J. Nutr.* **112**, 1320.

TANEJA, S. K. and NIRMAL (1980). Histopathology of testes of mice fed on zinc-deficient diet. *Ind. J. Exp. Biol.* **18**, 1411.

TERHUNE, M. W. and SANDSTEAD, H. H. (1972). Decreased RNA polymerase activity in mammalian zinc deficiency. *Science* **177**, 68.

THOMA, F., KOLLER, T. and KLUG, A. (1979). Involvement of histone H1 in the organization of the nucleosome and of the salt dependent superstructures of chromatin. *J. Cell Biol.* **83**, 403.

THOMAS, A. J., BUNKER, V. W., HINKS, L. J., SODHA, N., MULLEE, M. A. and CLAYTON, B. E. (1988). Energy, protein zinc and copper status of twenty-one elderly inpatients: Analyzed dietary intake and biochemical indices. *Brit. J. Nutr.* **59**, 181.

THORNALLEY, P. J. and VASAK, M. (1985). Possible role for metallothionein in protection against radiation-induced oxidative stress. Kinetics and mechanism of its reaction with superoxide and hydroxyl radicals. *Biochim. Biophys. Acta*, **827**, 36.

TODD, W. R., ELVEHJEM, C. A. and HART, E. B. (1934). Zinc in the nutrition of the rat. *Am. J. Physiol.* **107**, 146.

TUCKER, H. F. and SALMON, W. D. (1955). Parakeratosis or zinc deficiency disease in the pig. *Proc. Soc. Exp. Biol. Med.* **88**, 613.

TURNLAND, J. R., KING, J. C., GONG, B., KEYES, W. R. and MICHEL, M. C. (1984). A stable isotope study of zinc absorption in young men: Effects of phytate and alpha-cellulose. *Am. J. Clin. Nutr.* **40**, 1071.

TURNLAND, J. R., DURKIN, N., COSTA, F. and MARGEN, S. (1986). Stable isotope studies of zinc absorption and retention in young and elderly men. *J. Nutr.* **116**, 1239.

USDA—United States Department of Agriculture (1976–1988). *Composition of*

Foods: Raw, Processed, Prepared. Agric. Handb. No. 8: AH-8-1, Dairy and Egg Products (1976); *AH-8-2, Spices and Herbs* (1977); *AH-8-3, Baby Foods* (1978); *AH-8-4, Fats and Oil* (1979); *AH-8-5, Poultry Products* (1979); *AH-8-6, Soups, Sauces, and Gravies* (1980); *AH-8-7, Sausages and Luncheon Meats* (1980); *AH-8-8, Breakfast Cereals* (1982); *AH-8-9, Fruits and Fruit Juices* (1982); *AH-8-10, Pork and Pork Products* (1983); *AH-8-11, Vegetables and Vegetable Products* (1984); *AH-8-12, Nut and Seed Products* (1984); *AH-8-13, Beef Products* (1986); *AH-8-14, Beverages* (1986); *AH-8-16, Legumes and Legume Products* (1986); *AH-8-15, Finfish and Shellfish Products* (1987); *AH-8-18, Baked Products* (1988); *AH-8-20, Cereal Grains, Pastas, Snacks* (1988).

USDA—United States Department of Agriculture, Food and Consumer Services (1986). *Nutrition Monitoring in the United States.* A progress report from the Joint Nutrition Monitoring Evaluation Committee. US Department of Health and Human Services. Public Health Service, National Center for Health Statistics, Human Nutrition Information Service, Hyattsville, Maryland.

UNDERWOOD, E. J. and SOMERS, M. (1969). Studies of zinc nutriture in sheep. I. The relation of zinc to growth, testicular development, and spermatogenesis. *Austral. J. Agric. Res.* **20**, 889.

VALLEE, B. L., WACKER, W. E. C., BARTHOLOMAY, A. F. and ROBIN, E. D. (1956). Zinc metabolism in hepatic dysfunction. I. Serum zinc in Laënnec's cirrhosis and their validation by sequential analysis. *New Engl. J. Med.* **255**, 403.

VAN RENSBERG, S. J. (1981). Epidemiologic and dietary evidence for a specific nutritional predisposition to esophageal cancer. *J. Natl Cancer Instit.* **67**, 243.

WALLACE, E., CALVIN, H. I., SALGO, M. P., DENNIS, J. E. and PLOETZ, K. (1984). Normal levels of zinc and sulfhydryls in morphologically abnormal populations of spermatozoa from moderately zinc-deficient rats. *Gam. Res.* **9**, 375.

WALLWORK, J. C. (1987). Appraisal of the methodology and applications for measurement of the zinc content of blood components as indicators of zinc status. *Biol. Trace Element Res.* **12**, 335.

WALLWORK, J. C. and DUERRE, J. A. (1985). Effect of zinc deficiency on methionine metabolism, methylation reactions and protein synthesis in isolated perfused rat liver. *J. Nutr.* **115**, 252.

WALLWORK, J. C. and SANDSTEAD, H. H. (1990). Zinc. In *Nutrition and Bone Development* (D. J. Simmons, Ed.), p. 316. Oxford University Press.

WALLWORK, J. C., FOSMIRE, G. J. and SANDSTEAD, H. H. (1981). Effect of zinc deficiency on appetite and plasma amino acid concentrations in the rat. *Brit. J. Nutr.* **45**, 127.

WALLWORK, J. C., BOTNEN, J. H. and SANDSTEAD, H. H. (1982). Influence of dietary zinc on rat brain catecholamines. *J. Nutr.* **112**, 514.

WALRAVENS, P. A. and HAMBIDGE, K. M. (1976). Growth of infants fed a zinc supplemented formula. *Am. J. Clin. Nutr.* **29**, 1114.

WALRAVENS, P. A., HAMBIDGE, K. M., NELDER, K. H., SILVERMAN, A., VAN DOORNINCK, J. W., MIERAN, G. and FAVARA, B. (1978). Zinc metabolism in acrodermatitis enteropathica. *J. Pediatr.* **93**, 71.

WALRAVENS, P. A., KREBS, N. F. and HAMBIDGE, K. M. (1983). Linear growth of low income preschool children receiving a zinc supplement. *Am. J. Clin. Nutr.* **38**, 195.

WAPNIR, R. A., KHANI, D. E., BAYNE, M. A. and LIFSHITZ, F. (1983). Absorption of zinc by the rat ileum: effects of histidine and other low molecular-weight ligands. *J. Nutr.* **113**, 1346.

WARKANY, J. and PETERING, H. G. (1972). Congenital malformations of the central nervous system in rats produced by maternal zinc deficiency. *Teratology* **5**, 319.

WEINBERGER, C., THOMPSON, C. C., ONG, E. S., LEBO, R., GRUOL, D. J. and EVANS, R. M. (1986). The c-erb-A gene encodes a thyroid receptor. *Nature* **324**, 641.

WEISMANN, K. and FLAGSTAD, T. (1976). Hereditary zinc deficiency (Adema disease) in cattle, in animal models parallel to acrodermatitis enteropathica. *Acta Dermatol.* (*Stockholm*) **56**, 151.

WELLS, J. L., JAMES, D. K., LUXTON, R. and PENNOCK, C. A. (1987). Maternal leucocyte zinc deficiency at start of third trimester as a predictor of fetal growth retardation. *Brit. Med. J.* **294**, 1054.

WELSH, S. O. and MARSTON, R. M. (1982). Zinc levels of the US food supply 1909–1980. *Food Technol.* **36**, 70.

WENSINK, J., LENGLET, W. J. M., VIS, R. D. and VAN DEN HAMER, C. J. A. (1987). The effect of dietary zinc deficiency on the mossy fiber zinc content of the rat hippocampus. A microbeam PIXE Study. *Histochem.* **87**, 65.

WHITE, H. S. (1969). Inorganic elements in weighted diets of girls and young women. *J. Am. Diet. Assoc.* **55**, 38.

WILLSON, R. L. (1988). Zinc and iron in free radical pathology and cellular control. In *Zinc in Human Biology* (C. F. Mills, Ed.), p. 147. Springer-Verlag, London.

WOLMAN, S. L., ANDERSON, G. H., MARLISS, E. B. and JEEJEEBHOY, K. N. (1979). Zinc in total parenteral nutrition; Requirements and metabolic effects. *Gastroenterol.* **76**, 458.

WHO—World Health Organization (1973). Zinc. In *Trace Elements in Human Nutrition*, Technical Report, 532, p. 9.

WU, FY-H. and WU, C.-W. (1983). The role of zinc in DNA and RNA polymerases. In *Metals Ions in Biological Systems, Vol. 15, Zinc and its Role in Biology and Nutrition* (H. Siegel, Ed.), p. 157. Marcel Dekker, Inc., New York.

XUE-CUN, C., TAI-AN, Y., JIN-SHENG, H., QIU-YAN, M., ZHI-MIN, H. and LI-XIANG, L. (1985). Low levels of zinc in blood, pica, anorexia, and poor growth in Chinese preschool children. *Am. J. Clin. Nutr.*, **42**, 694.

10

Copper, Manganese, Cobalt, and Magnesium

PHYLLIS E. JOHNSON AND FORREST H. NIELSEN
USDA, ARS, Human Nutrition Research Center, University Station, Grand Forks, North Dakota, USA

I. COPPER

A. Metabolic Functions of Copper

Copper is an essential dietary nutrient for animals and humans. It is involved in numerous metabolic functions, including erythropoiesis, skeletal mineralization, synthesis of connective tissue, myelin formation, catecholamine metabolism, oxidative phosphorylation, antioxidant protection, lipid metabolism, immune function, cardiac function, and the regulation of glucose metabolism. The reader is referred to several comprehensive reviews on the metabolic functions of copper (Mason, 1979; Allen and Solomons, 1984; Solomons, 1985; Davis and Mertz, 1987). The most common manifestations of copper deficiency in humans are microcytic, hypochromic anemia and neutropenia. Copper deficiency has been found to cause elevation of serum cholesterol in both animals (Davis and Mertz, 1987) and humans (Klevay *et al.*, 1984). Serum triglycerides and phospholipids are also elevated. Copper deficiency in animals can lead to sudden death associated with aortic or cardiac rupture (Davis and Mertz, 1987), and thus has been suggested to play a role in the etiology of ischemic heart disease in humans (Klevay, 1975, 1983). Nutritional copper deficiency in humans has been observed in infants recovering from severe malnutrition and fed a diet of cow's milk (Cordano *et al.*, 1964; Graham and Cordano, 1969), in premature infants fed copper-deficient formulas (Al-Rashid and Spangler, 1971) or maintained on total parental nutrition (Sutton *et al.*, 1985) and in a few otherwise normal infants fed cow's milk from birth (Naveh *et al.*, 1981; Levy *et al.*, 1985). Signs of copper deficiency in these infants included anemia, neutropenia, osteoporosis, depigmentation, and neurological disturbances. Adult humans fed experimental diets low in copper have exhibited increases in cholesterol (Klevay *et al.*, 1984), abnormal cardiac function (Klevay *et al.*, 1984; Reiser *et al.*, 1985), decreased glucose tolerance (Klevay *et al.*, 1986), and impairment in autonomic cardiovascular function (Lukaski *et al.*, 1988). These changes have occurred at copper intakes of 0·7–1·0 mg/day. It should be noted that changes in serum cholesterol and in glucose tolerance, in particular, have been observed only in a very small number of subjects. The degree to which these signs are related to copper nutriture in humans needs further study.

B. Estimated Requirements for Dietary Copper

No Recommended Dietary Allowance for copper has been established (Food and Nutrition Board, 1980), but the Estimated Safe and Adequate Intake is set at 2–3 mg/day for adults and adolescents over 11 years of age. A large proportion of self-chosen diets in the United States are believed to contain less than 2 mg/day (White, 1969; Holden *et al.*, 1979; Klevay *et al.*, 1979).

Intakes of 1·1–1·25 mg copper/day by adult men (Johnson and Lykken, 1988) or postmenopausal women (Johnson *et al.*, 1988) were insufficient to maintain a non-negative copper balance if surface losses were taken into account. Women of child-bearing age were in negative copper balance with an intake of 2 mg/day (Crews *et al.*, 1980; Taper *et al.*, 1980). Balance, exclusive of surface losses, in elderly men fed semipurified liquid formula diets was 0·01–0·06 mg/day at a copper intake of 3·3 mg copper/day according to Turnlund *et al.* (1981). On the other hand, young men consuming 3·1–3·25 mg copper/day were in marked positive balance (Greger and Snedeker, 1980), and young men fed 1·3 mg/day were also in positive balance (Turnlund *et al.*, 1988). Adolescent girls fed diets containing 1·2–1·3 mg copper/day had an apparent balance of 0·3–0·4 mg copper/day, exclusive of surface losses (Greger *et al.*, 1978). Surface losses of copper were 0·34 ± 0·24 mg copper/day for men consuming 1·1–1·5 mg copper/day (Jacob *et al.*, 1981). However, these values may be high. Recent findings indicate surface losses of 0·08 ± 0·05 mg copper/day for men consuming 0·6–2·6 mg copper/day (D. B. Milne, personal communication). It is not known if surface losses in women differ. The results of a series of balance studies in men fed various forms of dietary fiber by Klevay *et al.* (1980) suggested the daily requirement for copper to be approximately 1·5 mg for adult men consuming mixed western diets. In general, it appears that the effects of age and sex on copper absorption need to be better characterized; requirements may not be the same for all adults. Moreover, additional studies of metabolic and physiological function at different intakes of copper, such as those cited above, are needed before the copper requirement can be reliably defined.

C. Sources of Dietary Copper

Copper is widely distributed in foods, but is most concentrated in liver, legumes, shellfish, meats, whole grains, and nuts (Gormican, 1970; Pennington and Calloway, 1973; Davis and Mertz, 1987). Approximately 10% of the copper in the average United States diet is contributed by meat, poultry, and fish (Sandstead, 1982). Reported copper concentrations in pork are higher than in beef (Table 10-1), and both beef and pork have higher copper concentrations than poultry (Table 10-2). Liver is the most concentrated source of copper, with beef liver containing as much as 16 mg/100 g (Davis and Mertz, 1987).

D. Copper Bioavailability

Copper bioavailability has not been studied as extensively as the bioavailability of other minerals. The advent of new isotopic tracer techniques has produced an upsurge in the amount of data on this topic in the past few years.

Although milk is low in copper and feeding of cow's milk has been associated with the development of copper deficiency in infants, the copper in human milk is highly available and is sufficient to maintain health in breast-fed infants according to studies by MacDonald *et al.* (1982) and Salim *et al.* (1986). Studies in this laboratory found that 3-month old infants absorbed $90 \pm 7\%$ of the copper from breast milk and $81 \pm 12\%$ of the copper from a cow's milk-based infant formula (Johnson and Canfield). High doses of ascorbic acid were found to be detrimental to copper status in monkeys, rats, and guinea pigs (Mason, 1979; Allen and Solomons, 1984; Solomons, 1985; Davis and Mertz, 1987), but have not been found to impair copper absorption in humans (Jacob *et al.*, 1987).

In balance studies in adolescent boys, addition of hemicellulose, but not cellulose or pectin, adversely affected copper retention (Drews *et al.*, 1979). Isotopic studies of copper absorption in the presence of cellulose by Turnlund *et al.* (1985) did not show any detrimental effect of cellulose on

TABLE 10-1
COPPER, MAGNESIUM AND MANGANESE CONTENT OF MEATS[a]
(mg/100 g cooked)

	Total edible			*Separable lean*		
	Cu	*Mg*	*Mn*	*Cu*	*Mg*	*Mn*
Beef						
Chuck roast	0·132	19	0·016	0·164	24	0·019
Rib roast	0·095	19	0·013	0·098	25	0·016
Prime rib	0·089	20	0·013	0·089	25	0·016
Ribeye steak	0·098	24	0·014	0·100	27	0·016
Round steak	0·097	24	0·015	0·107	28	0·016
T-bone steak	0·130	24	0·013	0·143	29	0·015
Hamburger	0·090	22	0·019	0·088	23	0·016
Liver, fried	2·822	23	0·423	—	—	—
Pork						
Pork chops, fried	0·080	26	0·009	0·089	32	0·012
Pork roast	0·118	18	0·012	0·129	20	0·014
Spareribs	0·142	24	0·014	—	—	—
Ham, canned	0·130	17	0·029	0·084	17	0·025
Ham, picnic	0·112	17	0·033	0·128	20	0·041
Liver, braised	0·634	14	0·300	—	—	—
Lamb						
Lamb chops	0·060	17	No values	0·060	22	No values

[a] Mn values were obtained from USDA (1976–87) except for lamb chops. Cu values are taken from Gormican (1970) and Mg values from USDA (1977–78).
— Means that no value was found.

copper absorption. Men fed eight slices of whole wheat bread per day absorbed 58–85% of the copper in their diets (Johnson and Lykken, 1988). Phytic acid, which is antagonistic to zinc, calcium, and iron absorption, did not affect copper absorption in adult men (Turnlund *et al.*, 1985). A diet high in fiber from fruits and vegetables resulted in a negative copper balance in men; but when fruits and vegetables were replaced by fruit juices and vegetable juices, copper balance was positive according to studies by Kelsay *et al.* (1979).

In rats, the form of the dietary carbohydrate was shown to have a profound effect on the manifestations of copper deficiency in studies carried out by Fields *et al.* (1984). Rats fed diets containing fructose or sucrose as the dietary carbohydrate exhibited more severe signs of copper

TABLE 10-2

COPPER, MAGNESIUM AND MANGANESE CONTENT OF CHICKEN AND TURKEY PARTS COOKED BY FRYING AND ROASTING WITH SKIN ON AND SKIN OFF
(mg/100 g cooked)[a]

	Total edible			*Skin on*						*Skinless*					
				Fried			*Roasted*			*Fried*			*Roasted*		
	Cu	*Mg*	*Mn*	*Cu*	*Mg*	*Mn*	*Cu*	*Mg*	*Mn*	*Cu*	*Mg*	*Mn*	*Cu*	*Mg*	*Mn*
Chicken															
Breast				0·057	30	0·026	0·050	27	0·018	0·054	31	0·021	0·049	29	0·017
Drumstick				0·080	23	0·026	0·077	23	0·021	0·080	24	0·021	0·079	24	0·021
Thigh				0·089	25	0·036	0·078	22	0·021	0·090	26	0·027	0·081	24	0·021
Wing				0·061	19	0·028	0·057	19	0·018	0·053	21	0·016	0·054	21	0·016
Liver, simmered	0·37	21	0·297												
Turkey															
Breast							0·076	28	0·024				0·070	29	0·024
Leg							0·233	24	0·025				0·242	25	0·026
Wing							0·154	20	0·024				0·166	22	0·027
Liver, simmered	0·560	15	0·253												

[a] Mn values were obtained from USDA (1976–87), Cu values from Gormican (1970) and Mg values from USDA (1977–78).

deficiency, including greater mortality, than rats fed starch. This apparently is the result of a metabolic interaction between copper and the carbohydrates, as copper absorption and rate of excretion are affected minimally, if at all, by the carbohydrate in the diet (Johnson, 1989). In humans, electrocardiogram abnormalities were found in a study involving feeding of low copper diets that contained fructose (Reiser *et al.*, 1985).

Raw beef contains copper that is poorly available to rats, and rats fed raw beef developed anemia in studies by Moore *et al.* (1964). Cooking the beef improved the availability of the copper. In rats, absorption of copper from plant and animal foods was found to be similar by Johnson *et al.* (1988). Rats absorbed less copper from liver than from other foods tested; the greatest percent copper absorption was from shrimp, beef, and sunflower seeds. In contrast, adult women absorbed more copper from goose liver than from goose breast meat, while copper absorption from peanut butter and sunflower seed butter was similar to that from the goose breast meat in recent studies by Johnson *et al.* (1988).

When compared to that in men fed 51 g protein/day, copper balance was improved in adult men fed 150 g protein/day and 3·1–3·2 mg copper/day (Greger and Snedeker, 1980). In another balance study by Turnlund *et al.* (1981), the amount of copper needed to achieve balance dropped from 1·50 mg/day to 1·33 mg/day when protein intake was increased from 40 g/day to 100 g/day. No changes in copper retention were found, however, when protein intake was varied between 25 and 46 g/day (Price *et al.*, 1970).

Women fed meat-containing diets absorbed 41% of the copper in the diet but only 34% from diets based on plant protein according to Turnlund *et al.* (1983). In pregnant women fed the same diets, there was no difference in absorption of copper from the two diets. However, there was greater net retention of copper from the plant protein diets by both pregnant and non-pregnant women, because of the greater copper content of the plant protein diet. In a study by Gibson *et al.* (1983), postmenopausal vegetarian women had greater intakes of copper than did non-vegetarian women, but copper status as reflected by hair copper did not differ between the two groups. In a balance study comparing male and female Asian Indian vegetarians, American vegetarians, and American non-vegetarians, copper intake by American vegetarians was greater than copper intake by Asian Indian vegetarians or by non-vegetarians, but copper balance did not differ among the three groups (Kelsay *et al.*, 1988). The results of these studies suggest that copper is less available from western-type vegetarian diets than from non-vegetarian western diets. Asian Indian vegetarian diets may differ in copper bioavailability from western-type vegetarian diets.

II. MANGANESE

A. Metabolic Functions of Manganese

Like copper, manganese is involved in many metabolic functions, although its biochemical role in these functions has not been characterized to the extent that has been done for copper. Manganese functions as an essential component of enzymes involved in protein and energy metabolism, and in the formation of mucopolysaccharides. Manganese is involved in the regulation of carbohydrate and lipid metabolism, in cartilage and bone matrix formation, and plays an important role in brain function. Manganese is assumed to be an essential nutrient for humans. Several comprehensive reviews (Utter, 1976; Hurley, 1982, 1984; Keen *et al.*, 1985; Hurley and Keen, 1987) provide details that will not be discussed herein.

Manganese deficiency has been produced in all species of animals studied. Skeletal abnormalities in manganese-deficient animals are common, and are characterized by defects in cartilage or bone matrix formation. Manganese deficiency during pregnancy of rats results in offspring with congenital, irreversible ataxia caused by abnormal development of the otoliths (Hurley, 1968; Erway *et al.*, 1970). Manganese deficiency also causes ultrastructural abnormalities of the rough endoplasmic reticulum in liver, kidney, heart, and pancreas which has been described by Bell and Hurley (1973).

The involvement of manganese in brain function is demonstrated by the tendency for manganese-deficient rats to have convulsions, and to manifest electroencephalographic abnormalities (Hurley *et al.*, 1963). Manganese toxicity causes symptoms similar to those of Parkinson's disease (Donaldson, 1987). Serum manganese levels have been reported to be low in patients with certain types of epilepsy (Papavasiliou *et al.*, 1979; Carl *et al.*, 1986).

Manganese has been reported to affect carbohydrate metabolism in animals (Hurley *et al.*, 1984) and humans. A diabetic patient, who did not respond to insulin injections, responded to oral manganese with decreased blood glucose levels (Rubenstein *et al.*, 1962). Patients with chronic manganese poisoning have hypoglycemia when given intravenous glucose tolerance tests according to Hassanein *et al.* (1966).

One possible case of manganese deficiency in a human was described by Doisy (1972) and involved a man who was fed a semipurified formula diet as a part of a study of vitamin K metabolism. He developed weight loss, depressed growth of hair and nails, dermatitis and hypocholesterolemia.

Also, his black hair developed a reddish tinge, and his clotting protein response to vitamin K supplementation was abnormal. The preceding symptoms are not signs of vitamin K deficiency. When it was realized that manganese had inadvertently been left out of the diet, the subject was treated by feeding a mixed hospital diet. Although the patient responded to the treatment, no supplementation with manganese alone was tried. Thus, it is impossible to say conclusively that this case represented manganese deficiency in a human.

Experimental manganese deficiency may have been produced in men fed a manganese-deficient diet containing 0·1 mg manganese/day by Friedman *et al.* (1987). These men exhibited decreased serum cholesterol and a fleeting dermatitis, *Miliaria crystallina.* Calcium, phosphorus, and alkaline phosphatase activity in the blood increased. However, short-term manganese supplementation did not reverse these changes.

B. Estimated Requirements for Dietary Manganese

No Recommended Dietary Allowance for manganese has been established by the Food and Nutrition Board (1980), but the Estimated Safe and Adequate Intake has been set at 2·5–5 mg/day for adults. Intakes of manganese from self-chosen diets in the United States tend to fall within this range.

The manganese requirement was estimated by Friedman *et al.* (1987) to be 0·74 mg/day for adult men from a balance study with three levels of manganese intake ranging from 0·1–2·5 mg/day in a formula diet. In a study using diets composed of conventional foods and with manganese intakes from 1·2–3·8 mg/day, however, Freeland-Graves *et al.* (1988) found the manganese requirement to be 3·5 mg/day for young men. The latter value for the manganese requirement is consistent with earlier recommendations of 3·7–5·5 mg/day (Basu and Malakar, 1940), 3·5–7 mg/day (Freeland-Graves *et al.*, 1987), 2·74 mg/day (De, 1949), and 3·72 mg/day (Rao and Rao, 1982). Earlier studies have yielded conflicting results as to the amount of manganese intake needed to achieve a positive balance. Positive balances were reported at intakes of 5·4–17·3 mg/day (Rao and Rao, 1980), and negative balances were reported at intakes of 2·1–17·3 mg/day (Spencer *et al.*, 1979; Johnson *et al.*, 1982; Patterson *et al.*, 1984; Schwartz *et al.*, 1986). Some of the variability among these balance studies is probably related to differences in manganese bioavailability from the diets studied, but of course, much of it may be caused by the inherent limitations of balance studies. Bioavailability effects are discussed in greater detail below.

C. Sources of Dietary Manganese

Manganese is found mainly in plant foods. Meat, fish, and poultry are poor sources. The highest concentrations of manganese occur in nuts, legumes, and whole grains (Hurley and Keen, 1987). Most of the manganese in grains is in the germ or whole bran fractions; refined flour is low in manganese. The manganese content of vegetables is variable. Tea is a very rich source of manganese, containing 350–900 μg/g on a dry basis (Wenlock *et al.*, 1979). The manganese concentrations in meat are low, typically 0·35–1·1 mg/kg (USDA, 1976–87). Manganese concentrations in beef, pork, and poultry are similar as shown in Table 10-1 and Table 10-2. Liver is the animal food containing the highest concentration of manganese, with approximately 0·3–0·4 mg Mn/100 g.

D. Manganese Bioavailability

The substance which has the greatest negative effect on manganese bioavailability apparently is dietary fiber. Young men were in negative or near zero balance with a manganese intake of 14–15 mg/day when the diet included 15 g of unprocessed wheat bran (Schwartz *et al.*, 1986). This level of manganese intake is 3 times greater than the maximum of the Estimated Safe and Adequate Intake (Food and Nutrition Board, 1980). Female American vegetarians with a manganese intake of 4·1 mg/day and consuming 5·9 g crude fiber and 12·8 g of neutral detergent fiber (NDF) per day were in significantly more negative balance than American non-vegetarians from the same community who consumed only 2·6 mg manganese/day with 3·5 g/day crude fiber and 6·3 g/day of NDF as shown by Kelsay *et al.* (1988); similar differences were found for men in the same study. Men fed eight slices of whole-wheat bread per day and consuming 10–11 mg manganese/day were in negative manganese balance (P. E. Johnson, unpublished data). Phytic acid, which occurs in many of the same food sources as dietary fiber, has an adverse effect on zinc and iron absorption. However, phytic acid does not consistently inhibit manganese absorption in rats (Davies and Nightingale, 1975; Lee and Johnson, 1989); but its effects on manganese metabolism in humans have not been studied.

Dietary calcium ranging from 200–1500 mg/day did not affect manganese balance in men (Spencer *et al.*, 1979). Likewise, in women fed 590 or 1400 mg calcium/day, manganese balance at intakes of 1 or 6 mg/day was unaffected by dietary calcium (Johnson and Lykken, 1989). In adolescent girls, manganese balance was unaffected by calcium intake ranging from 260–620 mg/day (Price *et al.*, 1970) or 300–1300 mg/day (Price and Bunce, 1972).

The availability of manganese from human milk, bovine milk, and bovine milk formula is similar (Keen *et al.*, 1986; Raghib *et al.*, 1986) but availability from soy formula is less than that from human milk for rats (Raghib *et al.*, 1986).

Iron is known to interact with manganese, and the two minerals have mutually inhibitory effects on absorption. Mild anemia in one subject markedly decreased the rate of manganese excretion (Mahoney and Small, 1968) and anemic subjects absorbed 7·5% of ingested manganese, which is higher than the 3·0% for normal subjects (Thomson *et al.*, 1971).

The amount of protein or nitrogen in the diet does not significantly affect manganese balance (Price *et al.*, 1970; Price and Bunce, 1972; Greger and Snedeker, 1980). Although meat contains relatively little manganese, the substitution of beef and tuna for soy isolate brought about a more positive manganese balance in women (Kies *et al.*, 1987). When diets containing soy, casein, beef, tuna, or chicken were formulated with an identical protein content and supplemental amino acids were added to meet minimum requirements of rats, manganese balance was most positive for the soy diets and was negative when tuna was fed (P. E. Johnson and E. Korynta, unpublished data). In another study with rats, manganese was more available from soy protein than from casein-based diets (Lee and Johnson, 1989). However, non-vegetarians were in less negative balance than vegetarians (Kelsay *et al.*, 1988) despite lower manganese intakes. Substitution of meat or fish for legumes in an Indian diet produced a more positive manganese balance (Rao and Rao, 1980). The conflicting results of these studies suggest that protein quality or amino acid composition may affect manganese availability.

III. COBALT

Among the trace elements required for human health, cobalt is unique because it is not required as an ion. The only known function for cobalt is as the metal ion at the center of the corrin ring of vitamin B_{12}. Vitamin B_{12} is a cofactor for at least three mammalian enzymes; these are methylmalonyl-CoA mutase, DL-5-methyltetrahydrofolate-homocysteine methyl-transferase (methionine synthase), and leucine 2,3-aminomutase.

Vitamin B_{12} is made in nature only by microorganisms. Among the microorganisms which synthesize vitamin B_{12} are those found in the rumen of ruminants. Thus, ruminants are the only animals which can have their vitamin B_{12} requirement fulfilled by the dietary intake of cobalt. Like all other animals, humans must get their requirement for cobalt by consuming foods rich in vitamin B_{12}. These foods include meat and meat products, and to a lesser extent, milk and milk products.

Because the discussion of cobalt in human health is essentially one centered around vitamin B_{12}, and because various aspects of vitamin B_{12} in human health are described in Chapter 15 of this volume, cobalt in human health will not be discussed further here.

IV. MAGNESIUM

Magnesium is the fourth most abundant cation in the body and is second only to potassium in its intracellular concentration. The adult human weighing 70 kg contains between 20–28 g of magnesium. Of the total, about 60–65% is in bone, 27% is in muscle, 6–7% in other cells, and only 1% is in extracellular fluid. Magnesium catalyzes or activates more than 300 enzymes in the body. Among the enzyme systems in which magnesium has a role are those involved in hydrolysis and transfer of phosphate groups, fatty acid degradation, protein synthesis, DNA synthesis and degradation, cardiac and smooth muscle contraction, and calcium ion transport and utilization. Because magnesium is crucial in so many life processes, it is not surprising that it has been the focus of numerous books, reviews, and symposia (Aikawa, 1976, 1981; Flink, 1976; Shils, 1976, 1988; Wacker *et al.*, 1977; Wacker, 1980; Altura *et al.*, 1987). The reader is referred to those sources for further information on the biochemical, physiological, pharmacological and toxicological aspects of magnesium. The present discussion will emphasize the clinical signs of deficiency and human nutritional requirements of magnesium only.

A. Magnesium Deficiency in Humans

(i) Experimental deficiency

Although magnesium deficiency can be induced with relative ease in young experimental animals, deficiency has been found to be difficult to induce in humans. In fact, efforts to produce symptomatic magnesium deficiency in humans simply by restricting dietary intake have been generally unsuccessful although some subjects became hypomagnesmic or retained large amounts of magnesium when repleted. According to Shils (1988), four groups of investigators have attempted to induce magnesium deficiency experimentally in human volunteers. The one study which was successful (Shils, 1969), involved seven subjects (six males and one female) who had undergone radical surgery of the head and neck for the treatment of carcinoma of some part of the oral cavity; consequently, they required feeding via nasoesophageal tube. The diet the subjects received was based on casein, dextrose, cornstarch, corn oil, and purified vitamins and minerals in water. This purified diet resulted in infrequent small stools, which caused adverse psychological reaction in some individuals, delayed the passing of fecal markers, and interfered with the clear-cut separation of stools by dietary period. The diet provided slightly less than 0·8 meq (10 mg) of magnesium/day. Thus, even in the one study in which a symptomatic magnesium deficiency was induced, the subjects were not healthy individuals consuming a relatively normal diet. Furthermore, the deficiency was acute and severe. Plasma magnesium fell to levels that were 10–30% of control periods. Urine and fecal magnesium decreased to extremely low levels within seven days.

Among the signs of deficiency found under the above conditions by Shils (1969) were the following: hypomagnesmia, hypocalcemia, and hypokalemia were consistently present; neuromuscular signs (positive Trousseau's signs, tremors, fasciculations, and gross muscle spasms) occurred in five of the subjects after 25–110 days on the deficient diet; some electrocardiographic changes occurred which were correlated with hypocalcemia and/or hypokalemia; anorexia, nausea, and apathy occurred frequently and usually preceded an exacerbation of the neurological changes. The findings from this study indicated that magnesium is essential for the normal metabolism of potassium and calcium, is essential for the mobilization of calcium from bone, and has deficiency signs, which are secondary consequences of complex electrolyte changes.

(ii) Clinical deficiency

Clinical magnesium deficiency is virtually always a conditioned deficiency. These conditioning factors are usually the consequence of some illness which probably interferes with the absorption or promotes the excretion of magnesium. Magnesium deficiency is indicated by a depression in some tissue or blood magnesium concentration. However, the description of magnesium deficiency signs in these situations must be considered with caution because complex and uncontrollable variables are usually present in these often quite ill individuals. Often present are nutritional inadequacies, metabolic abnormalities, electrolyte and fluid imbalances, manifestations of basic disease, infection, and administration of various medications. Among the pathologic settings in which hypomagnesmia may occur are alcoholism, cirrhosis, kidney disease, malabsorption syndromes, extensive bowel resection, gastroileal bypass, severe or prolonged diarrhea, protein-calorie malnutrition, acute pancreatitis, hyperaldosteronism, diabetes mellitus, thyroid gland disease, parathyroid gland disease, vitamin D-resistant rickets, pellagra, malignant osteolytic disease, burns, and diuretic therapy (Wacker, 1980).

Shils (1988) stated in his review that it may be useful to distinguish three types of magnesium depletion:

(1) Depletion caused by a failure to ingest, absorb or retain sufficient magnesium in the presence of normal glomerular function; this depletion is characterized by hypomagnesmia and deficiency signs similar to experimental deficiency.
(2) Depletion associated with other nutrient deficiencies that induce serious cellular catabolism, potassium depletion, and/or acidosis associated with tissue (including bone) loss of magnesium. However, serum magnesium is maintained near normal through some oral intake and from significant mining of tissue magnesium stores. The anticipated signs of experimental deficiency except for tissue depletion are absent in this type of deficiency.
(3) Depletion of either the above two types but of less severity, which is associated with glomerular dysfunction, thus resulting in normal or high serum magnesium concentrations.

Recently, magnesium deficiency has been suggested to be a contributor to some vascular disorders in humans. Instead of being based upon the experimental and clinical findings mentioned above, these suggestions come from epidemiologic findings, animal experiments, tissue magnesium measurements, and magnesium supplementation trials.

Magnesium deprivation has been associated with cardiovascular disease since 1957 when it was first determined that the incidence of cardiovascular disease was highest in areas where drinking water is soft and lowest where it is hard (Kobayashi, 1957). Reviews (Seelig and Heggveit, 1974; Durlach *et al.*, 1985; Neri *et al.*, 1985) have concluded that the most reliable water factor associated with cardiovascular risks or mortality is the magnesium content. In addition to the epidemiologic evidence, these reviews also cite other findings which suggest that a magnesium deficit might enhance cardiovascular mortality. Neri *et al.* (1985) reported that subpharmacologic doses of magnesium stabilize arryhthmias, lower blood pressure in hypertensives, increase cardiac output, reduce infarct size, and protect against cardiotoxic substances and stress. They concluded that the myocardium can become selectively depleted in magnesium and can thereby become impaired in its ability to respond to a sudden demand for increased cardiac output. Seelig and Heggtveit (1974) suggested that magnesium was beneficial in the prevention of ischemic heart disease through action at the cellular level; that is through (1) counteracting the adverse effects of excessive intracellular calcium; (2) maintaining the proper intracellular concentration of potassium; and (3) maintaining the integrity of subcellular structures. They stated that the long-term prophylactic use of magnesium for the inhibition of atherogenesis or the prevention of acute ischemic attacks, or both, required further study. Rayssiguier (1986) concluded from studies with magnesium-deficient rats that magnesium was necessary to prevent abnormalities in lipid metabolism and platelet function which could lead to atheroma and thrombotic complications. In contrast to the above, after reviewing the evidence for an inverse relationship between magnesium intake and coronary artery disease and its sequelae, Shils (1988) concluded that low magnesium intake is not a significant etiological factor in ischemic heart disease.

Magnesium status has also been associated with hypertension. High dietary magnesium (0·75% of diet) was found to inhibit the development of hypertension in young spontaneously hypertensive (SHR) rats and to reduce arterial blood pressure in mature SHR rats (Wolf *et al.*, 1987). The high dietary magnesium caused diarrhea, polyuresis and growth depression in the rats. In comparison to Wistar-Kyoto rats, SHR rats were found to have lower magnesium concentrations in selected organs (kidney, heart, lung and bone, but not serum) by Wallach and Verch (1986). Resnick *et al.* (1983) studied 102 normotensive and 98 hypertensive people and found those with low-renin hypertension had a mean serum magnesium concentration of 2·07 meq/liter, those with normal-renin hypertension had a mean of 1·94 meq/liter, and those with high-renin hypertension had a mean of 1·83 meq/liter. Each group was significantly different from the others, and the high- and low-renin groups differed significantly from the normotensive group which had a mean serum magnesium concentration of 1·91 meq/liter. Resnick *et al.* (1984) also found an inverse relationship between intracellular red cell free magnesium concentration and systolic blood pressure.

The role of magnesium in hypertension needs further clarification. Most likely any role magnesium has in hypertension will be found to be secondary or indirect in nature. If magnesium does have an effect in hypertension, it probably is through changes in intracellular calcium, which would in turn affect renin, parathyroid secretion and vascular tone (Shils, 1988).

In a recent review, Franz (1987) stated that there is an increasing amount of evidence which indicates that low magnesium status may be involved in several disorders that can occur during pregnancy. These disorders include hypertension, vasospasm, coagulation defects, premature delivery, intrauterine growth retardation, muscle cramping, and toxemia. Based upon epidemiologic findings, Franz (1987) concluded that the magnesium intake of pregnant women needs to be increased by either dietary means or supplements, especially among low-income women in soft-water areas.

The preceding study of Franz (1987) shows that much remains to be learned about the consequences of a low magnesium intake, and at what level of intake that adverse effects begin to appear. It is rather surprising that an element with so many critical essential functions has not been conclusively found to cause, upon low dietary intake, some distinct clinical disorder in otherwise apparently healthy individuals.

B. Magnesium Requirements of Healthy Individuals

Because the consequences of low dietary intake are unclear, it should not be surprising that there is uncertainty about the dietary requirement for magnesium. The variance in the suggestions for the requirement of magnesium is large. Marshall *et al.* (1976) used 14-day balance studies to obtain data which suggested that negative magnesium balance can be prevented by intakes of 100 mg/day, and thus concluded that the magnesium requirement must be below this value. After extensively reviewing the literature relating to human magnesium requirements, Seelig (1981) suggested magnesium intakes should be 6–10 mg/kg body weight/day for young adults and twice that much for those undergoing active anabolism, or under stress. This translates into total daily intakes of 450–700 mg for a 70-kg man, and as much as 600–1000 mg for a 100-kg man.

There are Recommended Dietary Allowances (RDA) for magnesium (Food and Nutrition Board, 1980). These RDAs are 40–70 mg/day for infants, and increase to 250 mg/day at age 10 years. Adolescent and adult males and non-pregnant and non-lactating females have RDAs in the range of 300–400 mg/day (5–6 mg/kg body weight/day). The RDA for pregnant and lactating women is 450 mg/day. It should be emphasized that these RDAs are based on consumption data, old balance studies, and human milk analyses published mainly from 1964 to 1969. Much of the old balance data is probably unreliable because of analytical and methodological problems. Spencer *et al.* (1980), pointed out that most of the balance studies were of short duration (less than 15 days), and were not performed on adults maintained on a constant diet in metabolic wards. Shils (1988) has stated:

> the fact that clinically significant hypomagnesmia is uncommon and the lack of verified reports of symptomatic magnesium deficiency in a healthy population raise the question about the reliability of the current RDA for magnesium.

Moreover, the Food and Nutrition Board (1986) of the National Research Council of the National Academy of Science posed the questions:

> Since few studies have been devoted exclusively to magnesium requirements and the reliability of many of the resultant data is questionable, should there be an RDA or should only a provisional intake be established for magnesium?

and

> Since there is no apparent evidence of magnesium deficiency in the general population, are data on the magnesium content of the average diet reliable enough to justify lowering the RDA?

There is no doubt that magnesium is required by humans. However, it is clear that more quantitative and precise data obtained under strictly controlled conditions are needed to set a reliable RDA. Studies designed to investigate magnesium requirements should be cognizant of the fact that the magnesium requirement is likely to be increased by diets high in fiber (Hallfrisch *et al.*, 1987) and protein (Mahalko *et al.*, 1983).

C. Magnesium in the Diet

The 1977–78 Nationwide Food Consumption Survey (US Department of Health and Human Services, 1986) found that over 38% of all individuals examined had daily intakes of less than 69% of the RDA for magnesium. Mean magnesium intakes in this survey were about 310 mg/day for adult males, and 230 mg/day for adult females. Actual analyses of contemporary diets also indicate that the magnesium intakes of many people do not meet the RDA. Srivastava *et al.* (1978) found that male and female students selected foods at a university cafeteria which supplied 247 and 224 mg magnesium/day, respectively. In Sweden, analyses of duplicate diets reported by Abdulla (1986) showed that male and female pensioners' mean magnesium intakes were 231 and 175 mg/day, respectively. However, the daily magnesium intake of vegetarians in the group was found to be much higher, 615 and 468 mg/day for men and women, respectively. Hallfrisch *et al.* (1987) found that the mean daily intake of magnesium in a self-selected daily diet for 20 men was 241 mg, for 19 premenopausal women was 183 mg, and for 12 postmenopausal women was 171 mg. Franz (1987) reviewed the literature and found six reports published between 1980 and 1983 on magnesium intake during pregnancy in the United States. The mean magnesium intakes ranged from 158–259 mg/day when no supplements were taken.

Foods richest in magnesium on a kcal basis include leafy vegetables, nuts, skim milk and grains (Franz, 1987). However, refining or processing of grains can remove the majority of magnesium. For example, Marier (1986) reported that on a kg dry weight basis, wheat contained 1586 mg magnesium; unpolished rice contained 1477 mg magnesium, whereas, polished rice contained 251 mg magnesium. Refined foods such as sugar, fats and oils are the lowest in magnesium density, usually less than 50 mg/1000 kcal (Holden *et al.*, 1979). Thus, it is not surprising that foods made from the above items, including most cakes, cookies, doughnuts and pastries, usually contain less than 50 mg/1000 kcal.

Meats, especially fatty types, are also relatively poor sources of magnesium. For example, bacon, sausage and frankfurters have a magnesium density similar to baked goods, 50 mg/1000 kcal. Lean meats (Table 10-1) and poultry (Table 10-2) are somewhat higher in magnesium density, ranging between 50–100 mg/1000 kcal. Although some types of meats can add significant amounts of magnesium to the diet, a diet high in meat is likely to contain less than 200 mg/1000 kcal unless it contains significant amounts of magnesium-dense foods. The magnesium concentrations of some meats are shown in Table 10-1.

V. SUMMARY

Findings from animal experiments have conclusively shown that copper, manganese, cobalt and magnesium are essential elements. Biochemical functions also have been described for these elements. However, the importance and requirements of these elements for humans are presently uncertain.

Although many people routinely consume less than the Estimated Safe and Adequate Intake of copper (2–3 mg/day), finding of a copper deficiency which impairs health in free-living adults has been elusive. Moreover, finding consistent signs of copper deficiency in adults fed experimental diets low in copper has been difficult. Nonetheless, copper is most likely necessary for optimal health and well-being. An excellent source of copper is liver. Red meat and poultry supply some copper, but are not especially good sources.

Signs of manganese deficiency have not been conclusively described for humans. Thus, whether manganese nutriture should be of concern for humans is unknown. Nonetheless, an Estimated Safe and Adequate Intake of 2·5–5·0 mg Mn/day for adults has been set. Meat, fish and poultry are poor sources for manganese.

Among the trace elements required for human health, cobalt is unique because it is not required as an ion. The only known function for cobalt is as the metal ion at the center of the corrin ring of vitamin B_{12}. Humans must get their requirement for cobalt by consuming foods rich in vitamin B_{12}. These foods include meat and meat products, and to a lesser extent, milk and milk products.

Although magnesium deficiency can be induced with relative ease in young experimental animals, deficiency has been found to be difficult to induce in humans. In one study in which symptomatic magnesium deficiency was induced, the subjects were not healthy individuals consuming a relatively normal diet. Furthermore, the deficiency was acute and severe which made the differentiation between deficiency signs of magnesium and electrolyte imbalance difficult. Recognized clinical magnesium deficiency is virtually always a conditioned deficiency. Describing signs of magnesium deficiency under these conditions is difficult because complex and uncontrollable variables are usually present in these often quite ill individuals. To date, it has not been conclusively demonstrated that the low dietary intake of magnesium causes some distinct clinical disorder in otherwise apparently healthy individuals. Nonetheless, an RDA of 300–400 mg/day has been set for adolescent and adult males, and non-pregnant and non-lactating females. Although the RDA may be questionable, there is no doubt that magnesium is required by humans. Meats, especially fatty types, are relatively poor sources of magnesium. Some types of lean meats can add significant amounts of magnesium to the diet. However, a diet high in meat should contain significant amounts of magnesium-dense foods.

VI. REFERENCES

ABDULLA, M. (1986). *Inorganic Chemical Elements in Prepared Meals in Sweden.* University of Lund, Lund, Sweden.

AIKAWA, J. K. (1976). Biochemistry and physiology of magnesium. In *Trace Elements in Human Health and Disease. Vol. 2. Essential and Toxic Elements* (A. S. Prasad and D. Oberleas, Eds), p. 47. Academic Press, New York.

AIKAWA, J. K. (1981). *Magnesium: Its Biologic Significance.* CRC Press, Boca Raton, FL.

ALLEN, L. H. and SOLOMONS, N. W. (1984). Copper. In *Absorption and Malabsorption of Mineral Nutrients* (N. W. Solomons and I. H. Rosenberg, Eds), p. 199. Alan R. Liss, Inc., New York.

AL-RASHID, R. A. and SPANGLER, J. (1971). Neonatal copper deficiency. *N. Engl. J. Med.* **285**, 841.

ALTURA, B. M., DURLACH, J. and SEELIG, M. S. (Eds) (1987). *Magnesium in Cellular Processes and Medicine.* Karger, Basel.

BASU, P. and MALAKAR, C. (1940). Iron and manganese requirements of human adults. *J. Indian Chem. Soc.* **17**, 317.

BELL, L. T. and HURLEY, L. S. (1973). Ultrastructural effects of manganese deficiency in liver, heart, kidney, and pancreas of mice. *Lab. Invest.* **29**, 723.

CARL, G. F., KEEN, C. L., GALLAGHER, B. B., CLEGG, M. S., LITTLETON, W. H., FLANNERY, D. B. and HURLEY, L. S. (1986). Association of low blood manganese concentrations with epilepsy. *Neurology* **36**, 1584.

CORDANO, A., BAERTL, J. M. and GRAHAM, G. G. (1964). Copper deficiency in infancy. *Pediatrics* **34**, 324.

CREWS, M. G., TAPER, L. J. and RITCHEY, S. J. (1980). Effects of oral contraceptive agents on copper and zinc balance in young women. *Am. J. Clin. Nutr.* **33**, 1940.

DAVIES, N. T. and NIGHTINGALE, R. (1975). The effects of phytate on intestinal absorption and secretion of zinc and whole-body retention of zinc, copper, iron, and manganese in rats. *Brit. J. Nutr.* **34**, 243.

DAVIS, G. K. and MERTZ, W. (1987). Copper. In *Trace Elements in Human and Animal Nutrition*, Vol. 1, 5th edn. (W. Mertz, Ed.), p. 301. Academic Press, New York.

DE, H. N. (1949). Copper and manganese metabolism with typical Indian dietaries and assessment of their requirement for the Indian adult. *Indian J. Med. Res.* **37**, 301.

DOISY, E. A., JR (1972). Micronutrient controls on biosynthesis of clotting proteins and cholesterol. In *Trace Substances in Environmental Health—VI* (D. D. Hemphill, Ed.), p. 193. University of Missouri Press, Columbia, MO.

DONALDSON, J. (1987). The physiopathologic significance of manganese in brain: Its relation to schizophrenia and neurodegenerative disorders. *NeuroToxicology* **8**, 451.

DREWS, L. M., KIES, C. and FOX, H. M. (1979). Effect of dietary fiber on copper, zinc, and magnesium utilization by adolescent boys. *Am. J. Clin. Nutr.* **32**, 1893.

DURLACH, G., BARA, M. and GUIET-BARA, A. (1985). Magnesium level in drinking water and cardiovascular risk factor: Ce hypotheses. *Magnesium* **4**, 5.

ERWAY, L., HURLEY, L. S. and FRASER, A. (1970). Congenital ataxia and otolith defects due to manganese deficiency in mice. *J. Nutr.* **100**, 643.

FIELDS, M., FERRETTI, R. J., REISER, S. and SMITH, J. C., JR (1984). The severity of copper deficiency in rats is determined by the type of dietary carbohydrate. *Proc. Soc. Exp. Biol. Med.* **175**, 530.

FLINK, E. B. (1976). Magnesium deficiency and magnesium toxicity in man. In *Trace Elements in Human Health and Disease. Vol. 2. Essential and Toxic Elements* (A. S. Prasad and D. Oberleas, Eds), p. 1. Academic Press, New York.

FOOD AND NUTRITION BOARD (1980). *Recommended Dietary Allowances*, 9th edn. National Academy of Sciences, Washington, DC.

FOOD AND NUTRITION BOARD (1986). Recommended dietary allowances: Scientific issues and process for the future. *J. Nutr.* **116**, 482.

FRANZ, K. B. (1987). Magnesium intake during pregnancy. *Magnesium* **6**, 18.

FREELAND-GRAVES, J. H., BALES, C. W. and BEHMARDI, F. (1987). Manganese requirements in humans. In *Nutritional Bioavailability of Manganese* (C. Kies, Ed.), p. 90. American Chemical Society, Washington, DC.

FREELAND-GRAVES, J. H., BEHMARDI, F., BALES, C. W., DOUGHERTY, V., LIN, P.-H., CROSBY, J. B. and TRICKETT, P. S. (1988). Metabolic balance of manganese in young men consuming diets containing five levels of dietary manganese. *J. Nutr.* **118**, 764.

FRIEDMAN, B. J., FREELAND-GRAVES, J. H., BALES, C. W., BEHMARDI, F., SHOREY-KUTSCHKE, R. L., WILLIS, R. A., CROSBY, J. B., TRICKETT, P. C. and HOUSTON, S. D. (1987). Manganese balance and clinical observations in young men fed a manganese-deficient diet. *J. Nutr.* **117**, 133.

GIBSON, R. S., ANDERSON, B. M. and SABRY, J. H. (1983). The trace metal status of a group of post-menopausal vegetarians. *J. Am. Dietet. Assoc.* **82**, 246.

GORMICAN, A. (1970). Inorganic elements in foods used in hospital menus. *J. Am. Dietet. Assoc.* **56**, 397.

GRAHAM, G. G. and CORDANO, A. (1969). Copper depletion and deficiency in the malnourished infant. *Johns Hopkins Med. J.* **124**, 139.

GREGER, J. L. and SNEDEKER, S. M. (1980). Effect of dietary protein and phosphorus levels on the utilization of zinc, copper, and manganese by adult males. *J. Nutr.* **110**, 2243.

GREGER, J. L., ZAIKIS, S. C., ABERNATHY, R. P., BENNETT, O. A. and HUFFMAN, J. (1978). Zinc, nitrogen, copper, iron, and manganese balance in adolescent females fed two levels of zinc. *J. Nutr.* **108**, 1449.

HALLFRISCH, J., POWELL, A., CARAFELLI, C., REISER, S. and PRATHER, E. S. (1987). Mineral balances of men and women consuming high fiber diets with complex or simple carbohydrate. *J. Nutr.* **117**, 48.

HASSANEIN, M., GHALEB, H. A., HAROUN, E. A., HEGAZY, M. R. and KHAYYAL, M. A. H. (1966). Chronic manganism: Preliminary observations on glucose tolerance and serum proteins. *Brit. Ind. Med.* **23**, 67.

HOLDEN, J. M., WOLF, W. R. and MERTZ, W. (1979). Zinc and copper in self-selected diets. *J. Am. Dietet. Assoc.* **75**, 23.

HURLEY, L. S. (1968). Approaches to the study of nutrition in mammalian development. *Fed. Proc.* **27**, 193.

HURLEY, L. S. (1982). Clinical and experimental aspects of manganese in nutrition. In *Clinical, Biochemical, and Nutritional Aspects of Trace Elements* (A. S. Prasad, Ed.), p. 369. Alan R. Liss, New York.

HURLEY, L. S. (1984). Manganese. In *Present Knowledge in Nutrition*, 5th edn, p. 558. The Nutrition Foundation, Washington, DC.

HURLEY, L. S. and KEEN, C. L. Manganese. In *Trace Elements in Human and Animal Nutrition*, 5th edn (W. Mertz, Ed.), p. 185. Academic Press, New York.

HURLEY, L. S., WOOLEY, D. E., ROSENTHAL, F. and TIMIRAS, P. S. (1963). Influence of manganese on susceptibility of rats to convulsions. *Am. J. Physiol.* **204**, 493.

HURLEY, L. S., KEEN, C. L. and BALY, D. L. (1984). Manganese deficiency and toxicity: Effects on carbohydrate metabolism in the rat. *Neurotoxicology* **5**, 97.

JACOB, R. A., SANDSTEAD, H. H., MUNOZ, J. M., KLEVAY, L. M. and MILNE, D. B. (1981). Whole body surface loss of trace metals in normal males. *Am. J. Clin. Nutr.* **34**, 1379.

JACOB, R. A., SKALA, J. H., OMAYE, S. T. and TURNLUND, J. R. (1987), Effect of varying ascorbic acid intakes on copper absorption and ceruloplasmin levels of young men. *J. Nutr.* **117**, 2109.

JOHNSON, M. A., BAIER, M. J. and GREGER, J. L. (1982). Effects of dietary tin on zinc, copper, iron, manganese, and magnesium metabolism of adult males. *Am. J. Clin. Nutr.* **35**, 1332.

JOHNSON, P. E. (1989). Effect of various dietary carbohydrates on absorption and excretion of copper in the rat as measured by isotope dilution. *J. Trace Elem. Exp. Med.* **1**, 143.

JOHNSON, P. E. and CRANFIELD, W. K. (1989). Stable zinc and copper absorption in free-living infants fed breast milk or formula. *J. Trace Elem. Exp. Med.* **2**, 285.

JOHNSON, P. E. and LYKKEN, G. I. (1988). Copper-65 absorption by men fed intrinsically and extrinsically labeled whole wheat bread. *J. Agric. Food Chem.* **36**, 537.

JOHNSON, P. E. and LYKKEN, G. I. (1989). Manganese and calcium balance and absorption in women fed two levels of Ca and Mn. *FASEB J.* **3**, A760.

JOHNSON, P. E., STUART, M. A. and BOWMAN, T. D. (1988). Bioavailability of copper to rats from various foodstuffs and in the presence of different carbohydrates. *Proc. Soc. Exp. Biol. Med.* **187**, 44.

JOHNSON, P. E., STUART, M. A., HUNT, J. R., MULLEN, L. and STARKS, T. L. (1988). ^{65}Copper absorption by women fed intrinsically and extrinsically labeled goose meat, goose liver, peanut butter, and sunflower butter. *J. Nutr.* **118**, 1522.

KEEN, C. L., LONNERDAL, B. and HURLEY, L. S. (1985). Manganese. In *Biochemistry of the Essential Ultratrace Elements* (E. Frieden, Ed.), p. 89. Plenum, New York.

KEEN, C. L., BELL, J. G. and LONNERDAL, B. (1986). The effect of age on manganese uptake and retention from milk and infant formulas in rats. *J. Nutr.* **116**, 395.

KELSAY, J. L., JACOB, R. A. and PRATHER, E. S. (1979). Effect of fiber from fruits and vegetables on metabolic responses of human subjects. III. Zinc, copper, and phosphorus balances. *Am. J. Clin. Nutr.* **32**, 2307.

KELSAY, J. L., FRAZIER, C. W., PRATHER, E. S., CANARY, J. J., CLARK, W. M. and POWELL, B. S. (1988). Impact of variation in carbohydrate intake on mineral utilization by vegetarians. *Am. J. Clin. Nutr.* **48**, 875.

KIES, C., ALDRICH, K. D., JOHNSON, J. M., CREPS, C., KOWALSKI, C. and WANG, R. H. (1987). Manganese availability for humans. Effect of selected dietary factors. In *Nutritional Bioavailability of Manganese.* (C. Kies, Ed.), p. 136. American Chemical Society, Washington, DC.

KLEVAY, L. M. (1975). Coronary heart disease: The zinc/copper hypothesis. *Am. J. Clin. Nutr.* **28**, 764.

KLEVAY, L. M. (1983). Copper and ischemic heart disease. *Biol. Trace Elem. Res.* **5**, 245.

KLEVAY, L. M., RECK, S. J. and BARCOME, D. F. (1979). Evidence of dietary copper and zinc deficiencies. *J. Am. Med. Assoc.* **241**, 1916.

Klevay, L. M., Reck, S. J., Jacob, R. A., Logan, G. M., Jr, Munoz, J. M. and Sandstead, H. H. (1980). The human requirement for copper. I. Healthy men fed conventional American diets. *Am. J. Clin. Nutr.* **33**, 45.

Klevay, L. M., Inman, L., Johnson, L. K., Lawler, M., Mahalko, J. R., Milne, D. B., Lukaski, H. C., Bolonchuk, W. and Sandstead, H. H. (1984). Increased cholesterol in plasma in a young man during experimental copper depletion. *Metabolism* **33**, 1112.

Klevay, L. M., Canfield, W. K., Gallagher, S. K., Henriksen, L. K., Lukaski, H. C., Bolonchuk, W., Johnson, L. K., Milne, D. B. and Sandstead, H. H. (1986). Decreased glucose tolerance in two men during experimental copper depletion. *Nutr. Rept Intl* **33**, 371.

Kobayashi, J. A. (1957). Geographical relationship between the chemical nature of river water and death rate from apoplexy. *Bev. Ohara Inst. Lansw. Biol.* **11**, 12.

Lee, D.-Y. and Johnson, P. E. (1989). ^{54}Mn absorption and excretion in rats fed soy protein and casein diets. *Proc. Soc. Exp. Biol. Med.* **190**, 211.

Levy, Y., Zeharia, A., Grunebaum, M., Nitzan, M. and Steinherz, R. (1985). Copper deficiency in infants fed cow milk. *J. Pediatr.* **106**, 786.

Lukaski, H. C., Klevay, L. M. and Milne, D. B. (1988). Effects of dietary copper on human autonomic cardiovascular function. *Eur. J. Appl. Physiol.* **58**, 74.

MacDonald, L. D., Gibson, R. S. and Miles, J. E. (1982). Changes in hair zinc and copper concentrations of breast fed and bottle fed infants during the first six months. *Acta Paediatr. Scand.* **71**, 785.

Mahalko, J. R., Sandstead, H. H., Johnson, L. K. and Milne, D. B. (1983). Effect of a moderate increase in dietary protein on the retention and excretion of Ca, Cu, Fe, Mg, P, and Zn by adult males. *Am. J. Clin. Nutr.* **37**, 8.

Mahoney, J. P. and Small, W. J. (1968). Studies on manganese III. The biological half-life of radiomanganese in man and factors which affect this half-life. *J. Clin. Invest.* **47**, 643.

Marier, J. R. (1986). Magnesium content of the food supply in the modern-day world. *Magnesium* **5**, 1.

Marshall, D. H., Nordin, B. E. C. and Speed, R. (1976). Calcium, phosphorus and magnesium requirement. *Proc. Nutr. Soc.* **35**, 163.

Mason, K. E. (1979). A conspectus of research on copper metabolism and requirements of man. *J. Nutr.* **109,** 1979.

Moore, T., Constable, B. J., Day, K. C., Impey, S. G. and Symonds, K. R. (1964). Copper deficiency in rats fed upon raw meat. *Brit. J. Nutr.* **18**, 135.

Naveh, Y., Hazani, A. and Berant, M. (1981). Copper deficiency with cow's milk diet. *Pediatrics* **68**, 397.

Neri, L. C., Johansen, H. L., Hewitt, D., Marier, J. and Langner, N. (1985). Magnesium and certain other elements and cardiovascular disease. *Sci. Total Environ.* **42**, 49.

Papavasiliou, P. S., Kutt, H., Miller, S. T., Rosal, V., Wang, Y. Y. and Aronson, R. B. (1979). Seizure disorders and trace metals: Manganese tissue levels in treated epileptics. *Neurology* **29**, 1466.

Patterson, K. Y., Holbrook, J. T., Bodner, J. E., Kelsay, J. L., Smith, J. C., Jr and Veillon, C. (1984). Zinc, copper, and manganese intake and balance for adults consuming self-selected diets. *Am. J. Clin. Nutr.* **40**, 1397.

PENNINGTON, J. T. and CALLOWAY, D. H. (1973). Copper content of food. *J. Am. Dietet. Assoc.* **63**, 143.
PRICE, N. O. and BUNCE, G. E. (1972). Effect of nitrogen and calcium on balance of copper, manganese, and zinc in preadolescent girls. *Nutr. Rept Intl* **5**, 275.
PRICE, N. O., BUNCE, G. E. and ENGEL, R. W. (1970). Copper, manganese, and zinc balance in preadolescent girls. *Am. J. Clin. Nutr.* **23**, 258.
RAGHIB, M. H., CHAN, W. Y. and RENNERT, O. M. (1986). Comparative biological availability of manganese from extrinsically labelled milk diets using sucking rats as a model. *Brit. J. Nutr.* **55**, 49.
RAO, C. N. and RAO, B. S. N. (1980). Absorption and retention of magnesium and some trace elements by man from typical Indian diets. *Nutr. Metab.* **24**, 244.
RAO, C. N. and RAO, B. S. N. (1982). Copper, manganese, and cobalt balance in adult men and estimation of a daily requirement of copper and manganese. *Nutr. Rept Intl* **26**, 1113.
RAYSSIGUIER, Y. (1986). Magnesium, lipids and vascular diseases. Experimental evidence in animal models. *Magnesium* **5**, 182.
RESNICK, L. M., LARAGH, J. H., SEALEY, J. E. and ALDERMAN, M. H. (1983). Divalent cations in essential hypertension. Relations between serum ionized calcium, magnesium and plasma renin activity. *New Engl. J. Med.* **309**, 888.
RESNICK, L. M., GUPTA, R. K. and LARAGH, J. H. (1984). Intracellular free magnesium in erythrocytes of essential hypertension: Relation to blood pressure and serum divalent cations. *Proc. Nat. Acad. Sci. USA* **81**, 6511.
REISER, S., SMITH, J. C., JR, MERTZ, W., HOLBROOK, J. T., SCHOLFIELD, D. J., POWELL, A. S., CANFIELD, W. K. and CANARY, J. T. (1985). Indices of copper status in humans consuming a typical American diet containing either fructose or starch. *Am J. Clin. Nutr.* **42**, 242.
RUBENSTEIN, A. H., LEVIN, N. W. and ELLIOT, G. A. (1962). Manganese-induced hypoglycemia. *Lancet* **ii**, 1348.
SALIM, S., FAHRQUARSON, J., ARNEIL, G. C., COCKBURN, F., FORBES, G. I., LOGAN, R. W., SHERLOCK, J. C. and WILSON, T. S. (1986). Dietary copper intake in artificially fed infants. *Arch. Dis. Child.* **61**, 1068.
SANDSTEAD, H. H. (1982). Cu bioavailability and requirements. *Am. J. Clin. Nutr.* **35**, 809.
SCHWARTZ, R., APGAR, B. J. and WIEN, E. M. (1986). Apparent absorption and retention of Ca, Cu, Mg, Mn and Zn from a diet containing bran. *Am. J. Clin. Nutr.* **43**, 444.
SEELIG, M. S. (1981). Magnesium requirements in human nutrition. *Magnesium Bull.* **3** (Suppl. 1a), 26.
SEELIG, M. S. and HEGGTVEIT, H. A. (1974). Magnesium interrelationships in ischemic heart disease: A review. *Am. J. Clin. Nutr.* **27**, 59.
SHILS, M. E. (1969). Experimental human magnesium depletion. *Medicine* **48**, 61.
SHILS, M. E. (1976). Magnesium deficiency and calcium and parathyroid hormone interrelations. In *Trace Elements in Human Health and Disease Vol. 2. Essential and Toxic Elements* (A. S. Prasad and D. Oberleas, Eds), p. 23. Academic Press, New York.
SHILS, M. E. (1988). Magnesium. In *Modern Nutrition in Health and Disease* (M. E. Shils and V. R. Young, Eds), p. 159. Lea & Febiger, Philadelphia, PA.

SOLOMONS, N. W. (1985). Biochemical, metabolic, and clinical role of copper in human nutrition. *J. Am. Coll. Nutr.* **4**, 83.

SPENCER, H., ASMUSSEN, C. R., HOLTZMAN, R. B. and KRAMER, L. (1979). Metabolic balances of cadmium, copper, manganese and zinc in man. *Am. J. Clin. Nutr.* **32**, 1867.

SPENCER, H., LESNIAK, M., KRAMER, L., COFFEY, J. and OSIS, D. (1980). Studies of magnesium metabolism in man. In *Magnesium in Health and Disease* (M. S. Seelig, Ed.), p. 911. Spectrum, New York.

SRIVASTAVA, U. S., NADEAU, M. H. and GUENEAU, L. (1978). Mineral intakes of university students: Magnesium content. *Nutr. Rept Intl* **18**, 235.

SUTTON, A. M., HARVIE, A., COCKBURN, F., FAHRQUARSON, J. and LOGAN, R. W. (1985). Copper deficiency in the preterm infant of very low birthweight. Four cases and a reference range for plasma copper. *Arch. Dis. Child.* **60**, 644.

TAPER, L. J., HINNERS, M. L. and RITCHEY, S. J. (1980). Effects of zinc intake on copper balance in adult females. *Am. J. Clin. Nutr.* **33**, 1077.

THOMSON, A. B. R., OLATUNBOSUM, D. and VALBERG, L. S. (1971). Interrelation of intestinal transport system for manganese and iron. *J. Lab. Clin. Med.* **78**, 642.

TURNLUND, J., COSTA, F. and MARGEN, S. (1981). Zinc, copper, and iron balance in elderly men. *Am. J. Clin. Nutr.* **34**, 2641.

TURNLUND, J. R., SWANSON, C. A. and KING, J. C. (1983). Copper absorption and retention in pregnant women fed diets based on animal and plant proteins. *J. Nutr.* **113**, 2346.

TURNLUND, J. R., KING, J. C., GONG, B., KEYES, W. R. and MICHEL, M. C. (1985). A stable isotope study of copper absorption in young men: Effect of phytate and α-cellulose. *Am. J. Clin. Nutr.* **42**, 18.

TURNLUND, J. R., WADA, L., KING, J. C., KEYES, W. R. and ACORD, L. L. (1988). Copper absorption in young men fed adequate and low zinc diets. *Biol. Trace Elem. Res.* **17**, 31.

USDA (1976–87). *Handbooks 8.1-16: Composition of Foods.* US Dept of Agriculture, Hyattsville, MD.

USDA (1977–78). *Nationwide Food Consumption Survey of Individuals.* US Dept of Agriculture, Hyattsville, MD.

US DEPARTMENT OF HEALTH AND HUMAN SERVICES (1986). US Department of Agriculture. *Nutrition Monitoring in the US*, DHHS Publ. #86-1255. Public Health Service, US Government Printing Office, Washington, DC.

UTTER, M. F. (1976). The biochemistry of manganese. *Med. Clin. N. Am.* **60**, 713.

WACKER, W. E. C. (1980). *Magnesium and Man.* Harvard University Press, Cambridge, MA.

WACKER, W. E. C., AIKAWA, J. K., DAVIS, G. K., HORRATH, D. J. and LINDSAY, W. L. (1977). Magnesium. In *Geochemistry and the Environment. Vol. 2. The Relation of Other Selected Trace Elements to Health and Disease*, p. 11. National Academy of Sciences, Washington, DC.

WALLACH, S. and VERCH, R. L. (1986). Tissue magnesium in spontaneously hypertensive rats. *Magnesium* **5**, 33.

WENLOCK, R. W., BUSS, D. H. and DIXON, E. J. (1979). Trace nutrients. 2. Manganese in British food. *Brit. J. Nutr.* **41**, 253.

WHITE, H. S. (1969). Inorganic elements in weighed diets of girls and young women. *J. Am. Dietet. Assoc.* **55**, 558.

WOLF, J. P., LUTHRINGER, C., BERTHELOT, A. and BERTHELAY, S. (1987). Blood pressure and plasma renin activity after magnesium supplementation in the spontaneously hypertensive rat: A study during developing and established hypertension. *Magnesium* **6**, 243.

11

Calcium, Phosphorus, Sodium and Potassium

NJERI KARANJA, TALASH A. LIKIMANI*
and DAVID A. MCCARRON
*Oregon Health Sciences University,
Division of Nephrology and Hypertension,
Portland, Oregon, USA*

I. INTRODUCTION

The amount of energy in the American diet derived from meat, poultry, and fish has risen steadily since the Second World War. With the exception of phosphorus (PO_4^-) and possibly potassium (K^+), the content of sodium (Na^+) and calcium (Ca^{2+}) in meat is low relative to other food sources. Nevertheless, research gathered over time has indicated that meat consumption is associated with significant alterations in metabolism of Ca^{2+}, PO_4^-, Na^+, and K^+.

This chapter will examine briefly the normal metabolism of Ca^{2+}, PO_4^-, Na^+, and K^+ and, where data are available, how meat consumption affects the manner in which these minerals are metabolized. We will then provide an overview of modern-day chronic illnesses whose etiology and/or progression has been linked to alterations in the metabolism of Ca^{2+}, PO_4^-, Na^+, and K^+. These include chronic renal failure, nephrolithiasis, hypertension, cancers of the gastrointestinal tract, and osteoporosis.

II. NORMAL METABOLISM AND REGULATION OF Ca^{2+}, PO_4^-, Na^+ AND K^+

A number of excellent and comprehensive reviews of the normal metabolism of each of the minerals covered in this chapter are available in the literature

* Present address: University of Nairobi, Department of Food Science and Nutrition, Faculty of Agriculture and Veterinary Science, Kabete, Kenya.

for the interested reader (Lee *et al.*, 1981; Allen, 1982; Bronner and Coburn, 1982; Papper, 1983; Whang, 1983).

A. Calcium

Calcium is one of the most important nutrients in the human diet. In addition to conferring structural integrity to mineralized tissue, it plays a diverse role in maintaining cellular function. Its most important roles include a second messenger in smooth and skeletal muscle contraction, mobilization of fuels, secretory function, and acting as a co-factor in a number of enzymatic reactions (Bronner and Coburn, 1982).

Dairy products supply approximately 75% of all dietary calcium of western cultures. The rest comes from green leafy vegetables and certain varieties of nuts. Consequently, meat is a relatively minor source of calcium except in cases where bone might be consumed along with the meat. The normal intake of calcium ranges from 400–1000 mg per day in the United States. Unlike minerals such as sodium and potassium, only 25–30% of the calcium ingested in the diet is absorbed. Intestinal absorption decreases with age and is generally enhanced or depressed by other dietary components. Accordingly, components such as oxalic and phytic acids, long-chain unsaturated fatty acids, and diphosphates decrease calcium absorption. In contrast, simple carbohydrates, especially lactose, and protein appear to enhance its absorption (Allen, 1982; Bronner and Coburn, 1982).

Extracellular calcium is maintained within very narrow limits. In humans, plasma concentrations are about 2·5 mmol/liter. Some 45% of this calcium exists in the ionized form, 40% is reversibly bound to plasma proteins, and 15% is complexed to anions such as citrate and phosphate (Bronner and Coburn, 1982).

Overall, calcium balance is hormonally regulated at three major sites: intestine, kidney, and bone. The most important hormones in the maintenance of calcium homeostasis are parathyroid hormone (PTH), vitamin D and calcitonin. Although the detailed mechanisms of how overall homeostasis is maintained are not yet known, a composite model has been formulated on the basis of experimental data. The model stipulates that a fall ($<2{\cdot}5$ mmol/liter) in serum ionized calcium levels results in the release of PTH. PTH functions either directly or indirectly at the three major control sites to restore serum calcium levels (Bronner and Coburn, 1982).

In the kidney, PTH directly enhances the fractional reabsorption of calcium from the glomerular filtrate. Similarly, PTH directly stimulates calcium mobilization from bone, largely through promoting the formation of lysosomal enzymes that enhance bone resorption. Stimulation of intestinal calcium absorption by PTH is indirect, being mediated by $1\alpha,25(OH)_2$ vitamin D. In the kidney, a satellite action of PTH is to increase the activity of the 1-α-hydroxylase enzyme, which hydroxylates the 25-OH vitamin D at the number one position. In turn $1\alpha,25(OH)_2$ vitamin D promotes the absorption of calcium from the gut (Allen, 1982; Bronner and Coburn, 1982).

Reduction of serum calcium is the most important action of calcitonin. When serum calcium levels exceed physiologic levels, calcitonin is secreted from the thyroid gland to lower calcium to appropriate levels. Unlike PTH, which acts at multiple sites to restore calcium homeostatis, it appears that calcitonin functions predominantly on bone where it lowers production of lysosomal enzymes and the rates of mineral release as well as producing alterations in collagen metabolism (Bronner and Coburn, 1982).

B. Phosphorus

Like calcium, phosphorus plays an important role in virtually all aspects of life. It is a major constituent of bone, and thus confers structural integrity to mineralized tissue. Additionally, phosphorus provides linkage between nucleotides that consist of ribose and deoxyribose nucleic acids. In this respect, then, it contributes to the structure of chromosomes and the process of growth and heredity. Phosphorus is a constituent of a large number of enzymes and metabolic intermediates involved in important functions, such as metabolism of carbohydrates, as well as many oxidation–reduction reactions (Lee *et al.*, 1981).

Phosphorus is widely distributed with higher amounts being found in high protein foods, including meat, and somewhat lower concentrations being found in fruits and some vegetables. Soft drinks also supply substantial amounts of phosphorus in societies where they are consumed in large quantities. The recommended dietary allowance for phosphorus is 800 mg per day. This recommendation is based on the need to supply a diet that contains a calcium:phosphorus ratio of 1. In western cultures it is estimated that phosphorus consumption greatly exceeds that of calcium such that the ratio may be as low as 0·3 (Lee *et al.*, 1981).

The dynamics of intestinal phosphorus absorption differ substantially from those of calcium. Net phosphorus absorption is 60–65% of dietary intake, an amount that is double that of calcium. Additionally, fractional intestinal absorption of phosphorus is a linear function of dietary intake. Thus, when phosphorus intake is high, more is absorbed and excreted in the feces and vice versa. The absorption of calcium, on the other hand, is curvilinear in nature and its fecal excretion tends to increase with lower dietary intakes. Intestinal absorption of phosphorus is enhanced by $1\alpha,25(OH)_2$ vitamin D, calcium, sodium, potassium, and calcitonin. PTH does not appear to have any direct effects on the intestinal absorption of phosphorus except as it may be influenced by PTH's effect on the renal synthesis of $1\alpha,25(OH)_2$ vitamin D (Lee *et al.*, 1981).

Phosphorus homeostasis is controlled much in the same manner as calcium by the kidney, bone, and gut. Accordingly, when plasma levels fall, PTH-mediated increases in $1\alpha,25(OH)_2$ vitamin D cause enhanced intestinal absorption of phosphorus along with PTH-induced bone resorption and enhanced renal reabsorption. When plasma concentrations rise above desirable levels, removal occurs through reduced intestinal transport, increased fecal excretion, bone accretion, and glomerular filtration combined with low renal reabsorption (Lee *et al.*, 1981).

C. Sodium

Sodium is the major extracellular cation in mammals. Its major function is the control of plasma osmolality along with the maintenance of water balance and osmotic pressure in the extracellular fluid compartment.

The normal human diet provides sufficient sodium to meet basic requirements for this cation, since it is widely distributed in foods. Normal intake in western societies ranges between 5–15 g (80–260 mmol) sodium chloride per day. This amount far exceeds the 1–2 mmol per day required to sustain life. Sodium is almost completely absorbed in the gastrointestinal tract with negligible amounts being excreted in feces (Papper, 1983; Vander, 1985).

Serum sodium levels are maintained at a constant level of 136–145 meq/liter, primarily as a result of renal reabsorption and excretion. Serum sodium levels may fall due to factors such as reduced sodium intake, excessive perspiration, or pathologic situations. A fall in serum sodium triggers a chain of events all designed to restore sodium homeostasis. Initial events include a fall in plasma volume and plasma oncotic pressure, which in turn prevent adequate venous return and subsequent fall in arterial pressure. A major consequence of decreased arterial pressure is generalized vasoconstriction and reduced resistance to blood flow from the renal artery to the glomerulus, thus lowering capillary blood pressure and the glomerular filtration rate (GFR). Because sodium excretion is a direct function of glomerular filtration rate and sodium reabsorption, a fall in the filtration rate results in a fall in sodium filtered and that which is excreted.

Conversely, when volume expansion occurs due to excess sodium consumption or disease states, GFR is increased to promote renal sodium loss and restore plasma volume (Vander, 1985).

About 60–70% of the filtered sodium load is reabsorbed in the proximal tubule. Another 20–30% is absorbed in the Loop of Henle and the remainder in the distal tubules. It is this latter amount of sodium that is controlled by the renin–angiotensin–aldosterone hormonal axis. Briefly, the axis is triggered by a fall in arterial pressure as a consequence of reduced serum sodium. When this happens, renin is secreted from the juxtaglomerular apparatus of the kidney. Renin in turn converts angiotensin I into angiotensin II which along with decreased plasma sodium concentrations directly stimulate aldosterone production from the adrenal gland. Aldosterone conserves sodium by promoting its reabsorption in the distal tubules and collecting duct. Angiotensin II itself has direct renal effects since it constricts blood vessels which leads to a fall in GFR and a subsequent fall in the amount of sodium filtered (Tannenbaum, 1976; Papper, 1983).

Other humoral agents that regulate sodium balance include cortisol, estrogen, growth hormone, insulin and catecholamines, all of which promote sodium reabsorption; whereas glucagon, progesterone and PTH decrease sodium reabsorption (Tannenbaum, 1976; Vander, 1985).

D. Potassium

Potassium is the major cation of the intracellular space. In this respect, then, its distribution is opposite to that of sodium as described earlier. The steep gradient that maintains low extracellular potassium in the face of relatively high intracellular potassium (as well as high extracellular sodium in the face of low intracellular sodium concentrations) is accomplished through the action of the ATP-dependent sodium/potassium pump (Na^+/K^+-ATPase). The pump is fueled by oxidative energy and continually transports potassium into the cell and sodium out of the cell against their respective concentration gradients. The pump is therefore critical in adjusting the ionic balance necessary for potassium to participate in a variety of cellular processes. The most important of these include transmission of nerve impulses and contractility of cardiac, skeletal and smooth muscle (Whang, 1983; Vander, 1985).

The major sources of potassium are fresh vegetables, fruits and fruit juices, milk, poultry, shellfish, other meats and grains in that order. The average intake in a normal diet varies between 40–90 meq/day (Whang, 1983).

The amount of extracellular potassium is governed by total body potassium, which is approximately 4200 meq, and its distribution between the intra- and extracellular space that is regulated by the Na^+/K^+ pump mentioned earlier. Total body potassium is a function of intake and excretion. Of the amount ingested, only minute quantities are excreted in the feces and sweat, indicating that, like sodium, potassium is almost completely absorbed in the gastrointestinal tract. Accordingly, the kidney is the major organ regulating potassium homeostasis, even though extrarenal factors play a minor role (Whang, 1983; Vander, 1985).

Plasma potassium is completely filtered at the glomerulus. Of this load, 50% is reabsorbed in the proximal tubule and 40% in the Loop of Henle. Hence, with a low potassium intake, the proximal tubule and the Loop of Henle reabsorb 90% of the net potassium filtered in the glomerulus. The remaining 10% is reabsorbed in the distal nephron. In the case of excess potassium consumption, the proximal tubule and the loop still reabsorb 90% of the filtered potassium load; however, the distal nephron secretes potassium back into the lumen rather than reabsorbing it. Clearly, then, it is in the distal parts of the nephron where renal potassium balance is controlled (Vander, 1985).

Potassium reabsorption, especially in the distal segments, is controlled by a variety of factors. One of the most important of these factors is aldosterone. Unlike its role in sodium homeostasis, aldosterone promotes potassium excretion rather than conserving it. An increase in plasma potassium above 4·5 meq/liter directly stimulates the production of aldosterone by the adrenal cortex. Aldosterone then stimulates the Na^+/K^+-ATPase located on the basolateral membrane of the cells of the distal nephron, causing these cells to accumulate potassium. As the intracellular potassium level rises, it creates a gradient that causes potassium to be re-excreted into the lumen (Vander, 1985).

Other factors that control potassium homeostasis are acid–base balance, sodium metabolism, and certain humoral factors. As a rule, alkalosis, whether respiratory or metabolic, causes potassium loss while acidosis tends to promote potassium retention. Similarly, alteration in renal sodium handling alters potassium homeostasis. Thus, under conditions of increased sodium excretion, there is a concomitant increase in potassium excretion. This loss is caused by an increase in fluid delivery to the lumen which lowers potassium concentration in the lumen, thereby collapsing the gradient necessary for potassium to enter the cell for subsequent reabsorption (Whang, 1983; Vander, 1985).

Humoral regulators of potassium homeostasis include insulin, which lowers serum potassium primarily through promoting its uptake in muscle, glucocorticoids, which generally increase renal potassium clearance, and catecholamines, which appear to have a biphasic influence on plasma potassium, i.e. an initial α-adrenoceptor mediated rise in plasma followed by a rapid β-adrenoceptor-mediated decline reflecting cellular uptake (Whang, 1983).

III. EFFECTS OF MEAT CONSUMPTION ON RENAL FUNCTION AND THE METABOLISM OF Ca^{2+}, PO_4^-, Na^+ AND K^+

With the exception of phosphorus and possibly potassium, meats as a group do not contain sufficient quantities of the minerals covered in this chapter to impact significantly on dietary intake of these minerals. Additionally, routine meat processing, cooking, or storage do not produce significant alterations in the mineral content of meat (Hultin, 1976). In some instances, however, the amount of sodium in meat can be altered during processes such as curing. Sodium nitrite normally added to maintain color during the curing process is itself too low to appreciably contribute to sodium intake. However, the curing process also involves addition of sodium chloride. Thus, persons consuming significant amounts of cured meats may have somewhat higher intakes of sodium. Similarly, mechanical deboning of meat, a process designed to recover edible meat from bone, can raise the calcium content of meat (Tso *et al.*, 1984). In general, mechanically deboned meat contains 0·50–0·75% calcium, while hand-deboned meat contains 0·008–0·0013% calcium (Kolbye and Nelson, 1977). While the actual content of Ca^{2+}, Na^+, and K^+ in meat does not influence their overall intake, meat consumption has a profound effect on the metabolism and overall body balance of these minerals. Over 60 years ago, Ambard (1920) noted that the consumption of protein, especially meat protein, aggravated the clinical manifestation of uremia. Subsequent studies in animals and humans have demonstrated that protein restriction retards the progression of some forms of renal disease (Brenner *et al.*, 1982; Klahr, 1989). Yet protein itself is not considered to be the primary initiator of renal disease. Rather, protein is thought to act synergistically with initiating factors to accelerate renal failure and/or to sustain its progression even after the initiating factors are removed.

Protein consumption is thought to worsen renal disease through its effect on renal hemodynamics, i.e. renal blood flow (RBF), glomerular filtration rate (GFR), and renal vascular resistance (RVR). In normal rats, consumption of a diet containing 20% casein yielded a GFR of 0·62 ml/min and kidney weight of 500 mg, while consumption of an 8% casein diet resulted in a GFR of 0·3 ml/min and kidney weight of 293 mg (Pennell *et al.*, 1975). Similar findings have been reported in dogs (Mitch, 1984) and sheep (Rabinowitz *et al.*, 1973). Thus, it appears that an increase in kidney mass is one of the factors responsible for the increased GFR.

In humans Ambard (1920) reported that patients receiving amino acids intravenously during hyperalimentation developed enlarged kidneys accompanied by significant alterations in renal hemodynamics. At the opposite end of the spectrum, adults and children with protein-calorie malnutrition experience a reduction in GFR and RBF that is restored upon protein repletion (Brenner *et al.*, 1982). In normal volunteers, the effect of three levels of protein on GFR and RBF was examined by Pullman *et al.* (1954). A progressive fall in both GFR and RBF was observed as protein intake was reduced from a range of 2·3–3·0 g protein/kg body weight/day to 0·1–0·4. Thus, in humans a meat-based meal appears to lower RVR, raise GFR and RBF, and enhance sodium excretion (Brenner *et al.*, 1982; Klahr, 1989).

The mechanisms through which protein consumption alters renal hemodynamics are poorly understood. Nevertheless, data collected over a number of years demonstrate that high protein consumption profoundly affects overall balance of calcium and perhaps sodium and phosphorus (Klahr and Alleyne, 1973). At any given level of calcium intake, increases in dietary protein enhance urinary calcium excretion. Accordingly, at a constant level of Ca^{2+} and PO_4^- intake, a twofold increase in protein causes a 50% increase in urinary Ca^{2+} (Zemel, 1988). At low levels of Ca^{2+} consumption (500 mg/day) protein-induced calciuria is not associated with a compensatory rise in intestinal absorption. A modest increase in dietary calcium tends to counteract the calciuretic effect of protein. However, Linkswiler *et al.* (1981) and Hegsted *et al.* (1981) have demonstrated that at protein intakes of 142 g/day, human subjects remain in negative calcium balance, even when dietary calcium intake is 1400 mg/day.

Although the majority of studies have shown a calciuretic effect of protein, not all studies support the view that increased dietary protein results in long-term negative Ca^{2+} balance. Spencer *et al.* (1988) have argued that the increased Ca^{2+} excretion seen with protein loading is transient in nature and tends to disappear over time. In these studies, a high protein diet in the form of meat did not alter overall calcium balance in the short-term (18–30 days) or long-term (78–132 days). There are several potential reasons for the discrepancy. First, meat contributes substantially to overall phosphorus intake. Phosphorus tends to reduce urinary calcium loss and may offset protein-induced hypercalciuria. Accordingly, in cases where a modest intake of PO_4^- occurs along with protein, CA^{2+} balance may remain unaltered as reported by Spencer *et al.* (1983) while Ca^{2+} loss may be significant when PO_4^- consumption remains low in the face of higher protein intakes as reported by Linkswiler *et al.* (1981). Ironically phosphorus supplied as phosphoric acid, as it is found in soft drinks, tends to promote calciuria and may aggravate protein-induced calciuria.

A second factor that may explain the discrepancy in the studies of protein's effect on Ca^{2+} balance is the constancy (or the lack thereof) of dietary sodium intake. As mentioned earlier, protein feeding results not only in hemodynamic changes but is also associated with a significant loss of sodium in urine. Additionally, when dietary sodium intake is high, renal reabsorption decreases accordingly to maintain its homeostasis. Since both sodium and Ca^{2+} are co-transported in certain segments of the nephron, a high protein intake by virtue of its ability to promote sodium excretion may also promote calcium excretion. If a high protein diet is also high in sodium, then calciuria may be significant enough to perturb overall calcium balance.

Taken collectively, these data indicate that protein consumption, especially meat-derived protein, is associated with significant changes in renal function. Under conditions of high sodium intake and/or high soft drink consumption, significant urinary calcium loss may occur to the extent that overall Ca^{2+} balance is perturbed. Even though protein consumption is associated with enhanced natriuresis, there are no experimental data that indicates this in itself is detrimental to overall sodium balance in healthy humans. Nevertheless, increased sodium excretion is associated not only with enhanced Ca^{2+} loss, but also with enhanced K^+ loss. To date, however, there is no evidence indicating that meat consumption affects potassium balance in any significant way.

IV. MEAT CONSUMPTION IN RELATION TO Ca^{2+}, PO_4^-, Na^+ AND K^+ METABOLISM AND HEALTH

The progression and/or the prognosis of several modern-day diseases has been linked to alterations in the metabolism of Ca^{2+}, PO_4^-, Na^+, and K^+. Inasmuch as protein intake can alter the metabolism of these minerals, an indirect link can be made between meat protein consumption and the development of these chronic diseases. For disorders such as chronic renal failure, nephrolithiasis and, to a certain extent, hypertension, the link is more direct. The association between protein intake and gastrointestinal cancer and osteoporosis, on the other hand, is less direct.

A. Chronic Renal Failure

Progressive renal failure is a significant public health problem in the US. Improvement in morbidity and mortality from end stage renal disease (ESRD) has occurred as a consequence of advances in renal transplantation and dialysis. It is estimated, however, that by 1990 the cost for these procedures in the US will be as high as \$3·5 billion, excluding lost productivity due to illness related to progressive renal failure (Zeller, 1987). These economic considerations have prompted health care workers to seek ways of delaying ESRD by reducing the rate at which renal failure progresses. Accordingly, there is a renewed interest in the role that animal protein, and specifically meat, plays in the progression of renal disease.

As reviewed earlier, evidence demonstrating that high protein intakes alter renal hemodynamics in laboratory animals is compelling, even though it is not yet clear how these changes contribute to progressive loss of renal function in humans. The most comprehensive model of how alterations in GFR, RBF, and RVR might contribute to progressive loss of renal function has been put forth by Brenner *et al.* (1982). In this model, an initial insult to the kidney may occur due to repeated infections, uncontrolled systemic hypertension, loss of cellular immunity, or a number of other causes (Klahr, 1989). The kidney responds to the loss of functional units caused by the initial injury with compensatory mechanisms that include a decrease in RVR which promotes arteriolar vasodilation, increased single nephron RBF and, by extension, GFR.

The major consequence of these hemodynamic changes is increased glomerular hydrostatic pressure, which ultimately precipitates glomerulosclerosis due to the destruction of the permselective properties of the nephron. As the injured nephrons lose their ability to function, healthy nephrons undergo adaptive hemodynamic changes, and the cycle for progressive loss of renal function is established (Brenner *et al.*, 1982). Viewed in the context of the evidence that protein consumption alters renal hemodynamics, one can see how a high protein intake might accelerate renal failure without initiating the process *per se*. The so-called Brenner model is well supported by studies in experimental models of uremia. Not only does protein restriction modify renal hemodynamics, it also changes the outcome of experimental renal disease (Brenner *et al.*, 1982; Zeller,

1987; Klahr, 1989). Although preliminary data have been reported in humans, the benefits of protein restriction remain to be verified with more prospective, randomized controlled studies (Zeller, 1987).

Deposition of calcium–phosphorus complexes at the site of renal injury is thought to accelerate glomerulosclerosis (Klahr, 1989). Since meat protein contains significant amounts of phosphorus, it has been proposed that the concomitant decrease in phosphorus that occurs with protein restriction accounts for a reduction in renal injury. A test of this hypothesis by Ibels *et al.* (1978) indicated that phosphorus restriction markedly reduces the amount of calcium deposited in the kidney, in addition to reducing other markers of progressive renal failure. In a study where both protein and PO_4^- were modified together, a protective synergism between reduced protein and phosphorus intake was reported with regard to survival and renal function in subtotally nephrectomized rats (Kikuchi *et al.*, 1983). Likewise, an additive improvement in creatinine clearance has been reported to occur in patients whose diets were modified to contain low protein and phosphorus intakes (Barsotti *et al.*, 1984). As with protein intake, however, a definitive role for phosphorus intake in the progression of renal disease needs to be explored more rigorously in prospective randomized trials in humans.

B. Nephrolithiasis

The prevalence of upper urinary tract stones usually consisting of calcium oxalate or phosphate (nephrolithiasis) is higher in affluent societies where consumption of animal protein is higher. Conversely, in societies where animal protein is low, there is a lower prevalence of nephrolithiasis (Andersen, 1969; Robertson *et al.*, 1979a). These observations suggest that the risk of stones in a given population is related to the consumption of animal protein. Several studies have demonstrated a positive association between protein consumption and urinary components that promote nephrolithiasis. These include urinary pH, calcium, oxalate, acidic mucopolysaccharides, and uric acid (Robertson *et al.*, 1979a). Robertson *et al.* (1979b) conducted a study in which animal protein consumption was varied from 1 to 92 g/day, and calcium and phosphorus were kept constant. There were significant increases in calcium, oxalate, and uric acid as the content of animal protein was raised. In the same study patients that were recurrent stone formers reported a higher animal protein intake than either single stone formers or normal subjects. In another study, Brockis *et al.* (1982) compared 30 meat-consuming subjects of the Mormon religion to an age- and sex-matched group of vegetarian Seventh Day Adventists. These workers found an increased excretion of calcium and uric acid but not oxalate in the Mormon group relative to the Seventh Day Adventists.

Despite these findings, it appears that a susceptibility to stone formation has to exist for animal protein to promote nephrolithiasis. Consequently, protein *per se* is not generally considered to be an etiologic factor in the development of nephrolithiasis. This view derives support from a recent report by Breslau *et al.* (1988) who examined the effect of different types of protein on calcium metabolism and propensity for renal stone formation in 15 young non-stone formers. The subjects received either a vegetarian diet, an ovo-vegetarian diet, or an omnivorous diet containing beef, fish, and chicken for 12 days. The diets were comparable with respect to Ca^{2+}, PO_4^-, Na^+, K^+ and magnesium, as well as in the amount of total protein and other energy yielding nutrients. Urinary calcium excretion increased significantly from $2{\cdot}6 \pm 0{\cdot}4$ to $3{\cdot}7 \pm 0{\cdot}3$ mmol/day when subjects were switched from the vegetarian diet to the omnivore diet. Similarly, the urinary uric acid content was higher on the animal protein diet than on the vegetarian diet. Oxalate excretion, however, was higher in the latter group than in the former. Despite the enhanced excretion of these stone forming constituents, crystallization studies revealed no propensity towards the formation of calcium oxalate or calcium phosphate stones. Similarly, uric acid excretion, though increased on the meat protein diet, did not result in formation or the propensity toward the formation of uric acid stones. The authors concluded that factors other than meat protein are responsible for the increased incidence of calcium stones (Breslau *et al.*, 1988).

Most of the studies reported to date have been short in duration. Consequently, little or no information exists regarding the effect of chronic high protein intake on the development of nephrolithiasis. It may well be that chronic high protein consumption is accompanied by chronic adaptation that prevents stone formation in non-stone formers, whereas these adaptations are absent in persons predisposed to nephrolithiasis. In any case, the available data are not sufficient to support the view that meat consumption promotes renal stone formation in normal individuals.

C. Hypertension

Lacto-ovo-vegetarians as a group experience lower blood pressures than non-vegetarians (Sacks *et al.*, 1974; Armstrong *et al.*, 1977). The exclusion of meat in the vegetarian diet has led to the speculation that animal proteins may be responsible for the higher blood pressures documented in non-vegetarians.

Intervention studies have generally failed to find any effect of dietary protein intake on blood pressure. Several controlled studies on blood pressure in normotensive subjects found no effect of raising or lowering dietary protein content (Sacks *et al.*, 1984; Prescott *et al.*, 1987). Curiously, there are no studies of dietary protein manipulation in patients with essential hypertension. The limited studies of dietary protein restriction in patients with renal disease have yet to identify a blood pressure effect.

There are several mechanisms by which dietary protein intake might raise blood pressure as outlined by McCarty (1981). These include increased intake of amino acid neurotransmitter precursors; stimulation of plasma renin activity; interference with pharmacologic antihypertensive therapy, which has been shown with methyldopa; and competition with endogenous tyrosine, which lowers blood pressure. Conversely, there are mechanisms by which dietary protein intake might lower blood pressure. These include stimulation of sympathetic nervous system vasodepressor pathways; decreased sensitivity to angiotensin II and norepinephrine; and the fact that tyrosine, tryptophan, and taurine are precursors of vasodepressor central nervous system (CNS) neurotransmitters. Each of these substances lowers blood pressure in the rat, but there is currently no evidence that they do so in human hypertension. Despite a lack of a direct association between blood pressure and animal protein consumption, meat may still impact on blood pressure by virtue of its ability to alter mineral metabolism, especially that of calcium, phosphorus, and sodium (Organizing Committee, 1988).

(i) Sodium

The notion that reduction of dietary sodium chloride either lowers blood pressure and/or prevents its rise has been advanced for many years. Dahl (1960) first reported that a direct linear relationship existed between salt intake and the prevalence of hypertension among five separate populations around the world. Later scrutiny of these data indicated that salt intake within each of the chosen populations was not uniform, methods of blood pressure measurement were not described, and the data were not adjusted for age and sex distributions (Prineas and Blackburn, 1985). The issue has been explored again in a recent international epidemiologic study, where these variables were controlled (The Intersalt Cooperative Research Group, 1988). The study consisted of 52 centers with 200 participants in 32 countries, for a total of 10 079 subjects. Sodium excretion ranged from 0·2–242 mmol/day. In 48 of the 52 centers, intake ranged from 100–242 mmol/day. When these 48 centers were considered separately, there was no relationship between urinary sodium excretion and the median blood pressure or the prevalence of hypertension. Instead, factors such as body mass index, alcohol, and age were strongly associated with blood pressure. Thus, epidemiologic data supporting the view that reduction of salt intake lowers blood pressure are weak (Swales, 1988).

Intervention trials of reduced salt intake as a treatment for hypertension have been reviewed by Grobbee and Hoffman (1986). In thirteen well-performed, prospective, randomized, controlled clinical trials of dietary salt restriction in patients with hypertension, reduction of salt intake was generally 80 mmol (2 g Na, 5 mg NaCl) per day. A significant decrease was observed in only three of the thirteen trials. The decreases in blood pressure were modest. Grobbee *et al.* (1986) also found that the fall in blood pressure was related to the height of the initial blood pressure. In addition, they identified a relationship between age and the fall in blood pressure. Older individuals were more likely to decrease their blood pressure with dietary salt restriction.

Similar observations concerning initial blood pressure and response to intervention were made by Morgan and Nowson (1986), who plotted the relationship between blood pressure and the logarithm of sodium excretion in over 40 trials on dietary salt restriction. The most impressive results of dietary salt restriction were reported by MacGregor *et al.* (1982) who performed a randomized, cross-over, placebo-controlled trial of dietary salt restriction in patients with hypertension. Mean blood pressure in their patients dropped by 8 mm Hg.

Dietary salt restriction trials have produced rather heterogeneous results. One explanation for this is the possibility that only a fraction of hypertensive individuals are sensitive to the blood pressure-raising effects of salt, while the rest may have hypertension related to other mechanisms. Weinberger *et al.* (1986) formulated a definition of salt sensitivity on the basis of responses to either acute salt loading and depletion, or to dietary intervention. They found that one-third of normal individuals were salt-sensitive according to their definition. Among hypertensive subjects, approximately half were salt-sensitive. Older individuals and black subjects were more likely to be salt-sensitive. These investigators have identified an influence of genetic variance on salt-sensitivity of blood pressure, and have proposed a possible genetic marker for the condition. Similar heterogeneous responses were also identified in normal individuals.

In summary, salt restriction lowers blood pressure in some individuals but not in all, and is generally more effective in older and in more severely hypertensive patients. Patients with renal insufficiency may also benefit from salt and protein restriction.

(ii) Calcium

A variety of epidemiologic reports have associated higher levels of dietary calcium with lower blood pressure or a reduced risk of developing hypertension. The reports encompass a broad age range, diverse geographic areas, and various ethnic and racial groups (Morris and McCarron, 1987). The relationship has not however been observed in all reports that have addressed this issue (Sempos *et al.*, 1986), and the potential magnitude, that is, impact on blood pressure, of increasing dietary calcium intake has been discounted by some observers (Feinstein, 1985).

The first National Health and Nutrition Examination Survey performed by the National Center for Health Statistics generated one of the largest databases that has been used to evaluate this relationship (McCarron *et al.*, 1984). This database has been assessed by several groups and the association between calcium intake and blood pressure has been reported either in the entire population sampled or in specific subgroups (Morris and McCarron, 1987). It has been suggested that there is a threshold of approximately 400–600 mg/day of dietary calcium. Below this level, the risk of elevated blood pressure increases sharply (McCarron *et al.*, 1984; Witteman *et al.*, 1987); above it, the antihypertensive effect of increasing calcium intake is modest. From a four-year prospective study of approximately 60 000 women participating in the Nurses Health Study, a 23% reduction in the risk of developing high blood pressure was associated with a regular calcium intake above 800 mg/day, compared to an intake below 400 mg/day (Witteman *et al.*, 1987).

Several lines of evidence indicate that calcium metabolism is subtly abnormal in a subset of individuals with essential hypertension. The data, however, are inconsistent and contain seemingly paradoxical findings. Parathyroid hormone levels are modestly increased in hypertensive individuals (McCarron *et al.*, 1980; Grobbee *et al.*, 1986). Serum ionized calcium values have been reported to be lower or not different in hypertensive as compared to normotensive persons (McCarron, 1982; Resnick *et al.*, 1983). Serum total calcium values are variable with lower, similar, or slightly higher levels being noted (McCarron, 1989). Reduced serum phosphorus levels have been consistently observed (McCarron, 1989). Increased urinary calcium excretion has been reported (McCarron *et al.*, 1980; Strazzullo *et al.*, 1983), but is most evident when indexed against sodium excretion (McCarron *et al.*, 1980).

In experimental models of hypertension, a variety of metabolic disturbances related to calcium have also been identified (McCarron *et al.*, 1981; Young *et al.*, 1986). The findings parallel much of what has been described in humans. There is evidence of increased parathyroid hormone function, decreased serum ionized calcium values, lower serum phosphate concentrations, low $1\alpha,25(OH)_2$ vitamin D (Kurtz *et al.*, 1986), impaired intestinal transport, abnormal renal reabsorption of calcium (McCarron *et al.*, 1981), and reduced bone mineral content (Izawa *et al.*, 1985). For the most part, these metabolic disturbances have been identified in the spontaneously hypertensive rat, but other animal models (including the Dahl sodium chloride-sensitive model, the DOCA saline model, and the two-kidney, one-clip renal model) have also been reported as exhibiting one or more of these calcium disturbances (Young *et al.*, 1986; Spencer *et al.*, 1988; McCarron, 1989).

A variety of calcium salts (carbonate, citrate, phosphate, gluconate and lactate) have been shown to lower blood pressure in some laboratory models. The observation that dietary calcium supplementation tends to lower blood pressure in diverse models of high blood pressure suggests that failure to maintain adequate calcium homeostasis may be a common contributing mechanism to the development of arterial hypertension in a variety of pathologic states. Preliminary observations indicating that adding intermediate amounts of calcium to the diet of one animal model, the Dahl-S rat, may raise blood pressure suggest that this is not a uniform effect.

More than twenty calcium intervention trials in humans employing a variety of intervention periods (2–48 weeks) and sample sizes (8–200 subjects) have been reported (McCarron and Morris, 1987; McCarron, 1989). Some were not placebo-controlled or randomized and many included relatively small sample sizes (McCarron and Morris, 1987). A number of different calcium salts as well as dietary calcium have been used. In general, a modest antihypertensive response was detected in approximately two-thirds of these trials, with average decreases of 4–7 mm Hg systolic and 2–4 mm Hg diastolic blood pressure (McCarron and Morris, 1985). A blood pressure-lowering effect of calcium has been reported in both male and female hypertensive subjects (McCarron and Morris, 1985), blacks as well as whites (Lyle *et al.*, 1987, Zemel *et al.*, 1988a,b), young adults (Grobbee and Hofman, 1986) as well as elderly, (Grobbee and Hofman, 1986b; Nelson, 1987; Zemel *et al.* 1988a,b) and in normotensive males (Lyle *et al.*, 1987). The blood pressure response in all these trials is heterogeneous; that is, while more individuals exhibit a reduction in blood pressure compared to placebo, there is a subset of individuals whose blood pressure may rise modestly when additional calcium is consumed (McCarron and Morris, 1985). This pattern of response is true of other dietary maneuvers including Na^+ restriction and K^+ supplementation.

There has been no consistent predictor of a blood pressure response to increased calcium intake in the human studies. A variety of potential predictors have been reported, including modestly higher parathyroid hormone levels, lower serum ionized calcium or total calcium concentration, older age, and lower renin activity. Urinary calcium excretion has increased modestly in several of the trials, but no increase in renal calculi formation has been noted.

The mechanism(s) by which dietary calcium lowers blood pressure is unclear. Various explanations have been proposed, including a direct action of calcium on resistance arteries, changes in calcium regulating hormones, natriuresis, phosphate depletion, and modulation of central nervous system sympathetic function (McCarron, 1989).

(iii) Phosphorus

There is some epidemiologic evidence suggesting a possible relationship between dietary phosphorus and hypertension. In normotensive humans, serum levels of inorganic phosphorus have been found to be inversely related to blood pressure (Ljunghall and Hedstrand, 1977). In patients with hypertension, serum levels of inorganic phosphorus are significantly decreased compared to those in normotensive persons (McCarron, 1982).

Although severe phosphorus depletion decreases blood pressure by decreasing high energy phosphate stores and myocardial and vascular contractility, it is conceivable that moderate phosphorus depletion could exacerbate hypertension. Given that energy in the form of ATP is required for many ion transport systems that regulate cellular electrolyte homeostasis, it has been proposed that moderate phosphorus depletion, by impairing the function of such ion transport systems, may induce alterations in cellular calcium metabolism, which increase vascular resistance. Phosphorus depletion is also associated with increased urinary excretion of calcium and may contribute to calcium deficiency. Furthermore, decreased circulating levels of inorganic phosphorus induce increases in circulating levels of $1,25(OH)_2$ vitamin D. Some investigators have proposed that increased circulating levels of $1,25(OH)_2$ vitamin D may increase blood pressure, but this point is controversial (Resnick, 1987).

Bindels *et al.* (1987) have reported that in the spontaneously hypertensive rat, administration of supplemental phosphorus as potassium phosphate attenuates hypertension. In their study, hypertensive rats were given either a normal diet, supplemental potassium as potassium chloride, or supplemental potassium as potassium phosphate. Blood pressure was lower in the rats given the phosphate salt than in the other two groups. These findings are preliminary and will require confirmation with different phosphorus salts. There are no well-controlled studies examining the effects of supplemental phosphorus on blood pressure in humans with essential hypertension.

(iv) Potassium

In the absence of clear-cut data that meat consumption has a significant effect on K^+ metabolism, it is difficult to assess whether meat consumption *per se* can be linked to potassium's effect on regulation of blood pressure. Nevertheless, epidemiologic studies suggest an inverse relationship between blood pressure, stroke, and potassium intake. Data from intervention studies in both humans and animals suggest that potassium has modest antihypertensive properties, which may be mediated by the natriuretic and diuretic properties of potassium.

D. Gastrointestinal Cancer

Energy-yielding nutrients and some vitamins, particularly A and C, have long been implicated in preventing some cancers, such as those of the colon, rectum and breast. Extensive research in this area, however, has yielded inconsistent data regarding the association between these nutrients and certain types of cancer. Consequently, researchers have turned to other nutrients as possible mediators of some cancers. Among the macrominerals, calcium, sodium, and potassium have been implicated to the greatest extent in the pathogenesis of colon cancer (Nelson, 1987).

A protective role for dietary Ca^{2+} in the pathogenesis of colon cancer was suggested by epidemiologic observations that an inverse relationship exists between milk intake and the incidence of colon cancer in Japan and Sweden, and in Seventh Day Adventists (Nelson, 1987). In a 19-year prospective follow-up of 3102 men, the incidence of colon cancer was reported to be inversely related to dairy product consumption (Garland *et al.*, 1985). More recently, Slattery *et al.* (1988) conducted a population-based case-control study of 231 cases and 391 controls in Utah. In this study, calcium was found to protect against colon cancer in both males and females. Upon adjustment for calories, protein, and fat, calcium was still negatively related to cancer with the level of protection being somewhat lower in women (Slattery *et al.*, 1988). Thus, epidemiologic data have consistently demonstrated that increased calcium consumption reduces the risk of colon cancer in humans.

Studies in experimental animals have not been as conclusive as the epidemiologic evidence. Studies by Nelson (1987) compared milk-based diets to high dietary calcium diets and standard chow. In spite of a somewhat lower incidence of tumors in the rats consuming milk-based diets, no statistical differences were found between the three diets. In a study by Nutter *et al.* (1983) the ability of dimethylhydrazine to induce colonic tumors was compared in mice fed either high or low fat diets combined with diets containing powdered milk or beef as the protein source. In this study milk-based diets augmented dimethylhydrazine's ability to induce colonic tumors irrespective of the fat content of the diets. Other studies in rats and mice have demonstrated that supplemental dietary calcium and/or vitamin D decrease intestinal epithelial cell proliferation, a process associated with decreased susceptibility to gastrointestinal cancer (Wargovich *et al.*, 1983, 1984; Pence and Buddingh, 1987).

Data gathered in humans is more in line with the epidemiologic findings. A number of intervention studies have demonstrated that calcium protects against gastrointestinal cancer (Lipkin and Newmark, 1985; Buset *et al.*, 1986; Rozen *et al.*, 1987). Lipkin *et al.* (1985) examined the frequency and distribution of epithelial cell proliferation in colonic crypts obtained from patients with a family history of colon cancer before and after oral Ca^{2+} supplementation (1·25 g/day). After 2–3 months of supplementation colonic epithelial cell proliferation was significantly reduced to levels approaching those of persons at low risk for colonic cancer. In a follow-up study this same group (Lipkin *et al.*, 1989) reported that exposure of colonic epithelial cells to calcium either *in vivo* or *in vitro* decreased the rate of thymidine incorporation into these cells. Thus, calcium appears to arrest progressive cellular proliferation and enhance terminal differentiation in a manner consistent with reduced tumor growth. The molecular mechanisms of how calcium might affect the carcinogenetic process, however, have yet to be examined.

Data implicating sodium and potassium in the initiation and/or progression of gastrointestinal cancers are less extensive and limited to epidemiologic studies and a small number of animal experiments. Examination of the relationship between cancer rates and diet has revealed that a positive association exists between sodium intake and cancers of the esophagus, stomach, and colon (Jansson, 1986). In a worldwide study of this phenomenon, the ratio of K^+/Na^+ was reported to be negatively correlated with esophageal and colon cancer in Iran, Japan, Norway, and France and with the overall cancer mortality in Evans County, Georgia.

Only a limited number of studies have been conducted in animals to support the role of Na^+ and/or the K^+/Na^+ ratio in the pathogenesis of gastrointestinal cancer. In the two studies reported to date, reduced sodium intake and/or increased potassium consumption have been shown to counteract the tumor-promoting capabilities of dimethylhydrazine. (Jacobs, 1983; Takahashi *et al.*, 1983). In the absence of intervention data in humans, the implications of these data are uncertain at the present time. Nevertheless, given the role that meat protein appears to play in overall metabolism of sodium and calcium as reviewed earlier, it would seem prudent to avoid excessive protein intake especially in situations where sodium intake and soft drink consumption is higher while calcium consumption is below 800 mg/day.

E. Osteoporosis

Age-related loss of bone mass (osteoporosis) represents a significant public health problem in the elderly. It is estimated that 25–30% of all women in the US above 65 years old have osteoporosis (Marcus, 1982; Lindsay and Dempster, 1985). The central role played by calcium, phosphorus, and to some extent sodium in bone structure has prompted extensive work focusing on the relationship between consumption of these nutrients and osteoporosis.

Dietary calcium restriction predictably produces osteoporosis in animals (Marcus, 1982). In humans, however, a definite link between low calcium intakes and osteoporosis has not always been demonstrated in cross-sectional epidemiologic studies. As an example, Nordin (1966) was able to correlate bone density with calcium intake in Japan and Finland, but not in Gambia and Jamaica. Similarly, Matkovic *et al.* (1979) demonstrated a higher incidence of osteoporosis in a Yugoslavian population with an average calcium intake of 500 mg/day compared to a similar population with a calcium intake of 1100 mg/day in the same country. These findings are diametrically opposed to those of Garn (1970), who examined this relationship in 382 Ohio residents. In this study, calcium intakes ranging from 300–2000 mg/day bore no relationship to metacarpal cortical thickness. Thus, epidemiologic evidence does not strongly support the tenet that dietary calcium during adult life influences the extent and/or the rate of bone loss.

Given the complex nature by which calcium is metabolized, it is not surprising that the data relating intake alone to bone loss remain ambiguous. As reviewed earlier, calcium homeostasis is determined not only by its intake, but also by the efficiency with which it is metabolized. Thus, its absorption, skeletal turnover, and renal handling are as important as intake. Additionally, other nutrients, notably meat protein, phosphorus, and sodium, impact significantly on overall calcium balance in relatively healthy persons.

Protein consumed in the form of animal flesh has been implicated in osteoporosis. Epidemiologic data in north Alaskan Eskimos appear to indicate that they sustain rates of bone loss that are 10–15% higher than those of age-matched white Alaskans (Mazess and Mather, 1974). Yet the Eskimos adhere to a lifestyle generally considered beneficial to skeletal integrity, i.e. they remain active through most of their lives and generally consume substantial quantities of calcium and phosphorus. The major distinguishing characteristic of the Eskimo diet is its reliance on animal protein, which was estimated to be between 200 and 400 g/day by Mazess and Mather (1974). Viewed in the context of the extensive body of data showing that high protein intakes produce significant calciuria, it is conceivable that the higher incidence of osteoporosis in this population is a consequence of their high meat consumption. As documented by Linkswiler *et al.* (1981) protein-induced calciuria is not adequately compensated for by increased intestinal calcium absorption. Under conditions of extended periods of urinary calcium loss, the body relies on bone to act as a reservoir for calcium. This in turn can cause extensive demineralization over a lifetime of high protein intake. These views are supported by studies in vegetarians who generally have higher bone densities than omnivores (Ellis *et al.*, 1972). Nevertheless, a direct link between meat consumption and osteoporosis has as yet to be established in humans on a longitudinal basis.

Dietary phosphorus has also been implicated in osteoporosis. The theory has been advanced that as western diets have changed to include more processed foods, the overall consumption of phosphorus including that contained in meats has increased substantially. In western societies, the phosphorus contained in beverages represents the largest increase. It has been postulated that as the $Ca^{2+}:PO_4^-$ ratio falls below 1, with increased PO_4 intake, a transient suppression of serum ionized Ca^{2+} occurs which stimulates PTH secretion that in turn promotes bone resorption. This phenomenon commonly termed nutritional hyperparathyroidism was indirectly demonstrated by Bell *et al.* (1977). While interesting, these data are not supported by other studies in primates (Anderson *et al.*, 1977) and humans (Spencer *et al.*, 1965; Goldsmith *et al.*, 1976). Thus, a direct role for increased phosphorus including that derived from meats in the pathogenesis of osteoporosis has not been conclusively demonstrated.

There are suggestions in the literature that excessive sodium in the diet may also cause nutritional hyperparathyroidism and, by extension, a reduction in bone mineral content. As reviewed earlier, both calcium and sodium are co-transported in some segments of the nephron. Additionally it has long been known that sodium loading increases urinary calcium excretion (Kleeman *et al.*, 1964). The effects of protein loading on renal hemodynamics predict that an increase in sodium excretion would occur as a consequence of the increased GFR (Vander, 1985). The resultant loss of calcium decreases serum ionized calcium, which in turn activates the PTH–vitamin D axis which restores Ca^{2+} balance in part by resorbing bone. That these mechanisms may underlie the sodium-induced bone de-mineralization is supported by a number of studies in animals and humans. Goulding and Campbell (1984) have examined the effect of oral sodium loads on bone mineral metabolism. In albino rats a diet containing 8% sodium chloride caused significant calciuria, increased urinary cyclic AMP and hydroxyproline, and reduced bone content of Ca^{2+} and PO_4^-. Goulding and Lim (1983) have reported similar findings in humans using only hydroxyproline as a measure of bone resorption. Because hydroxy-proline is at best a crude measure of bone de-mineralization, the relevance of these findings to human osteoporosis is uncertain.

V. SUMMARY

In summary, it is well recognized that meat does not contribute significantly to the amount of calcium in the diet, except for deboned meat and poultry, which contains appreciable amounts. Although fresh meat is relatively low in sodium, cured and processed meat contains a relatively large amount and may play a role in development of hypertension in some individuals. Meat is not a good source of potassium, but still may make a small but important contribution to total potassium intake. Data gathered over the last 40 years demonstrate that meat consumption can alter the metabolism of these minerals, primarily through its effect on the renal handling of them. Thus, excessive meat consumption alters renal hemodynamics and, by extension, the rate at which calcium, sodium and perhaps potassium and phosphorus are excreted. Consequently, high meat consumption over extended periods of time may cause sustained mineral loss resulting in an imbalance in these minerals. Such imbalances have been implicated in osteoporosis, some forms of gastrointestinal cancer, nephrolithiasis and hypertension in susceptible individuals. Similarly, protein-induced elevation of renal blood flow, glomerular filtration rate and renal vasodilatation may accelerate the destruction of glomeruli, contributing significantly to progressive renal failure. Despite these observations, linkages between meat protein consumption and the diseases reviewed in this chapter still need to be demonstrated unequivocally in prospective randomized studies in humans. In the interim, it would seem prudent to practice moderation with regard to meat protein consumption.

VI. ACKNOWLEDGEMENTS

This work was supported by a grant from the National Dairy Promotion and Research Board. The authors are also indebted to Anita Kay for the preparation of the manuscript and to Molly Reusser for editorial assistance.

VII. REFERENCES

ALLEN, L. H. (1982). Calcium bioavailability and absorption: a review. *Am. J. Clin. Nutr.* **35**, 783.

AMBARD, L. (1920). *Physiologie Normale et Pathologique de Reins*. Paris, Masson et cie.

ANDERSEN, D. A. (1969). Historical and geographical differences in the pattern of incidence of urinary stones considered in relation to possible aetiological factors. *Proc. Renal Stone Res. Symp.*, p. 7. Churchill, London.

ANDERSON, M. P., HUNT, R. D. and GRIFFITHS, D. (1977). Long-term effect of low dietary calcium: phosphate ratio on the skeleton of cebus albifrons monkeys. *J. Nutr.* **107**, 834.

ARMSTRONG, B., VAN MERWYK, A. J. and COATES, H. (1977). Blood pressure in Seventh-Day Adventist vegetarians. *Am. J. Epidem.* **105**, 444.

BARSOTTI, G., GIANNONI, A., MORELLI, E., LAZZERI, M., VLAMIS, I., BALDI, R. and GIOVANNETTI, S. (1984). The decline of renal function slowed by very low phosphorus intake in chronic renal patients following a low nitrogen diet. *Clin. Nephrol.* **21**, 54.

BELL, R. R., DRAPER, H. H. and TZENG, D. Y. M. (1977). Physiological responses of human adults to foods containing phosphate additives. *J. Nutr.* **107**, 42.

BINDELS, R. J. M., VAN DEN BROEK, L. A. M., HILLEBRAND, S. J. W. and WOKKE, J. M. P. (1987). A high phosphate diet lowers blood pressure in spontaneously hypertensive rats. *Hypertension* **9**, 96.

BRENNER, B. M., MEYER, T. W. and HOSTETTER, T. H. (1982). Dietary protein intake and the progressive nature of kidney disease: The role of hemodynamically mediated glomerular injury in the pathogenesis of progressive glomerular sclerosis in aging, renal ablation and intrinsic renal disease. *N. Engl. J. Med.* **307**(11) 652.

BRESLAU, N. B., BRINKLEY, L., HILL, K. D. and PAK, C. Y. C. (1988). Relationship of animal protein-rich diet to kidney stone formation and calcium metabolism. *J. Clin. Endocrinol. Metab.* **66**, 140.

BROCKIS, J. G., LEVITT, A. J. and CRUTHERS, S. M. (1982). The effect of vegetable and animal protein diets on calcium, urate and oxalate excretion. *Brit. J. Urol.* **54**, 590.

BRONNER, F. and COBURN, J. W. (1982). Calcium physiology. In *Disorders of Mineral Metabolism* (F. Bronner and J. W. Coburn, Eds), Volume II, p. 43. Academic Press, London.

BUSET, M., LIPKIN, M., WINAWER, S., SWAROOP, S. and FRIEDMAN, E. (1986). Inhibition of human colonic epithelial cell proliferation *in vivo* and *in vitro* by calcium. *Cancer Res.* **46**, 5426.

DAHL, L. K. (1960). Possible role of salt intake in the development of essential hypertension. In *Essential Hypertension.* (K. D. Bock and P. T. Cottier, Eds), p. 53. Springer Verlag, Berlin.

ELLIS, F. R., HOLESH, S. and ELLIS, J. W. (1972). Incidence of osteoporosis in vegetarians and omnivores. *Am. J. Clin. Nutr.* **25**, 555.

FEINSTEIN, A. R. (1985). Tempest in a P-Pot? *Hypertension* **7**, 313.

GARLAND, C., BARRETT-CONNOR, E., ROSSOF, A. H., SHEKELLE, R. B., CRIQUI, M. H. and PAUL, O. (1985). Dietary vitamin D and calcium and risk of colorectal cancer: A 19-year prospective study in men. *Lancet* **1**, 307.

GARN, S. M. (1970). *The Earlier Gain and Later Loss of Cortical Bone in Nutritional Perspective.* C. C. Thomas. Springfield, Illinois.

GOLDSMITH, R. S., JOWSEY, J. and DUBE, W. J. (1976). Effect of phosphorus supplementation on serum parathyroid hormone and bone morphology in osteoporosis. *J. Clin. Endocrinol. Metabl.* **43**, 523.

GOULDING, A. and LIM, P. E. (1983). Effects of varying dietary salt intake on the fasting urinary excretion of sodium calcium and hydroxyproline in young women. *NZ Med. J.* **96**, 853.

GOULDING, A. and CAMPBELL, D. R. (1984). Effects of oral loads of sodium chloride on bone consumption in growing rats consuming ample dietary calcium. *Min. Electr. Metab.* **10**, 58.

GROBBEE, D. E. and HOFMAN, A. (1986a). Does sodium restriction lower blood pressure? *Brit. Med. J.* **293**, 27.

GROBBEE, D. E. and HOFMAN, A. (1986b). Effects of calcium supplementation on diastolic blood pressure in young people with mild hypertension. *Lancet* **2**, 703.

GROBBEE, D. E., HACKENG, W. H. L., BIRKENHAGER, J. C. and HOFMAN, A. (1986). Intact parathyroid hormone (I-84) in primary hypertension. *Clin. Exp. Hypertens.* **A8**, 299.

HEGSTED, M., SCHUETTE, S. A., ZEMEL, M. B. and LINKSWILER, H. M. (1981). Urinary calcium and calcium balance in young men as affected by level of protein and phosphorus intake. *J. Nutr.* **111**, 553.

HULTIN, H. O. (1976). Characteristics of muscle tissue. In *Principles of Food Science. Part 1. Food Biochemistry* (O. R. Fennema, Ed.), p. 578. Marcel Dekker, Inc. New York.

IBELS, L. S., ALFREY, A. C., HAUT, L. and HUFFER, W. E. (1978). Preservation of function in experimental renal disease by dietary restriction of phosphate. *N. Engl. J. Med.* **298**, 122.

IZAWA, Y., SAGARA, K., KADOTA, T. and MAKITA, T. (1985). Bone disorders in spontaneously hypertensive rat. *Calcif. Tissue Int.* **37**, 605.

JACOBS, M. M. (1983). Trace element inhibition of carcinogenesis and angiogenesis. *Biol. Trace Elements Res.* **5**, 375.

JANSSON, B. (1986). Inverse relationship between the intracellular K/Na ratio and cancer. *Cancer Bull.* **38**(1), 62.

KLAHR, S. (1989). Effects of protein intake on the progression of renal disease. *Ann. Rev. Nutr.* **9**, 87.

KLAHR, S. and ALLEYNE, G. A. O. (1973). Effects of chronic protein-calorie malnutrition on the kidney. *Kidney Int.* **3**, 129.

KIKUCHI, H., MATSUSHITA, T. and HIRATA, K. (1983). Improved dietary treatment with low protein and phosphorus restriction in uremic rats. *Kidney Int.* **24** (Suppl. 16), 254.

KLEEMAN, C. R., BOHANNA, J., BERNSTEIN, D., LING, S. and MAXWELL, M. H. (1964). Effects of variations in sodium intake on calcium excretion in normal humans. *Proc. Soc. Exp. Biol. Med.* **115**, 29.

KOLBYE, A. and NELSON, M. A. (1977). Health and safety aspects of the use of mechanically deboned meat. *Meat Poultry Inspection Program*, Vol. II. Food Safety and Quality Service, US Department of Agriculture, Washington, DC.

KURTZ, T. W., PORTALE, A. A. and MORRIS, R. C., JR (1986). Evidence for a difference in vitamin D metabolism between spontaneously hypertensive and Wistar-Kyoto rats. *Hypertension* **8**, 1015.

LEE, D. B. N., BRAUTBAR, N. and KLEEMAN, C. R. (1981). Disorders of phosphorus metabolism. In *Disorders of Mineral Metabolism*, Vol. III (F. Bronner and J. W. Coburn, Eds), p. 283. Academic Press, Inc., London.

LINDSAY, R. and DEMPSTER, D. W. (1985). Osteoporosis—Current concepts. *Bull NY Acad. Med.* **61**(4), 307.

LINKSWILER, H. M., ZEMEL, M. B., HEGSTED, M. and SCHUETTE, S. (1981). Protein-induced hypercalciuria. *Fed. Proc.* **40**, 2429.

LIPKIN, M. and NEWMARK, H. (1985). Effect of added dietary calcium on colonic epithelial cell proliferation in subjects at high risk for familial colon cancer. *New Engl. J. Med.* **313**, 1381.

LIPKIN, M., FRIEDMAN, E., WINAWAR, S. J. and NEWMARK, H. (1989). Colonic epithelial cell proliferation in responders and nonresponders to supplemental dietary calcium. *Cancer Res.* **49**, 248.

LJUNGHALL, S. and HEDSTRAND, H. (1977). Serum phosphate inversely related to blood pressure. *Brit. Med. J.* **1**, 553.

LYLE, R. M., MELBY, C. L., HYNER, G. C., EDMONDSON, J. W., MILLER, J. Z. and WIENBERGER, M. H. (1987). Blood pressure and metabolic effects of calcium supplementation in normotensive white and black men. *JAMA* **257**, 1772.

MACGREGOR, G. A., MARKANDU, N. D. and BEST, F. E. (1982). Double-blind randomized cross-over trial of moderate sodium restriction in essential hypertension. *Lancet* **1**, 351.

MARCUS, R. (1982). The relationship of dietary calcium to the maintenance of skeletal integrity in man—An interface of endocrinology and nutrition. *Metabolism*, **31**(1), 93.

MATKOVIC, V., KOSTIAL, K. and SIMONOVIC, I. (1979). Bone status and fracture rates in two regions of Yugoslavia. *Am. J. Clin. Nutr.* **32**, 540.

MAZESS, R. B. and MATHER, W. (1974). Bone mineral content of North Alaskan eskimos. *Am. J. Clin. Nutr.* **27**, 916.

MCCARRON, D. A. (1982). Lower serum concentrations of ionized calcium in patients with hypertension. *New Engl. J. Med.* **307**, 226.

MCCARRON, D. A. (1989). Calcium metabolism and hypertensive cardiovascular disease. *Kidney Int.* **35**, 717.

McCarron, D. A. and Morris, C. D. (1985). Blood pressure response to oral calcium in persons with mild to moderate hypertension: A randomized, double-blind, placebo-controlled, crossover trial. *Ann. Intern. Med.* **103**, 825.
McCarron, D. A. and Morris, C. D. (1987). The calcium deficiency hypothesis of hypertension. *Ann. Intern. Med.* **107**, 919.
McCarron, D. A., Pingree, P. A., Rubin, R. J., Gaucher, S. M., Molitch, M. and Krutzik, S. (1980). Enhanced parathyroid function in essential hypertension: A homeostasis response to a urinary calcium leak. *Hypertension* **2**, 162.
McCarron, D. A., Yung, N. N., Ugoretz, B. A. and Krutzik, S. (1981). Disturbances of calcium metabolism in the spontaneously hypertensive rat (SHR): Attenuation of hypertension by calcium supplementation. *Hypertension* **3** (Suppl I), I162.
McCarron, D. A., Morris, C. D., Henry, H. J. and Stanton, J. L. (1984). Blood pressure and nutrient intake in the United States. *Science* **224**, 1392.
McCarty, M. F. (1981). Prospects for nutritional control of hypertension. *Med. Hypotheses* **7**, 271.
Mitch, W. E. (1984). The influence of the diet on the progression of renal insufficiency. *Ann. Rev. Med.* **35**, 246.
Morgan, T. and Nowson, C. (1986). The role of sodium restriction in the management of hypertension. *Can. J. Physiol. Pharmacol.* **64**, 786.
Morris, C. D. and McCarron, D. A. (1987). Dietary calcium intake in hypertension. *Hypertension* **10**, 350.
Nelson, R. L. (1987). Dietary minerals and colon carcinogenesis. *Anticancer Res.* **7**, 259.
Nordin, B. E. C. (1966). International patterns of osteoporosis. *Clin. Orthop.* **45**, 17.
Nutter, R. L., Gridley, D. S., Kettering, J. D., Goude, A. G. and Slater, J. M. (1983). BALB/C mice fed milk or beef protein: Differences in response to 1,2,dimethylhydrazine carcinogenesis. *JNCI* **71**, 867.
Organizing Committee (1988). Education Program on Nonpharmacologic Management of Hypertension: Summary of Papers and Selected Bibliographies. National Kidney Foundation, Inc., New York.
Papper, S. (1983). Sodium: its biologic significance. In *CRC Series on Cations of Biologic Significance* (J. K. Aikawa, Ed.). CRC Press, Boca Raton.
Pence, B. C. and Buddingh, F. (1987). Inhibition of dietary fat promotion of colon carcinogenesis by supplemental calcium or vitamin D. *Proc. Am. Assoc. Cancer Res.* **28**, 154.
Pennell, J. D., Sanjand, V., Frey, N. R. and Jamison, R. L. (1975). The effect of urea infusion on the urinary concentrating mechanisms in protein depleted rats. *J. Clin. Invest.* **55**, 399.
Prescott, S. L., Jenner, D. A., Beilin, L. J., Margetts, B. M. and Vandongen, R. (1987). Controlled study of the effects of dietary protein on blood pressure in normotensive humans. *Clin. Exp. Pharmacol. Physiol.* **14**, 159.
Prineas, R. J. and Blackburn, H. (1985). Clinical and epidemiologic relationships between electrolytes and hypertension. In: *NIH Workshop on Nutrition and Hypertension* (J. J. Horan, M. Blaustein, J. B. Dunbar, W. Kachadorian, N. M. Kaplan and A. P. Simouplous Eds). p. 63. New York: Biomedical Information Corporation.
Pullman, T. N., Alving, A. S., Dern, R. J. and Landowne, M. (1954). The influence

of dietary protein intake on specific renal functions in normal man. *J. Lab. Clin. Med.* **44**, 320.

RABINOWITZ, L., GUNTHER, R. A., SHOJI, E. S., FREEDLAND, R. A. and AVERY, E. H. (1973). Effects of high and low protein diets on sheep renal function and metabolism. *Kidney Int.* **4**, 188.

RESNICK, L. M. (1987). Uniformity and diversity of calcium metabolism in hypertension. A conceptual framework. *Am. J. Med.* **82** (Suppl 1B), 16.

RESNICK, L. M., LARAGH, J. H., SEALEY, J. E. and ALDERMAN, M. H. (1983). Divalent cations in essential hypertension: Relations between serum ionized calcium, magnesium and plasma renin activity. *New Engl. J. Med.* **309**, 888.

ROBERTSON, W. G., PEACOCK, M. and HODGKINSON, A. (1979a). Dietary changes and the incidence of urinary calculi in the UK between 1958 and 1976. *J. Chron. Dis.* **32**, 469.

ROBERTSON, W. G., PEACOCK, M., HEYBURN, P. J., HANES, F. A., RUTHERFORD, A., CLEMENTSON, E., SWAMINATHAN, R. and CLARK, P. B. (1979b). Should recurrent oxalate stone formers become vegetarians? *Brit. J. Urol.* **51**, 427.

ROZEN, P., FIREMAN, Z., WAX, Y. and RON, E. (1987). Oral calcium suppresses increased colonic mucosal proliferation of persons at risk for colorectal neoplasia. *Gastroenterology* **92(II)**, 1603.

SACKS, F. M., ROSNER, B. and KASS, E. H. (1974). Blood pressure in vegetarians. *Am. J. Epidemiol.* **100**, 390.

SACKS, F. M., WOOD, P. G. and KASS, E. H. (1984). Stability of blood pressure in vegetarians receiving dietary protein supplements. *Hypertension*, **6**, 199.

SEMPOS, C., COOPER, R., KOVAR, M. G., JOHNSON, C., DRIZD, T. and YETLEY, E. (1986). Dietary calcium and blood pressure in National Health and Nutrition Examination Surveys I and II. *Hypertension*, **8**, 1067.

SLATTERY, M. L., SORENSON, A. W. and FORD, M. H. (1988). Dietary calcium intake as a mitigating factor in colon cancer. *Am. J. Epidemiol.* **128**, 504.

SPENCER, H., MENCZEL, J. and LEWIN, I. (1965). Effect of high phosphorus intake on calcium and phosphorus metabolism in man. *J. Nutr.* **86**, 125.

SPENCER, H., KRAMER, L., DEBARTOLO, M., NORRIS, C. and OSIS, D. (1983). Further studies of the effect of a high protein diet as meat on calcium metabolism. *Am. J. Clin. Nutr.* **37**, 924.

SPENCER, H., KRAMER, L. and OSIS, D. (1988). Do protein and phosphorus cause calcium loss? *J. Nutr.* **118**, 657.

STRAZZULLO, P., NUNZIATA, P. and CIRILLO, M. (1983). Abnormalities of calcium metabolism in essential hypertension. *Clin. Sci.* **65**, 137.

SWALES, J. D. (1988). Salt saga continued. Salt has only small importance in hypertension. *Brit. Med. J.* **297**, 307.

TAKAHASHI, M., KOKUBO, T. and FURUKAWA, J. (1983). Effect of high salt diet on rat gastric carcinogenesis induced with *n*-methyl-*N'*-nitro-*N*-Nitrosoguanidine. *Gan.* **74**, 28.

TANNENBAUM, S. R. (1976). Vitamins and minerals. In *Principles of Food Science. Part I. Food Biochemistry* (O. R. Fennema, Ed.), p. 347. Marcel Dekker, Inc., New York.

THE INTERSALT COOPERATIVE RESEARCH GROUP (1988). Intersalt: An international study of electrolyte excretion and blood pressure. Results for 24-hour urinary sodium and potassium. *Brit. Med. J.* **297**, 319.

TSU, T. N., MCLAUGHLIN, K., MAHONEY, A. J. and HENDRICKS, D. G. (1984). Bioavailability of calcium in meat products prepared from hand or mechanically deboned beef shank. *J. Nutr.* **114**, 946.

VANDER, A. J. (1985). *Renal Physiology*, 3rd edn, McGraw-Hill, New York.

WARGOVICH, M. J., ENG, V. W. S., NEWMARK, H. L. and BRUCE, W. R. (1983). Calcium ameliorates the toxic effect in deoxycholic acid on colonic epithelium. *Carcinogenesis* (*Lond.*) **4**, 1205.

WARGOVICH, M. J., ENG, V. W. S., NEWMARK, H. L. and BRUCE, W. R. (1984). Calcium inhibits the damaging and compensating proliferative effects of fatty acids on mouse colon epithelium. *Cancer Lett.* **23**, 253.

WEINBERGER, M. H., MILLER, J. Z., LUFT, F. C., GRIM, C. E. and FINEBERG, N. S. (1986). Definitions and characteristics of sodium sensitivity and blood pressure resistance. *Hypertension*, **8** (Suppl. II), II-127.

WITTEMAN, J. C. M., WILLETT, W. C. and STAMPFER, M. J. (1987). Dietary calcium and magnesium and hypertension: a prospective study (abstract). *Circulation*, **76** (Suppl IV), 35.

YOUNG, E. W., BUKOSKI, R. D. and MCCARRON, D. A. (1986). Calcium metabolism in essential hypertension. *Proc. Soc. Exp. Biol. Med.* **8**, 45.

ZELLER, K. R. (1987). Effects of dietary protein and phosphorus restriction on the progression of chronic renal failure. *Am. J. Med. Sci.* **294**, 328.

ZEMEL, M. B. (1988). Calcium utilization: Effect of varying level and source of dietary protein. *Am. J. Clin. Nutr.* **48**, 880.

ZEMEL, M. B., GUALDONI, S. M. and SOWERS, J. R. (1988a). Reduction in total and extracellular water associated with calcium-induced natriuresis and the antihypertensive effect of calcium in blacks. *Am. J. Hypertens.* **1**, 70.

ZEMEL, M. B., KRANIAK, J. K., STANDLEY, P. R. and SOWERS, J. R. (1988b). Erythrocyte cation metabolism in salt-sensitive hypertensive blacks is affected by dietary sodium and calcium. *Am. J. Hypertens.* **1**, 386.

WHANG, R. (1983). Potassium: Its biologic significance. In *CRC Series on Cations of Biologic Significance*, (J. K. Aikawa, Ed.) p. 25. CRC Press, Boca Raton.

12

Role of Meat as a Source of Protein and Essential Amino Acids in Human Protein Nutrition

PETER L. PELLETT

Department of Human Nutrition, University of Massachusetts at Amherst, Amherst, Massachusetts, USA

AND

VERNON R. YOUNG

School of Science, Massachusetts Institute of Technology, Cambridge, Massachusetts, USA

I. INTRODUCTION

While the term 'meat' has been used in an archaic sense for food in general i.e. anything used as nourishment for men or animals, a more specific definition is the edible flesh, organs, and glands of animals used for food. Meat by-products includes all products, both edible and inedible, other than the carcass meat. In a broad sense, the term 'meat' may mean the flesh of poultry, fish or other seafoods and game. Because of the similarity in the amino acid composition of these protein sources the term will be used here to include poultry but will exclude particular consideration of fish and fish products.

An assessment of the role of meat proteins in meeting the nitrogen needs of human subjects in order to provide the nutritionally indispensable (essential) amino acids, under various conditions, requires that we give some attention first to the estimates of requirements for total protein (nitrogen) and for the specific indispensable amino acids. This subject has been reviewed by us (Young and Scrimshaw, 1978; Young and Pellett, 1988) and by many others (Williams *et al.*, 1974, FAO/WHO/UNU, 1985). Hence, only a brief summary of some of the more important issues will be presented here in order to permit a more useful consideration, given below, of the potential, protein nutritional quality of different meats and meat products in human nutrition.

II. PROTEIN AND AMINO ACID REQUIREMENTS

The requirements for total protein, at various stages during the life cycle of humans, have been reviewed recently by FAO/WHO/UNU (1985). In Table 12-1, the safe levels of intake of high quality proteins, defined in FAO/WHO/UNU (1985) report, as those from eggs, meat and milk, are given for different age groups. These have been derived largely from growth and metabolic nitrogen balance studies, and they reveal an age-related decline in protein needs (when expressed per kg body weight) to maintain an adequate protein nutritional status.

Second, the requirement for dietary protein consists of two components; (a) a requirement for the nutritionally indispensable (essential) amino acids

TABLE 12-1
SAFE LEVELS OF PROTEIN INTAKE (g protein/kg/body wt/day) AS PROPOSED BY FAO/WHO/UNU (1985)[a]

Age group	*Males*	*Females*
3–6 months	1·85	1·85
6–9 months	1·65	1·65
9–12 months	1·5	1·5
1–2 years	1·2	1·2
2–3 years	1·15	1·15
3–5 years	1·1	1·1
5–7 years	1·0	1·0
7–10 years	1·0	1·0
10–12 years	1·0	1·0
12–14 years	1·0	0·95
14–16 years	0·94	0·9
16–18 years	0·88	0·8
Adults	0·75	0·75
Pregnancy		+6 g[b]
Lactation 0–6 months		+17·5 g[b]
6 months		+13 g[b]

[a] Uncorrected for nutritional value (amino acid scores) of mixed dietary proteins for infants and children and digestibility for all groups.
[b] Total daily addition per subject.

TABLE 12-2

A LISTING OF THE INDISPENSABLE AMINO ACIDS, CONDITIONALLY INDISPENSABLE AMINO ACIDS AND DISPENSABLE AMINO ACIDS IN HUMAN NUTRITION

Indispensable	*Conditionally indispensable*	*Dispensable*
Histidine	Cystine	Aspartic Acid
Isoleucine	Tyrosine	Asparagine
Leucine	Taurine	Glutamic Acid
Lysine	Glycine?	Glutamine
Methionine		Alanine
Phenylalanine		Proline
Threonine		Arginine
Tryptophan		Serine
Valine		

(Table 12-2) and for other amino acids (conditionally indispensable) under specific physiological and pathological conditions, and (b) the need to meet the requirement for non-specific nitrogen in order to supply the nitrogen necessary for synthesis of the nutritionally dispensable amino acids (Table 12-2) and other physiologically important nitrogen-containing compounds, such as nucleic acids, creatine and the porphyrins. In reference to the first of these two major components, it is usually accepted that the concentration and availability of the individual indispensable amino acids are major factors responsible for the differences in the nutritive values of various food protein sources. Hence, the efficiency with which the intake of a given source of food protein is capable of supporting an adequate state of nutritional health will depend on: (a) the physiological requirements for the individual indispensable amino acids and for total nitrogen, and (b) the concentration of specific amino acids in the particular source of food protein of interest.

Based on current international estimates for the requirements for specific indispensable amino acids in various age groups (Table 12-3) it can be seen, and is shown graphically in Fig. 12-1, that the human infant and young child require a source, or mixture, of food proteins that is relatively high in the concentration of indispensable amino acids. In addition, as also shown here, with growth and development the currently accepted values of the need for the indispensable amino acids decline more rapidly than that for total protein, so that in the adult the relative concentration of indispensable amino acids needed for maintenance of nutritional adequacy is much lower than in the infant or young child. Because of these changes in specific amino

TABLE 12-3
SOME ESTIMATES OF AMINO ACID REQUIREMENTS IN PRE-SCHOOL AND SCHOOL-AGE CHILDREN, AND IN ADULTS[a]

Amino acid	*Pre-school (2–5 years old)*		*School children*[b] *(10–12 years old)*		*Adults (18 years +)*	
	(mg/kg/day)	*(mg/g prot.)*	*(mg/kg/day)*	*(mg/g prot.)*	*(mg/kg/day)*	*(mg/g prot.)*
Histidine	?		?		8–10	16
Isoleucine	31	28	28	28	10	13
Leucine	73	66	44	44	14	19
Lysine	64	58	44	44	12	16
Methionine and cystine	27	25	22	22	13	17
Phenylalanine and tyrosine	69	63	22	22	14	19
Threonine	37	34	28	28	7	9
Tryptophan	12·5	11	3·3	9	3·5	5
Valine	38	35	25	25	10	13
Total (−His)	352	320	216	222	84	111

[a] From Tables 4 and 38 in FAO/WHO/UNU (1985).
[b] Based on summary by Williams *et al.* (1974).

acid requirements relative to the requirements for total protein (nitrogen), Arroyave (1974), among others, has concluded, that the nutritional quality of the protein needed will vary according to the age of the individual consumer.

Before proceeding, however, with a more detailed assessment of the nutritional quality of meat proteins it is worth making some additional comments about current knowledge of the amino acid requirements of humans. Thus, as summarized in Table 12-3, the current, internationally accepted requirements for the individual indispensable amino acids, expressed per unit of body weight, in the adult are not only substantially lower than those in infants and pre-school children but they are also considerably lower, as indicated above, when the requirements are expressed per unit of the total protein need. Hence, when the FAO/WHO/UNU (1985) amino acid requirement estimates for the adult, expressed per unit of protein need, are compared (Table 12-4) with the amino acid pattern of various plant and animal protein sources, it is evident that the level of all of the amino acids in these food sources is much higher (per unit of protein)

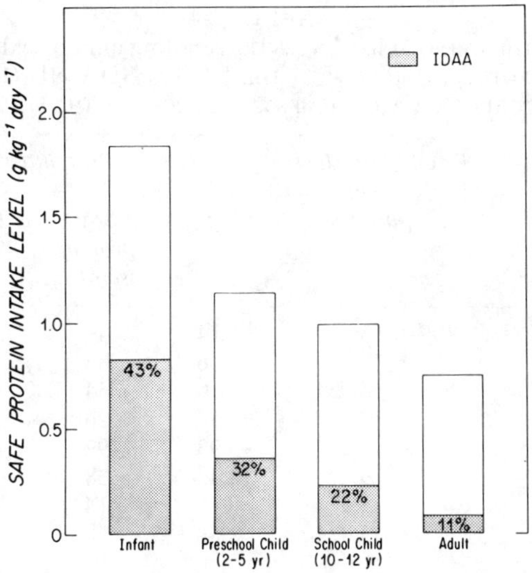

FIG. 12-1. Relationship between the requirement for the total of the indispensable amino acids (IDAA) and safe protein intakes for various age groups. Drawn from data and recommendations of FAO/WHO/UNU (1985).

than for the amino acid pattern required by the adult. On this basis all of the indispensable amino acids, including the sulfur amino acids, in beef, for example, as well as in other sources such as soy proteins, are in considerable excess of adult needs. Thus, all usual food proteins would readily meet and, indeed, exceed the requirement for the indispensable amino acids when the dietary protein was at least equal to the safe protein intake levels listed in Table 12-1.

From the above, there should be little reason to be further concerned with an assessment of the nutritional quality of meat proteins in adults. It also follows that the focus of attention need only be on protein nutrition in children and infants and, particularly, in the latter group where they might be given diets containing a single protein source or limited number of protein sources, as in the case of feeding infants with a proprietary formula, possibly supplemented with strained foods. In contrast to this generalization, however, there is increasing evidence that the current international (FAO/WHO/UNU, 1985) and national (Williams *et al.*, 1974) estimates of the requirement for most indispensable amino acids in the adult are far too low (Young *et al.*, 1981, 1985). If this evidence is correct, and further substantiated, then this has important implications for the approaches that

TABLE 12-4

COMPARISON OF THE AMINO ACID CONCENTRATION (mg amino acid per g protein) IN VARIOUS FOOD PROTEIN SOURCES WITH THE FAO/WHO/UNU (1985) AMINO ACID SCORING, OR REQUIREMENT, PATTERN FOR THE ADULT

Amino acid	*FAO/WHO/UNU adult pattern*	*Protein source*			
		Egg[a]	*Soy protein isolate*[b]	*Beef*[a]	*Wheat*[c]
Isoleucine	13	54	49	48	34
Leucine	19	86	82	81	61
Lysine	16	70	64	89	27
Met + Cys (SAA)	17	57	26	40	36
Phe + Tyr	19	93	92	80	81
Threonine	9	47	38	46	27
Tryptophan	5	17	14	12	11
Valine	13	66	48	50	51
Total	111	490	413	446	328

[a] Composition taken from FAO/WHO/UNU (1985).
[b] Composition taken from Young *et al.* (1984a).
[c] Composition taken from Table 10 in Young and Pellett (1985).

should be taken to assess, comprehensively, the role of various food protein sources, including meat, in human protein nutrition.

The probable inadequacy of most current estimates of amino acid requirements in adults has been discussed by us previously (Young *et al.*, 1981, 1985). However, on the basis of theoretical and metabolic considerations (Young *et al.*, 1989), as well as from results of ^{13}C-tracer studies involving estimates of minimum intakes of specific indispensable amino acids required to maintain body amino acid balance (Young, 1987), we conclude that the requirements for leucine, lysine, threonine, and valine in the adult are probably about two-to-three times higher than the values proposed by FAO/WHO/UNU (1985) (Table 12-3). Furthermore, the requirements for the other indispensable amino acids, that we have not so far reassessed by direct experimental study, can be predicted from new knowledge about the dynamic status of protein and amino acid metabolism (Young *et al.*, 1989). Thus, from the available data, principally that obtained in our laboratories, we have arrived at a new set of tentative estimates for the amino acid needs of the adult. These are shown in Table 12-5, and they are compared here with the estimates by FAO/WHO/UNU

TABLE 12-5

NEWLY REVISED ESTIMATES OF AMINO ACID REQUIREMENTS IN ADULTS AND A PROPOSED NEW AMINO ACID SCORING PATTERN FOR THIS AGE GROUP

Amino acid	*FAO/WHO/UNU requirement*[a] *(mg/kg/day)*	*New revised estimates*[b]	
		Requirement (mg/kg/day)	*Pattern (mg/g prot.)*
Isoleucine	10	23	38
Leucine	14	39	65
Lysine	12	30	50
Met + Cys (SAA)	13	15	25
Phe + Tyr	14	39	65
Threonine	7	15	25
Tryptophan	3·5	6	10
Valine	10	20	35

[a] Estimates from FAO/WHO/UNU (1985).
[b] See Young *et al.* (1989) for discussion of the development of the new requirement estimates and Pellett and Young (1988b) for the new amino acid scoring pattern.

(1985). From these data a new amino acid requirement *pattern* (amino acid scoring pattern) for the adult has now been proposed (Table 12-5).

It can be seen that the proposed new adult pattern is quite similar to that recommended by FAO/WHO/UNU (1985) for the pre-school and early school-age child (2–5 years) (see Table 12-3 for comparison), except for a lower threonine and slightly lower lysine content in the newly proposed adult pattern. If these revised estimates of amino acid requirements in adults are rational, as we believe they are, for reasons discussed elsewhere (Young, 1987; Young *et al.*, 1989), the nutritional value of different protein sources would not be affected as markedly by the age of the consumer, in contrast to the suggestion made by Arroyave (1974) or as stated in FAO/WHO/UNU (1985). Indeed, based on the revised estimations of amino acid requirements that we have proposed (Young *et al.*, 1989), it follows that for an evaluation of dietary protein quality, it may only be necessary to use two amino acid requirement (or scoring) patterns; one for the infant, which according to FAO/WHO/UNU (1985) should be based on the amino acid composition of breast milk and the other, as shown in Table 12-5, for all groups above about two years of age.

In view of the current, but still inadequate, state of our knowledge about the quantitative aspects of the amino acid requirements in humans it now appears to us that there is probably little, if any, age-dependent change in the requirements for indispensable amino acids, when they are expressed per unit of protein required, above age about two years. Thus, the pattern of change in amino acid requirements shown in Fig. 12-1 should not be accepted, at least not without critical analysis and evaluation. In any case, it is our view that it would be prudent to explore and to assess critically the nutritional value of meat proteins in all of the major age group categories (i.e. infants, pre-school and school-age children, adolescents and adults), based on the proposal that a single scoring pattern be used for all individuals of about two years and older.

A. Protein Quality Evaluation in Humans

Finally, before our attention is specifically directed to the protein nutritional value of meats in human nutrition, it is to be recognized that it is not always practical to measure the value of a food protein directly for human nutrition purposes. Thus, a number of laboratory indices of protein quality have been used (Table 12-6). Chemical methods, although analytically precise, are subject to a number of limitations (Pellett and Young, 1984). Hence, an alternative, or preliminary, approach, prior to conduct of direct experiments in humans, involves a biological assessment, usually involving the laboratory rat.

Clinical methods for the evaluation of protein quality are based on the same principles applied to the corresponding animal assays, but require

TABLE 12-6

SOME LABORATORY METHODS FOR EVALUATING PROTEIN QUALITY[a]

Approach based on:	*Example(s)*
Nitrogen retention	Nitrogen balance index
Weight gain	Protein efficiency ratio (PER)
	Relative protein value (RPV)
Biochemical measures	Plasma protein regeneration
	Blood urea concentration
	Cysteine dioxygenase
	Plasma amino acids
Rapid biological methods	Tetrahymena
	Insects
Other	Available lysine
	Enzyme digestion

[a] Based on Bender (1983).

TABLE 12-7
METHODS THAT HAVE OR MAY BE USED TO ASSESS PROTEIN QUALITY IN HUMAN SUBJECTS[a]

Approach	*Comments*
Nitrogen balance	Commonly used, difficult to measure and affected by many factors
Growth	Applies to young, ethical concerns
Measurement on blood	
Free amino acids	Potential for estimating limiting amino acid
Urea	Of possible value (children)
Albumin	For a quantitative index more investigation required
Protein (enzymes, transport proteins)	
Measurements on urine	
N compounds (urea, NH_4, 3-MeHis)	Perhaps useful for qualitative purposes
Body composition	
^{40}K, IVNAA,[b] Body water (^2H_2O)	Precision and/or availability of technique a limiting factor

[a] From Young and Pellett (1985).
[b] In-vivo neutron activation analysis.

some modification for application to human subjects (Pellett and Young, 1980). The major procedures and criteria that may be used are shown in Table 12-7. These include growth or nitrogen balance techniques, alone or in combination with biochemical analysis of serum protein and amino acids, hemoglobin, blood urea nitrogen, the urinary excretion of creatinine, sulfur compounds and other metabolites. The majority of studies so far conducted in humans for determining the nutritional value of food proteins have been based on measures of growth, N balance and dietary N utilization in the case of infants and children or indices of N balance in adolescents and adults.

(i) Meat protein as a predominate source of dietary protein: nitrogen (N) balance studies

In Table 12-1 the intakes of high quality protein sources that would be adequate for the support and maintenance of host protein status are given but it is known that food proteins differ in their capacity to maintain protein status at the same levels of protein intake. However, because of the generally accepted high quality of meat proteins only brief consideration needs to be given here to direct metabolic studies and in much of the remaining part of this chapter we will emphasize the amino acid composition of meats and its significance under various dietary situations.

Measurements of the least amount of different proteins that will maintain adult human subjects in body N balance or support normal growth in young children provide the basis for assessing the comparative nutritional value of different food proteins. This particular topic has been reviewed extensively by various expert groups (Pellett and Young, 1980), and more recently by the 1981 FAO/WHO/UNU Expert Consultation on Energy and Protein Requirements (FAO/WHO/UNU, 1985).

Unfortunately, there are limited metabolic data on the protein nutritional value of meat and meat-products in human subjects. However, the results of short-term nitrogen balance studies carried out in adult humans confirm the fact that beef and egg are essentially identical in their capacity to maintain N balance and both are superior to that of wheat proteins, for example (Young *et al.*, 1975). Additional studies also conducted in human adults confirm these observations (Wayler *et al.*, 1983) and the results of a long-term metabolic study by Young *et al.* (1986) further underscore the fact that the nutritional value of lean beef, as the test protein source, is high and fully capable of meeting physiological requirements. Indeed it seems more useful, for purposes of the present review to consider the amino acid composition of meats and, particularly, how the amino acids of meat contribute to and complement the overall amino acid pattern of different diets. To do this we will focus our attention in the following section on the proteins in meat and their amino acid composition. Their relationship to human amino acid requirements will then be discussed.

III. AMINO ACID COMPOSITION OF MEATS AND MEAT BY-PRODUCTS

The broad overall chemical composition of typical adult mammalian muscle is shown in Table 12-8. Of the total protein, which represents about one-fifth of the wet weight, some 60% is that associated with the myofibrillar fraction while 30% is of sarcoplasmic origin. Of the other soluble nitrogenous constituents (less than 2% of total weight), about one-third consists of creatinine (Greaser, 1986) and about one-fifth each come from free amino acids and from the combined histidine derivatives, carnosine and anserine. While the other free amino acids present in muscle

TABLE 12-8

CHEMICAL COMPOSITION OF A TYPICAL ADULT MAMMALIAN MUSCLE[a]

Component		*Wet weight (%)*
Water		75·0
Protein		19·0
(a) Myofibrillar[b]	(11·5)	
(b) Sarcoplasmic[c]	(5·5)	
(c) Connective tissue[d] and organelle	(2·0)	
Lipid[e]		2·5
Carbohydrate[f]		1·2
Soluble non-protein		
(a) Nitrogen[g]		1·65
(b) Inorganic[h]		0·65
(c) Vitamins[i]		<0·10

[a] Adapted from Lawrie (1979).
[b] Myosin, actin, tropomyosins, troponins and actinins.
[c] Mainly soluble enzymes and extracellular proteins, such as myoglobin and hemoglobin.
[d] Collagen, elastin and insoluble enzymes such as cytochromes.
[e] Neutral lipids, phospholipids and fatty acids.
[f] Lactic acid, glucose-6-phosphate, glycogen and glucose.
[g] Creatine, inosine monophosphate, free amino acids, carnosine and anserine and nucleotides.
[h] Phosphorus, potassium and trace minerals in nutritionally significant amounts.
[i] Fat soluble and water soluble; small quantities but nutritionally significant.

can be used in meeting nutritional requirements, it can be seen from Table 12-8 that, in quantitative terms, they are not a nutritionally significant source when compared to the amino acids that are derived from the breakdown of the various protein fractions during digestion and absorption within the intestinal tract.

The majority of meat consumed, particularly in the more developed regions of the world, is that from skeletal muscle. The structure of muscle fiber in meat has been discussed by Cassens (1978) and the chemistry of these tissues, with particular relevance to their proteins, has been reviewed by various investigators (Bodwell and McClain, 1978; Bechtel, 1986; Bodwell and Anderson, 1986). Also the physical and biochemical changes occurring in muscle during storage and preservation have been reviewed recently by Pearson (1986). Briefly, therefore, the proteins that give structural rigidity to muscle and also function in the transduction of chemical energy into the mechanical energy of contraction collectively constitute the myofibrillar proteins. Myosin is the most abundant of the muscle proteins and constitutes some 50–60% of the myofibrillar protein component of muscle or comprises about one-third of the total muscle protein. Myosin has a molecular weight of approximately 500 000 daltons and is a long asymmetrical molecule with two identical long polypeptide chains and two light chains. The long chains (each an α-helix which coil around each other in a further α-helix) both contain about 1800 amino acids. The amino acid composition of myosin is shown in Table 12-9 where it can be seen to be particularly rich in the amino acid lysine. Myofibrillar proteins also contain some 20% of actin, in the form of a single polypeptide chain containing about 450 amino acids with a molecular weight of 42 000. Actin, has lower levels of lysine but is relatively high in tryptophan. Tropomyosin constitutes about 7% of the myofibrillar protein fraction and contains especially high levels of lysine. The remaining 23% of protein in the myofilaments is largely accounted for by a large number of different proteins, including titin, C-protein, nebulin, myomesin, desmin, X-protein, troponin, α-actinin and β-actinin among others.

The remaining approximately two-thirds of the muscle protein is associated with the sarcoplasm, the connective tissues and various intracellular organelles. The sarcoplasmic proteins can be easily extracted with cold water and include all of the glycolytic enzymes and myoglobin. Myoglobin is a conjugated protein, which gives the red color to muscles, and serves as the storage site for oxygen. The amount of myoglobin present is generally a function of the extent and type of muscle activity of the tissue involved, the extent of the blood supply, the general oxygen availability, and/or the age of the animal (Bodwell and McClain, 1978). Myoglobin is present in relatively large quantities in heart tissue because of the heavy oxygen demand, although, in contrast, the wing muscles of birds are lower in myoglobin than the rest of their skeletal muscles. Here the increased oxygen demand of these tissues is supplied by a highly efficient blood supply. Of all mammals, whales have the highest skeletal muscle myoglobin concentrations, which account for their ability to remain submerged in water for long periods. The amino acid composition of whale myoglobin is shown also in Table 12-9. The amino acid composition of the actinins also are broadly similar to those of the various actins in the muscles of different species (Table 12-9).

The protein, collagen, is the major fibrous element of the connective tissues and is the most abundant single protein of the body. Collagen fibers are widely distributed in skin, bone, cartilage, tendon and arterial walls, as well as in the sarcolemma. Collagen constitutes over one-third of the total protein of the body with a significant proportion of it being found in bone.

TABLE 12-9

AMINO ACID COMPOSITION (mg amino acid per g protein) OF MUSCLE PROTEINS, CONNECTIVE TISSUE COMPONENTS AND OF SELECTED MEAT PRODUCTS[a]

	Beef	*Pork*	*Lamb*	*Cured processed meats*	*MDM*	*Actin*	*Myosin*	*Tropo-myosin*	*Bovine collagen*	*Bovine elastin*	*Whale myoglobin*
Aspartic acid	88	89	85	91	88	107	115	117	43	9	60
Threonine	40	51	49	49	32	77	54	31	18	9	33
Serine	38	40	39	42	38	58	41	40	35	7	36
Glutamic acid	144	145	144	129	142	140	229	320	99	19	157
Proline	54	46	48	52	61	50	25	6	114	106	26
Glycine	71	61	67	80	82	43	26	9	187	189	47
Alanine	64	63	63	64	67	58	59	89	74	158	85
Valine	57	50	50	52	61	49	47	29	23	140	53
Methionine	23	25	23	22	28	42	33	25	8	Tr	16
Cystine	14	13	13	15	15	12	11	9	—	—	—
Total SAA	37	38	36	37	43	43	54	44	34	8	16
Isoleucine	51	49	48	49	39	84	55	39	15	31	67
Leucine	84	75	74	74	80	82	108	121	28	72	132
Tyrosine	32	30	32	29	25	67	33	29	67	13	31
Phenylalanine	40	41	39	40	43	48	47	9	21	52	56
Total aromatic amino acids	72	71	71	69	68	115	80	38	88	65	87
Histidine	29	32	27	28	30	27	24	10	8	1	104
Lysine	84	78	76	74	78	70	146	184	30	4	156
Arginine	66	64	69	66	77	74	79	75	75	11	40
Tryptophan	11	13	13	10	5	20	9	—	—	—	22

[a] Adapted from Pellett and Young (1984) where original citations are presented. MDM = mechanically deboned meat.
Tr = trace.

Furthermore, collagen differs from most other proteins in that it has a distinctive distribution of amino acids. Bodwell and McClain (1978) indicate that the presence of both hydroxylysine and hydroxyproline is required for including a protein in the collagen class. These hydroxy-amino acids are formed by a post-translational process where lysine and proline residues are hydroxylated during the synthesis of large polypeptide precursors of collagen. One-third of the amino acid content of collagen is due to glycine, and it is also rich in proline. However, it contains no tryptophan or cysteine. Collagen fibers undergo thermal shrinkage to a fraction of their original length when heated, but the extent varies from one species to another (Bodwell and McClain, 1978). At higher temperatures collagen is converted, in large part, to soluble gelatin. Elastin is another connective tissue protein, which can be differentiated from collagen by the absence of a well defined X-ray diffraction pattern and also by its different amino acid composition. While glycine is high in both collagen and in elastin, the latter protein has lower levels of hydroxyproline, hydroxylysine and lysine (Table 12-9). Since less expensive cuts of meat would tend to contain higher levels of connective tissue, as also would mechanically deboned meats, the protein nutritional value of such meats has been the subject of attention and particularly in relation to the regulation of the nutritional value of such protein sources (Bodwell, 1984). In Table 12-9 the amino acid composition of various meats (beef, pork, lamb, processed meats and mechanically deboned meats) are shown for purposes of comparison with the composition of the major muscle protein fractions. The distinctly different amino acid pattern present in the connective tissue proteins is especially obvious.

Before the amino acid composition of the various cuts of meat and poultry tissues is examined, brief mention might be given to the content of protein, fat and food energy in various selected raw and cooked portions of meat and poultry (Table 12-10). The composition of meat depends upon the species source, the degree of fatness of the animal, the specific cut used, the degree of cutting and trimming, the curing and/or processing treatments and methods used for packaging and storage. Hence, individual cuts of meat will vary greatly in composition, and precise values can be assigned only by analysis of that particular cut (Rice, 1978). However, for illustrative purposes, some selected data on various cuts of raw and cooked meat and poultry products are presented in Table 12-10.

While poultry meat is often higher in protein and lower in fat than other meats, species differences are generally less significant than the cut and whether the analysis applies to the cooked or raw food. The protein content

TABLE 12-10

PROTEIN, FAT, FOOD ENERGY AND AMINO ACID COMPOSITION OF SELECTED RAW AND COOKED MEAT AND POULTRY PORTIONS (per 100 g)[a]

Meat cut	*R/C*[b]	*Prot.* (%)	*Fat* (%)	*Food energy* (*kcal*)	*Pcal* (%)	*Lys* (*mg*)	*SAA*[c] (*mg*)	*Thr* (*mg*)	*Try* (*mg*)
Beef									
Chuck	R	18·7	19·6	257	29·1	1 630	700	830	220
Sirloin	R	14·5	38·8	412	14·1	1 270	540	640	170
Hamburger lean	R	20·7	10·0	179	46·3	1 730	680	870	255
Hamburger	C	27·4	11·3	219	50·0	2 280	900	1 150	340
Tenderloin	C	27·8	20·8	307	36·2	2 430	1 040	1 230	330
Corned beef	C	22·9	30·4	372	24·6	2 000	860	1 010	270
Heart	C	13·5	3·8	93	58·0	1 110	460	620	180
Liver	C	25·9	10·6	229	45·1	1 940	930	1 230	390
Pork									
Loin chop	C	29·4	25·6	357	32·9	2 870	1 090	1 360	380
Ham	C	23·0	30·6	374	24·6	1 970	870	1 030	260
Boston butt	R	15·5	24·5	287	21·6	1 510	570	710	200
Lamb									
Leg	R	17·8	16·2	222	32·1	1 440	660	820	230
Loin	C	22·0	29·4	359	24·5	1 780	820	1 010	290
Veal									
Flank	R	16·5	27·0	314	21·0	1 380	570	720	220
Flank	C	23·2	32·3	390	23·8	1 940	810	1 010	300
Round	R	19·5	9·0	164	47·6	1 630	680	850	260
Chicken									
Breast	C	29·8	7·8	197	60·5	2 530	1 200	1 240	340
Broiler	C	27·3	13·6	239	45·7	2 320	1 100	1 140	310
Drumstick	C	27·1	11·2	215	50·4	2 300	1 100	1 150	320

[a] Rice (1978) and USDA (1976–86).
[b] R = raw, C = cooked.
[c] SAA = sulfur amino acids.

can range from about 13 to almost 30%, while fat can vary from 4 to approximately 40%. Hence, protein-energy concentration (Pcal %) values range very widely from about 14% in raw sirloin (it can be as low as 4% in raw bacon) to over 60% in cooked chicken breast. Amino acid composition data for four indispensable amino acids, lysine, total sulfur amino acids, threonine, and tryptophan, are also shown in Table 12-10. These are the amino acids most likely to be limiting in usual diets in various areas of the world (FAO/WHO/UNU, 1985). In the present case the amino acid values are presented in absolute terms (mg/100 g of meat) to emphasize the point that the amino acid supply is determined to a major extent by the amount of protein present in the particular product. Furthermore, the importance of meat, as a source of lysine, should be noted from these data; 100 g of meat, supplying between about one-third and one-half of daily total protein needs for an adult, would supply 60–100% of estimated lysine needs, even when compared to the higher amino acid requirement estimates proposed above (Table 12-5).

The effects of cooking on the composition of meats are considerable and these have been well discussed by Rice (1978). Protein is denatured by heat so that the soluble proteins become insoluble and there is a loss of water. Raw meats, thus, have higher moisture content than cooked meats. To some extent, the water loss is proportional to the length of time and the temperature used in cooking. For broiling or roasting, surface evaporation adds a dehydration effect to the denaturation effect and the juices that are lost carry with them some water-soluble nutrients including proteins. These amounts, however, are relatively small in comparison with the total nutrients present. In contrast to the protein which becomes more firm as it is heated, fat melts and drains from the surface. This again is proportional to the intensity of heat and the duration of cooking. Fat losses from meat can occur, even in deep fat frying because the lean muscle portions are hydrophobic and will not take up fat. However, at the same time, substantial amounts of cooking fat may adhere to the surface, especially if 'breading' mixtures are used (Rice, 1978). An illustration of changes that can occur as a result of cooking is given in Table 12-11. A variety of cooking methods were used in the generation of these data, including simmering, broiling and roasting but the effects are broadly similar. For certain cuts (mainly muscle meat) protein concentration increases by about 6–8 g/100 g while water decreases between about 10–12 g/100 g. Fat and food energy contents increase, on average, to a smaller extent than does that for protein, giving a modest increase in Pcal %. A statistical analysis on this data showed the changes to be highly significant ($P < 0{\cdot}001$). Similar effects of cooking occur with organ meats, such as heart, kidney, liver, lung and pancreas, but they seem to be more variable.

Raw meat, when purchased, contains bone, cover fat, gristle and tendons, which may or may not be removed prior to cooking. In the more wealthy regions of the world these components are not ordinarily eaten. The amount of bone, however, is a significant component defining the amount of edible meat and, therefore, the amino acids that can be obtained from a particular cut. A food group code has been developed by the USDA (1979) and is now widely used in the organization of food composition data banks. Mean compositions of some of the major meat categories, with the

TABLE 12-11

CHANGES IN THE COMPOSITION OF MEATS CAUSED BY COOKING

Meat		*Protein* (*g/100 g*)	*Water* (*g/100 g*)	*Fat* (*g/100 g*)	*kcal* (*per 100 g*)	*Pcal %*
Retail cuts:						
	Beef	6.3 ± 1.3^{a}	-10.6 ± 1.4^{a}	4.2 ± 1.8^{a}	65 ± 14^{a}	2.5 ± 0.8^{a}
	Pork	7.0 ± 0.5^{a}	-11.8 ± 0.9^{a}	4.6 ± 1.0^{a}	72 ± 9^{a}	3.5 ± 0.6^{a}
	Lamb	6.2 ± 1.1^{b}	-10.5 ± 0.4^{a}	4.0 ± 1.2^{b}	62 ± 6^{a}	3.1 ± 1.1^{c}
	Veal	7.9 ± 0.8^{a}	-11.1 ± 1.0^{a}	2.7 ± 1.8^{b}	62 ± 9^{a}	2.9 ± 0.5^{a}
Variety meats:						
	Beef	5.4 ± 6.4^{c}	-11.0 ± 8.1^{b}	3.8 ± 3.3^{b}	68 ± 44^{b}	-0.2 ± 6.0^{d}
	Pork	7.4 ± 4.5^{b}	-9.4 ± 6.0^{b}	2.1 ± 2.4^{b}	47 ± 38^{b}	0.5 ± 6.5^{d}
	Lamb	7.2 ± 4.0^{b}	-9.2 ± 6.9^{b}	4.8 ± 3.2^{b}	54 ± 39^{b}	-0.3 ± 5.7^{d}
	Veal	8.2 ± 5.2^{b}	-9.9 ± 6.6^{b}	1.9 ± 2.7^{d}	52 ± 38^{b}	1.0 ± 5.7^{d}

Values shown are changes with cooking (Rice, 1978).
Paired '*t*' tests used for testing differences between means; $^{a}P < 0.001$; $^{b}P < 0.01$; $^{c}P < 0.05$; ^{d}Non-significant.

coefficients of variation (CV%), are shown in Table 12-12. Considerable compositional variation occurs, however, for both raw and cooked cuts even within these categories. The data for protein, fat and food energy are those presently tabulated in the Massachusetts Nutrient Data Bank (Hoover, 1987). Not surprisingly the coefficients of variation are large, being often in excess of 50%. The increase that occurs in protein and in Pcal % following cooking can also be observed from Table 12-12 and this summary amplifies further the data shown in Table 12-10. The potential, high degree of variability emphasizes the importance of accurately identifying meat cuts, if realistic estimates of protein, fat and food energy values are desired. Amino acid composition data are also shown in Table 12-12. Here coefficients of variation cannot be given because frequently only one or two analyses, expressed as mg/g protein, served as the basis for calculating data expressed as mg per 100 g of meat product of interest. Nevertheless, these data reflect the general similarity in the amino acid composition of muscle meat among the various economically important meat-producing species. This point is further illustrated in Table 12-13 where it can be seen that only for blood and skin are the differences in amino acid composition of these protein sources significant in comparison with those of the other meat products listed. The tryptophan levels appear to be somewhat more variable than those for other amino acids, which probably more reflects the poor analytical quality of the tryptophan data rather than indicating true differences in the amino acid composition of the products shown here. The generally high levels for the major indispensable amino acids, lysine, total sulfur amino acids, threonine and tryptophan, also should be noted. In our view, meats are of major or potential importance in meeting daily lysine needs, as we discuss below.

From the foregoing, it is to be concluded that the amino acid composition of meat protein is relatively constant regardless of the cut or organ from which the meat is obtained. A notable exception is for meats containing large amounts of connective tissue, because of the distinctly different amino acid composition of collagen and elastin. We have discussed this point more extensively elsewhere (Pellett and Young, 1984), in relation to the nutritional quality of mechanically-deboned meats and poultry, that are likely to be high in connective tissue proteins.

Finally, with reference to the amino acid composition of meats, it appears that the amino acids of meats are quite resistant to the effects of cooking. However, tests with experimental animals have shown that extended heat processing (16 h in steam at 121°C) can lead to reduced availability of lysine, methionine and tryptophan (Rice, 1978) and so severe

TABLE 12-12

COMPOSITION OF MEATS IN MAJOR USDA CATEGORIES

USDA categories	*Raw/cooked*	*N*[a]	*Protein (per 100 g)*	*Fat (g per 100 g)*	*Kcal (per 100 g)*	*Pcal %*	*(mg/g protein)*			
							Lys	*SAA*	*Thr*	*Try*
21 Beef										
211 Beef steak + bone	R	45	18·7 (15)[b]	19·4 (65)	255 (40)	36·3 (50)	87	37	44	12
	C	47	26·4 (16)	21·4 (63)	306 (34)	40·3 (44)	87	37	44	12
212 Beef steak w/o bone	R	14	19·2 (14)	16·9 (74)	234 (43)	40·9 (51)	87	37	44	12
	C	13	27·4 (15)	17·6 (75)	276 (37)	46·3 (42)	87	37	44	12
22 Pork										
221 Pork chops	R	13	19·3 (11)	15·1 (61)	218 (34)	40·9 (44)	98	37	46	13
	C	44	27·0 (14)	20·9 (36)	304 (19)	37·4 (29)	98	37	46	13
223 Ham	C	31	21·1 (18)	14·0 (67)	218 (37)	43·5 (34)	88	38	45	12
226 Bacon	R	7	6·3 (58)	69·7 (30)	656 (26)	4·7 (85)	80	27	35	8
	C	9	18·0 (59)	52·9 (59)	539 (45)	23·6 (91)	79	31	37	9
23 Lamb/veal/game										
231 Lamb	R	30	17·1 (13)	18·5 (60)	240 (38)	34·6 (49)	81	37	46	13
	C	24	24·7 (14)	19·2 (62)	279 (33)	40·7 (41)	81	37	46	13
232 Veal	R	22	18·6 (7)	15·0 (46)	214 (27)	37·2 (27)	84	35	43	13
	C	12	23·8 (16)	13·0 (58)	219 (34)	46·3 (46)	84	35	43	13
24 Poultry										
241 Chicken	R	38	18·5 (19)	12·7 (96)	194 (50)	46·7 (44)	82	39	42	11
	C	86	26·2 (14)	12·5 (41)	231 (20)	47·4 (27)	82	40	42	11
242 Turkey	R	53	20·3 (13)	8·1 (104)	160 (41)	57·2 (32)	90	39	43	11
	C	60	26·8 (14)	8·1 (64)	190 (23)	59·0 (23)	91	39	43	11
25 Organ meats/sausages, etc.										
251 Organ meats	R	54	16·6 (15)	9·4 (86)	160 (41)	48·2 (37)	78	36	44	12
	C	46	24·3 (24)	11·4 (75)	213 (34)	51·0 (35)	76	37	44	12
252 Sausages, luncheon meats	C	93	15·6 (22)	22·2 (44)	277 (31)	256 (49)	81	37	42	10

Composition taken from Massachusetts Nutrient Data Bank.

[a] *N*-number of food items in category.

[b] Coefficient of variation (%).

TABLE 12-13
AMINO ACID COMPOSITION (mg/g protein) OF VARIOUS MEATS AND MEAT PRODUCTS

	His	*Iso*	*Leu*	*Lys*	*SAA*	*AAA*	*Thr*	*Trp*	*Val*
Beef (various cuts)	35	52	82	87	37	75	44	12	56
Steak	34	45	79	83	37	72	44	11	49
Corned beef	32	43	73	76	36	68	39	9	44
Beef blood	88	18	128	149	44	101	59	7	97
Beef heart	26	51	89	82	34	82	46	13	58
Beef liver	27	52	92	75	36	88	48	15	63
Beef tongue	25	48	78	83	34	74	43	12	51
Sausage	32	43	73	77	36	69	38	9	44
Veal	32	53	73	84	35	77	43	13	52
Salami pork/beef	31	42	76	80	37	69	42	9	47
Pork (various cuts)	51	48	81	89	37	76	47	13	54
Cured ham	32	50	77	84	40	77	41	10	52
Fresh ham	48	47	81	98	37	74	46	13	54
Canned ham	39	43	78	86	38	71	45	11	45
Canadian bacon	36	38	70	79	40	63	40	10	40
Pork sausage	32	50	77	84	40	77	41	10	52
Pork lunch meat	29	46	77	76	44	72	40	10	53
Pork spam	33	51	76	81	35	74	49	14	52
Lamb (various cuts)	28	52	77	81	37	75	46	13	49
Duck	25	47	78	79	41	74	41	12	49
Turkey	30	50	78	90	39	77	44	11	52
Chicken meat	31	49	73	80	40	71	41	11	49
Chicken skin	19	32	59	60	37	56	36	8	42
Chicken leg	29	50	73	82	40	71	41	11	49
Chicken breast	31	53	75	85	40	73	42	12	50
Goose	26	51	84	86	42	80	43	14	52

Source: Massachusetts Nutrient Data Bank (Hoover, 1987) and USDA (1976–86).

processing conditions should thus be avoided. Some of the general effects of processing on nutritive value of proteins have been reviewed by Ford (1973) and Tannenbaum (1974) and for meat proteins by Hamm (1970). Also the possible importance of protein digestibility and bioavailability of amino acids in mechanically deboned meats have been discussed by Carpenter (1984). There is little evidence that processing, such as canning, and careful dehydration have significant effects on digestibility and nutritive value of meat proteins. Rapid freezing methods and lyophilization of meat products also do not result in significant changes in their protein nutritional value. This is also true in the case of ionizing radiation used for the preservation of meats (Rice, 1978). This is not to say that changes do not occur, but rather that careful treatment does not cause significant deleterious effects. It should be noted however, that under conditions sufficient to cause major browning (Maillard reaction), including long term storage at elevated temperatures, there can be a deterioration in nutritional value, especially with respect to lysine availability. This, however, is more likely to be a problem with milk-based products which contain both high levels of lactose and lysine-rich proteins (Finot, 1983).

IV. GLOBAL ASPECTS OF MEAT PROTEIN PRODUCTION AND CONSUMPTION IN RELATION TO PROTEIN AND AMINO ACID NUTRITION

Having considered above the protein and amino acid needs in humans and the protein and amino acid composition of meats, it is now appropriate to attempt to interrelate these two areas. Hence, we will consider in this section the diets, and contribution made by meat proteins to protein and amino acid intakes and requirements, in various populations.

Food consumption patterns differ considerably in different regions of the world. In Table 12-14, using data from the Fifth World Food Survey (FAO, 1985) we illustrate the share of the total dietary energy supplied by the major food groups in different geographical regions of the world. In the economically richer regions of the world, those with developed market economies, some 30% of the food energy is supplied from animal products with 70% from vegetable products. In contrast, in the poorer regions of the world, such as Africa and the Far and Near East, more than 90% of the food energy may be provided from vegetable products, with less than 10% originating from animal foods. The situation with regard to the place of meat in the diet is even more extreme; some 15% of the food energy is provided from meat products is available in developed market economies but less than 3% from these products in Africa and the Far East (Table 12-14). This uneven distribution throughout the world, with respect to meat availability, is also illustrated in Fig. 12-2, based on food balance data for 145 countries (FAO, 1984). For 45 of these countries average meat availability is less than 50 g a day with, values for India, Indonesia and Sri Lanka, being as little as or lower than 10 g daily. At the other extreme, for example, the United States, New Zealand, Argentina and, perhaps, surprisingly Mongolia, averages of more than 300 g per day of meat are available for consumption. Estimated 'consumption' data based on USDA (1988a) information for the United States gives a value of 275 g a

TABLE 12-14

SHARE OF THE MAJOR FOOD GROUPS IN TOTAL DIETARY ENERGY SUPPLY BY REGION AND ECONOMIC GROUP[a]

	Developed market economies	*E. Europe USSR*	*Africa*	*Far East*	*Latin America*	*Near East*	*Asian CPEs*[b]	*Developing market economies*	*LDCs*[c]	*World*
Vegetable products	68·3	72·9	93·5	94·2	82·9	89·3	90·0	91·4	93·3	83·7
Cereals	26·4	37·5	46·7	67·4	40·2	58·2	66·9	57·7	65·0	50·2
Pulse, nuts	2·4	1·4	7·0	5·9	4·9	3·8	3·5	5·6	6·5	3·9
Root, tubers	3·7	6·0	19·8	3·0	5·6	1·8	12·0	6·2	8·3	6·9
Sugar	13·0	13·0	5·2	8·4	17·2	9·9	1·8	9·7	3·8	9·1
Vegetable, fruits	4·8	3·6	4·8	3·3	5·4	6·4	2·2	4·4	3·8	4·0
Other[d]	18·0	11·4	10·0	6·2	9·6	9·2	3·6	7·8	5·9	9·6
Animal products	31·7	27·1	6·5	5·8	17·1	10·7	10·0	8·6	6·7	16·3
Meat, offal	15·3	9·9	2·8	1·2	8·1	4·0	7·4	3·1	2·7	7·6
Milk	8·5	8·5	2·0	2·5	5·5	3·7	0·5	3·1	2·5	4·4
Eggs	1·6	1·5	0·3	0·2	0·8	0·4	0·7	0·4	0·2	0·9
Fish	1·6	1·4	0·8	0·7	0·7	0·3	0·5	0·7	0·5	0·9
Animal oils and fats	4·7	5·8	0·7	1·1	2·0	2·3	0·9	1·3	0·8	2·5

[a] FAO (1985), data for 1979–81.

[b] Centrally planned economies.

[c] Less developed countries.

[d] Other comprises, vegetable oils and fats, stimulants, spices and alcoholic beverages.

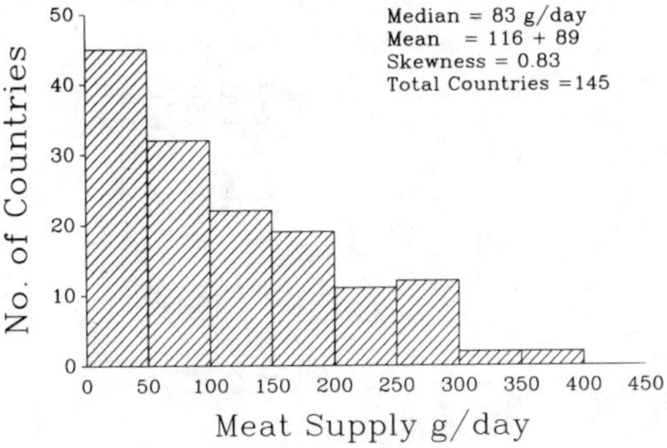

FIG. 12-2. Distribution frequency of daily meat supply in 145 countries. Data source: FAO (1984).

day, which is similar to those of FAO (1984). These values are based on 'availability' data.

The variable distribution of meat availability or consumption in the different regions are emphasized further in Table 12-15 where health, wealth and dietary data for 130 countries have been tabulated. From the broad relationships illustrated here, it can be seen that as wealth (indicated by *per caput* gross national product (GNP)) increases, health indicators such as the mortality rate of children under five years and the prevalence of births of low weight infants decline. Dietary differences associated with these changes are increases in total protein per day, in animal, meat and milk protein per day, and in the percentage of animal and meat protein in relation to total dietary protein. Other associated dietary changes involve total fat and retinol intakes. A further elaboration of these relationships is shown in Table 12-16, where we have summarized the results of linear regression analysis performed on the data from the same countries used in constructing Table 12-15. All correlation coefficients shown in Table 12-16 are highly significant ($P < 0{\cdot}001$). Other correlates such as social and health variables have been discussed elsewhere (Pellett, 1987) but we feel that it is worth pointing out that as *per caput* GNP increases, total protein, animal protein, milk protein and dietary lysine concentration all increase. In addition, as total dietary protein availability increases, there is a rise in the amount and proportion of the total protein from animal protein foods and, particularly, from meat proteins. The lysine concentration of the protein of mixed diets also increases as more protein, more animal protein and more meat protein are available. It must be emphasized that while the significant relationships presented here between health data and dietary factors

TABLE 12-15

HEALTH, WEALTH AND DIETARY DATA FOR 130 COUNTRIES GROUPED ON THE BASIS OF THEIR UNDER-FIVE MORTALITY RATES

Group	*No. of countries*	*Population (million)*	*GNP per caput (US $)*	*Under-five mortality rate*	*% of children <5 yrs*	*Low birth weight (%)*	*Total prot. (g/d)*	*Animal prot. (%)*	*Meat prot. (g/d)*	*Meat prot. (%)*	*Milk prot. (%)*	*Fat (g/d)*	*Retinol (μg/d)*	*Food energy (% of req.)*
1	32	462	295	227	18	16	53	21	6	11	6	33	140	91
2	32	1 498	1 623	130	17	13	62	25	8	12	7	51	190	101
3	30	1 032	2 207	58	14	11	70	37	15	19	10	63	260	111
4	36	1 165	7 817	15	8	6	94	57	26	27	19	126	620	129

Source of data: FAO (1984) and UNICEF (1987).

TABLE 12-16

CORRELATION MATRIX BETWEEN WEALTH, DEMOGRAPHIC AND DIETARY DATA FOR 130 COUNTRIES[a]

	IMR	*Under 5 years (%)*	*Prot. (g/d)*	*Animal prot. (g/d)*	*Animal prot. (%)*	*Meat prot. (g/d)*	*Meat prot. (%)*	*Milk prot. (g/d)*	*Fat (g/d)*	*Lysine*[b] *(m/g prot.)*
GNP US$ *per caput*	−0·61	−0·59	0·68	0·78	0·73	0·67	0·62	0·72	0·78	0·73
Infant mortality rate		0·78	−0·70	−0·75	−0·75	0·66	−0·62	−0·65	−0·70	−0·74
Percentage of population under 5 years			−0·67	−0·74	−0·69	−0·64	−0·56	−0·66	−0·74	−0·69
Protein (g/day)				0·88	0·74	0·83	0·69	0·81	0·85	0·73
Animal protein (g/day)					0·95	0·92	0·86	0·90	0·91	0·93
Animal protein (%)						0·87	0·88	0·85	0·83	(0·98)[c]
Meat protein (g/day)							0·96	0·76	0·83	0·85
Meat protein (%)								0·68	0·74	0·85
Milk protein (g/day)									0·88	0·84
Fat (g/day)										0·81

[a] Number of data pairs vary between 109–130, depending on the variable. All R values $P < 0{\cdot}001$. Data from FAO (1984) and UNICEF (1987).

[b] Lysine (mg/g protein) calculated from multiple regression equation—Lys = 0·57 AP% + 0·33 PP% + 31·3, derived from data for 20 countries ($R^2 = 0{\cdot}86$) AP% and PP% are percentages of total protein from animal protein and pulse protein (includes soybean) respectively.

[c] Animal protein % is the major component in the prediction equation.

TABLE 12-17

WORLD POPULATION AND MEAT PRODUCTION IN VARIOUS REGIONS

Countries	Population 1985 (millions)	Meat production					
		Total Million (metric tons)	Per capita (kg)	Approximate percentages			
				Cattle	Sheep	Pigs	Poultry
Developed							
North America	264·2 (1·0)	28·2 (1·4)	106·8	43	1	25	30
Western Europe	377·4 (0·4)	31·0 (2·4)	82·0	32	4	46	20
Oceania	19·0 (1·4)	3·7 (1·2)	196·0	50	31	9	10
Eastern Europe and USSR	392·4 (0·8)	27·1 (2·5)	69·0	36	5	44	15
Developing							
Africa	449·0 (3·0)	5·0 (2·4)	11·2	48	15[a]	9	28
Far East	1 379·4 (2·3)	6·3 (3·9)	4·6	15[b]	13[a]	57	16
Latin America	406·2 (2·4)	15·3 (2·8)	37·6	56	3	19	22
Near East	240·2 (2·8)	4·4 (4·2)	18·2	37	28	<1	35
Developing countries	3 632·8 (2·2)	52·1 (4·0)	14·3	44	12	22	23
Developed countries	1 210·5 (0·8)	94·8 (2·2)	78·3	37	4	37	21

Source: FAO (1986), USDA (1988*b*).

[a] Includes goat.

[b] Includes buffalo.

Note: Values in parentheses for population and production data are the annual rates of change.

including protein source and lysine content are of interest, they must not be considered causal, since all are directly or indirectly related with wealth as expressed as GNP. The point being made is simply that meat proteins are major contributors to the availability of total protein and lysine in diets, particularly in those of populations that are more affluent and where infant and childhood mortality rates are low.

The large differences in the presence of meat in diets among various regions are also illustrated in Table 12-17, where production data shows a 5-fold greater value for the developed countries, considered as a group, as compared to developing countries. Nevertheless, for all regions in the world, it appears that meat production is generally increasing at a faster rate than population growth. One exception, that is all too common for many food and health related statistics, is the continent of Africa. Also shown here are approximate estimates of the total meat production contributed separately by cattle, sheep, pigs and poultry. These data indicate a slight excess in cattle as compared to pig production, but other data (USDA, 1988b) are somewhat at variance with this and show about 42% of world meat production originating from pigs with 32% from cattle. In the United States over the last decade (Table 12-18) there has been a dramatic increase in poultry production. Parallel changes can also be shown for Nigeria, which we give here as an example of a developing country. Of course the changes in this latter country begin from a much lower base level than is the case of the US. Beef production in the United States has declined to a small extent over the same time period, but in contrast, beef production has increased in Nigeria.

TABLE 12-18

CHANGES IN MEAT PRODUCTION (MILLION METRIC TONS) 1976–1986 FOR UNITED STATES AND NIGERIA

	United States			*Nigeria*		
	1976	*1986*	*% change*	*1976*	*1986*	*% change*
Beef	11·7	11·3	−4	0·17	0·23	+35
Lamb	0·15	0·15	0	0·15	0·18	+20
Pork	5·9	6·4	+8	0·04	0·05	+25
Poultry	5·6	8·3	+48	0·13	0·22	+69
Total	23·4	26·1	+12	0·49	0·68	+39

Source: USDA (1988b).

TABLE 12-19

FOOD ENERGY, PROTEIN AND INDISPENSABLE AMINO ACIDS IN DIETS OF TWENTY SELECTED COUNTRIES COMPARED WITH GNP AND THE UNDER-FIVE MORTALITY RATE (MR)

Country	Under-five MR	GNP (US$)	Dietary energy (kcal/day)	Protein (g/day)	Animal protein (g/day)	Percentage of total protein					(mg/g protein)				Lys (mg/d)
						Animal	Meat	Milk	Cereal	Pulse	Lys	SAA	Thr	Try	
Sierra Leone	302	310	1 938	42	10	24	5	3	52	11	54	41	42	12	2 270
Rwanda	214	280	2 274	54	4	6	5	2	12	48	52	29	34	11	2 810
Yemen Arab Rep.	210	550	2 475	77	17	22	10	8	63	10	44	34	35	12	3 390
Bangladesh	116	130	1 837	40	5	13	4	3	79	2	44	36	34	12	1 760
Nigeria	182	730	2 178	55	11	19	8	2	50	10	42	36	37	12	2 480
Pakistan	174	380	2 180	56	13	24	6	16	66	5	40	34	33	11	2 240
Ghana	153	350	1 769	41	13	32	11	1	37	10	48	34	35	11	1 970
Indonesia	126	540	2 372	49	6	12	3	1	67	11	46	42	41	44	2 250
Tunisia	110	1 270	2 763	76	17	22	8	9	61	16	44	34	32	12	3 340
Guatemala	109	1 160	2 138	58	13	24	13	9	58	12	46	33	38	10	2440
Ecuador	92	1 150	2 114	50	26	51	21	16	31	6	62	37	40	12	3 100
Syria	71	1 620	3 005	85	22	26	10	13	51	7	46	34	33	12	3 910
Paraguay	64	1 240	2 839	80	33	41	32	6	27	18	61	34	37	11	4 800
Thailand	55	860	2 330	47	12	26	11	2	59	3	51	44	43	11	2 400
Yugoslavia	31	2 100	3 550	103	39	37	20	13	51	4	52	35	35	12	5 360
Portugal	22	1 970	3 204	85	35	41	22	8	43	3	59	36	38	11	5 020
Hungary	21	2 110	3 484	95	49	52	30	15	35	<1	65	36	38	12	6 180
Greece	28	3 770	3 668	108	52	49	23	17	35	4	60	35	36	12	6 480
Austria	13	9 140	3 575	91	57	63	36	19	24	1	68	36	39	12	6 190
United States	13	15 390	3 641	106	72	68	39	21	18	1	70	36	40	12	7 420

Note: Mortality rates (MR) for under five-year-old children and infants, GNP taken from UNICEF (1987). Energy and protein data from FAO (1984). Pulse protein percentages were calculated by including soybean from the nut and oilseed category.

As already alluded to above, the pattern of dietary consumption, especially the amount of animal protein, is a significant determinant of dietary amino acid supply, which is illustrated in Table 12-19, using data for 20 countries. For present purposes, we selected these countries, except for the US, at random from the stratified UNICEF (1987) tabulation of 130 countries. Thus, we chose five countries from each of four groups classified on the basis of the mortality rate of children under five years. This also, in effect, classified them on economic status, since child mortality rates and GNP show a high correlation (Table 12-16). Between 35 and 70 food items were used to generate the values given in Table 12-19. These items reflect the major contributors to the protein in diets as judged from food balance sheets (FAO, 1984).

From the data for 20 countries it is possible to describe the broad relationships between dietary pattern and *per caput* GNP, which expand to some degree on the conclusions drawn earlier by Perissé *et al.* (1969). Thus, as wealth increases, so does total protein availability, the percentage of that protein derived from animal foods and especially the availability of meat (Tables 12-15 and 12-16). These relationships are extended here, however, to considerations of the concentrations of indispensable amino acids and, in particular, of lysine in the diet. Thus, in the US 68% of the dietary protein is derived from animal sources, with 39% coming from meat (Table 12-19). In contrast, in Bangladesh nearly 80% of protein is derived from cereals with only 13% from animal sources (4% from meat products). As total protein, animal protein and meat protein availability decrease so also does the dietary lysine concentration ($P < 0{\cdot}001$). Furthermore, it appears that lysine is the amino acid whose supply could perhaps be marginal, from a nutritional health standpoint, in the poorer countries, at least in relation to our proposed amino acid requirement pattern of 50 milligram lysine per gram protein (Pellett and Young, 1988a). (See also Table 12-5).

The important role of animal foods in supplying a significant proportion of total lysine intake is further evident from the use of multiple regression analysis shown in Table 12-20. Using lysine (mg/g protein) as the dependent variable, the simple prediction equation:

$$\text{Lysine (mg/g prot.)} = 0{\cdot}57\,\text{AP}\,\% + 0{\cdot}33\,\text{PP}\,\% + 31{\cdot}3$$

can be derived, where AP % and PP % are the percentages of the total protein provided by animal foods and pulses (including soybean), respectively. About 76% of the correlation was due to the animal protein percentage and this increased to 86% by including pulse protein percentages. We then dissected the animal protein into its individual

TABLE 12-20

MULTIPLE REGRESSION ANALYSIS OF DATA FOR TWENTY COUNTRIES RELATING DIETARY PROTEIN COMPONENTS AND LYSINE VALUE

Dependent variable lysine: mg/g protein

Animal	*Meat*	*Milk*	*Pulse*	*Cereal*	*Residual*	*Constant*	*R*	*F*
	(*Protein per cent*)							
0·47[a]						37·5[a]	0·87	56·9
0·57[a]			0·33[b]			31·3[a]	0·93	52·5
0·51[c]			0·25[d]	−0·05[d]		36·3[d]	0·93	33·1
	0·72[a]					41·2[a]	0·89	68·5
	0·55[a]			−0·16[c]		51·3[a]	0·92	47·4
	0·55[a]			−0·15[c]	0·34[c]	48·4[a]	0·94	40·3
	0·65[b]		0·09[d]	−0·09[d]	0·41[d]	42·8[b]	0·94	28·8
	0·76[b]	0·32[d]	0·38[d]	0·06[d]	0·71[d]	26·4[d]	0·95	23·7

Dependent variable lysine: mg/day

Animal	*Meat*	*Milk*	*Pulse*	*Cereal*	*Residual*	*Constant*	*R*	*F*
	(*Protein g/day*)							
87·0[a]						1 588[a]	0·97	268·3
92·0[a]			47·9[b]			1 214[a]	0·98	199·1
93·1[a]			64·8[a]	22·0[b]		443[b]	0·99	253·3
	140·2[a]					1 975[a]	0·96	203·5
	105·3[a]	73·9[c]				1 875[a]	0·97	134·4
	101·9[a]	88·3[b]	28·4[c]			1 664[a]	0·97	97·2
	111·0[a]	71·6[c]	38·3[c]	17·4[d]		1 102[b]	0·98	87·0
	92·5[a]	89·0[b]	75·7[b]	25·0[b]	125·7[b]	286[d]	0·99	117·4

From original data in Table 12-19.
[a] $P<0{\cdot}001$; [b] $P<0{\cdot}01$; [c] $P<0{\cdot}05$; [d] Non-significant.

components of meat, milk, and residual (fish and egg) protein and these values were used for multiple regression analysis, together with pulse and cereal proteins. The results of this analysis (Table 12-20) showed that meat protein percentage (MP%) could also be used as an efficient predictor ($R^2 = 0{\cdot}79$) of dietary lysine concentration. This equation was:

$$\text{Lysine (mg/g prot.)} = 0{\cdot}72\ \text{MP}\ \% + 41{\cdot}2$$

An equation involving meat protein percentage and cereal protein percentage appeared also to be an excellent predictor of lysine value ($R^2 = 0{\cdot}85$) but further complexity did not add greatly to prediction ability. If the dependent variable was changed to lysine expressed in milligrams per day, animal protein and meat protein, expressed in grams per day, were efficient predictors of dietary lysine availability (Table 12-20: bottom). While more dietary detail improved prediction ability, the gains were not practically significant.

The ability of both animal protein concentration and meat protein concentrations to predict the dietary lysine value can be explained by the rather similar content of lysine in all major animal protein foods coupled with the distinctly different concentration of lysine in cereal foods. This point is illustrated in Table 12-21, using data in the Massachusetts Nutrient Data Bank. The information on the variability in amino acid composition within the different food protein groups is shown here for lysine only. These standard deviations should, however, be treated with considerable reservation since the amino acid compositions for the more than 2400 food items in the Data Bank are not all based on individual analytical determinations. Many, in fact, represent values (mg/100 g) for prepared foods that were calculated from a limited number of analytical values obtained for the original meat source, such as beef. Despite the limitations in the available analytical data, the mean amino acid composition data for animal foods in Table 12-21 might be compared with those given earlier in Table 12-13 for the different meat products. It will be noted from this comparison that there is a close relationship between the lysine content of animal protein foods, aggregated as a broad group (Table 12-21), and the lysine content of individual meat and meat products shown in Table 12-13. Indeed this remains true for the majority of the indispensable amino acids in these food protein sources.

TABLE 12-21

INDISPENSABLE AMINO ACID COMPOSITION (mg per g protein) OF SELECTED FOOD GROUPS FROM MASSACHUSETTS NUTRIENT DATA BANK[a]

	No. of items	*Lysine*[b]	*SAA*	*Thr*	*Try*	*Iso*	*Leu*	*AAA*	*Val*
Animal foods	1 233	85 ± 9	38	44	12	50	81	78	55
Legumes	85	65 ± 7	25	40	12	51	79	82	52
Cereals	260	29 ± 7	36	33	10	43	78	80	49
Others	887	48 ± 14	26	36	12	40	62	67	48

[a] Amino acid composition data originate from FAO (1970) and USDA (1976–86).
[b] Mean $\pm$ SD (see text).

V. MEAT AND PROTEIN CONSUMPTION IN THE UNITED STATES

Considerable changes have taken place over the last two decades in the consumption pattern of animal foods. As shown in Fig. 12-3, *per caput* consumption of poultry, fish and dairy products increased and that for red meat and eggs decreased in the US between 1967 and 1986. Total consumption of animal foods and meat, on a *per capita* basis has, however, increased with an estimated 276 g per head per day of meat being consumed in 1988. The increase in pork and poultry has, therefore, more than offset the decline in beef consumption (USDA, 1988a).

Average intakes of meat, poultry and fish for individuals within a given age and sex group in the United States, based on the USDA nationwide food consumption survey (USDA, 1983), are shown in Fig. 12-4. Although these data include fish, the amount consumed is relatively small, being less than 6% of the total average daily consumption and it is generally below 20 g per day. Hence, the data depicted in Fig. 12-4 essentially represent meat and poultry intakes. It can be seen that males between the age of 15 and 50 were the major consumers of meat and poultry products, with female daily consumption levels being considerably lower. These same data, from USDA (1983), but showing a more comprehensive breakdown into the various meat categories, are given in Table 12-22. It can be seen that for

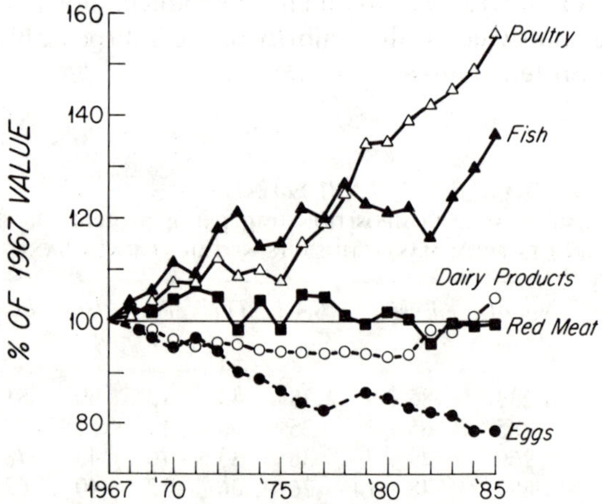

FIG. 12-3. *Per capita* consumption of animal protein foods in the US. Changes between 1967 and 1985 (USDA, 1988a).

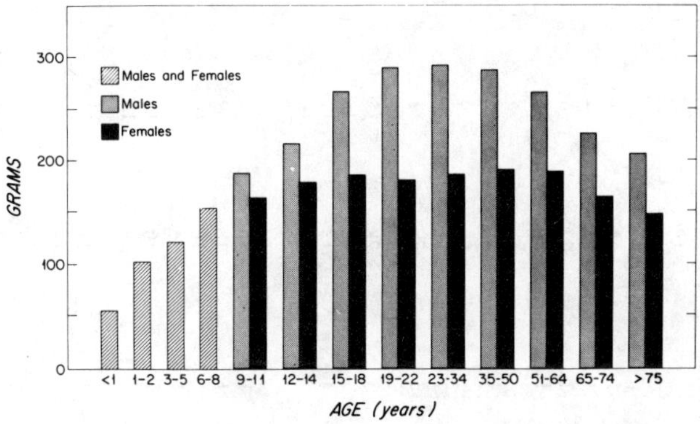

FIG. 12-4. Meat, poultry and fish consumption in the US (average intake per individual per day) (USDA, 1983).

young adult females (age 19–22 years) meat intake is only about 60% of that compared to males within the same age group. Although not shown in Table 12-22, surveys on low income women performed at the same time showed (for the age group 19–22 years) a slightly lower consumption of 174 g of meat products per day. These data originate from a survey for 1977–1978 (USDA, 1983). A more recent survey (USDA, 1986) for data collected during the Spring of 1985 (Table 12-23), still shows essentially similar consumption data for economically disadvantaged women (19–34 years), with the value being 179 g meat, poultry and fish. Hence meat consumption is still relatively high in this less economically privileged sector of the US population.

We have used the 1983 survey data (USDA, 1983) to calculate the protein and amino acid values of diets consumed by various groups within the US population. These estimates are shown in Table 12-24. Some 40 food items were used to calculate the amino acid compositional data for each of the 22 age and sex categories. Also shown in Table 12-24 are amino acid data arranged for various income levels and race. The estimated level of food energy and total protein consumption varies considerably with age and with sex, as would be expected. Nevertheless, a striking feature of this analysis is the constancy of the overall dietary amino acid pattern, as a function of age, sex and income. Furthermore, while the dietary amino acid pattern remained almost constant there was considerable variation in the consumption of different protein foods among the various age and sex groupings. For example, although not shown in Table 12-24, milk consumption was over 600 g per day in 12–18 year old males, but only 230 g

TABLE 12-22

AVERAGE INTAKE[a] PER INDIVIDUAL PER DAY[b] OF MEAT, POULTRY, FISH[a] IN 48 STATES FOR THE PERIOD 1977–78

Sex and age (Years)	*Indiv. no.*	*Total*	*Beef*	*Pork*	*Lamb, veal, game*	*Poultry*		*Organ meat mixtures*	*Franks, sausages, luncheon meats*	*Fish, shellfish*	*Mixtures, mainly meat, fish poultry*
						Total	*Chicken*				
Male and females											
Under 1	421[c]	55	6	3	2	6	5	1	2	—	35
1–2	1 035[c]	103	20	8	1	14	12	1	15	4	40
3–5	1 719	122	27	11	1	16	15	1	17	6	44
6–8	1 841	154	34	13	1	20	18	1	18	7	60
Males											
9–11	939	189	43	16	2	23	20	2	19	8	76
12–14	1 150	216	52	18	1	26	23	1	22	9	84
15–18	1 394	267	66	25	2	30	26	2	25	10	07
19–22	1 030	290	76	25	1	32	28	3	29	14	09
23–34	2 716	292	75	28	3	30	26	2	30	16	07
35–50	2 571	288	78	30	3	31	27	3	28	15	01
51–64	2 161	266	71	29	3	30	27	5	26	18	84
65–74	1 049	226	51	24	4	28	24	4	18	17	79
75 and over	465	206	54	27	4	21	19	3	16	10	70
Females											
9–11	1 011	164	40	14	1	20	18	1	18	6	65
12–14	1 148	179	42	16	1	21	19	1	18	9	71
15–18	1 473	186	45	16	2	22	20	1	16	11	73
19–22	1 317	183	43	19	1	24	22	1	16	11	69
23–34	3 879	187	46	17	2	23	21	2	16	11	69
35–50	3 759	191	51	19	2	24	20	3	14	13	65
51–64	2 936	190	46	19	3	25	22	3	14	14	67
65–74	1 376	165	38	17	4	24	22	3	11	12	55
75 and over	751	148	34	16	3	22	20	3	12	8	51
All individuals	36 142[c]	204	51	20	2	24	22	2	19	12	74

Source: USDA (1983).

[a] Quantities given are for foods as ingested (g/day); no inedible parts are included.

[b] Based on 3 consecutive days of dietary intake.

[c] Excludes breast-fed infants.

TABLE 12-23

MEAT AND POULTRY CONSUMPTION AND PROTEIN-ENERGY VALUE OF LOW INCOME HOUSEHOLDS

Age (years)	*Total (g/d)*	*Beef (g/d)*	*Poultry (g/d)*	*Frank-furters, sausages (g/d)*	*Mixtures: mainly meat, poultry, fish (g/d)*	*Energy (kcal)*	*Protein (g)*	*Food fat (g)*	*Pcal %*	*Fcal %*
Children										
1–3	107	13	16	15	45	1 330	52·8	53·3	15·9	36·1
4–5	119	17	14	18	51	1 523	56·6	60·7	14·9	35·9
All	112	15	15	16	48	1 404	54·3	56·2	15·5	36·0
Women										
19–34	179	26	21	16	80	1 669	65·5	66·8	15·7	36·0
35–50	165	28	21	13	66	1 395	56·4	56·1	16·2	36·2
All	174	26	21	15	75	1 574	62·4	63·1	15·9	36·1

Source: USDA (1986).

per day in elderly females. Consumption of meat foods was 55 g daily for children younger than one year but more than 290 g per day for males in the 19–50 year category. Thus, in the United States, both the amounts and types of protein foods consumed can vary widely in the various age and sex groups, but the amino acid pattern (mg/g protein) remains almost unchanged.

Although amino acid composition data for low income families surveyed in the United States in 1985 were not calculated, the broad similarities between the consumption patterns of animal foods shown in Tables 12-22–12-24 lead to the conclusion that there would be no major problems in amino acid supply even for low income women and children. From this analysis, a major cause of potential concern is not in relation to the dietary protein intake but in reference to the apparently very low levels of food energy intakes for adult females.

Based on these considerations of the amino acid composition of meat proteins and of the impact of these sources of food protein on the amino acid pattern of diets it should be evident that relatively small quantities of animal foods in the diets of children would have a favorable effect on the supply of indispensable amino acids. This point has also been discussed by us previously (Pellett and Young, 1988a) and it is again illustrated in Table 12-25. Thus, the daily consumption of 200 ml milk would supply 8–14% of the daily food energy needs, depending on the age of the child, but could

TABLE 12-24

FOOD ENERGY, PROTEIN, MEAT AND AMINO ACID COMPOSITION OF UNITED STATES DIETS BASED ON USDA DATA

	kcal (per/d)	*Prot. (g/d)*	*Pcal %*	*Fcal %*	*Meat poultry (% prot.)*	*Amino acids mg/g prot.*			
						Lys	*SAA*	*Thr*	*Try*
Males and females (years)									
<1	950	42	17·5	34·0	11·3	69	31	40	12
1–2	1 240	51	16·2	36·9	24·6	71	35	40	12
3–5	1 440	56	15·5	36·7	27·6	70	35	40	12
6–8	1 770	68	15·4	35·3	27·6	69	35	40	12
Males (years)									
9–11	1 950	77	15·7	37·0	30·2	70	35	40	12
12–14	2 170	86	15·9	37·2	30·4	70	35	40	12
15–18	2 440	99	16·1	37·8	33·6	71	35	40	12
19–22	2 240	95	16·9	38·4	38·6	72	35	40	12
23–34	2 320	95	16·3	37·7	38·5	72	35	40	12
35–50	2 200	94	17·0	38·8	41·0	72	35	39	12
51–64	2 100	90	17·2	38·7	40·2	71	35	39	12
65–74	1 890	80	16·9	37·1	36·1	70	34	39	12
75 and over	1 870	77	16·4	37·3	36·8	69	35	39	12
Females (years)									
9–11	1 790	70	15·7	36·9	29·2	70	34	40	12
12–14	1 770	70	15·8	37·2	31·1	71	34	40	12
15–18	1 670	68	16·2	37·5	33·6	71	35	40	12
19–22	1 560	64	16·5	37·4	35·9	72	35	39	12
23–34	1 580	64	16·1	38·2	37·1	71	34	39	12
35–50	1 490	65	17·4	38·3	39·4	71	34	39	12
51–64	1 500	65	17·3	37·3	33·5	70	34	39	12
65–74	1 450	62	17·1	36·5	35·6	69	34	39	12
75 and over	1 460	59	16·2	36·8	34·1	68	34	38	12
Race—all ages, both sexes									
Blacks	1 640	72	17·5	35·0	40·0	71	35	40	12
Whites	1 760	73	16·7	39·0	34·9	71	35	39	12
Income—all ages, both sexes (in thousand $)									
<$6 000	1 610	68	16·9	36·2	35·4	70	35	40	12
$6–10	1 750	73	16·6	37·4	34·6	70	35	39	12
$10–16	1 780	73	16·4	37·9	35·5	71	35	39	12
$16>	1 830	76	16·5	38·6	36·5	71	35	40	12

Calculated from USDA (1983).

TABLE 12-25

ESTIMATED CHILD REQUIREMENTS FOR PROTEIN AND OTHER NUTRIENTS IN RELATION TO INTAKES OF MILK AND MEAT

Age group	*Daily requirement*					*Approximate percentage of daily requirement supply by:*									
						200 ml whole milk					*25 g cooked lamb*				
	Energy (kcal)	*Protein (g)*	*Lysine (mg)*	*Calcium (mg)*	*Vitamin B_{12} (μg)*	*Energy (kcal)*	*Protein (g)*	*Lysine (mg)*	*Calcium (mg)*	*Vitamin B_{12} (μg)*	*Energy (kcal)*	*Protein (g)*	*Lysine (mg)*	*Calcium (mg)*	*Vitamin B_{12} (μg)*
9–12 months	950	14	900	600	0·5	14	46	59	40	>100	5	50	63	<1	80
1–2 years	1 150	14	800	700	0·7	10	46	66	34	100	4	50	71	<1	57
2–4 years	1 350	16	900	800	1·0	9	41	58	30	70	3	44	63	<1	40
4–6 years	1 550	18	1 000	800	1·0	8	37	53	30	70	3	39	56	<1	40

Source: Protein, food energy, and lysine requirements FAO/WHO/UNU (1985); calcium and vitamin B_{12} requirements, NAS–NRC (1980); milk and lamb composition; Pellett and Shadarevian (1970), and Pennington and Church (1985).

supply some 40% of the protein, over 50% of the lysine, 35% of the calcium, and more than 70% of the vitamin B_{12}. Similarly, while 25 g meat would supply less than 5% of the food energy it could provide 45% of daily protein needs, 60–70% of the lysine, and 40–80% of the vitamin B_{12}. Thus, on this basis, meat is of considerable importance, in even small quantities, in supplying lysine to complement predominantly cereal diets that might well be limiting in this amino acid.

VI. SUMMARY AND CONCLUSIONS

In this chapter we have attempted to highlight the value of meat proteins in relation to human protein nutrition. We began with a brief consideration of the requirements for protein and for indispensable amino acids in humans at various ages and then gave an account of the amino acid composition of different meats and meat products. From this treatment it is to be concluded that meat proteins serve as a complete and well-balanced source of amino acids for effectively meeting human physiological requirements. Indeed mixed proteins from beef or meat in general are considered to be among those with the highest protein nutritional value and they serve along with proteins from milk and eggs as a basis for establishing the protein requirements of humans beyond the age of weaning (FAO/WHO/UNU, 1985). We then considered the contribution made by meat proteins to the protein component of diets on a world wide basis and also within the United States. Clearly, there is a very large variation in the contribution made by meat proteins to the availability and intake of total dietary protein among populations in the technically advanced and developing regions of the world. However, it can be shown, from considerations of the amino acid composition of the major food protein sources, that animal proteins and meat protein, in particular, are a major determinant of the lysine content of diets. This indispensable amino acid might well be limiting or marginal in diets of some countries where cereals, such as wheat for example, are the predominant source of the total dietary energy supply. Thus, modest amounts of animal protein foods, including meat, can have a potentially favorable impact on the protein nutritional quality of such diets. Indeed, on this basis alone we (Pellett and Young, 1988a) have concluded that increases in the availability of animal foods, and here we include meat, would be desirable from a nutritional standpoint in a number of developing countries, given the appropriate political will and economic considerations.

In contrast to the foregoing conclusions, there are those that write from a very committed viewpoint and maintain that eating of meat is morally wrong. Admittedly, arguments can be made in favor of a decline in the consumption of certain contemporary meat products, at least in individuals at risk for certain degenerative diseases within affluent populations of western nations, but Wynne-Tyson (1988) goes too far in claiming that there is no medical, nutritional or social justification for the practice of eating meat. We disagree, based on the foregoing, and further point out that the nutritional justification for meat consumption lies in the concentrated package of protein, amino acids, as well as the bioavailable micronutrients, that it provides. Indeed this characteristic allows for meeting human protein nutritional needs within a relatively low dietary volume, a consideration of particular importance in relation to the bulky diets of populations in many developing regions.

While there is no absolute nutritional requirement for meat proteins *per se*, and the same is true for all other food protein sources, meats are in general, not only of high protein nutritional value but also they are supplied by foods, that for many populations, are attractive to human tastes and enjoyable to eat. Their positive nutritional characteristics should not be minimized by the fact that poor dietary habits carry with them actual or potential health risks. Prudent dietary choices, that include meat and meat products are consistent with meeting physiological requirements and supporting long-term health maintenance.

VII. REFERENCES

ARROYAVE, G. (1974). Amino acid requirements by age and sex. In *Nutrients in Processed Foods: Proteins* (P. L. White and D. C. Fletcher, Eds), p. 15. Publishing Sciences Group, Inc., Acton, Mass.

BECHTEL, P. J. (Ed.) (1986). *Muscle as Food.* Academic Press, Orlando, Florida.

BENDER, A. E. (1983). Protein evaluation. Role of Milk Proteins in Human Nutrition (W. Kaufmann, Ed.), Kieler Milchwirtschaftliche Forschungsberichte **35**, 267.

BODWELL, C. E. (1984). The protein nutritional quality of meat and poultry products: Scientific basis for regulation. *Am. J. Clin. Nutr.* **40** (Supplement), 671.

BODWELL, C. E. and ANDERSON, B. A. (1986). Nutritional composition and value of meat and meat products. In *Muscle as Food* (P. J. Bechtel, Ed.), p. 321. Academic Press, Orlando, Florida.

BODWELL, C. E. and MCCLAIN, P. E. (1978). Proteins. In *The Science of Meat and Meat Products*, 2nd edn (J. F. Price and B. S. Schweigert, Eds), p. 78. Food and Nutrition Press, Inc., Westport, CT.

CARPENTER, K. J. (1984). Background paper 2: Possible importance of protein digestibility and bioavailability of amino acids. *Am. J. Clin. Nutr.* **40**, 704.

CASSENS, R. G. (1978). Microscopic structure of animal tissues. In *The Science of Meat and Meat Products*, 2nd edn (J. F. Price and B. S. Schweigert, Eds), p. 11. Food and Nutrition Press, Inc., Westport, CT.

FAO (1970). *Amino Acid Content of Foods and Biological Data on Proteins.* FAO Nutr. Mtg Rep. Ser. No. 37, Food and Agriculture Organization, Rome.

FAO (1984). *Food Balance Sheets 1979–81.* Food and Agriculture Organization, Rome.

FAO (1985). *The Fifth World Food Survey.* Food and Agriculture Organization, Rome.

FAO (1986). *Country Tables : Basic Data on the Agricultural Sector.* Economic and Social Policy Department, Food and Agriculture Organization, Rome.

FAO/WHO/UNU (1985). *Energy and Protein Requirements.* Report of a Joint FAO/WHO/UNU Expert Consultation. Technical Report Series No. 724. World Health Organization, Geneva.

FINOT, P. A. (1983). Chemical modifications of the milk proteins during processing and storage: Nutritional, metabolic and physiological consequences. Role of Milk Proteins in Human Nutrition (W. Kaufman, Ed.), *Kieler Milchwirt. Forschberichte* **35**, 357.

FORD, J. E. (1973). Some effects of processing on nutritive value. In *Proteins in Human Nutrition* (J. W. G. Porter and B. A. Rolls, Eds), p. 515. Academic Press, New York.

GREASER, M. L. (1986). Conversion of muscle to meat. In *Muscle as Food* (P. J. Bechtel, Ed.), p. 37. Academic Press, Orlando, Florida.

HAMM, R. (1970). Properties of meat proteins. In *Proteins as Human Food* (R. A. Lawrie, Ed.), p. 167. AVI Publishing, Westport, CT.

HOOVER, L. W. (1987). *Nutrient Data Bank Directory.* 6th edn. 12th Annual Nutrient Data Book Conference, Houston, Texas, April 1987. University of Missouri Press, Columbia, Missouri.

LAWRIE, R. A. (1979). *Meat Science*, 3rd edn. Pergamon Press, Oxford.

NAS–NRC (National Academy of Sciences–National Research Council) (1980). *Recommended Dietary Allowances*, 9th edn. National Academy of Sciences, Washington, DC.

PEARSON, A. M. (1986). Physical and biochemical changes occurring in muscle during storage and preservation. In *Muscle as Food* (P. J. Bechtel, Ed.), p. 103. Academic Press, Orlando, Florida.

PELLETT, P. L. (1987). Determinants of nutritional status. *Food and Nutrition* **13**(1), 2, FAO, Rome.

PELLETT, P. L. and SHADAREVIAN, S. (1970). *Food Composition Tables for Use in the Middle East*, 2nd edn. American University of Beirut, Beirut, Lebanon.

PELLETT, P. L. and YOUNG, V. R. (1980). *Nutritional Value of Protein Foods.* United Nations University, World Hunger Program; Food and Nutrition Bulletin, Supplement 4. United Nations University, Tokyo.

PELLETT, P. L. and YOUNG, V. R. (1984). Background paper 4: Evaluation of the use of amino acid composition data in assessing the protein quality of meat and poultry products. *Am. J. Clin. Nutr.* **40**, 718.

PELLETT, P. L. and YOUNG, V. R. (1988a). The contribution of livestock products to human dietary needs with special reference to West Asia and North Africa. *Workshop on Small Ruminants in Mediterranean Areas* (E. F. Thomson and

F. S. Thomson, Eds), p. 3. Kluwer Academic Publishers, Dordrecht and International Center for Agricultural Research in Dry Areas—ICARD, Aleppo, Syria.

PELLETT, P. L. and YOUNG, V. R. (1988b). Commentary: Protein and amino acid needs for adults. *Ecol. Food Nutr.* **21**, 321.

PENNINGTON, J. A. T. and CHURCH, H. N. (1985). *Bowes and Church's Food Values of Portions Commonly Used*, 14th edn. J. B. Lippincott Co., Philadelphia.

PERISSÉ, J., SIZARET, F. and FRANCOIS, P. (1969). The effect of income on the structure of the diet. *Nutr. Newsletter* (FAO) **3**, 1.

RICE, E. E. (1978). The nutritional content and value of meat and meat products. In *The Science of Meat and Meat Products*, 2nd edn (J. F. Price and B. S. Schweigert, Eds), p. 287. Food and Nutrition Press, Inc., Westport, CT.

TANNENBAUM, S. (1974). Industrial processing. In *Nutrients in Processed Foods: Proteins* (P. L. White and D. C. Fletcher, Eds), p. 131. Publishing Sciences Group, Inc., Acton, Mass.

UNICEF (United Nations International Children's Emergency Fund) (1987). *The State of the World's Children 1987*. UNICEF, New York, USA.

USDA (1976–86). *Agricultural Handbook No. 8-1* (1976); *8-2* (1977); *8-5* (1979); *8-6* (1980); *8-7* (1980); *8-8* (1982); *8-10* (1983); *8-11* (1984); *8-12* (1986); *8-13* (1986) and *8-14* (1986). Agriculture Research Service, United States Department of Agriculture, Washington, DC.

USDA (1979). *Manual of Food Codes and Conversions of Measurements to Gramweight For Use With Individual Food Intake Data from 1977–78*. Nationwide Food Consumption Survey. US Department of Agriculture, Science and Education Administration, Human Nutrition Center, Consumer and Food Economics Institute, Washington, DC.

USDA (1983). *Food Intakes: Individuals in 48 States, year 1977–1978*. Consumer Nutrition Division Human Nutrition Information Service, US Dept of Agriculture, Hyattsville, JD 20782. Nationwide Food Consumption Survey 1977–78. Report I-1.

USDA (1986). *Nationwide Food Consumption Survey: Low-income Women 19–50 Years and Their Children 1–5 years, 1 Day—1985*. USDA, HNIS, NFCS, CSFII Report No. 85-2, USDA, Hyattsville, MD.

USDA (1988a). *Agricultural Chartbook, US Department of Agriculture, Agriculture Handbook No.* 673. USDA/ARS, Washington, DC.

USDA (1988b). *World Indices of Agricultural and Food Production 1977–86*. Economic Research Service, Statistical Bulletin No. 759. United States Department of Agriculture, Washington, DC.

WAYLER, A., QUEIROZ, E., SCRIMSHAW, N. S., STEINKE, F. H., RAND, W. M. and YOUNG, V. R. (1983). Nitrogen balance studies in young men to assess the protein quality of an isolated soy protein in relation to meat proteins. *J. Nutr.* **113**, 2485.

WILLIAMS, H. H., HARPER, A. E., HEGSTED, D. M., ARROYAVE, G. and HOLT, L. E., JR (1974). Nitrogen and amino acid requirements. In *Improvement of Protein Nutriture*, p. 23. US Food and Nutrition Board, National Academy of Sciences, Washington, DC.

WYNNE-TYSON, J. (1988). *Food for a Future: How World Hunger Could be Ended by the Twenty-First Century*. Thorsons Publishers Ltd, Wellingborough, England.

YOUNG, V. R. (1987). 1987 McCollum Award Lecture: Kinetics of human amino acid metabolism: Nutritional implications and some lessons. *Am. J. Clin. Nutr.* **46**, 709.

YOUNG, V. R. and PELLETT, P. L. (1985). Wheat proteins in relation to protein requirements and availability of amino acids. *Am. J. Clin. Nutr.* **42**, 1077.

YOUNG, V. R. and PELLETT, P. L. (1988). How to evaluate dietary protein. In *Milk Proteins: Nutritional, Clinical, Functional and Technological Aspects* (C. A. Barth and E. Schlimme, Eds), p 7. Springer-Verlag, New York.

YOUNG, V. R. and SCRIMSHAW, N. S. (1978). Nutritional evaluation of proteins and protein requirements. In *Protein Resources and Technology* (M. Milner, N. S. Scrimshaw and D. I. C. Wang, Eds), p. 136. AVI Publishing Co., Westport, CT.

YOUNG, V. R., PUIG, M., QUEIROZ, E., SCRIMSHAW, N. S. and RAND, W. M. (1984a). Evaluation of the protein quality of an isolated soy protein in young men: Relative nitrogen requirements and effect of methionine supplementation. *Am. J. Clin. Nutr.* **39**, 16.

YOUNG, V. R., WAYLER, A., GARZA, C., STEINKE, F. H., MURRAY, E., RAND, W. M. and SCRIMSHAW, N. S. (1984b). A long-term metabolic balance study in young men to assess the nutritional quality of an isolated soy protein and beef proteins. *Am. J. Clin. Nutr.* **39**, 8.

YOUNG, V. R., FAJARDO, L., MURRAY, E., RAND, W. M. and SCRIMSHAW, N. S. (1975). Protein requirements of man: Comparative nitrogen balance response within the submaintenance-to-maintenance range of intakes of wheat and beef proteins. *J. Nutr.* **105**, 534.

YOUNG, V. R., MEQUID, M., MEREDITH, C., MATTHEWS, D. E. and BIER, D. M. (1981). Recent developments in knowledge of human amino acid requirements. In *Nitrogen Metabolism in Man* (J. C. Waterlow and J. M. L. Stephens, Eds), p. 133. Applied Science Publishers, London.

YOUNG, V. R., MEREDITH, C., HOERR, R., BIER, D. M. and MATTHEWS, D. E. (1985). Amino acid kinetics in relation to protein and amino acid requirements: The primary importance of amino acid oxidation. In *Substrate and Energy Metabolism in Man* (J. S. Garrow and D. Halliday, Eds), p. 119. John Libbey, London.

YOUNG, V. R., PELLETT, P. L. and BIER, D. M. (1989). A theoretical basis for increasing current estimates of the amino acid requirements in adult man, with experimental support. *Am. J. Clin. Nutr.* **50**, 80.

13

Fat-Soluble Vitamins: Vitamins A, E, D and K

JOHN EDGAR SMITH
Nutrition Department, Pennsylvania State University, Pennsylvania, USA

I. INTRODUCTION

The vitamins are one of the six essential types of foods. Specifically, they are a group of organic compounds which are required in the diet in milligram or microgram amounts. Although the vitamins are only required in micro-amounts, their omission from the diet can have catastrophic effects. Even today, vitamin deficiencies remain a leading cause of blindness and death in children of third world countries. Traditionally, the vitamins have been divided into two groups based on how they are partitioned in an ether/ethanol–water extraction system. The vitamins that accumulate in the ether phase are known as the fat-soluble vitamins, while those that partition into the ethanol–water phase are called the water-soluble vitamins. The compounds that comprise the fat-soluble vitamins have been divided into four classes based on their biological activity. These classes have been designated as vitamin A activity, vitamin D activity, vitamin E activity, and vitamin K activity. Each of these activities is expressed by more than one compound. Due to their hydrophobic nature the fat-soluble vitamins are present in the fatty portion of the foods. The practice of trimming the fat from meat slightly reduces the content of the fat-soluble vitamins. Nevertheless, most animal fats have low fat-soluble vitamin/calorie ratios, so the net effect of trimming meat fat on fat-soluble vitamin intake may be beneficial.

II. VITAMIN A

A. Compounds with Vitamin A Activity

The compounds that exhibit vitamin A activity belong to two different chemical classifications, the retinoids and the carotenoids. The retinoids are defined as a group of compounds with structures that resemble retinol, while carotenoids resemble *β*-carotene. Only a very few compounds in either of these classifications have vitamin A biological activity. The carotenoids are widely distributed in plants, particularly the green and orange vegetables. *β*-Carotene is the carotenoid with the highest provitamin A activity, and it is the most abundant of the provitamin A carotenoids. Most of the naturally occurring retinoids have vitamin A activity, and they are found in foods of animal origin.

Of the compounds that exhibit full vitamin A activity, retinol and the retinyl esters have the highest biological activity on a molar basis. The activity of retinol is defined as 100% as a reference point. As shown in Fig. 13-1, the main structural features of retinol are a cyclohexene ring, a side chain with four conjugated double bonds, and a terminal alcohol group. In general retinol exists as the all-*trans*-isomer which has the highest biological activity of the various *cis-trans* isomers when given orally.

The retinyl esters are the most abundant retinoids found in nature. While retinyl palmitate is the most plentiful of the retinyl esters, retinyl stearate and retinyl oleate are also present in substantial amounts. A few other long chain retinyl esters are present, but in much smaller amounts.

Retinaldehyde is an important metabolite of vitamin A. The conversion

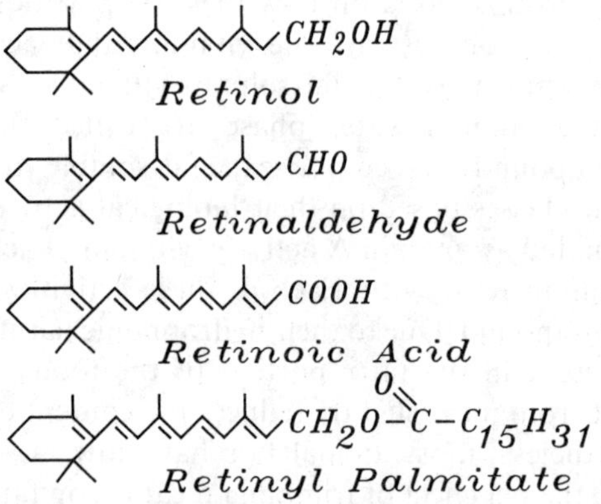

FIG. 13-1. The retinoids with vitamin A activity.

of 11-*cis*-retinaldehyde to the all-*trans* form is the initial event involving it in vision. The biological activity of retinaldehyde is 91% of that observed for retinol (Smith and Borchers, 1972). Retinol and retinaldehyde are freely interconverted enzymatically, but about 9% of the retinaldehyde is converted to retinoic acid.

Retinoic acid is responsible for many of the vitamin A activities. However, retinoic acid does not support the full spectrum of vitamin A activities. It will maintain tissue differentiation and growth, and animals given retinoic acid as their sole source of vitamin A will remain in good health. Nonetheless, it will not support reproduction (Thompson *et al.*, 1964) or vision (Dowling and Wald, 1960) in mammalian species. Recently, retinoic acid has been shown to be produced from retinol in animal tissues in very small, but significant quantities (Napoli and Race, 1987). Retinoic acid is about 10 times more active than retinol in an in-vitro hamster tracheal tissue culture assay (Sporn *et al.*, 1976). In the intact animal the results are a bit less clear. Retinoic acid is rapidly excreted from the animal and is not stored to any significant extent. Thus, when it is given daily it is only about 14% as active as retinol in a growth bioassay (Goodman *et al.*, 1974). In contrast, retinoic acid is equally as active as retinol, if it is given at frequent intervals (6 h or less) (Zile and DeLuca, 1968).

B. Deficiency

In most parts of the world a dormant season exists in which plants do not readily grow. Thus, carotenoids are largely available in the diet on a seasonal basis. Mammalian species have adapted to this environmental challenge by storing vitamin A in the liver during the periods of abundance. Adult humans typically have a liver vitamin A reserve that would last 1–2 years. In contrast young children frequently do not store sufficient vitamin A to carry them through the dormant season. Young children are also more susceptible to diseases, such as diarrhea, measles, and respiratory disease which rapidly deplete their modest vitamin A reserves (Campos *et al.*, 1987; Sommer *et al.*, 1987). By the time they reach school age most of the children have sufficient vitamin A reserves to handle the environmental stresses. In Europe and North America young children rarely develop vitamin A deficiency. In large part, this is due to the animal products in their diets. These products are also available in the diet for the whole year, so the child does not experience a period of extremely low vitamin A intake.

On a world-wide basis vitamin A deficiency remains the leading cause of blindness in children. In Asia alone 5 million children will show some sign of vitamin A deficiency (Tielsch and Sommer, 1984). The problem is most prevalent in children between two and four years of age. The first symptom of vitamin A deficiency to appear is usually nightblindness (Oomen, 1976). Nightblindness is distinguished by the inability to recognize forms or shapes when first placed in a dark environment. It is caused by the loss of vitamin A from the visual pigments of the retina. As the deficiency progresses, conjunctival xerosis (drying) of the eye occurs. The production of tears becomes greatly reduced, and frequently a white foamy conjunctival lesion known as a Bitot's spot appears. When children with xerosis experience stressful conditions such as diarrhea or measles, corneal ulcers frequently develop. This ulceration may be so severe that the lens may protrude from the eye. While the xerosis is readily corrected by the administration of vitamin A, the ulcerations almost always result in the development of a corneal scar which causes blindness.

The immune system is also compromised by mild vitamin A deficiency, so deficient children are much more susceptible to infection. Sommer *et al.* (1986) have shown that at least one-third of deaths in preschool children in Sumatra could be prevented by vitamin A supplementation.

C. Metabolic Function

Vitamin A activity is expressed by two, and possibly more, entirely separate mechanisms. In vitamin A deficiency cellular differentiation is significantly altered (Hayes *et al.*, 1968). Epithelial cells fail to differentiate into the highly-differentiated mucus-secreting cells characteristic of many tissues, and flat squamous cells appear instead. Likewise, mesenchymal cells are arrested in the blast (or synthetic) stage of differentiation. The thick, poorly formed bones that develop in severe vitamin A deficiency are the direct result of the lack of osteoclasts. The osteoblasts synthesize bone matrix at a nearly normal rate, but the essential resorption and remodeling associated with normal bone growth does not occur. When vitamin A is given, osteoclasts appear, and the remodeling process begins. Retinoic acid is the active form of vitamin A in controlling differentiation. Two nuclear receptors that specifically bind retinoic acid have been identified (Giguere *et al.*, 1987; Brand *et al.*, 1988). The exact functions of these receptors have not been defined on a biochemical basis, but some degree of overlap with the thyroxine receptor has been demonstrated (Umesono *et al.*, 1988). Clearly, the process of cellular differentiation is controlled through these nuclear receptors.

The mechanism by which vitamin A supports vision is entirely different. As shown in Fig. 13-2, the all-*trans*-retinol taken up from the plasma is converted to 11-*cis*-retinol and then subsequently to 11-*cis*-retinaldehyde

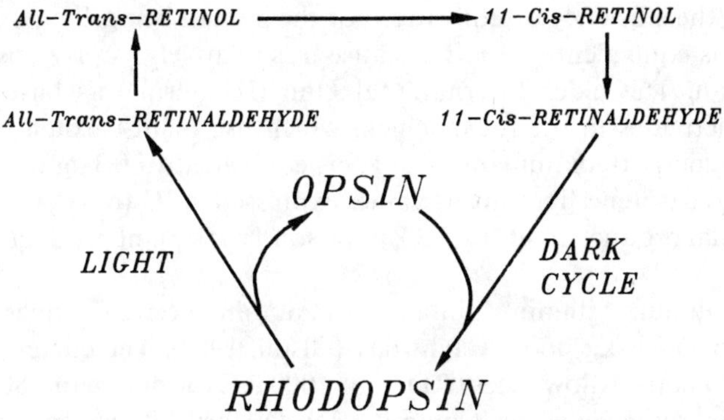

FIG. 13-2. The visual cycle. This figure is based on the classical work of Wald (1968), but also incorporates the newer findings of Bernstein *et al.*, (1987).

in the pigment epithelial cells of the retina (Bernstein *et al.*, 1987). The 11-*cis*-retinaldehyde is transported to the outer segment of the rod cells where it specifically forms a Schiff's base with the lysine at position 297 on the protein rhodopsin (Dratz and Hargrave, 1983). The initial response in vision is the conversion of the 11-*cis*-retinaldehyde to all-*trans*-retinaldehyde. This can be induced by a single photon of light. The 'excited' rhodopsin activates a cascade of events which lowers cyclic GMP and elevates GMP levels within the cell (Zurer, 1983). The change in this ratio closes the sodium channels of the outer segment membrane. The change in sodium permeability of the membrane and the consequent hyper-polarization of the cell generate the nerve impulse, which is sent to the brain. The all-*trans*-retinaldehyde is then released from the rhodopsin and transferred back to the pigment epithelial cells, where it can be converted to all-*trans*-retinol and recycled.

Other mechanisms of vitamin A action may also be possible. Vitamin A deficient rats maintained on diets supplemented with retinoic acid suffer testicular atrophy or fetal resorption (Thompson *et al.*, 1964). These conditions may be the result of some unknown action of vitamin A, or they may reflect the presence of a barrier that retinoic acid does not cross.

D. Vitamin A Requirements

Dietary vitamin A activity is currently expressed in terms of the Retinol Equivalent (RE). One RE is equal to the activity of 1 μg of retinol (Committee on Dietary Allowances, 1980). Other retinoid or carotenoid concentrations are expressed in terms of the equivalent retinol activity, based on the efficiency of utilization for the human being. Thus, 6 μg of β-carotene is equivalent to 1 RE, because it is relatively poorly absorbed in the human. The older International Unit (IU) term was based on the relative activities in the rat or chick, which use plant carotenoids much more efficiently than humans. The IU is equivalent to 0·3 μg of retinol or 0·6 μg of β-carotene. To convert values expressed in IU to RE, if the source is an animal product divide by 3·33, if the source is a plant product divide by 10.

The minimum vitamin A intake to maintain acceptable liver stores is roughly 6·66 RE/kg body weight/day (Olson, 1987). The current Recommended Dietary Allowances (RDA) of 1000 RE for males and 800 RE for females are quite generous (Committee on Dietary Allowances, 1980), and it has been suggested that these should be lowered to 700 RE for males and 600 RE for females (or 9·3 RE/kg body weight) (Olson, 1987). These values are more in line with the median vitamin A intake of the American population.

E. Meat as a Source of Vitamin A

Typical values for the vitamin A content of several meat and fish products are listed in Table 13-1. Quite clearly, liver and fish-liver oils are the richest sources of vitamin A. Fish-liver oils are so rich in vitamin A and D that they have been recognized as a nutritional supplement for over a century. But, they should only be used in very limited amounts due to their very high vitamin content. The value of liver as a source of vitamin A in the diet was conclusively demonstrated by the NHANES II survey data (Block *et al.*, 1985). Although only 1·7% of the test population consumed liver in the 24 h recall survey, it represented 12·5% (or 20% if calculated based on RE) of the total vitamin A activity consumed by the whole population. This was twice the level obtained from any other food. Unfortunately, a large percentage of the population does not eat liver. Exact estimates of the number of people who do not eat liver are not readily available, but a crude estimate can be made. The USDA Nationwide Food Consumption Survey in 1977, found that only 1·2% of the population consumed liver on any given day (Pao *et al.*, 1982). Thus, if the average individual consumes liver about once a month, liver is eaten by about 36% of the population. So, roughly 60% of the population never consumes liver. This is a very crude estimate that may be in error by 10–20%. Liver consumption is also related to family income. Liver was purchased by 9% of US households on a weekly basis (US Department of Agriculture, 1982), with households in the lowest 40th percentile of income purchasing about twice as much liver as

TABLE 13-1

THE VITAMIN A CONTENT OF MEAT AND FISH PRODUCTS[a]

Product	*Vitamin A RE/100 g*	*Type of assay*	*Reference*
Beef steak	10	HPLC	Sivell *et al.* (1984)
Liver, beef	10 728	Source not specified	US Department of Agriculture (1976–1984)
Chicken breast	37	HPLC	Sivell *et al.* (1984)
Chicken leg	60	HPLC	Sivell *et al.* (1984)
Liver, chicken	6 165	Source not specified	US Department of Agriculture (1976–1984)
Loin, pork	3	Source not specified	US Department of Agriculture (1976–1984)
Ham	2	Source not specified	US Department of Agriculture (1976–1984)
Lard	34	Carr–Price; bioassay	Ames and Harris (1954)
Liver, pork	5 399	Source not specified	US Department of Agriculture (1976–1984)
Mackerel	43	HPLC	Sivell *et al.* (1984)
Salmon	33	HPLC	Sivell *et al.* (1984)
Rainbow trout	29	HPLC	Sivell *et al.* (1984)
Cod-liver oil	134 000	Carr–Price	Pugsley *et al.* (1945)

[a] The values are expressed as retinol equivalents (RE). One RE is equal to 1 μg of retinol.

the higher income groups. Much of the liver produced in the United States is exported, so an ample supply exists to expand American consumption of liver. Excessive consumption of liver (more than once every other week) should be avoided, because of its very high vitamin A content. Vitamin A toxicity can develop from eating liver too frequently.

Although liver is a major source of vitamin A, vitamin A is also contained in adipose tissue. The well documented 'lard factor', which has been reported to have a sparing effect on the vitamin A requirement was shown to be simply retinyl esters or retinol present in lard. Using an elaborate analysis system, Ames and Harris (1954) found lard to contain from 15–75 RE/100 g. Since the lipids contained in low vitamin A containing meat products comprise approximately 15% of the caloric intake (Welsh and Marston, 1982), these products may contribute 1–2% of the daily vitamin A intake.

The accurate analysis of biological samples with a high lipid content, relative to the vitamin A content, is extremely difficult and requires elaborate procedures similar to those used by Ames and Harris (1954). Because of difficulties in analysis most of the low vitamin A meat products have not been analyzed for vitamin A by procedures that yield accurate results.

Although meats contain only negligible amounts of the provitamin A carotenoids, the lipids and proteins in meats aid in the absorption of plant carotenoids. For instance, children consuming vegetarian diets have developed symptoms characteristic of vitamin A deficiency. By adding lipids to the diet carotene absorption was increased (Roels *et al.*, 1958). High quality dietary protein has also been shown to improve the utilization of carotene (Berger *et al.*, 1962). Many plants, that are very rich sources of the provitamin A carotenoids, contain almost no triglyceride and only modest amounts of low quality protein. Without dietary triglycerides, the lipid globules and micelles are not formed in the intestine to dissolve the carotenoids and aid in their absorption.

III. VITAMIN E

A. Vitamin E Activity

Vitamin E is known as the antioxidant vitamin. The main identified activity of vitamin E is in the protection of other nutrients and cellular constituents. In fact vitamin E is recognized as 'nature's best fat-soluble antioxidant' (Scott, 1978). The name vitamin E is now used as a general term to describe the biological activity associated with α-tocopherol. Eight naturally occurring compounds exhibit this antioxidant activity. These are divided among two groups: the tocopherols and the tocotrienols. The tocopherols have a phytyl side chain that is entirely saturated, while the tocotrienols have three double bonds in the side chain. The tocopherols have higher biological activities than the corresponding tocotrienols (Leth and Sondergaard, 1977). Four separate vitamers have been identified for both the tocopherols and the tocotrienols. These vitamers differ in the number of methyl groups attached to the aromatic ring. In reality two of these compounds, α-tocopherol and γ-tocopherol, account for most of the vitamin E activity in the typical human diet (Fig. 13-3). α-Tocopherol has the highest biopotency of any of the E vitamers (Joffe and Harris, 1943). However, the shift in the American diet to more corn oil and soybean oil has resulted in higher intakes of γ-tocopherol (Bieri and Evarts, 1974). These oils are quite rich in γ-tocopherol relative to α-tocopherol. However, the biopotency of γ-tocopherol is only about 10% of that of α-tocopherol (Bieri and Evarts, 1974), with the low biopotency of γ-tocopherol being related to its rapid disposal rate. α-Tocopherol is preferentially retained in

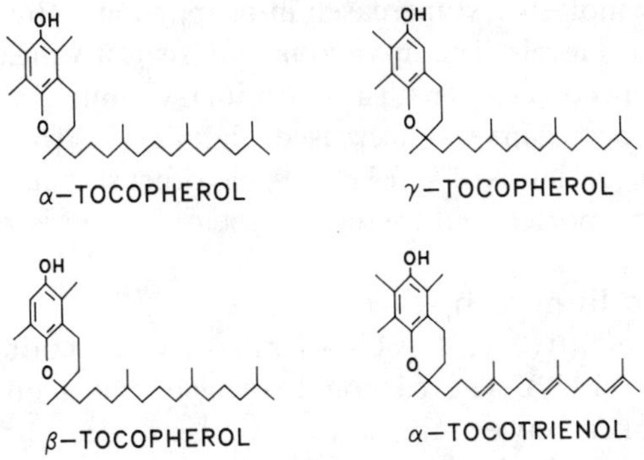

FIG. 13-3. The major compounds with vitamin E activity found in the diet. If the biopotency of α-tocopherol is set at 100%, on a molar basis the activity of β-tocopherol will be 40% (Joffe and Harris, 1943), γ-tocopherol will be 10% (Bieri and Evarts, 1974), and α-tocotrienol will be 16% (Leth and Sondergaad, 1977).

the tissues, which is reflected in the high ratio of α-tocopherol to the other tocopherols in meat products.

B. Deficiency

The clinical symptoms of vitamin E deficiency are quite rare and are mainly observed in individuals with fat absorption problems. Vitamin E deficiency quite commonly develops in children with chronic cholestasis (Sokol, 1988), abetalipoproteinemia (Muller and Lloyd, 1982), or cystic fibrosis (Farrell *et al.*, 1977), unless they are supplemented with very large doses (30–90 mg/kg body weight/day) of vitamin E. These children typically exhibit neurological problems including the loss of deep tendon reflexes, the loss of vibratory sensation in the arms and legs, and ataxia. If the deficiency remains untreated, pigmentary retinopathy and muscular problems develop. Vitamin E deficiency is not the primary cause of any of these diseases, but the deficiency, which occurs secondary to fat malabsorption, does cause some of the more severe problems associated with these conditions. Premature infants also show symptoms of vitamin E deficiency.

Adult humans not suffering from fat absorption problems do not exhibit clinical symptoms of deficiency. However, the serum vitamin E levels of about 5% of the Canadian population were below 0·5 mg/dl according to Desai (1968). Values below 0·5 mg/dl are indicative of a suboptimal vitamin E status.

Horwitt *et al.* (1963) kept a group of adult human subjects on a vitamin E restricted diet (~4 mg of RRR-α-tocopherol per day) for six years. The in-vitro red cell hemolysis test increased in proportion to the decrease in the serum tocopherol levels. The in-vitro hemolysis test values obtained after the first year were consistent with a suboptimal vitamin E status. In the fifth year, the erythrocyte survival decreased slightly. This was associated with serum α-tocopherol levels of $<0{\cdot}3$ mg/dl. No other significant symptoms of deficiency were reported, but these were the only criteria really examined.

C. Metabolic Function

Polyunsaturated fatty acids (PUFA) are very susceptible to oxidative damage (Chow, 1979). The carbon–hydrogen bonds on the methylene carbons positioned between the double bonds are weak, and the hydrogen can be dislodged easily. As shown in Fig. 13-4, the resulting free radicals are vulnerable to oxygen attack. Two major problems are created by the oxidation of these fatty acids. First, the peroxides formed are unstable and

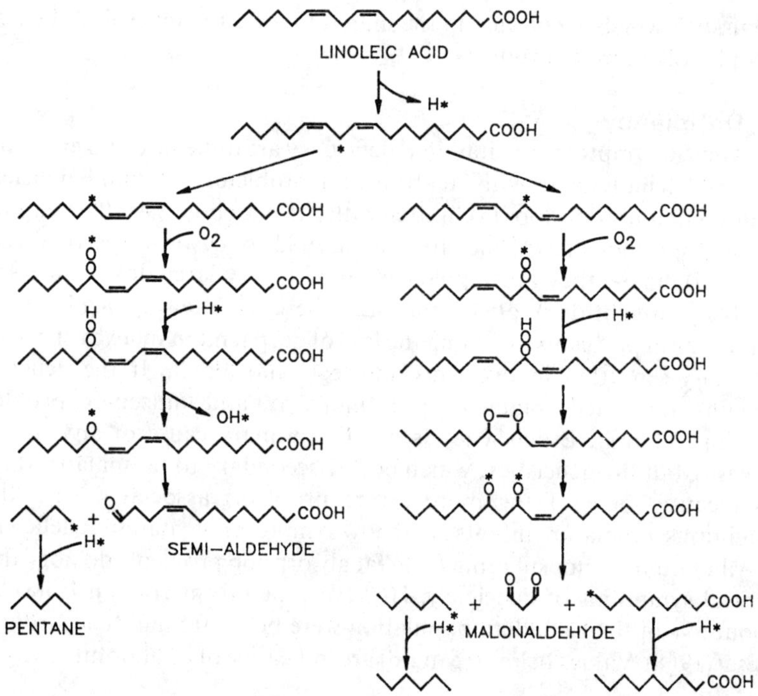

FIG. 13-4. A possible scheme for the autoxidation of linoleic acid. This scheme is based on the scheme of Chow (1979) for the autoxidation of linolenic acid.

break down to very toxic compounds, such as malonaldehyde. Malonaldehyde damages other cellular components, such as proteins and lipids, by forming random cross-linkages between the molecules. The cross-linked regions of these molecules are not biodegradable, so these materials accumulate in the lysosomes of the cell. The second problem created by the oxidation is that the peroxide radicals formed after the oxygen attack are very reactive and will abstract hydrogen from adjacent PUFA. Thus, a series of chain reactions are initiated that will destroy most of the other PUFA. This means that a large amount of malonaldehyde will be formed which will cause substantial tissue damage.

The tocopherols prevent this damage by terminating the chain reactions. As shown in Fig. 13-5, the tocopherols can very easily donate a hydrogen complete with the electron to satisfy the free radicals. After donating the hydrogen the tocopheryl radical can be converted back to tocopherol by ascorbic acid. Alternately the tocopheryl radical can be converted to stable metabolites such as tocopheryl quinone (Csallany *et al.*, 1962). In either event the products formed are stable, and the destruction of additional fatty acids is prevented.

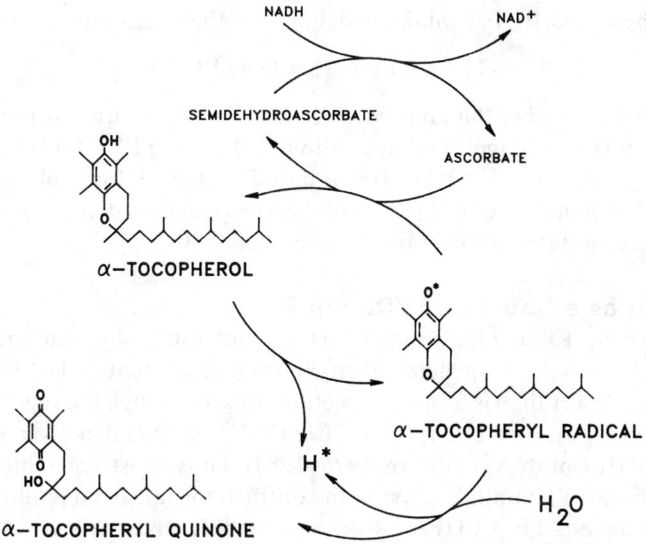

FIG. 13-5. The relationship of vitamin E and ascorbic acid in the prevention of oxidation of polyunsaturated fatty acids. The scheme is based on the studies of Diliberto and Allen (1980), Bascetta *et al.* (1983), and Kunert and Tappel (1983).

In animal studies many of the symptoms of vitamin E deficiency have been prevented by feeding lipid-soluble food grade antioxidants such as butylated hydroxytoluene (Marthedal, 1973). The antioxidant-responsive symptoms can become worse after the level of PUFA in the diet is increased. Many of the symptoms, such as fetal resorption, in-vitro red cell hemolysis, degenerative changes in the cerebellum, and formation of lipofuscins and ceroid pigments appear to be entirely due to the lack of antioxidant activity. Other symptoms which occur in severe deficiency, such as testicular atrophy and anemia, may be related to other functions of vitamin E.

D. Vitamin E Requirements

Total vitamin E activity is expressed in terms of the RRR-α-tocopherol equivalent (α-TE) (Committee on Dietary Allowances, 1980). One α-TE is equivalent to 1 mg of RRR-α-tocopherol. In the older literature vitamin E activity was expressed in International Units (IU). One IU of vitamin E activity was equal to the activity of 1 mg of all-*rac*-α-tocopheryl acetate. To convert IU to α-TE divide by 1·49.

The daily requirement for vitamin E is a function of the intake of PUFA. Horwitt (1986) has suggested that the relationship between the vitamin E requirement and PUFA intake is defined by the equation:

$$\alpha\text{-TE required} = 5 + 0{\cdot}5(\text{g PUFA})$$

This is slightly higher than has been recommended by other workers. Bieri and Evarts (1973) suggested that a ratio of 0·4 α-TE/g PUFA for the whole diet was satisfactory. The RDA for vitamin E is 10 α-TE for adult males and 8 α-TE for females, with higher intakes recommended for high PUFA intakes (Committee on Dietary Allowances, 1980).

E. Meat as a Source of Vitamin E

As shown in Table 13-2, animal fats are not especially rich sources of vitamin E activity. In general, their vitamin E content is 1–2 orders of magnitude lower than is found in vegetable oils. Although the vegetable oils have higher levels of PUFA, the α-TE/g PUFA ratios range from 0·36–2·6 (US Department of Agriculture, 1976–1984). Thus, most vegetable oils are good sources of vitamin E activity. In contrast, the fats from poultry, pork, and fish have α-TE/g PUFA ratios around 0·1, which is well below the recommended ratio for the whole diet. Because beef fat has a very low content of PUFA, it has a more favorable ratio of 0·6. However, the vitamin E content of beef is so low that it alone cannot meet the vitamin E

TABLE 13-2

THE VITAMIN E CONTENT OF MEAT AND FISH PRODUCTS[a]

Product	*Vitamin E α-TE/100 g*	*Type of assay*	*Reference*
Bacon	0·54	Emmerie–Engle	Bunnell *et al.* (1965)
Ham	0·30	Emmerie–Engle	Bunnell *et al.* (1965)
Pork sausage	0·18	Emmerie–Engle	Bunnell *et al.* (1965)
Pork chops	0·20	Emmerie–Engle	Bunnell *et al.* (1965)
Lard	1·2	Source not specified	US Department of Agriculture (1976–1984)
Ground beef	0·40	Emmerie–Engle	Bunnell *et al.* (1965)
Beef steak	0·17	Emmerie–Engle	Bunnell *et al.* (1965)
Liver, beef	0·73	Emmerie–Engle	Bunnell *et al.* (1965)
Chicken breast	0·39	Emmerie–Engle	Bunnell *et al.* (1965)
Cod	1·00	HPLC	Syvaoja *et al.* (1985)
Salmon	2·23	HPLC	Syvaoja *et al.* (1985)
Rainbow trout	1·66	HPLC	Syvaoja *et al.* (1985)
Whitefish	2·67	HPLC	Syvaoja *et al.* (1985)

[a] The vitamin E activity is expressed as α-tocopherol equivalents (α-TE, mg α-tocopherol). In fish, the value is the actual α-tocopherol content as other forms of vitamin E activity were negligible. In meats, α-tocopherol was separated from all other forms of vitamin E, but the other forms were not separated. Since γ-tocopherol is usually the main other form of vitamin E, the α-TE were calculated as the α-tocopherol + (other tocopherols × 0·1).

requirement (Horwitt, 1986). Assuming that animals fats represent 15% of the total caloric intake, they would contribute only 7–8% of the dietary vitamin E intake.

IV. VITAMIN D

A. Vitamin D Activity

Vitamin D is unique among the fat-soluble vitamins in that it can be synthesized in the skin in amounts sufficient to meet the entire metabolic need. When the skin is irradiated with ultraviolet light with a wavelength between 280–320 nm, 7-dehydrocholesterol in the skin is converted to vitamin D_3 (Webb and Holick, 1988). In fact exposure of the face and arms to the direct summer sun for 10–15 min two or three times a week should provide adequate amounts of vitamin D. In winter, sunlight contains less ultraviolet energy so a much longer exposure time is required. Also the body is usually covered with clothing, so the net effect is that much less vitamin D is formed during the winter. Other factors such as atmospheric pollution or the application of sunscreens reduce vitamin D synthesis (Matsuoka *et al.*, 1988).

Although the major source of vitamin D for most people is from synthesis in the skin, exposure to sunlight does not meet the metabolic demands of all of the people all of the time. The main dietary forms of vitamin D are vitamin D_3 (or cholecalciferol) and vitamin D_2 (or ergocalciferol). Several other compounds have been synthesized with vitamin D activity but these are largely laboratory curiosities. Vitamin D_3 and its metabolites are the main naturally occurring forms of the vitamin. However, most foods contain negligible amounts of vitamin D, unless they have been fortified.

B. Deficiency

In vitamin D deficiency intestinal absorption of calcium and phosphorus is impaired, and renal reabsorption of calcium is less efficient (DeLuca, 1978). As a result serum levels of calcium and phosphorus decrease. To maintain other functions essential for life, calcium and phosphorus are removed from the bones. The consequences of depletion of bone minerals are different for people of different ages. The three groups that most commonly exhibit clinical symptoms of vitamin D deficiency are young children, women who have given birth to several children, and the elderly (Haussler and McCain, 1977; Omdahl *et al.*, 1982).

In young children the condition known as rickets develops which is characterized by major deformation of the skeleton. The organic matrix of bone continues to be formed, but the mineral crystals that give bone strength and rigidity are not deposited. As a result, the bones become rubbery and bend to abnormal shapes under the stress of weight bearing. The classical skeletal deformities include: bowlegs or knock-knees, curvature of the spine, and deformities of the pelvis. Typically, the ends of bones, especially at the knees, wrists, ankles, and ribs, become enlarged. Although some correction may occur with therapy, many of these deformities are permanent and may cause problems later in life. A deformed pelvis can prove fatal to a young woman when she becomes pregnant if expert medical care is not available.

In the United States rickets has been brought under control by adding 10 μg of vitamin D to each quart of commercially processed milk. Vitamin D deficiency rickets now mainly occurs in large crowded cities such as Hong Kong and London where the milk is not fortified. Although rickets is quite common in Africa most of this is really due to a dietary calcium deficiency rather than a simple vitamin D deficiency (Lawson *et al.*, 1987). Vitamin D cannot stimulate calcium absorption if calcium is not available in the diet.

In adults vitamin D deficiency causes the condition known as osteomalacia (Barzel, 1983). Although, in adults, the long bones have closed and are not increasing in size at the same rate as in children, the bones are continually undergoing the process of remodeling. After the osteoclasts resorb an area of bone the osteoblasts move in and reform new bone tissue. In osteomalacia calcium and phosphorus are not available to calcify the matrix formed in the remodeling process. This weakens the bone and results in formation of many hairline fractures, which are very painful. Because they are in constant pain the individual develops a waddling gait and a stooped posture that makes them appear quite old.

The elderly population is also at risk to develop osteomalacia (Omdahl *et al.*, 1982; Barzel, 1983). Several studies have shown that many elderly people have serum 25-hydroxyvitamin D levels below those associated with optimal vitamin D status. A number of factors are associated with this suboptimal vitamin D status. Many elderly people do not drink vitamin D fortified milk. The elderly are frequently confined inside and do not have adequate exposure to sunlight. Also, in old people the skin tends to synthesize less vitamin D because it contains less 7-dehydrocholesterol (Webb and Holick, 1988).

C. Metabolic Function

The initial step in activation of vitamin D occurs in the liver parenchymal cells, where vitamin D_3 is converted to 25-hydroxyvitamin D_3 (25-OHD_3 or Calcidiol) (Fig. 13-6). The microsomal enzyme, calciferol-25-hydroxylase, apparently catalyzes the reaction, and the synthesis of 25-OHD_3 is regulated to some limited extent (Delvin *et al.*, 1978).

The active form of vitamin D is synthesized in the kidney by the conversion of 25-OHD_3 to 1,25-dihydroxyvitamin D_3 (1,25-$(OH)_2D_3$ or Calcitriol) (Ghazarian *et al.*, 1973). The production of 1,25-$(OH)_2D_3$ is tightly regulated by the serum levels of phosphate and parathyroid hormone (PTH) (DeLuca, 1978). Since the secretion of parathyroid hormone is controlled by the serum calcium level, the synthesis of 1,25-$(OH)_2D_3$ and the serum calcium levels are inversely related. When serum calcium and phosphate levels are in the normal range 24(R),25-dihydroxyvitamin D_3 (24,25-$(OH)_2D_3$) is the major metabolite of vitamin D formed in the kidney rather than 1,25-$(OH)_2D_3$. While 24,25-$(OH)_2D_3$ is essential to prevent parathyroid hypertrophy (Henry *et al.*, 1977), no clear role in the regulation of calcium or phosphorus metabolism has been given to this metabolite.

The regulation of intestinal calcium absorption is the most extensively

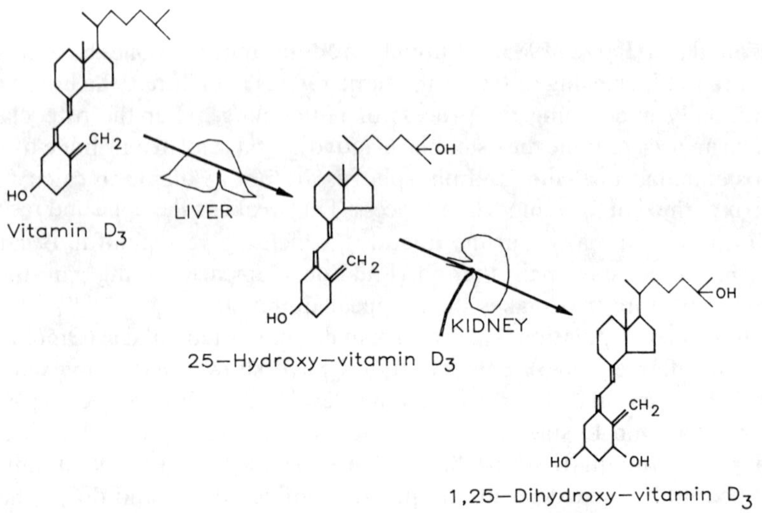

FIG. 13-6. The formation of the active metabolites of vitamin D. This scheme is based on the findings of Ponchon *et al.* (1969) and Lawson *et al.* (1971).

studied function of vitamin D. Intestinal calcium absorption occurs in two ways (Bronner, 1987). The simple passive diffusion of calcium between the cells (through the cell junctions) is not controlled by vitamin D. The energy to drive this process comes strictly from the high level of Ca^{2+} in the intestine. At a calcium intake of 1000 mg per day approximately 255 mg will be absorbed by the passive route (Sheikh *et al.*, 1988). At a lower intake of 500 mg per day passive diffusion will decrease to about 95 mg. However, if the individual has adapted to the level of calcium intake, the total calcium absorbed will be roughly the same with the two diets. The process of active calcium absorption, which is controlled by the level of circulating 1,25-$(OH)_2D_3$ in the bloodstream, will make up the difference.

1,25-$(OH)_2D_3$ exerts its control of calcium absorption through a specific receptor that reacts with the nuclear DNA to stimulate the synthesis of specific proteins (Baker *et al.*, 1988). Several proteins have been shown to be synthesized in response to 1,25-$(OH)_2D_3$ including calbindin (possibly involved in the movement of calcium across the cell) (Wasserman *et al.*, 1968), alkaline phosphatase (Wilson and Lawson, 1982), integral membrane calcium-binding protein (IMCAL) (present in the brush border and may increase calcium uptake) (Kowarski *et al.*, 1987), and enzymes involved in the synthesis of membrane phospholipids (O'Doherty, 1979).

The administration of vitamin D to deficient rats results in an increased incorporation of essential fatty acids in the plasma membrane phospholipids. However, if the rats are also deficient in the essential fatty acids, administration of vitamin D will not increase calcium absorption (Hay *et al.*, 1980). Changes in the phospholipid composition of the plasma membrane occur very rapidly and make the cells more permeable to calcium.

The mobilization of calcium and phosphorus from bone is controlled by the concerted actions of both 1,25-$(OH)_2D_3$ and PTH. The action of 1,25-$(OH)_2D_3$ is mediated through a specific receptor in the osteoblasts. However, the actual dissolving of calcified bone is executed by the osteoclasts rather than the osteoblasts. In response to 1,25-$(OH)_2D_3$ the osteoblasts produce a soluble factor that stimulates osteoclast activity (McSheehy and Chambers, 1987).

1,25-$(OH)_2D_3$ has a role in the regulation of bone formation. Osteoblasts that are treated with high levels of 1,25-$(OH)_2D_3$ produce less collagen, which is the main structural protein of bone (Lichtler *et al.*, 1989). In contrast, the synthesis of two other major bone proteins, osteocalcin and matrix γ-carboxy-glutamic acid containing protein (MGP), are increased by 1,25-$(OH)_2D_3$ (Price, 1988). One or possibly both of these proteins inhibit the random crystallization of the collagen matrix of bone.

Both of these proteins contain γ-carboxy-glutamic acid. The γ-carboxy-glutamic acid residues are formed by the post-translational carboxylation of certain specific glutamic acid residues through a vitamin K dependent process. Thus, two fat-soluble vitamins are required for the formation of these proteins. In rats that are treated with Warfarin to block the formation of γ-carboxy-glutamic acid, the epiphyseal growth plate becomes calcified and eventually closes. Normally, the epiphyseal growth plate does not close in rats. When both 1,25-$(OH)_2D_3$ and PTH are high, the net effect is increased resorption of bone combined with an inhibition of synthesis and calcification of the collagen matrix.

In contrast, when PTH is low, very modest levels of 1,25-$(OH)_2D_3$ stimulate the synthesis of collagen (Franceschi *et al.*, 1988). Thus, modest levels of 1,25-$(OH)_2D_3$ appear to increase the formation of bone (Gallagher *et al.*, 1986). At the same time the 1,25-$(OH)_2D_3$ stimulates the intestinal absorption of calcium and phosphorus making them available for the formation of bone crystals. The regulation of bone metabolism is a very complex process that involves the interplay of at least a dozen hormones and growth factors. The process is made even more complex by the different effects of high and low levels of the various factors.

D. Vitamin D Requirements

Vitamin D activity is expressed as the equivalent μg of vitamin D_3 (Committee on Dietary Allowances, 1980). Under the old terminology, one International Unit (IU) was equal to 25 ng of vitamin D_3. No official factors have been approved to express the relative activity of vitamin D and its more active metabolites.

The exact human requirement for vitamin D has not been determined. However, an estimate of the minimum requirement can be made. The major plasma metabolite, 25-OHD_3, has a relatively constant turnover regardless of the vitamin D status. Weber *et al.* (1976) found a turnover of about 37 ng/kg body weight/day (range 24·8–48·4) in men. For the ideal 70 kg man this would be 2·6 μg per day. However, kinetic studies using tritium-labeled vitamin D_3 show that 25-OHD_3 is not the only metabolite formed from vitamin D_3 (Mawer *et al.*, 1971; Smith and Goodman, 1971), and the efficiency of absorption of vitamin D from the intestine is only around 77% (Hollander *et al.*, 1971). Assuming that these factors account for half of the dietary vitamin D, the minimum vitamin D requirement would be 5–7 μg per day. The current RDA for vitamin D is 5 μg of vitamin D_3 for the adult human (Committee on Dietary Allowances, 1980). This is less than the projected requirement for many individuals assuming that vitamin D is only available from dietary sources. However, most adults will have sufficient exposure to sunlight to provide some additional vitamin D from synthesis in the skin.

E. Meat as a Source of Vitamin D

The vitamin D content of several meat and fish products are presented in Table 13-3. Vitamin D is not widely found in the foods naturally consumed by man, and plant materials are almost completely devoid of vitamin D activity. Meat and liver contain small amounts of vitamin D, but these are not adequate to meet the vitamin D requirement. If we assume that all meat fats have vitamin D activity equivalent to beef drippings, and that these fats comprise 15% of the total caloric intake, meat fats could contribute between 4–6% of the vitamin D requirement. Although liver contains slightly higher amounts of vitamin D, the level is nowhere near the magnitude of the vitamin A content. Since liver is rarely consumed, it is not a major contributor to vitamin D requirements.

Salt-water fish are the major naturally occurring source of vitamin D. A single serving (117 g) of most fish will provide more than the daily requirement for vitamin D. But, on a given day only about 8% of the American population consumes fish (Pao *et al.*, 1982), so fish alone do not provide an adequate supply of vitamin D.

TABLE 13-3
THE VITAMIN D CONTENT OF MEAT AND FISH PRODUCTS[a]

Product	*Vitamin D μg/100 g*	*Type of assay*	*Reference*
Beef drippings	0·58–1·1	Rat-bioassay	Henry *et al.* (1941)
Beef	0·25–0·3	Source not specified	DeLuca (1978), Burton (1976)
Liver, beef	1·2	Rat-bioassay	DeVaney and Munsell (1935)
Liver, lamb	0·4	Rat-bioassay	DeVaney and Munsell (1935)
Liver, pork	1·1	Rat-bioassay	DeVaney and Munsell (1935)
Mackerel	15·5	HPLC	Egaas and Lambertsen (1979)
Albacore	6·5	HPLC	Takeuchi *et al.* (1986)
Skipjack	3·5	HPLC	Takeuchi *et al.* (1986)
Salmon, canned	10·5	Rat-bioassay	DeVaney and Putney (1935)
Cod-liver oil	258–880	HPLC	Egaas and Lambertsen (1979)

[a] Values are expressed as μg of vitamin D_3. The fish products contain almost exclusively vitamin D_3. The mammalian tissues probably contain about equal amounts of vitamin D_3 and 25-OHD_3 as outlined by Mawer *et al.* (1972).

Until the present century, man has depended on synthesis of vitamin D in the skin as his major source of vitamin D. With the development of inexpensive techniques to synthesize vitamin D, fortified foods have become a major source of vitamin D. Milk is routinely fortified with 10 μg of vitamin D per quart, and approximately half of the major margarine manufacturers fortify their product with 1·5 μg of vitamin D per serving (14 g).

V. VITAMIN K

A. Vitamin K Activity

The most evident function of vitamin K is its role in blood clotting. The antihemorrhagic activity of vitamin K is exhibited by phylloquinone (vitamin K_1), which is widely distributed among green plants (Shearer *et al.*, 1980), and by a series of menaquinones (vitamin K_2), which are produced by microorganisms. The menaquinones differ in structure from phylloquinone in that each of the isoprenoid units of the side chain is unsaturated (Fig. 13-7). The various menaquinones differ from each other by the number of repeating isoprenoid units in the side chain. The menaquinones with 4–7 isoprenoid units in the side chain have slightly greater biological activity than phylloquinone (Matschiner and Doisy, 1966a). As the side chain becomes longer, there is a proportionate drop in the biological activity. The decline in biopotency seems to be related to the reduced absorption of the

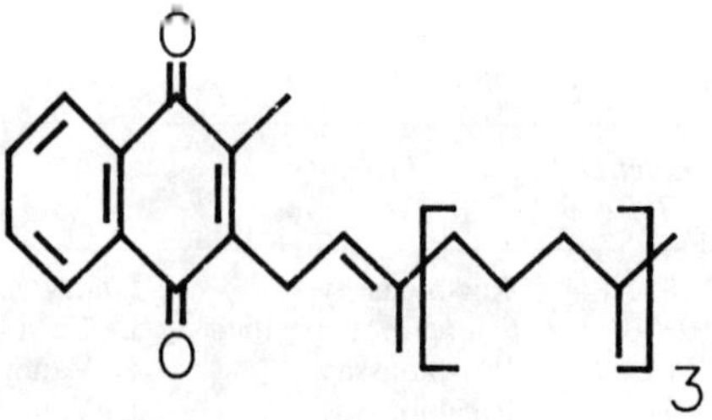

Phylloquinone

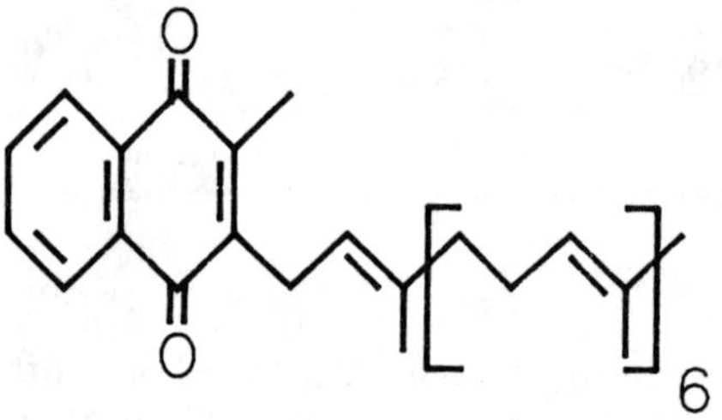

Menaquinone–7

FIG. 13-7. The compounds with vitamin K activity.

larger more hydrophobic compounds, as menaquinone-9 has 25 times the activity of phylloquinone when given by intracardial injection (Matschiner and Taggart, 1968).

B. Deficiency

The clinical symptoms of vitamin K deficiency are rarely seen, because many green plants contain very high levels of vitamin K activity. The problems mainly occur in individuals with complications in fat absorption or in newborn infants.

When fat absorption problems occur, such as obstruction of the bile duct, serious internal bleeding problems may begin within one to two months (Savage and Lindenbaum, 1983). When compared to the other fat-soluble vitamins, the reserves of vitamin K are very modest (Shearer *et al.*, 1988). Thus, vitamin K reserves are rapidly depleted when anything interferes with vitamin K absorption.

In newborn infants the plasma levels of vitamin K are very low, probably because the vitamin is not efficiently transported across the placenta (Shearer *et al.*, 1982). If the infants do not receive adequate vitamin K, the classical newborn hemorrhagic disease can occur. This is characterized by cutaneous and mucosal membrane bleeding as well as by intracranial hemorrhaging which can often prove fatal. Since human milk is very low in vitamin K, the intracranial hemorrhage may occur at a later age in breast fed infants whose mothers are in marginal status (Chaou *et al.*, 1984).

Although it is frequently stated that individuals treated with antibiotics show bleeding problems, complications are rarely observed (Savage and Lindenbaum, 1983). Prolonged clotting times or bleeding problems are only observed when other stress factors are coupled with antibiotic therapy. Intestinal bacteria have undoubtedly synthesized some of the vitamin K that is absorbed from the small intestine. However, the largest population of intestinal bacteria reside in the colon, with a much smaller population being present in the small intestine. The bile salts are known to be required for the absorption of the menaquinones, but the bile salts are almost completely absorbed in the ileum. Thus, the bile salt concentration in the colon is very low, and it can be reasoned that the absorption of menaquinones in the colon is negligible. Since the human liver contains about half of its vitamin K activity as the menaquinones, they are clearly absorbed from the small intestine (Shearer *et al.*, 1988).

C. Metabolic Function

The only function of vitamin K that has been defined is its role in the formation of γ-carboxy-glutamic acid (GLA) (Stenflo *et al.*, 1974). GLA is a structural component of four proteins of the blood clotting cascade, including prothrombin, proconvertin (Factor VII), the Christmas factor (Factor IX), and the Stuart–Prower factor (Factor X) (Davie, 1980). Two proteins that down-regulate blood clotting by inactivating Factor V and Factor VIII also contain GLA. These are Protein S and Protein C. In addition to the blood clotting proteins, tissue proteins that contain GLA have been detected in kidney, lung and bone. The bone proteins, osteocalcin and MGP, were discussed in the vitamin D section. GLA provides an excellent calcium-binding site for these proteins, and in all cases this binding site is critical to the function of the protein.

The blood clotting factors form a calcium linkage with membrane phospholipids via GLA. The association with calcium and phospholipid is essential in order for the vitamin K-dependent blood clotting factors to become activated. In vitamin K deficiency, GLA is not formed so blood clotting does not occur. The actual formation of GLA in the blood clotting factors occurs in the liver, and vitamin K has no direct function in the blood (Suttie, 1984).

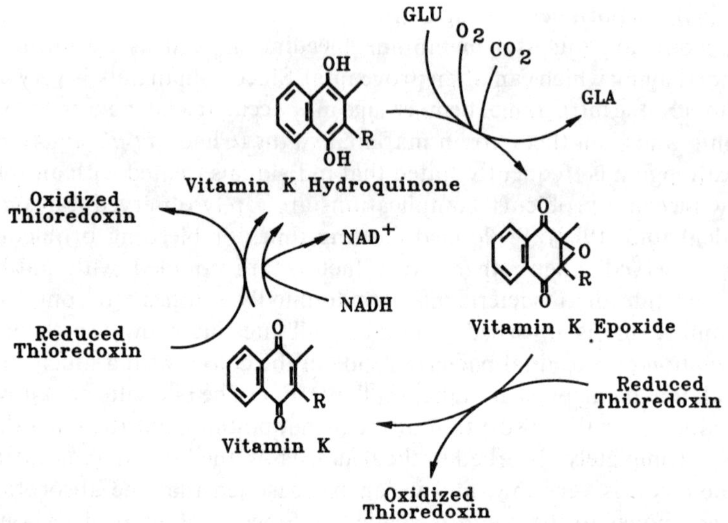

FIG. 13-8. The vitamin K cycle. This scheme was adapted from a scheme presented by Suttie (1984) and reflects the findings of Vermeer and Soute (1988) and Silverman and Nandi (1988).

GLA is formed by the post-translational modification of glutamic acid residues already incorporated into a protein chain. In prothrombin the first 10 glutamic acids from the amino terminal end of the protein are converted to GLA (Magnusson *et al.*, 1974). The other blood clotting factors are modified in a similar manner.

The role of vitamin K in the formation of GLA is the abstraction of a hydrogen, complete with its electron, from the γ-carbon of a glutamic acid residue (Dubois *et al.*, 1983). The resulting free-radical attacks carbon dioxide to form the GLA residue. Phylloquinone and the menaquinones all function in the same manner. Vitamin K undergoes several metabolic transformations during synthesis of GLA (Fig. 13-8). As GLA is formed, vitamin K epoxide is produced. The vitamin K cycle is completed by the reduction of vitamin K epoxide back to vitamin K. Several of the safer anticoagulants, such as Warfarin, block the conversion of vitamin K epoxide to vitamin K. If an overdose of anticoagulant is given, it can be counteracted by giving a very large dose of vitamin K.

D. Vitamin K Requirements

Vitamin K activity is generally expressed in terms of equivalent phylloquinone activity. Suttie *et al.* (1988) found that the dietary requirement for vitamin K was approximately 1 μg/kg body weight/day. A sensitive assay, which detects abnormal plasma prothrombin (prothrombin that lacks GLA), was used as the criterion in this study. The contribution of the intestinal bacteria to overall vitamin K nutriture was not assessed, but it was not sufficient to prevent the appearance of abnormal prothrombin with intakes of ~0·7 μg/kg body weight/day. This study is in agreement with the findings of Frick *et al.* (1967), who used starvation and antibiotic treatment to produce vitamin K deficiency. Based on a less sensitive blood clotting time assay, they reported that the requirement was between 0·3–1·5 μg/kg body weight/day. Thus, the requirement for the 'ideal 70 kg man' is about 70 μg/day. Since the vitamin K intake is typically greater than 100 μg/day, deficiency problems are rare in normal adults (Suttie *et al.*, 1988). An RDA has not been established for vitamin K (Committee on Dietary Allowances, 1980).

E. Meat as a Source of Vitamin K

Data on the vitamin K content of foods is very scarce, which is especially true with meat products. Many of the values presented in Table 13-4 were obtained from Olson (1980), in which he cites personal communications for the original sources. While meats are not recognized as the richest sources of vitamin K, they probably contribute enough to comprise 10% of the requirement.

Although the menaquinones were originally detected in *putrefied* fish meal, the emphasis should be strongly placed on the putrefied. Many of the early diets that were used to produce vitamin K deficiency contained 20%

TABLE 13-4

THE VITAMIN K CONTENT OF MEAT PRODUCTS[a]

Product	*Vitamin K μg/100 g*	*Type of assay*	*Reference*
Ground beef	7	Rat-bioassay	Matschiner and Doisy (1966b)
Liver, beef	92	Chick-bioassay	Matschiner and Doisy (1966a)
Beef fat	15	Source not specified	Olson (1980)
Liver, veal	27	Chick-bioassay	Matschiner and Doisy (1966a)
Liver, pork	25	Chick-bioassay	Matschiner and Doisy (1966a)
Liver, chicken	8	Chick-bioassay	Matschiner and Doisy (1966a)
Ham	15	Source not specified	Olson (1980)
Pork tenderloin	11	Source not specified	Olson (1980)
Bacon	46	Source not specified	Olson (1980)

[a] Values are expressed in terms of phylloquinone, but about half of the activity is apparently present as the menaquinones (Matschiner and Amelotti, 1968).

fish meal and 1% cod-liver oil (Almquist and Stokstad, 1935). Thus, fish products appear to be very low in vitamin K activity.

VI. SUMMARY

Meat, fish, and poultry are significant sources of the fat-soluble vitamins. Liver and liver products represent the largest source of vitamin A in the diet. Consuming a single serving of liver once a month will provide 20–30% of the recommended vitamin A intake for the month. Other meats contain less vitamin A, but they typically provide about 1–2% of the recommended intake. The meat, fish, and poultry food group along with eggs comprise most of the natural dietary sources of vitamin D. Meats and poultry will provide 4–6% of the recommended vitamin D intake. Fish, however, are quite rich in vitamin D, and a single serving will provide enough vitamin D to meet the requirement for 1–2 days. The meat, fish and poultry food group will typically supply 7–8% of the recommended vitamin E intake. Unfortunately, the ratio of vitamin E to polyunsaturated fatty acids is quite low in most meats. So, the vitamin E supplied does not compensate for the increase in the vitamin E requirement caused by the polyunsaturated fatty acids. Information about the vitamin K content of meats is quite limited. However, meats and poultry appear to provide about 10% of the vitamin K requirement. In contrast, the vitamin K activity in fish is apparently very low.

VII. REFERENCES

Almquist, H. J. and Stokstad, E. L. R. (1935). Hemorrhagic chick disease of dietary origin. *J. Biol. Chem.* **111**, 105.

Ames, S. R. and Harris, P. L. (1954). Identification of the so-called 'lard factor' as vitamin A. *Science* **120**, 391.

Baker, A. R., McDonnell, D. P., Hughes, M., Crisp, T. M., Mangelsdorf, D. J. Haussler, M. R., Pike, J. W., Shine, J. and O'Malley, B. W. (1988). Cloning and expression of full-length cDNA encoding human vitamin D receptor. *Proc. Natl Acad. Sci.* (*USA*) **85**, 3294.

Barzel, U. S. (1983). Vitamin D deficiency: A risk factor for osteomalacia in the aged. *J. Am. Ger. Soc.* **31**, 598.

Bascetta, E., Gunstone, F. D. and Walton, J. C. (1983). Electron spin resonance study of the role of vitamin E and vitamin C in the inhibition of fatty acid oxidation in a model membrane. *Chem. Phys. Lipids* **33**, 207.

Berger, S., Rechcigl, M., Jr, Loosli, J. K. and Williams, H. H. (1962). Protein quality and carotene utilization. *J. Nutr.* **77**, 174.

BERNSTEIN, P. S., LAW, W. C. and RANDO, R. R. (1987). Biochemical characterization of the retinoid isomerase system of the eye. *J. Biol. Chem.* **262**, 16848.

BIERI, J. G. and EVARTS, R. P. (1973). Tocopherols and fatty acids in American diets. *J. Am. Diet. Assoc.* **62**, 147.

BIERI, J. G. and EVARTS, R. P. (1974). Gamma tocopherol: Metabolism, biological activity and significance in human vitamin E nutrition. *Am. J. Clin. Nutr.* **27**, 980.

BLOCK, G., DRESSER, C. M., HARTMAN, A. M. and CARROLL, M. D. (1985). Nutrient sources in the American diet: Quantitative data from the NHANES II survey. I. Vitamins and minerals. *Am. J. Epidemol.* **122**, 13.

BRAND, N., PETKOVICH, M., KRUST, A., CHAMBON, P., DE THE, H., MARCHIO, A., TIOLLAIS, P. and DEJEAN, A. (1988). Identification of a second human retinoic acid receptor. *Nature* **332**, 850.

BRONNER, F. (1987). Intestinal calcium absorption: Mechanisms and applications. *J. Nutr.* **117**, 1347.

BUNNELL, R. H., KEATING, J., QUARESIMO, A. and PARMAN, G. K. (1965). Alpha-tocopherol content of foods. *Am. J. Clin. Nutr.* **17**, 1.

BURTON, B. T. (1976). *Human Nutrition.* McGraw-Hill, New York.

CAMPOS, F. A. C. S., FLORES, H. and UNDERWOOD, B. A. (1987). Effect of an infection on vitamin A status of children as measured by the relative dose response (RDR). *Am. J. Clin. Nutr.* **46**, 91.

CHAOU, W.-T., CHOU, M.-L. and EITZMAN, D. V. (1984). Intracranial hemorrhage and vitamin K deficiency in early infancy. *J. Pediat.* **105**, 880.

CHOW, C. K. (1979). Nutritional influence on cellular antioxidant defense systems. *Am. J. Clin. Nutr.* **32**, 1066.

COMMITTEE ON DIETARY ALLOWANCES (1980). *Recommended Dietary Allowances*, 9th edn. Food and Nutrition Board, National Research Council, National Academy of Sciences, Washington, DC.

CSALLANY, A. S., DRAPER, H. H. and SHAH, S. N. (1962). Conversion of d-α-tocopherol-C^{14} to tocopheryl-*p*-quinone *in vivo. Arch. Biochem. Biophys.* **98**, 142.

DAVIE, E. W. (1980). Structural properties of the vitamin K-dependent plasma proteins. In *Vitamin K Metabolism and Vitamin K-Dependent Proteins* (J. W. Suttie, Ed.), p. 3. University Park Press, Baltimore.

DELUCA, H. F. (1978). Vitamin D. In *The Fat-Soluble Vitamins* (H. F. DeLuca, Ed.), p. 69. Plenum, New York.

DELVIN, E. E., ARABIAN, A. and GLORIEUX, F. H. (1978). Kinetics of liver microsomal cholecalciferol 25-hydroxylase in vitamin D-depleted and repleted rats. *Biochem. J.* **172**, 417.

DESAI, I. D. (1968). Plasma tocopherol levels in normal adults. *Canad. J. Physiol. Pharmacol.* **46**, 819.

DEVANEY, G. M. and MUNSELL, H. E. (1935). Vitamin D content of calf, beef, lamb, and hog liver. *J. Home Econ.* **27**, 240.

DEVANEY, G. M. and PUTNEY, L. K. (1935). The vitamin A and D content of canned salmon. *J. Home Econ.* **27**, 658.

DILIBERTO, E. J., JR and ALLEN, P. L. (1980). Semidehydroascorbate as a product of the enzymatic conversion of dopamine to norepinephrine. Coupling of semidehydroascorbate reductase to dopamine-β-hydroxylase. *Mol. Pharm.* **17**, 421.

DOWLING, J. E. and WALD, G. (1960). The biological function of vitamin A acid. *Proc. Natl Acad. Sci. (USA)* **46**, 587.

DRATZ, E. A. and HARGRAVE, P. A. (1983). The structure of rhodopsin and the rod outer segment disk membrane. *Trend. Biochem. Sci.* **8**, 128.

DUBOIS, J., GAUDRY, M., BORY, S., AZERAD, R. and MARQUET, A. (1983). Vitamin K-dependent carboxylation. Study of the hydrogen abstraction stereochemistry with γ-fluoroglutamic acid-containing peptides. *J. Biol. Chem.* **258**, 7897.

EGAAS, E. and LAMBERTSEN, G. (1979). Naturally occurring vitamin D_3 in fish products analysed by HPLC, using vitamin D_2 as an international standard. *Internat. J. Vit. Nutr. Res.* **49**, 35.

FARRELL, P. M., BIERI, J. G., FRATANTONI, J. F., WOOD, R. E. and DI SANT'AGNESE, P. A. (1977). The occurrence and effects of human vitamin E deficiency. A study in patients with cystic fibrosis. *J. Clin. Invest.* **60**, 233.

FRANCESCHI, R. T., ROMANO, P. R. and PARK, K.-Y. (1988). Regulation of type I collagen synthesis by 1,25-dihydroxyvitamin D_3 in human osteosarcoma cells. *J. Biol. Chem.* **263**, 18938.

FRICK, P. G., RIEDLER, G. and BROGLI, H. (1967). Dose response and minimal daily requirement for vitamin K in man. *J. Appl. Physiol.* **23**, 387.

GALLAGHER, J. A., BENETON, M., HARVEY, L. and LAWSON, D. E. M. (1986). Response of rachitic rat bones to 1,25-dihydroxyvitamin D_3: Biphasic effects on mineralization and lack of effect on bone resorption. *Endocrinol.* **119**, 1603.

GHAZARIAN, J. G., SCHNOES, H. K. and DELUCA, H. F. (1973). Mechanism of 25-hydroxycholecalciferol 1α-hydroxylation. Incorporation of oxygen-18 into the 1α position of 25-hydroxycholecalciferol. *Biochemistry* **12**, 2555.

GIGUERE, V., ONG, E. S., SEGUI, P. and EVANS, R. M. (1987). Identification of a receptor for the morphogen retinoic acid. *Nature* **330**, 624.

GOODMAN, D. S., SMITH, J. E., HEMBRY, R. M. and DINGLE, J. T. (1974). Comparison of the effects of vitamin A and its analogs upon rabbit ear cartilage in organ culture and upon growth in the vitamin A-deficient rat. *J. Lipid Res.* **15**, 406.

HAUSSLER, M. R. and MCCAIN, T. A. (1977). Basic and clinical concepts related to vitamin D metabolism and action. *N. Eng. J. Med.* **297**, 974.

HAY, A. W. M., HASSAM, A. G., CRAWFORD, M. A., STEVENS, P. A., MAWER, E. B. and JONES, F. S. (1980). Essential fatty acid restriction inhibits vitamin D-dependent calcium absorption. *Lipids* **15**, 251.

HAYES, K. C., NIELSON, S. W. and EATON, H. D. (1968). Pathogenesis of the optic nerve lesion in vitamin A-deficient calves. *Arch. Ophthalmol.* **60**, 777.

HENRY, H. L., TAYLOR, A. N. and NORMAN, A. W. (1977). Response of chick parathyroid glands to the vitamin D metabolites, 1,25-dihydroxycholecalciferol and 24,25-dihydroxycholecalciferol. *J. Nutr.* **107**, 1918.

HENRY, K. M., GOODWIN, T. W., KON, S. K. and MORTON, R. A. (1941). Vitamin A and D in dripping. *Lancet* **I**, 311.

HOLLANDER, D., ROSENSTEICH, S. J. and VOLWILER, W. (1971). Role of the duodenum in vitamin D_3 absorption in man. *Am. J. Dig. Dis.* **16**, 145.

HORWITT, M. K. (1986). Interpretations of requirements for thiamin, riboflavin, niacin–tryptophan, and vitamin E plus comments on balance studies and vitamin B_6. *Am. J. Clin. Nutr.* **44**, 973.

HORWITT, M. K., CENTURY, B. and ZEMAN, A. A. (1963). Erythrocyte survival time and reticulocyte levels after tocopherol depletion in man. *Am. J. Clin. Nutr.* **12**, 99.

JOFFE, M. and HARRIS, P. L. (1943). The biological potency of the natural tocopherols and certain derivatives. *J. Am. Chem. Soc.* **65**, 925.

KOWARSKI, S., COWEN, L. A., TAKAHASHI, M. T. and SCHACHTER, D. (1987). Tissue distribution and vitamin D dependence of IMCAL in the rat. *Am. J. Physiol.* **253**, G411.

KUNERT, K.-J. and TAPPEL, A. L. (1983). The effect of vitamin C on in vivo lipid peroxidation in guinea pigs as measured by pentane and ethane production. *Lipids* **18**, 271.

LAWSON, D. E. M., FRASER, D. R., KODICEK, E., MORRIS, H. R. and WILLIAMS, D. H. (1971). Identification of 1,25-dihydroxycholecalciferol, a new kidney hormone controlling calcium metabolism. *Nature* **230**, 228.

LAWSON, D. E. M., COLE, T. J., SALEM, S. I., GALAL, O. M., EL-MELIGY, R., ABDEL-AZIM, S., PAUL, A. A. and EL-HUSSEINI, S. (1987). Aetiology of rickets in Egyptian children. *Hum. Nutr.: Clin. Nutr.* **41C**, 199.

LETH, T. and SONDERGAARD, H. (1977). Biological activity of vitamin E compounds and natural materials by the resorption-gestation test and chemical determination of the vitamin E activity of foods and feeds. *J. Nutr.* **107**, 2236.

LICHTLER, A., STOVER, M. L., ANGILLY, J., KREAM, B. and ROWE, D. W. (1989). Isolation and characterization of the rat α1(I)collagen promoter: Regulation by 1,25-dihydroxyvitamin D. *J. Biol. Chem.* **264**, 3072.

MAGNUSSON, S., SOTTRUP-JENSEN, L. and PETERSEN, T. E. (1974). Primary structure of the vitamin K-dependent part of prothrombin. *FEBS Lett.* **44**, 189.

MARTHEDAL, H. E. (1973). Encephalomalacia in chicks, with special reference to frequency and the occurrence of pathological and anatomical changes. *Acta Agric. Scand.* **Suppl. 19**, 58.

MATSCHINER, J. T. and AMELOTTI, J. M. (1968). Characterization of vitamin K from bovine liver. *J. Lipid Res.* **9**, 176.

MATSCHINER, J. T. and DOISY, E. A., JR (1966a). Bioassay of vitamin K in chicks. *J. Nutr.* **90**, 97.

MATSCHINER, J. T. and DOISY, E. A., JR (1966b). Vitamin K content on ground beef. *J. Nutr.* **90**, 331.

MATSCHINER, J. T. and TAGGART, W. V. (1968). Bioassay of vitamin K by intracardial injection in deficient adult male rats. *J. Nutr.* **94**, 57.

MATSUOKA, L. Y., WORTSMAN, J., HANIFAN, N. and HOLICK, M. F. (1988). Chronic sunscreen use decreases circulating concentrations of 25-hydroxyvitamin D. *Arch. Dermatol.* **124**, 1802.

MAWER, E. B., LUMB, G. A., SCHAFER, K. and STANBURY, S. W. (1971). The metabolism of isotopically labelled vitamin D_3 in man: The influence of the state of vitamin D nutrition. *Clin. Sci.* **40**, 39.

MAWER, E. B., BACKHOUSE, J., HOLMAN, C. A., LUMB, G. A. and STANBURY, S. W. (1972). The distribution and storage of vitamin D and its metabolites in human tissues. *Clin. Sci.* **43**, 413.

MCSHEEHY, P. M. J. and CHAMBERS, J. T. (1987). 1,25-dihydroxyvitamin D_3 stimulates rat osteoblastic cells to release a soluble factor that increases osteoclastic bone resorption. *J. Clin. Invest.* **80**, 425.

MULLER, D. P. R. and LLOYD, J. K. (1982). Effect of large doses of vitamin E on the neurological sequelae of patients with abetalipoproteinemia. *Ann. NY Acad. Sci.* **393**, 133.

NAPOLI, J. L. and RACE, K. R. (1987). The biosynthesis of retinoic acid from retinol by rat tissues in vitro. *Arch. Biochem. Biophys.* **255**, 95.

O'DOHERTY, P. J. A. (1979). 1,25-dihydroxyvitamin D_3 increases the activity of the intestinal phosphatidylcholine deacylation-reacylation cycle. *Lipids* **14**, 75.

OLSON, J. A. (1987). Recommended dietary intakes (RDI) of vitamin A in humans. *Am. J. Clin. Nutr.* **45**, 704.

OLSON, R. E. (1980). Vitamin K. In *Modern Nutrition in Health and Disease*, 6th edn. (R. S. Goodhart and M. E. Shils, Eds), p. 170. Lea & Febiger, New York.

OMDAHL, J. L., GARRY, P. J., HUNSAKER, L. A., HUNT, W. C. and GOODWIN, J. S. (1982). Nutritional status of a healthy elderly population: Vitamin D. *Am. J. Clin. Nutr.* **36**, 1125.

OOMEN, H. A. P. C. (1976). Vitamin A deficiency, xerophthalmia and blindness. In *Present Knowledge in Nutrition*, 4th edn (D. M. Hegsted *et al.*, Ed.), p. 73. The Nutrition Foundation, Washington, DC.

PAO, E. M., FLEMING, K. H., GUENTHER, P. M. and MICKLE, S. J. (1982). Foods commonly eaten by individuals: Amount per day and per eating occasion. *US Dept Agric., Home Economics Research Report* No. 44.

PONCHON, G., KENNAN, A. L. and DELUCA, H. F. (1969). 'Activation' of vitamin D by the liver. *J. Clin. Invest.* **48**, 2032.

PRICE, P. A. (1988). Role of vitamin K-dependent proteins in bone metabolism. *Ann. Rev. Nutr.* **8**, 565.

PUGSLEY, L. I., MORRELL, C. A. and KELLY, J. T. (1945). A survey of the vitamins A and D potencies of the liver oil of Atlantic cod (*Gadus morrhua* L.). *Canad. J. Res.* **23F**, 243.

ROELS, O. A., TROUT, M. and DUJACQUIER, R. (1958). Carotene balances of boys in Ruanda where vitamin A deficiency is prevalent. *J. Nutr.* **65**, 115.

SAVAGE, D. and LINDENBAUM, J. (1983). Clinical and experimental human vitamin K deficiency. In *Nutrition in Hematology* (J. Lindenbaum, Ed.), p. 271. Churchill Livingstone, New York.

SCOTT, M. L. (1978). Vitamin E. In *The Fat-Soluble Vitamins* (H. F. DeLuca, Ed.), p. 133. Plenum, New York.

SHEARER, M. J., ALLAN, V., HAROON, Y. and BARKHAM, P. (1989). Nutritional aspects of vitamin K in the human. In *Vitamin K Metabolism and Vitamin K-Dependent Proteins* (J. W. Suttie, Ed.), p. 317. University Park Press, Baltimore.

SHEARER, M. J., RAHIM, S., BARKHAM, P. and STIMMLER, L. (1982). Plasma vitamin K_1 in mothers and their newborn babies. *Lancet* **II**, 460.

SHEARER, M. J., MCCARTHY, P. T., CRAMPTON, O. E. and MATTOCK, M. B. (1988). The assessment of human vitamin K status from tissue measurements. In *Current Advances in Vitamin K Research* (J. W. Suttie, Ed.), p. 437. Elsevier, New York.

SHEIKH, M. S., RAMIEZ, A., EMMETT, M., SANTA ANA, C., SCHILLER, L. R. and FORDTRAN, J. S. (1988). Role of vitamin D-dependent and vitamin D-independent mechanisms in absorption of food calcium. *J. Clin. Invest.* **81**, 126.

SILVERMAN, R. B. and NANDI, D. L. (1988). Reduced thioredoxin: A possible physiological cofactor for vitamin K epoxide reductase. Further support for an active site disulfide. *Biochem. Biophys. Res. Commun.* **155**, 1248.

SIVELL, L. M., BULL, N. L., BUSS, D. H., WIGGINS, R. A., SCUFFAM, D. and JACKSON, P. A. (1984). Vitamin A activity in foods of animal origin. *J. Sci. Food Agric.* **35**, 931.

SMITH, J. E. and BORCHERS, R. (1972). Environmental temperature and the utilization of β-carotene by the rat. *J. Nutr.* **102**, 1017.

SMITH, J. E. and GOODMAN, D. S. (1971). The turnover and transport of vitamin D and of a polar metabolite with the properties of 25-hydroxycholecalciferol in human plasma. *J. Clin. Invest.* **50**, 2159.

SOKOL, R. J. (1988). Vitamin E deficiency and neurologic disease. *Ann. Rev. Nutr.* **8**, 351.

SOMMER, A., TARWOTJO, I., DJUNAEDI, E., WEST, K. P., JR, LOEDEN, A. A., TILDEN, R., MELE, L. AND THE ACEH STUDY GROUP (1986). Impact of vitamin A supplementation on childhood mortality. A randomized controlled community trial. *Lancet* **I**, 1169.

SOMMER, A., TARWOTJO, I. and KATZ, J. (1987). Increased risk of xerophthalmia following diarrhea and respiratory disease. *Am. J. Clin. Nutr.* **45**, 977.

SPORN, M. B., DUNLOP, N. M., NEWTON, D. L. and HENDERSON, W. R. (1976). Relationships between structure and activity of retinoids. *Nature* **263**, 110.

STENFLO, J., FERNLUND, P., EGAN, W. and ROEPSTORFF, P. (1974). Vitamin K dependent modifications of glutamic acid residues in prothrombin. *Proc. Natl Acad. Sci. (USA)* **71**, 2730.

SUTTIE, J. W. (1984). Vitamin K. In *Handbook of Vitamins. Nutritional, Biochemical, and Clinical Aspects* (L. J. Machlin, Ed.), p. 147. Marcel Dekker, New York.

SUTTIE, J. W., MUMMAH-SCHENDEL, L. L., SHAH, D. V., LYLE, B. J. and GREGER, J. L. (1988). Vitamin K deficiency from dietary vitamin K restriction in humans. *Am. J. Clin. Nutr.* **47**, 475.

SYVAOJA, E.-L., SALMINEN, K., PIIRONEN, V., VARO, P., KEROJOKI, O. and KOIVISTOINEN, P. (1985). Tocopherols and tocotrienols in Finnish foods: Fish and fish products. *J. Am. Oil Chem. Soc.* **62**, 1245.

TAKEUCHI, A., OKANO, T., SAYAMOTO, M., SAWAMURA, S., KOBAYASHI, T., MOTOSUGI, M. and YAMAKAWA, T. (1986). Tissue distribution of 7-dehydrocholesterol, vitamin D_3 and 25-hydroxyvitamin D_3 in several species of fishes. *J. Nutr. Sci. Vitaminol.* **32**, 13.

THOMPSON, J. N., HOWELL, J. M. and PITT, G. A. J. (1964). Vitamin A and reproduction in rats. *Proc. Roy. Soc. Ser. B* **159**, 510.

TIELSCH, J. M. and SOMMER, A. (1984). The epidemiology of vitamin A deficiency and xerophthalmia. *Ann. Rev. Nutr.* **4**, 183.

UMESONO, K., GIGUERE, V., GLASS, C. K., ROSENFELD, M. G. and EVANS, R. M. (1988). Retinoic acid and thyroid hormone induce gene expression through a common responsive element. *Nature* **336**, 262.

US DEPARTMENT OF AGRICULTURE (1976–1984). *Composition of Foods*, Consumer and Food Economics Institute. Agricultural Handbook No. 8 (revisions 8.1–8.12), US Gov. Print. Office, Washington, DC.

US DEPARTMENT OF AGRICULTURE (1982). Food consumption: Households in the United States, Spring 1977. *NFCS 1977–78*, report no. H-1, Human Nutrition Information Service.

VERMEER, C. and SOUTE, A. M. (1988). In vitro vitamin K dependent carboxylation of exogenous protein substances. In *Current Advances in Vitamin K Research* (J. W. Suttie, Ed.). p. 25. Elsevier, New York.

WALD, G. (1968). Molecular basis of visual excitation. *Science* **162**, 230.

WASSERMAN, R. H., CORRADINO, R. A. and TAYLOR, A. N. (1968). Vitamin D-dependent calcium binding protein. Purification and some properties. *J. Biol. Chem.* **243**, 3978.

WEBB, A. R. and HOLICK, M. F. (1988). The role of sunlight in the cutaneous production of vitamin D_3. *Ann. Rev. Nutr.* **8**, 375.

WEBER, H. P., GRAY, R. W., DOMINGUEZ, J. H. and LEMANN, J., JR (1976). The lack of effect of chronic metabolic acidosis on 25-OH-vitamin D metabolism and serum parathyroid hormone in humans. *J. Clin. Endocrinol. Metab.* **43**, 1047.

WELSH, S. O. and MARSTON, R. M. (1982). Review of trends in food use in the United States, 1909 to 1980. *J. Am. Diet. Assoc.* **81**, 120.

WILSON, P. W. and LAWSON, D. E. M. (1982). Incorporation of labelled leucine into alkaline phosphatase in response to 1,25-dihydroxycholecalciferol in chick intestinal brush border. *Eur. J. Biochem.* **125**, 555.

ZILE, M. and DELUCA, H. F. (1968). Retinoic acid: Some aspects of growth-promoting activity in the albino rat. *J. Nutr.* **94**, 302.

ZURER, P. S. (1983). The chemistry of vision. *Chem. Eng. News* Nov. 28, p. 24.

14

Thiamin, Riboflavin, Niacin, and Pantothenic Acid

CAROL T. WINDHAM, BONITA W. WYSE* AND R. GAURTH HANSEN

Department of Nutrition and Food Sciences, Utah State University, Logan, Utah, USA

I. INTRODUCTION

Interest in the American diet has been stimulated in recent years by research that suggests overconsumption of certain dietary factors may be involved in the development of chronic diseases, which are among the nation's primary health problems. As increasing attention has been given to the problems of overnutrition, nutrition policy has shifted toward emphasizing moderation of American dietary patterns and limitation of various food and food constituents (Hegsted, 1979).

The shift of emphasis toward greater concern about overconsumption of certain foods or food constituents does not mean less attention should be given to ensuring adequate intake of essential nutrients. Balance and variety in diets have been central themes of nutrition education programs for many years (Light and Cronin, 1981; National Advisory Committee on Nutrition Education, 1983; Krebs-Smith *et al.*, 1987), with the assumption that an appropriate mixture of food items will form the foundation of an adequate diet with respect to certain 'indicator' nutrients, namely, protein, calcium, iron, vitamins A and C and the B vitamins, thiamin, riboflavin and niacin. These three B vitamins, along with pantothenic acid, are central to the metabolism of all cells. They are coenzymes in specific reactions along the glycolytic, citric acid, and pentose phosphate pathways, as well as in subsidiary pathways of energy metabolism. As methods of food processing

* Present address: Office of the Dean, College of Family Life, Utah State University, Logan, Utah, USA.

change and as new foods appear on the market, the thiamin, riboflavin, niacin, and pantothenic acid content of available foods needs continual monitoring to assure the nutritional quality of the diet for these and other nutrients is maintained.

II. BIOCHEMICAL AND PHYSIOLOGICAL ROLES

A. Metabolism and Utilization

(i) Thiamin

The vitamin thiamin was first isolated in crystallized form by Jansen and Donath (1926) and synthesized by Roger R. Williams and his colleagues (Williams and Cline, 1936) (Fig. 14-1). The thiamin molecule consists of a pyrimidine ring and a thiazole component linked by a methylene bridge; it contains a quarternary N atom. The stability of thiamin is good, even in heat, when it is in the crystallized state or in an acid solution (pH less than 5·0). In a neutral or alkaline solution thiamin is readily ruptured at the methylene bridge into pyrimidine and thiazole. Thiamin can be converted by controlled oxidation into an inactive product, thiochrome, which is strongly fluorescent in ultraviolet light (Hennessy and Cerecedo, 1939). This property is the basis for the official standard method used for chemical estimation of the vitamin in biologic materials (Association of Official Agricultural Chemists, 1960; Association of Vitamin Chemists, 1966; Association of Official Analytical Chemists, 1980). Thiamin is also measured using microbiological (Baker *et al.*, 1964) and high-pressure liquid chromatography techniques (Walker *et al.*, 1981).

The total amount of thiamin in the human body is 25–30 mg, with 80% as thiamin pyrophosphate (Ferrenbee *et al.*, 1942). High concentrations are found in skeletal muscle, and in the heart, liver, kidney, and brain. Except in the sense that it is attached to enzymes, thiamin is not stored in the body. Excesses are excreted in the urine either as free thiamin or its metabolites; thus, no benefit is derived from consuming large doses (Neal and Pearson,

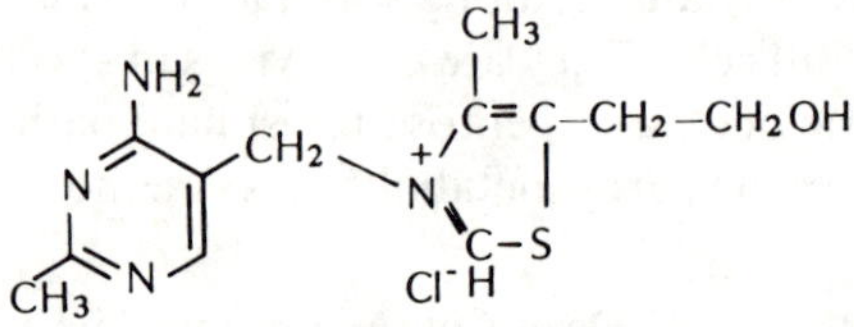

FIG. 14-1. Structure of thiamin.

1964; Balaghi and Pearson, 1966). Thiamin is found in foods in both the free vitamin and phosphate forms. Thiamin in plants is non-phosphorylated, whereas that in animal products occurs in the phosphate forms.

The active form of the vitamin is the coenzyme, thiamin pyrophosphate (TPP). There are two general reactions in humans when TPP functions as the Mg^{2+}-coordinated enzyme for active aldehyde transfers. These are the oxidative decarboxylation of α-keto acids catalyzed by dehydrogenase complexes and the formation of ketoses as catalyzed by transketolase. The three known enzyme reactions involving thiamin pyrophosphate as a coenzyme in human metabolic systems are pyruvate dehydrogenase, α-ketoglutarate dehydrogenase, and transketolase in the pentose–phosphate shunt. The thiamin-dependent decarboxylation reactions catalyzed by the dehydrogenase complexes are necessary for entry of pyruvate into the citric acid cycle as acetyl CoA (Lohman and Schuster, 1937; Gubler, 1968) and for production of succinyl CoA from α-ketoglutarate (Kochetov, 1982). The reactions catalyzed by transketolase are not directly in the main glycolytic pathway for carbohydrate metabolism. Instead, transketolase is essential in the pentose–phosphate pathway, which is the primary source of pentoses for the cell and a major source of reduced nicotinamide adenine dinucleotide phosphate (NADPH) for fatty acid and other biosyntheses. Enzyme-bound thiamin pyrophosphate functions as an aldehyde transferase in all these reactions. Accumulation of the intermediary products of metabolism when the necessary thiamin-containing enzyme is absent is believed to cause typical thiamin deficiency symptoms.

TPP appears to have a specific role in nerve transmission separate from its coenzyme function in the citric acid cycle and the pentose pathway (von Muralt, 1945; Pincus *et al.*, 1973; Matsuda and Cooper, 1981). It is still not clear whether TPP or thiamin triphosphate (TTP) is the neurophysiologically active form, because the two thiamin phosphates are rapidly interconvertible (Tanphaichitr and Wood, 1984). It is believed to function at the nerve cell membrane to allow transport of sodium and potassium ions freely across the membrane during nerve impulse transmission (Gubler, 1968; Itokawa and Cooper, 1970; Plaitakis *et al.*, 1982).

(ii) Riboflavin

Riboflavin was discovered as a heat-stable fraction, named vitamin B_2, in the search for the anti-beriberi factor (Emmett and Luros, 1920). Separate work (Warburg and Christian, 1932) on the properties of naturally occurring flavoproteins culminated in the discovery of a substance, later called riboflavin, effective for promoting growth in the rat. Riboflavin was first isolated from milk by Kuhn and colleagues and synthesized by Kuhn *et al.* (1935) and Karrer *et al.* (1935).

The chemical formula for riboflavin is 7,8-dimethyl-10-(1′-ribityl)-isoalloxazine (International Union of Nutrition Sciences, 1966) (Fig. 14-2). The alloxazine ring is linked to the alcohol, ribitol, derived from the pentose sugar, ribose. In plant and animal tissues riboflavin is linked via the ribitol with phosphoric acid to form riboflavin 5′-phosphate or flavin mononucleotide (FMN). This compound with the addition of adenosine monophosphate forms flavin adenine dinucleotide (FAD). These two most important derivatives of riboflavin are the prosthetic groups of the flavoprotein enzymes involved in oxidation–reduction reactions.

The free vitamin is a weak base, normally isolated or synthesized as an orange-yellow, needle-shaped, crystalline cluster, with an intense greenish-yellow fluorescence in water solutions (Shah, 1985). It is highly soluble in alkaline solution and slightly soluble at neutral or acidic pH. Riboflavin is relatively heat stable, except under alkaline conditions. In solution at any pH, but especially in acidic solutions, riboflavin is very unstable to both visible and ultraviolet light (Williams and Cheldelin, 1942; DeMerre and Brown, 1944). Special precautions are therefore needed during laboratory analysis to avoid light exposure of the vitamin.

The riboflavin content of tissues and biological fluids is primarily determined by either fluorometric or microbiological assay. Chemical assay of riboflavin relies upon the fact that the fluorescence of riboflavin is proportional to its concentration under controlled conditions of salt concentration, pH, and temperature. The natural yellow-green fluorescence in light of wavelength 440–550 nm is the basis for the fluorometric assay (Bursch, 1957; Koziol, 1971; Association of Official Analytical Chemists, 1980). Riboflavin is measured in terms of the difference between the fluorescence before and after chemical reduction (Shah, 1985). Both FMN and FAD, the enzymatic forms of riboflavin in tissues, are bound to protein

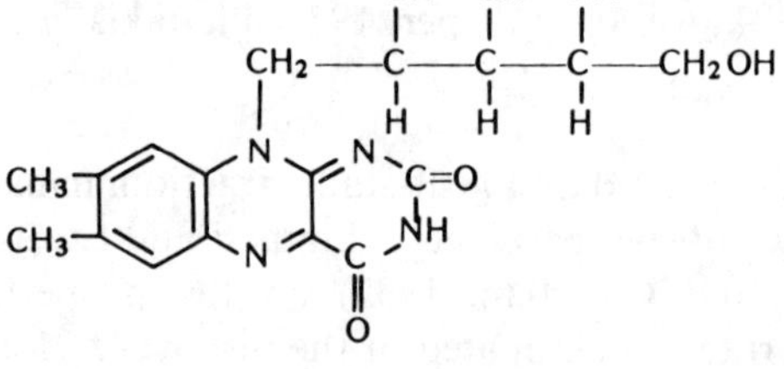

FIG. 14-2. Structure of riboflavin.

and must be liberated before analysis by either enzymatic or acid treatment (Koziol, 1971).

The microbiological assay of riboflavin is more sensitive than fluorometry but requires one to three days for completion. Riboflavin has also been quantified using animal growth assays (Clark, 1940; Wagner *et al.*, 1940; Street, 1941). Although animal assays best reflect riboflavin bioavailability, they are the most time-consuming, expensive, and the least accurate (Shah, 1985). The most commonly used microorganism is *Lactobacillus casei* (Snell and Strong, 1939; Cooperman and Lopez, 1984); while *Leuconostoc mesenteroides* and *Tetrahymena pyriformis* are used less frequently (Shah, 1985).

Riboflavin and its derivatives may also be determined by spectrophotometric (Fazekas and Kokai, 1971) and polarographic methods (Knobloch, 1971). The spectrophotometric measurement of riboflavin is often satisfactory for assaying pharmaceutical preparations, but because of its low sensitivity and the presence of interfering substances, it is not used as an assay method in foods (Shah, 1985). Recently, high-performance liquid chromatography (HPLC) has been reported as a method of riboflavin assay (Van de Weedrdjof *et al.*, 1973; Richardson *et al.*, 1978; Rueckemann and Ranifft, 1978; Kamman *et al.*, 1980).

The total amount of riboflavin in the body is thought to be about 15 mg. The liver, which is the major site of storage, contains about one-third of the total body flavins and, along with the kidney and heart, has the greatest concentration. Seventy to 90% is stored as FAD complexed with numerous flavoprotein dehydrogenases and oxidases; lesser amounts are stored as FMN, and less than 5% as free riboflavin (Cerletti and Ipata, 1960). FAD in tissues can be hydrolyzed to FMN and free riboflavin by phosphatases and nucleotides. Flavins bound to protein are resistant to hydrolysis, which probably accounts for the fact that significant stores of flavins remain in the livers of animals that die of riboflavin deficiency (Cooperman and Lopez, 1984). Riboflavin occurs in foods in the underivatized form and as FMN and FAD complexed to proteins, all of which can fulfil the human requirement.

Biosynthesis of the active forms of riboflavin appears to be tightly regulated and dependent on riboflavin status (Lee and McCormick, 1983). The first step is conversion to the coenzyme FMN by flavokinase or riboflavin kinase, primarily in the intestine and liver (Merrill *et al.*, 1978). Riboflavin and FMN are converted to FAD by FAD synthetase, which is widely distributed in tissues (McCormick, 1975), mostly in the cytosol (DeLuca and Kaplan, 1958).

In bound coenzyme form, riboflavin catalyzes oxidation–reduction reactions by acting as an intermediary in the transfer of electrons in numerous metabolic pathways, many of which are essential for the metabolism of carbohydrates, protein and lipids. Flavoprotein functions include electron transfers, dehydrogenation reactions, reactions with sulfur-containing compounds, hydroxylations, oxidative decarboxylations, dioxygenations, and reduction of oxygen to hydrogen peroxide (Merrill *et al.*, 1982). The riboflavin coenzymes are reversibly oxidized and reduced with ease by a shifting of double bonds in the isoalloxazine ring, a property which makes them particularly useful in biological systems. They are stronger oxidizing agents than NAD^+ and can participate in one- or two-electron processes, and thus in reactions with free radicals or metal ions; in reduced form, they can react directly with oxygen (Metzler, 1977).

Specifically, FMN is a component of the L-amino acid oxidase system that participates in enzymes that oxidize L-amino acids and L-α-hydroxy acids to α-keto acids. FAD participates in many enzyme systems, including succinic dehydrogenase (which links the Krebs cycle directly to oxidative phosphorylation), xanthine oxidase, glycine oxidase, lipoyl dehydrogenase, NAD^+-cytochrome c reductase, and D-amino acid oxidase. FAD is also a required coenzyme for glutathione reductase, the enzyme most commonly used to determine riboflavin status (Sauberlich *et al.*, 1973). Flavoproteins are necessary for both the synthesis and degradation of fatty acids, and both FMN and FAD participate in the mixed-function oxidase system. Riboflavin has an effect on the utilization of other B vitamins in that it is needed for the conversion of folic acid to its reduced coenzyme form, as well as to convert pyridoxine phosphate to pyridoxamine phosphate (Wada and Snell, 1961), a necessary coenzyme in the conversion of tryptophan to niacin. Riboflavin is thus an enzyme cofactor fundamental to most areas of metabolism, particularly anabolic and energy-yielding processes.

(iii) Niacin

Niacin is the official name for the vitamin that includes both nicotinic acid and nicotinamide. Nicotinic acid was first isolated as an oxidation product of nicotine, from which its name is derived (Hankes, 1984). Funk (1911) isolated it from rice polishings when he was searching for an anti-beriberi factor, but did not recognize its nutritional significance. The nutritional role of nicotinic acid was firmly established when it was isolated from liver concentrates and shown by Elvehjem and colleagues (1938) to cure black tongue in dogs. In the 1920s, Goldberger and colleagues (Goldberger *et al.*, 1926; Goldberger and Wheeler, 1928) of the US Public Health Service recognized that human pellagra and black tongue in dogs responded to treatment with animal protein and to boiled extracts of yeast almost devoid of protein. The biological function of nicotinic acid in hydrogen transport, suggesting that the compound was of metabolic importance, was discovered by Warberg and Christian (1935). The classification of nicotinic acid as a vitamin was fully established when Elvehjem *et al.* (1938) showed that the active component in the liver extracts they used to cure black tongue in dogs was nicotinamide. Subsequent treatment of pellagrous humans with nicotinic acid confirmed niacin as the pellagra-preventative factor (Spies *et al.*, 1938).

Nicotinic acid and nicotinamide are pyridine-3-carboxylic acid and pyridine-3-carboxamide, respectively, with nicotinamide being the active form (Fig. 14-3). The term 'niacin' is a generic descriptor of nicotinic acid and its derivatives that exhibit similar nicotinamide biological activity (American Institute of Nutrition, 1979). Both nicotinic acid and nicotinamide are odorless, white crystalline solids, readily soluble in water and alcohol but not in ether. They are stable in the dry state at temperatures below 50°C and in solution at temperatures not exceeding 120°C. When treated with acid or alkali, nicotinamide is converted to nicotinic acid (Hankes, 1984).

The most sensitive method for the determination of niacin in most samples is the microbiological assay using the organism *Lactobacillus arabinosis* (Snell and Strong, 1939). Samples of serum, urine, food, or tissues may be analyzed by this method (Hankes, 1984). Methods for chemical determination of niacin depend upon the reaction of the pyridine ring with cyanogen bromide to give a pyridimium compound that undergoes rearrangement to derivatives that couple with aromatic amines to produce colored compounds. The Association of Vitamin Chemists (1966) recognizes two methods that utilize *p*-methylaminophenol sulfate as the aromatic amine employed for color development. One method uses acid hydrolysis, and the other basic hydrolysis for liberating niacin. The Association of Official Agricultural Chemists (1960) adopted a method that utilizes sulfanilic acid for color development. These methods are less

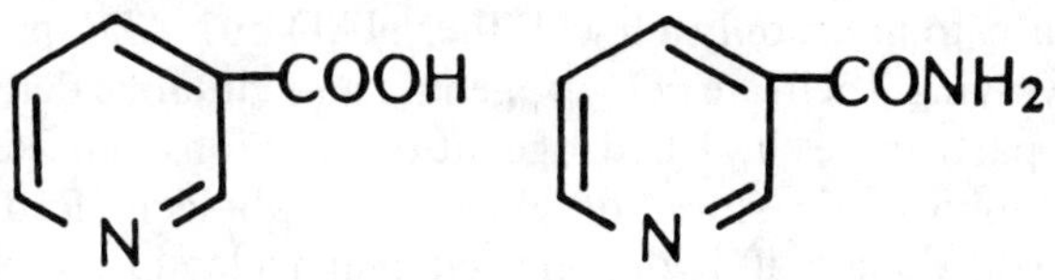

FIG. 14-3. Structure of nicotinic acid and nicotinamide.

sensitive than microbiological procedures and generally require extensive extraction, purification steps, and blank determinations (Hankes, 1984). Methods using fluorometry (Clark, 1980) and high-performance liquid chromatography (Shaik *et al.*, 1977; Hengen *et al.*, 1978; DeVries *et al.*, 1980) have emerged more recently as tools to determine nicotinamide.

In the tissues, most of the niacin is present as nicotinamide in NAD and NADP, for which there is continuous turnover (Hankes, 1984). Although the liver may contain a significant fraction of the free vitamin, in other tissues there is little storage of niacin as such (Knox, 1976; Hankes, 1984). Nicotinamide is primarily released from catabolism of tissue coenzymes by NAD glycohydrolase (Henderson, 1983).

In uncooked foods of animal origin the major forms of niacin are the cellular pyridine nucleotides, nicotinamide adenine dinucleotide NAD(H) and nicotinamide adenine dinucleotide phosphate NADP(H) (Henderson, 1983). Niacin-containing compounds in plant sources, especially cereals, are in bound form, some of which are not nutritionally available (Ghosh *et al.*, 1963). Two forms of bound niacin have been characterized: (1) peptides, which were called niacinogens; and (2) a carbohydrate complex which was called niacytin. Niacinogens are biologically available (Rao and Gopalan, 1984), but the niacytin form, found in maize, is unavailable and has been implicated in the etiology of pellagra among maize eaters (Kodicek and Wilson, 1960). Treatment of maize with alkali (Kodicek *et al.*, 1956) and roasting of sweet corn (Kodicek *et al.*, 1974) release niacin from the bound form.

A major source of niacin is dietary tryptophan which is converted in the liver to nicotinic acid. Certain bacteria can synthesize niacin from the amino acid tryptophan. Consequently, the dietary supply of this vitamin may be supplemented by intestinal bacterial synthesis in the presence of adequate provision of proteins rich in tryptophan (Heidelberger *et al.*, 1949; Latner, 1975).

NAD(H) and NADP(H) function in many metabolic pathways, especially those of anaerobic glycolysis, the citric acid cycle–electron transport chain, and fatty acid synthesis and oxidation. NAD-dependent enzyme systems include alcohol dehydrogenase, glycerol–phosphate dehydrogenase, lactic dehydrogenase, and glyceraldehyde-3-phosphate dehydrogenase, to name only a few. Either NAD or NADP participates in reactions involving isocitrate dehydrogenase and glutamic dehydrogenase. NADP also participates in dehydrogenation reactions, particularly in the hexose monophosphate shunt of glucose metabolism. Reduced NAD (NADH) usually donates its hydrogens to flavin nucleotides, and thus, to the electron transport chain for energy conservation in the oxidative phosphorylation process. Reduced NADP has an important role in synthesis of fats and steroids, giving up its hydrogens in cellular biosynthetic reactions. Synthesis of fatty acids specifically requires NADPH.

(iv) Pantothenic acid

Williams *et al.* (1933) identified an unknown substance in diverse biological sources that was a potent growth factor for yeast. Because of its widespread occurrence and acidic properties, it was called 'pantothenic' acid, derived from the Greek word for 'from everywhere'. When both the chick antidermatitis factor (Woolley *et al.*, 1939) and the liver filtrate factor of rats (Subbarow and Hitchings, 1939) were found to be pantothenic acid, its importance in animal nutrition warranted its inclusion as a vitamin. Studies on its isolation and chemical structure eventually led to its synthesis (Williams and Major, 1940). Although it was assumed that pantothenic acid functioned as part of a coenzyme like other vitamins, no pantothenate coenzyme was found until 14 years after the initial discovery of the vitamin.

Lipmann (1945) found acetylation of sulfanilamide to depend on an enzyme–coenzyme system present in liver homogenates. The coenzyme of acetylation, or 'coenzyme A' (CoA), was later shown to be a pantothenate derivative (Lipmann *et al.*, 1947; DeVries *et al.*, 1950) that is also widely distributed (Kaplan and Lipmann, 1948). The structure of CoA was determined enzymatically (Novelli *et al.*, 1954), and it was eventually chemically synthesized (Moffatt and Khorana, 1961).

The pantothenic acid molecule is a condensation product of pantoic acid and β-alanine (Fig. 14-4), scientifically known as D-*N*-(2,4-dihydroxy-3,3-dimethyl-butyryl)-β-alanine (McCormick, 1988). The vitamin is a pale yellow viscous oil, fairly stable at a neutral pH (between 5·0–7·0) but labile to acid, base and heat. Synthetic pantothenic acid is a white crystalline calcium or sodium salt, soluble in water.

The measurement of pantothenic acid in biological tissues was carried out by early researchers using growth responses of chicks to *Saccharomyces carlsbergensis* yeast (Pennington *et al.*, 1940). Snell *et al.* (1937) described the use of 13 species of lactic acid bacteria for assay purposes, with *L. debruckii*

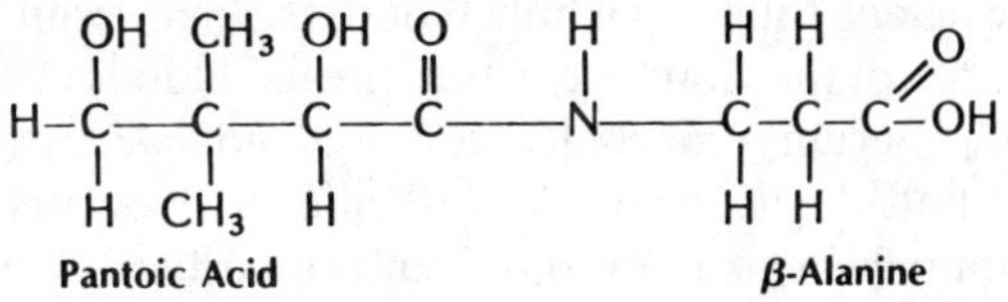

FIG. 14-4. Structure of pantothenic acid.

and *L. casei* being employed most routinely. Another lactic acid organism, *L. plantarum*, was discovered by Skeggs and Wright (1944) and is currently the most commonly used organism in the microbiological assay for pantothenic acid.

Early comparisons between bioassays and microbiological assays were disparate (Jukes, 1941, 1947), with greater available pantothenic acid on bioassay than that determined microbiologically. These discrepancies were partially explained when Ives and Strong (1946) recognized that biological samples must be treated hydrolytically to increase the total measurable pantothenic acid. Extensive research in enzymatic hydrolysis led eventually to the use of pigeon liver extract and an intestinal phosphatase (Novelli *et al.*, 1949). The ability of the two enzymes to liberate pantothenic acid from coenzyme A involves two cleavage points. The phosphatase cleaves pantotheine (the sulfhydral form) from its diphosphoesterase linkage to adenine, and the pigeon liver enzymes cleave the peptide linkage between pantethenate and β-mercaptoethylamine (Novelli *et al.*, 1954). Wittwer *et al.* (1983) later purified a pantetheine hydrolysis enzyme from pig kidney which substitutes well for the pigeon liver enzyme. Appropriate activity of either hydrolytic enzyme with the phosphatase releases any pantothenic acid from coenzyme A, phosphopantetheine, phosphopantothenic acid, dephospho coenzyme A, pantetheine, pantethine (the disulfide form), and other forms of the vitamins (Wittwer *et al.*, 1982). Microbiological assay of the pantothenate content of CoA correlates well with the bioassay after this 'dual enzyme' treatment (Lipmann *et al.*, 1950).

A radioimmunosssay (RIA) was developed for measuring pantothenic acid in blood (Wyse and Hansen, 1977; Wyse *et al.*, 1979) and compares favorably with values determined by microbiological assay using *Lactobacillus plantarum*. The assay has been modified and used successfully for quantifying pantothenic acid in urine, human breast milk, and foods (Wyse *et al.*, 1979; Walsh *et al.*, 1980; 1981a, b; Srinivasan *et al.*, 1981; Song *et al.*, 1984, 1985). An indirect enzyme-linked immunosorbent assay (Song *et al.*, 1990) and high-performance liquid chromatography (Halvorsen and Skrede, 1980) have recently been developed for quantifying pantothenic acid and CoA derivatives.

Pantothenic acid is found in whole blood, plasma, serum, and red blood cells. The majority of the vitamin exists in the red blood cells as coenzyme A (Hatano, 1962). Serum reportedly contains no coenzyme A but does contain free pantothenic acid. Pantothenic acid occurs in all tissues, especially in brain, heart, kidney and liver, primarily in CoA form, but also as phosphopantetheine and phosphopantothenate. Pantothenic acid is found largely as part of two coenzymes (coenzyme A and phosphopantethiene) in food sources as well as in animal tissues. The exception is blood plasma, where it is found primarily as pantothenic acid. Pantothenic acid occurs in food in both the bound and free form, although most is in the form of coenzyme A.

Pantothenic acid in active form functions as an integral component of 4′-phosphopantetheine, which serves as a covalently attached prosthetic group of acyl carrier protein (ACP) and as a component of the structure of coenzyme A. In each case, the peptide-linked β-mercaptoethylamine derivative of pantothenic acid, with its high-energy SH group, serves as the site for acyl attachment and activation. The S-acyl derivatives of these pantothenate coenzymes are formed on oxidation of aldehydes, on oxidative decarboxylation of α-keto acids, and from organic acids activated by ATP or GTP. The activated acyl groups may be transferred to other acceptors or modified by oxidation–reduction, carboxylation–decarboxylation, hydration–dehydration, racemization, carbon skeleton rearrangement, or formation of new carbon to carbon bonds. The versatility of the acylated coenzymes arises in part from the extended configuration of pantetheine and in part from the reactivity conferred by the thioester bond.

More than 70 enzymes are known to use CoA or ACP. Generally, pantothenate derivatives mediate the metabolism of carbohydrates, lipids and amino acids. Specifically, in the citric acid cycle CoA functions as an acyl acceptor for the pyruvate and α-ketoglutarate dehydrogenase complexes, forming acetyl CoA and succinyl CoA, respectively. These CoA thioesters are also formed on oxidative degradation of several amino acids. The acetyl group from acetyl CoA is the carbon source for the biosynthesis of fatty acids, prostaglandins, ketone bodies, cholesterol, steroid hormones, and other compounds. Succinyl CoA is an essential precursor for porphyrins, and hence, hemoglobin and cytochromes. In fatty acid synthesis and degradation, pantothenate coenzymes carry the acids as acyl groups through repetitive synthetic or degradative cycles. A CoA thioester is a necessary intermediate in the degradation of cholesterol to bile acid. Coenzyme A thioesters are the acyl donors for many acceptors, including choline and cholesterol.

B. Requirements and Standards

(i) Thiamin

Various biochemical tests based on thiamin metabolism or the biochemical functions of TPP have been developed to detect thiamin deficiency and establish thiamin adequacy in humans (Sauberlich, 1967). The most specific test involves the stimulation of erythrocyte transketolase by in-vitro addition of thiamin pyrophosphate and measurement of transketolase activity in whole blood or erythrocytes with and without TPP (Brin, 1962). An enhancement by greater than 16–25% in enzymatic activity with added TPP indicates a thiamine deficiency.

Many studies have been conducted to determine human thiamin requirement by experimental deficiency or nutrition surveys (Food and Nutrition Board, 1980). While there is a relationship between the utilization of thiamin and the amount of carbohydrate in the diet, it is more practical to relate thiamin intake to total dietary energy. Most experimental studies have examined the effects of varying levels of dietary thiamin on the occurrence of clinical signs of deficiency, on the excretion of thamin or its metabolites, and on erythrocyte transketolase activity. Subjects have generally been fed diets with ratios of carbohydrate and fat similar to those commonly consumed in the United States, as determined by national food consumption and diet and health surveys. On the basis of these studies the minimum requirement appears to be between 0·12 and 0·35 mg per 1000 kilocalories. In order to allow a factor of safety, the value of 0·50 mg per 1000 kcal has been recommended as adequate for most adults. However, many factors influence the requirement for thiamin and must be considered for individual cases or physiological groups.

Studies of urinary excretion of thiamin, blood thiamin levels, and erythrocyte transketolase activity indicate that the requirement for thiamin in women increases during pregnancy (Food and Nutrition Board, 1980). The increase appears to occur early in pregnancy and to remain constant throughout. Therefore, an allowance of 0·6 mg of thiamin per 1000 kcal or about an additional 0·4 mg/day is recommended throughout pregnancy. The thiamin requirement also increases during lactation. The lactating woman secretes approximately 0·1–0·2 mg of thiamin per day in milk. To account for both the thiamin loss in milk and the increased energy consumption during lactation, an allowance of 0·6 mg/1000 kcal is recommended, an additional 0·5 mg/day.

Information on the thiamin requirement of infants is limited. Studies of the thiamin requirement of infants in relation to the thiamin content of human milk suggest that the minimum daily requirement is about 0·03 mg/kg of body weight, or approximately 0·27 mg/1000 kcal. Although the thiamin content of human milk is considered sufficient to protect against deficiency, the allowance recommended to provide a margin of safety in milk formulas is 0·5 mg/1000 kcal. There are few studies of the thiamin requirement of children and adolescents. The thiamin allowance recommended for children and teenagers is 0·5 mg/1000 kcal.

It is now generally recognized that elderly persons have an increased requirement for the B vitamins, including thiamin. Because there is some evidence that older persons use thiamin less efficiently, it is recommended that they maintain an intake of 1 mg/day, even if they consume less than 2000 kcal daily (Food and Nutrition Board, 1980).

Requirements may be influenced by some dietary factors or practices that influence thiamin status and increase the risk of deficiency. A high intake of carbohydrate may increase the need for thiamin, particularly if the carbohydrate has been refined or processed to remove much of the thiamin, as in polished rice, overmilled wheat flour, and refined sugar. Excessive consumption of thiamin antagonists present in tea, coffee, blueberries, Brussels sprouts, red cabbage, and some types of raw seafood may tie up thiamin or destroy it, thus making it unavailable (Hilker and Somogyi, 1982; Murata, 1982; Vimokesant *et al.*, 1982). Groups who subsist largely on snack foods and unbalanced fad diets may also be at increased risk (Gubler, 1984). In the US, however, the chief group at risk of thiamin deficiency are those who consume excessive amounts of alcohol.

The thiamin content per 1000 kcal of selected meat products and other foods, compared to the RDA per 1000 kcal for adults, is presented in Fig. 14-5. The richest dietary sources of thiamin are pork products. The profiles were developed, using the National Live Stock and Meat Board (NLSMB, 1988), Dietary Analysis and Food Comparison System, developed at Utah State University.

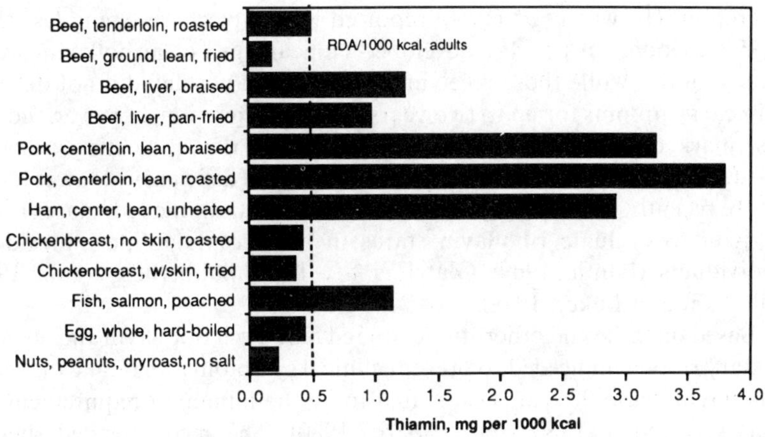

FIG. 14-5. Thiamin content of selected meats and other food products, mg per 1000 kcal.

(ii) Riboflavin

Several methods, including clinical signs, blood and urine levels, and enzyme activity, are used to determine riboflavin nutritional status. Clinical signs, such as cheilosis, stomatitis, and seborrheic dermatitis, are often non-specific, and thus difficult to attribute to lack of riboflavin (Interdepartmental Committee on Nutrition for National Defense, 1963). Urinary riboflavin excretion reflects recent dietary intake and thus has limited use as an indicator of deficiency, because it does not reflect flavin stores (Horwitt *et al.*, 1950). Blood levels of riboflavin tend to be variable and reflect current intake and are useful only in determining an individual's risk of developing a riboflavin deficiency (Tillotson and Sauberlich, 1971). Thus, blood levels of riboflavin have been shown to be somewhat unreliable indicators of nutritional status. Erythrocyte riboflavin levels are sometimes used because they provide a riboflavin storage site not dependent on current intake (Cooperman and Lopez, 1984).

An established, sensitive and specific test for quantifying any functional effect of riboflavin deficiency in the tissues is the measurement of activity of glutathione reductase (an FAD-containing enzyme) in erythrocytes, with and without added FAD (Sauberlich *et al.*, 1972; Tillotson and Baker, 1972). An activation coefficient of over 1·30 with added FAD indicates inadequate riboflavin in the tissues (Sauberlich *et al.*, 1972; Thurnham and Rathaketle, 1982).

Requirements for riboflavin have been determined from experimental studies on adults and infants, with minimum requirement defined as levels which prevent clinical signs of deficiency and provide for normal urinary excretion. Horwitt *et al.* (1950) reported that subjects receiving less than 0·55 mg riboflavin per day developed clinical signs of ariboflavinosis by four months, while those receiving 0·75–0·85 mg per day did not develop clinical symptoms for up to two years. Urinary excretion, however, did not rise markedly until intakes exceeded 1·1 mg per day, indicating a lack of tissue saturation and the possibility of subclinical deficiency at lower levels. More recently, studies have used erythrocyte glutathione reductase (EGR) activity to evaluate riboflavin status in adolescents, adult, and elderly individuals (Bamji, 1969; Glatzl *et al.*, 1970; Sauberlich *et al.*, 1972; Tillotson and Baker, 1972).

Based on these and other studies on red blood cell riboflavin and levels of dietary riboflavin needed to prevent clinical symptoms, an intake of 0·5 mg riboflavin per 1000 kcal is estimated to be the minimum requirement for adults (Food and Nutrition Board, 1980). The recommended dietary allowance, with a margin of safety factored in for healthy people of all ages, is 0·6 mg riboflavin per 1000 kcal. Elderly individuals and those consuming less than 2000 kcal/day are advised to consume a minimum of 1·2 mg daily. In contrast to thiamin, riboflavin requirements are not considered to increase when energy intake increases. There have, however, been reports that the level of riboflavin intake to maintain normal activity of EGR may be higher for athletes (Belko *et al.*, 1983). Use of oral contraceptive agents have been associated with stimulation of EGR, suggesting an increased requirement for women using these drugs (Briggs and Briggs, 1974; Sanpitak and Chayutimonkul, 1974; Admed *et al.*, 1975; Prasad *et al.*, 1975; Newman *et al.*, 1978; Roe *et al.*, 1982).

Studies of urinary excretion have shown that pregnant women excrete less riboflavin and require more energy than non-pregnant women (Brzezinski *et al.*, 1952; Jansen and Jansen, 1954). FAD stimulation of EGR activity indicates that the riboflavin requirement for women increases during pregnancy (Cooperman *et al.*, 1973; Heller *et al.*, 1974). The recommended dietary allowance is increased by 0·3 mg per day to meet the additional requirements of pregnancy. Riboflavin requirements also increase during lactation. The estimated amount of riboflavin secreted in human milk is 0·34 mg per day, with an efficiency of utilization for milk production of about 70%. Thus, an additional daily intake of 0·5 mg is recommended (Food and Nutrition Board, 1980).

The amount of riboflavin provided per 1000 kcal of selected meats and other foods, compared to the RDA per 1000 kcal, is illustrated in Fig. 14-6. Protein-rich foods are important sources of the vitamin, which is little affected by usual methods of food preparation.

(iii) Niacin

Assessment of the niacin requirement is complicated by the fact that dietary tryptophan can be converted to nicotinate mononucleotide (NMN) and then to NAD in the body. Quinolinic acid, synthesized from tryptophan, appears to be the immediate precursor for *de novo* synthesis of nicotinic acid and is the primary source of NMN (Gholson, 1966). The efficiency of conversion, which depends on a number of factors, is an important consideration in meeting the body's need for niacin. Protein, energy, pyridoxine and riboflavin nutritional status affect the efficiency of enzymes in the conversion sequence and thus may influence the amount of NAD available from tryptophan (Horwitt *et al.*, 1956; Goldsmith *et al.*, 1961; Consolazio *et al.*, 1972; Satyanarayana and Rao, 1977).

Because dietary tryptophan contributes to niacin nutriture, the term 'niacin equivalents' was introduced to facilitate the calculation of the

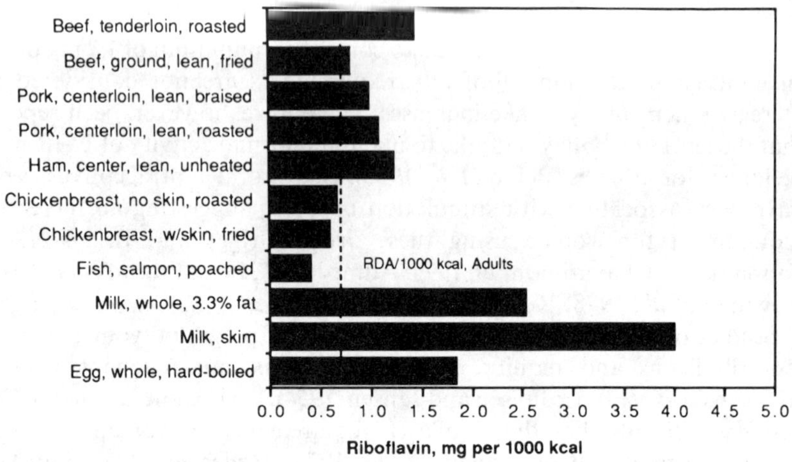

FIG. 14-6. Riboflavin content of selected meats and other food products, mg per 1000 kcal.

combined effects of nicotinic acid and tryptophan in the diet (Horwitt, 1955). Approximately 60 mg of dietary tryptophan is estimated to be equivalent to 1 mg niacin, based upon studies of the amounts of tryptophan converted to nicotinate mononucleotide (NMN) and its metabolites in human subjects (Horwitt *et al.*, 1956; Goldsmith, 1958). Because niacin deficiency syndromes are complicated by factors influencing the conversion of tryptophan into niacin, as well as by the questionable biological availability of bound forms of niacin in food, these factors must be carefully considered and intakes estimated in terms of niacin equivalents, or results of clinical or survey assessments may be misleading.

Biochemical assessment of niacin nutritional status is usually based on measurement of urinary metabolites. Measurement of N^1-methylnicotinamide is often employed in population surveys; it was the method used by the Interdepartmental Committee on Nutrition for National Defense (1963) for evaluation of niacin nutrition. The excretion ratio of N^1-methyl-2-pyridone-5-carboxylamide (2-pyridone) to N^1-methylnicotinamide is now considered to be the best index of niacin nutritional status (Sauberlich *et al.*, 1973). The ratio ranges from 1·3–4·0 under normal conditions; a ratio of less than 1·0 is indicative of niacin deficiency (deLange and Joubert, 1964). However, estimation of 2-pyridone is tedious and time-consuming and thus not readily adaptable as a field method. Determination of cellular or blood serum levels of nucleotides of nicotinamide has not proven to be a reliable method for evaluating niacin status, nor has a functional biochemical test for assessing body reserves been developed (Hankes, 1984).

Niacin requirements of humans are expressed in terms of niacin equivalents. Goldsmith (1958) and colleagues (Goldsmith *et al.*, 1956, 1961) first showed in human studies that 34–86 mg tryptophan, or an average of 55 mg, are equivalent to 1 mg niacin in preventing deficiency symptoms. Horwitt *et al.* (1956) obtained values of 46–86 mg tryptophan to 1 mg niacin and Wertz *et al.* (1958) reported a ratio that varied from 45:1 to 69:1. Some evidence indicates that pregnant women can convert tryptophan to niacin more efficiently than other adults (Wertz *et al.*, 1952). For the purposes of establishing niacin intake standards, a dietary intake of 60 mg tryptophan is considered equivalent to 1 mg niacin, and one niacin equivalent is considered equal to either of these amounts (Food and Nutrition Board, 1980).

Recommended dietary allowances for niacin are related to energy expenditure because of the role of the coenzymes NAD and NADP in respiration. Based on human depletion repletion studies, the minimum adult requirement of niacin has been reported as 4·4 mg niacin equivalents per 1000 kcal (Horwitt *et al.*, 1956; Horwitt, 1958). The Joint Food and Agriculture Organization/World Health Organization Expert Group (Joint FAO/WHO Expert Group, 1967) has suggested a safe intake of 6·6 mg niacin equivalents per 1000 kcal for all age groups. Recommended dietary allowances for the United States are based upon this value. The allowance recommended for adults, expressed as niacin equivalents, is 6·6 niacin equivalents per 1000 kcal and not less than 13 niacin equivalents at caloric intakes of less than 2000 kcal (Food and Nutrition Board, 1980).

In pregnancy (Wertz *et al.*, 1958) and on administration of estrogens and oral contraceptives (Horwitt *et al.*, 1975), larger than normal amounts of nicotinamide metabolites are excreted in the urine. It appears that estrogens induce the first enzyme, tryptophan dioxygenase, in the tryptophan-to-niacin conversion pathway. This may suggest that more tryptophan is converted to NAD during pregnancy, so that 60 mg tryptophan in the diet may be equivalent to more than 1 mg niacin. Alternatively, more tryptophan may be diverted through this pathway, or methylation of niacin may be increased during pregnancy, resulting in an increased niacin requirement (Food and Nutrition Board, 1980). The allowance recommended provides an increase of 2 niacin equivalents daily during pregnancy, based on the recommended increase in energy intake of 300 kcal daily. Use of oral contraceptive drugs appears to impair the tryptophan to niacin conversion secondary to vitamin B_6 deficiency

(Leklem *et al.*, 1975). The Food and Nutrition Board (1980) suggests, however, that the adult recommended allowance appears to provide an adequate degree of safety to meet these conditions.

With a recommended increase of 500 kcal to support lactation, an additional intake of 3·3 niacin equivalents is suggested (Food and Nutrition Board, 1980), based upon average levels of niacin in breast milk (Wertz *et al.*, 1958). Therefore, a total additional intake of 5 niacin equivalents per day is recommended during lactation.

Niacin therapy has been shown to be effective in increasing the ratio of high-density to low-density lipoproteins, increasing coronary blood flow, reducing serum cholesterol and triglyceride levels, and increasing brain circulation, and thus may have beneficial effects on these conditions of aging. Elderly individuals should ensure that their intakes of niacin meet the recommended allowance for adults.

The amount of preformed niacin found in selected meat items and other food products is presented in Fig. 14-7. The data are presented in mg preformed niacin per 1000 kcal and compared to the adult niacin RDA per 1000 kcal. Meat and poultry are the richest sources of the vitamin; milk is low in preformed niacin, but contains high amounts of tryptophan, and thus has a high niacin equivalent.

(iv) Pantothenic acid

At present, pantothenic acid status is determined by measuring urinary excretion of the vitamin, alone or in combination with whole blood levels. Numerous studies have shown urinary excretion to respond to changes in dietary intake (Fox and Linkswiler, 1961; Srinivasan *et al.*, 1981; Kies *et al.*, 1982; Song *et al.*, 1984, 1985; Eissenstat *et al.*, 1986). The normal range of excretion is 1–15 mg per day, with a mean of 4 mg (Sauberlich and Logan, 1983). Urinary excretion of less than 1 mg per day is considered abnormally low.

Normal ranges in whole blood are from 103–183 μg per dl (Sauberlich and Logan, 1983). Whole blood levels less than 100 μg per dl are also considered indicative of subnormal status. Serum levels of the vitamin seem to be less sensitive to dietary levels than urinary excretion, but they do respond to extreme changes in intake (Kies *et al.*, 1982). In a study of elderly subjects, Srinivasan *et al.* (1981) found that blood pantothenic acid levels did not correlate with unsupplemented dietary intake but did so when subjects were given a dietary supplement.

Biochemical means for detecting and evaluating pantothenic acid deficiency are limited. Even though CoA functions in over 70 different

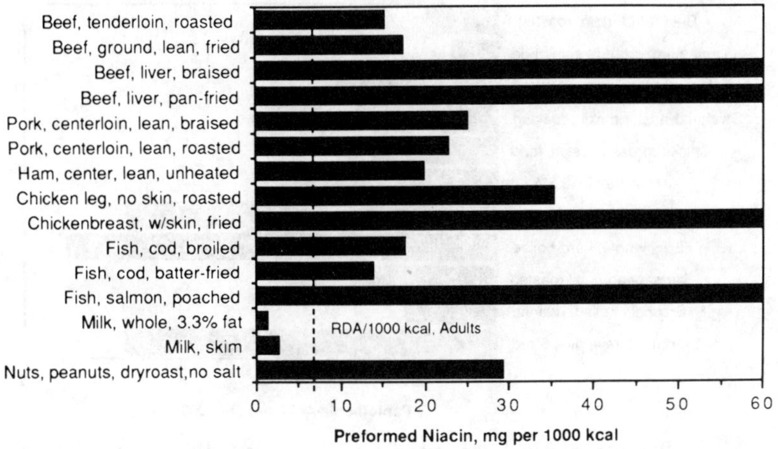

FIG. 14-7. Preformed niacin content of selected meats and other food products, mg per 1000 kcal.

metabolic reactions and is present in all human tissues, it has not been easy to isolate a metabolic step that can sensitively reflect nutritional status of the nutrient. Functional tests have been proposed based on acetylation of sulfanilamide by red blood cells (Ellestad *et al.*, 1970) and urinary excretion of acetylated *p*-aminobenzoic acid after a load test of pantothenate (Sarma *et al.*, 1949). Findings from dietary histories often do not correlate well with biochemical changes, thus the utility of these tests in reflecting pantothenic acid nutritional status is unknown.

Further research is needed to establish the relationship of pantothenic acid intake to urinary excretion and blood levels in order to provide suitable measures for evaluating status and establishing dietary recommendations. At present, dietary recommendations for various age and sex groups are based on estimates of normal intakes, along with limited research on urinary excretion in relation to intake. The Food and Nutrition Board (1980) has not set a recommended dietary allowance for pantothenic acid but has established a provisional allowance of 4–7 mg/day for adults. While estimates of intakes of adults in the US average 10–15 mg/day, the allowance is based on research demonstrating that consumption of 7 mg per day on a normal diet is associated with normal urinary excretion levels (Fox and Linkswiler, 1961).

Slightly higher intakes may be warranted during pregnancy and lactation (Ishiguro, 1962; Cohenour and Calloway, 1972; Song *et al.*, 1984,

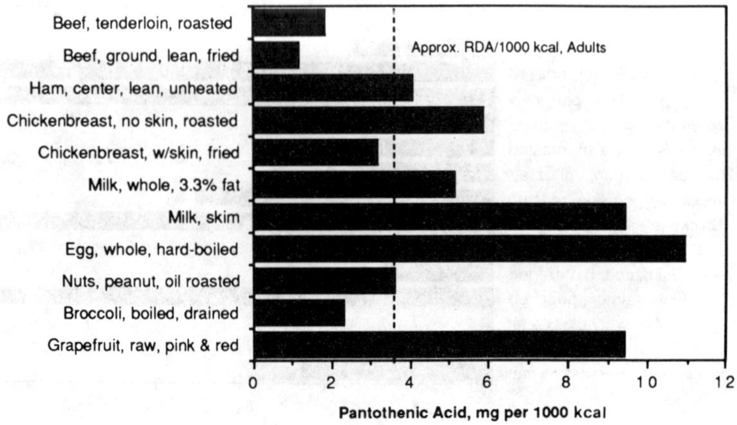

FIG. 14-8. Pantothenic acid content of selected meats and other food products, mg per 1000 kcal.

1985). The pantothenic acid content of human milk has been shown to reflect the level in the diet (Johnston *et al.*, 1981; Song *et al.*, 1984, 1985), with a correlation of 0·62 between dietary pantothenic acid and milk content. Human milk averages about 2·0–2·5 mg of pantothenic acid per liter (Song *et al.*, 1984, 1985). Recommended intakes of pantothenic acid for infants and children are presently based on proportional energy needs, with 2 mg per day being recommended for infants and 4–5 mg per day for adolescents (Food and Nutrition Board, 1980).

Figure 14-8 illustrates the amount of pantothenic acid per 1000 kcal in selected meats and other food products. These data were compared to a standard for adults of 3·5 mg pantothenic acid per 1000 kcal. This value was derived from 7 mg pantothenic acid, the upper limit of the Estimated Safe and Adequate Daily Dietary Intake (Food and Nutrition Board, 1980), assuming an average 2000 kcal diet. Pantothenic acid is a component of all living tissue, and all food groups make a significant contribution to dietary intake.

C. Deficiency and Excess

(i) Thiamin

Beriberi is the disease resulting from thiamin deficiency in humans. The most prominent clinical signs of beriberi are expressed as a triad of symptoms: (1) loss of appetite, nausea, and associated weight loss; (2) cardiovascular involvement; and (3) neurological symptoms. The signs and symptoms vary, depending on age, individual, diet, duration and severity of the deficiency, and abruptness of onset, but all three symptoms are generally present to some degree. Although the clinical syndrome of thiamin deficiency and biochemical function of the vitamin are well defined, the precise biochemical defect responsible for the pathophysiological manifestation of thiamin deficiency is not established.

In humans, no toxic effects, other than possibly some gastric upset, have been reported even with high oral doses of thiamin (Hayes and Hegsted, 1973). Few if any toxic effects have been noted with thousands of injections by subcutaneous, intramuscular, and intravenous routes of doses as high as 100–200 times the estimated daily requirements. Most of the reported instances of toxic reactions have occurred at dosages several hundred times the RDA (Dipalma and Ritchie, 1977). Neuromuscular and cardiovascular system effects, such as headache, convulsions, weakness, paralysis, vasodilatation, tachycardia, and cardiac arrhythmias, have been most evident (Miller and Hayes, 1982). Hypersensitivity reactions producing anaphylactic shock have occurred following repeated parenteral injections (Tetreault and Beck, 1956; Falk and Protheroe, 1979). For this reason, parenteral administration of thiamin is now used only in special cases (Gubler, 1984), and few cases of thiamin toxicity have been reported in recent years (Miller and Hayes, 1982).

(ii) Riboflavin

Signs of riboflavin deficiency appear in individuals who subsist on nutritionally poor diets for extended periods of time. The symptoms observed under these conditions may not necessarily be specific for riboflavin deficiency, since the diet may be lacking in several B vitamins. In experimental studies in which human subjects were fed diets lacking only in riboflavin or fed riboflavin antagonists, clinical signs most likely specific for riboflavin deficiency were observed (Sebrell and Butler, 1938). These included angular stomatitis, cheilosis, and nasolabial seborrhea, which responded to the administration of riboflavin. Other clinical features included magenta tongue with central atrophy of the lingual papillae (geographic tongue), dermatitis and pruritis of the scrotum and vulva (Horwitt *et al.*, 1949; Hills *et al.*, 1951), and numerous eye changes, including invasion of the cornea by capillary blood vessels, reduced tearing, and photophobia (Sydenstricker *et al.*, 1940).

In humans, toxicity from riboflavin is unknown (Miller and Hayes, 1982; Cooperman and Lopez, 1984). This may be due to its relatively low solubility, or because the transport system required for absorption of riboflavin is easily saturated, limiting the amount that can be absorbed. In fact, the absorptive capacity for orally administered riboflavin may be less than 20 mg in a single dose (Mayersohn *et al.*, 1969). While there is little risk of harm from megavitamin doses, likewise there is no apparent benefit, as any excess riboflavin absorbed is rapidly excreted in the urine of normal adults.

(iii) Niacin

The disease pellagra has been known to western Europe from the time of the introduction of maize as a food plant in the early 1700s. Through their classical experiments on human volunteers, Goldberger (1916) and associates (Goldberger and Wheeler, 1915) established that pellagra is a dietary deficiency disease. Usually the early symptoms of pellagra are weakness, lassitude, anorexia and indigestion (Elvehjem, 1940). This is followed by the classic 'three Ds': dermatitis, diarrhea and dementia. The beneficial effects of niacin in preventing pellagra were subsequently demonstrated (Spies *et al.*, 1938).

Although pellegra once was common in the southern United States and Europe, where maize was commonly consumed in poor communities, the disease has been eliminated there (Rao and Gopalan, 1984). Africa appears to be the only continent where there are areas in which pellagra remains an important public health threat, particularly in southern Africa where it remains endemic.

Large doses of nicotinic acid have been reported to reduce serum levels of cholesterol (Altschul *et al.*, 1955; Grundy *et al.*, 1981) and of very-low-density, intermediate-density, and low-density lipoproteins in patients with type-III hyperlipoproteinemia (Blum *et al.*, 1977; Patsch *et al.*, 1977). The Coronary Drug Project Research Group (1975) concluded that nicotinic acid is a safe drug, that it lowers plasma cholesterol by 9%, and that it reduces the recurrence rate of non-fatal myocardial infarction by 29%, but that it does not reduce mortality. The beneficial effects on serum lipid levels must be weighed against potential toxic effects of prolonged treatment with high doses.

Gram doses of nicotinic acid, but not nicotinamide, cause transient vasodilatation resulting in flushing, burning, and tingling, especially of the face, neck, and hands (Mosher, 1970; Hayes and Hegsted, 1973); transient heartburn, nausea, vomiting, and diarrhea (Hawkins, 1968; Gokal *et al.*, 1978; Russell and Oliver, 1978); and hyperpigmentation and bulbous dermatitis (Wittenborn *et al.*, 1974). The greatest concerns over possible toxicity from chronic niacin therapy comes from several reports of jaundice and liver dysfunction (Christensen *et al.*, 1961; Mosher, 1970; Winter and Boyer, 1973; Einstein *et al.*, 1975). Liver function tests for bilirubin, transaminase, and alkaline phosphatase have been found to be abnormal with niacin therapy. Severe jaundice may occur at dosages as low as 750 mg per day (Sugerman and Clark, 1974). Liver biopsy indicates cholestatic hepatitis, portal fibrosis, and parenchymal cell necrosis. The jaundice usually subsides after therapy is discontinued, but in some cases the abnormal liver function tests persist and hepatitis recurs, indicating irreversible liver damage. This evidence indicates a direct hepato-toxic effect of niacin, although risks are uncertain and vary with the individual. Most investigators consider niacin to be relatively harmless at moderate doses for limited periods of treatment; but there are toxic risks involved, and caution should be used when prescribing high doses of niacin to women of childbearing age and to patients with histories of ulcers, diabetes, and liver disease (Miller and Hayes, 1982).

(iv) Pantothenic acid

Research on pantothenic acid nutriture in human beings has been limited for several reasons. Since pantothenic acid is ubiquitous in nature a deficiency has been rare, except as an accompaniment to general, severe malnutrition. Deficiency was reported to cause the 'burning foot syndrome' among prisoners in Japan and the Philippines during World War II (Glusman, 1947). Symptoms included abnormal skin sensations of the feet and lower legs, increased by warmth and decreased by cold. Current concern about pantothenic acid status partly stems from increased intake of processed and refined foods, from which losses can be significant.

An overt dietary deficiency has not been clinically recognized in humans except when a metabolic antagonist, ω-methylpantothenic acid, was administered (Hodges *et al.*, 1959) or when a pantothenic acid-free semi-synthetic diet was given (Bean and Hodges, 1954; Bean *et al.*, 1955; Hodges *et al.*, 1958, 1959; Fry *et al.*, 1976). Subjects receiving the antagonist experienced a burning sensation in the feet, tenderness in the heels, muscle weakness, postural hypotension, rapid heart rate on exertion, epigastric distress with anorexia and constipation, depression, fatigue, and insomnia. Accompanying biochemical changes included decreased eosinopenic response to ACTH, change in glucose tolerance with increased sensitivity to insulin, and loss of antibody production. Subjects who received only a deficient diet without the antagonist developed fatigue and listlessness, but clinical symptoms did not emerge.

While overt deficiency of pantothenic acid is thought to be extremely rare, the methodology for determining pantothenic acid status has been so tedious and time-consuming that consistency for results of biochemical levels across laboratories has not been good. The radioimmunoassay (RIA) developed by Wyse *et al.* (1979) provides a superior method for determining pantothenic acid status. The RIA can be used alone or as a check on microbiological techniques. Using the RIA, researchers have determined that some population groups, particularly the elderly, adolescents, and pregnant or lactating women, may be at risk for suboptimal pantothenic acid status (Wyse and Hansen, 1977; Srinivasan *et al.*, 1981; Walsh *et al.*, 1981b; Song *et al.*, 1985; Eissenstat *et al.*, 1986). There are also indications that pantothenic acid metabolism may be impaired in alcoholics (Tao and Fox, 1976) and users of oral contraceptives (Lewis and King, 1980). Patients with chronic ulcerative and granulomatous colitis (Ellestad-Sayed *et al.*, 1976) are more likely than normal individuals to develop pantothenic acid deficiency.

High doses of pantothenic acid have been recommended in cases of burn and dermatitis, to relieve postoperative paralytic ileum, to prevent the graying of hair, and to protect against stress. However, the effectiveness of these treatments has not been substantiated (Miller and Hayes, 1982). There is no evidence of pantothenic acid toxicity in humans, although ingestion of 10–20 g of the calcium salt have caused occasional diarrhea and minor gastrointestinal disturbances (Harris and Lepkovsky, 1954; Hayes and Hegsted, 1973).

III. STATUS OF FOOD COMPOSITION DATA

A. Nutrient Composition

Increased demands by scientists, dietitians, the food industry, and government agencies for information on the nutrient content of foods derive from the awareness and importance being placed on the role of nutrition in public health problems. The Nutrient Data Research Branch of the Human Nutrition Information Service (HNIS), US Department of Agriculture (USDA) operates the National Nutrient Data Bank (NDB) and compiles and releases nutrient composition data in both published and machine-readable form (USDA, 1988a). In addition to reference data and tables, nutrient data bases are created to interpret results of food consumption surveys conducted by the Nutrition Monitoring Division of HNIS and by the National Center for Health Statistics.

The USDA Nutrient Data Bank is a computer-based management

system which stores nutrient data (Rizek *et al.*, 1984) and descriptive information about the data (Hepburn, 1982, 1987a). The data are obtained from both published sources and private communications. Published sources consist of the scientific and technical literature, numerous special bulletins, research reports, and other documents containing data or relevant material. Sources of unpublished data include industry, government agencies, and academic institutions. USDA personnel evaluate these data on the basis of sampling techniques, analytical methodology, and replication procedures to ensure the statistical validity of average or representative values which are incorporated into USDA-released data (Stewart, 1983; Rizek *et al.*, 1984; Hepburn, 1987a).

Some values in released data are calculated in standard ways from analytical values. Protein, for example, is not analyzed directly but is calculated from the average nitrogen content of each food. Nutrient content of food mixtures is calculated from analytical values for the raw products, adjusted for yield (fat and water changes) and for retention of vitamins and minerals. Accuracy of calculated values depends upon the accuracy of the analytical procedures upon which they are based (Rizek *et al.*, 1984).

Selected USDA food and nutrient data sets are discussed below. Users of computerized data sets should be familiar with the supplementary information in corresponding printed publications (USDA, 1988a). Considerable variation may occur between printed and computerized versions of USDA data bases because computerized tapes contain more current data and give imputed or estimated nutrient values where missing values appear in publications (Hoover and Pelican, 1984). Imputed values are flagged on the data tapes to indicate that data entries are not based on analytical values (Rizek *et al.*, 1984).

(i) Agriculture Handbook No. 8, *Data Base for Standard Reference*

The standard published nutrient data reference is *Agriculture Handbook No. 8, Composition of Foods: Raw, Processed, Prepared (AH-8)*, last completely revised in 1963 (USDA, 1963). The corresponding machine-readable data set is the USDA Nutrient Data Base for Standard Reference. Most current nutrition-related projects use one of these two reference sources or a data base derived primarily from one of them (Rizek *et al.*, 1984).

The USDA is conducting a major revision of *AH-8* to provide current nutrient information on foods. The revision of *Agriculture Handbook No. 8* is being issued in sections in order to expedite release of data to the public.

Each section contains a table of nutrient data for a major food group. The entire series will cover a wide range of food products. Published handbooks of meat and meat products include *No. 8-5, Poultry Products* (USDA, 1979), *No. 8-7, Sausages and Luncheon Meats* (USDA, 1980), *No. 8-10, Pork and Pork Products* (USDA, 1983), *No. 8-13, Beef Products* (USDA, 1986a), *No. 8-15, Fish and Shellfish* (USDA, 1987a) and *No. 8-21, Fast Foods* (USDA, 1988b). Meat and meat-related sections to be published are *8-17, Lamb, Veal and Game* and *8-22, Mixed Dishes* (Hepburn, 1987a).

The nutritive values contained in revised *Handbook No. 8* reflect the increasing information available on nutrients and food products. Data for individual food items may include 60 or more nutrients or food components, the number of samples from which the values were derived, and, where possible, the standard error, as indicators of the confidence that can be placed on the mean values (Hepburn, 1982, 1987b; Rizek *et al.*, 1984). The nutrient values in these revisions supersede data for those specific foods as given in the 1963 edition of *Handbook No. 8* and in other previous publications of the USDA. Descriptions of foods and data, taken from the published handbooks of meat, poultry, fish, and related products, are provided below.

The fifth in the series of publications, *Handbook No. 8-5*, serves as a basic reference for data on nutrients in poultry products (USDA, 1979). The number of poultry products for which data are tabulated was extended to 304, more than twice the number in the 1963 edition of the handbook. Some of the items in the previous edition were omitted. The nutritive values in the revision are based on an extensive review of over 1000 documents published since 1963. Much of the data for broiler-fryer chickens and for turkeys was obtained from studies conducted under contract with the former Agricultural Research Service (now part of the Science and Education Administration) between 1970 and 1975. Laboratory research on broiler-fryer chickens and turkeys, carried out under sponsorship of the Science and Education Administration, supplied much of the information on weights, physical composition, and tissue content of thiamin, riboflavin, and niacin. The research on chicken was conducted at Virginia Polytechnic and State University, Blacksburg. The study on turkey was made at the University of Nebraska, Lincoln. Most of the data for thiamin were determined by the fluorometric thiochrome procedure. Riboflavin was most frequently analyzed by fluorometry. Niacin data were obtained both chemically and microbiologically. The values for niacin do not include the niacin that could be contributed by tryptophan, a niacin precursor. The term 'niacin equivalent' applies to the potential niacin value, that is, to the sum of the preformed niacin and the amount that could be derived from tryptophan. In estimating the amount of niacin available from foods, the average value of 60 mg of tryptophan is considered equivalent to 1 mg of niacin.

The seventh in the *Handbook No. 8* series serves as a basic reference for data on nutrients in sausages and luncheon meats (USDA, 1980). The number of sausages and luncheon meats for which data are tabulated has been extended to 80, about twice the number in the 1963 edition of the handbook. All items in this revision are marketed products. Much of the nutrient data was obtained from analyses conducted since 1973 for nutritional labeling. The values for almost every food item in the 1963 handbook have been changed to incorporate more recent findings, thus the nutrient values in this revision supersede data for these specific foods given in the previous edition. The data used in this handbook were obtained primarily from private communications. Only limited data are included from the scientific and technical literature. Sources of unpublished data are industry, government agencies, and studies conducted under contract with the Science and Education Administration. Values for poultry products are from *Agriculture Handbook No. 8-5*.

The tenth in the series of *Handbook No. 8* publications provides data on nutrients in pork products (USDA, 1983). Data are presented for 132 fresh pork products and 54 cured products. For the purposes of this publication the term 'fresh' means uncured. Three fat classes of fresh pork cuts are not presented, as in the 1963 edition of this handbook, because pork is not currently marketed as such. The nutritive values in the revisions are based on an extensive review of the documents published since 1960. Much of the data for fresh pork cuts was obtained from studies conducted in 1979 and 1980 by the Agricultural Research Service. The nutrient data for the cured products were obtained primarily from analyses conducted since 1973 for nutritional labeling. Values for almost every food item in the 1963 handbook were changed to incorporate more recent findings. Laboratory research on pork, carried out under the sponsorship of the Agricultural Research Service, supplied a large portion of the information on cooking yields, physical composition, and content of vitamins. This research was conducted by the Meat Science Research Laboratory of the Animal Science Institute and the Nutrient Composition Laboratory of the Beltsville Human Nutrition Research Center. The National Live Stock and Meat Board and the National Pork Producers Council also assisted with developing the project plan, retail cut fabrication, and cooking procedures. Most of the values for fresh and cured sausages and luncheon meat products are from *Agriculture Handbook No. 8-7*. In this handbook most of the data for thiamin were determined by the fluorometric thiochrome procedure. Riboflavin and niacin data were obtained both chemically and microbiologically. Pantothenic acid was determined microbiologically.

Handbook No. 8-13 serves as a basic reference on nutrients in beef products. Data are presented for 360 beef products (USDA, 1986a). Much of the data for the retail cuts were obtained from studies conducted since 1977. The nutrient data for cured products were obtained since 1973 for nutritional labeling. Values for many of the beef items in the 1963 handbook have been changed to incorporate more recent findings, and new items have been added. The nutrient values in this revision supersede data for these specific foods given in the 1963 edition. Laboratory research on beef, carried out under the sponsorship of USDA's Agricultural Research Service, supplied a large portion of the information on cooking yields, physical composition, and content of vitamins for the retail cuts. This research was conducted by two ARS laboratories (the Meat Science Research Laboratory of the Animal Science Institute and the Nutrient Composition Laboratory of the Beltsville Human Nutrition Research Center), the University of Kentucky, and Michigan State University. The National Live Stock and Meat Board also assisted in developing the project plan, retail cut fabrication, and cooking procedures for the research. Additional laboratory research sponsored by the Human Nutrition Information Service provided much of the information on variety meats and part of the nutrient composition and yield information on ground beef and some retail cuts. Again, most of the data for thiamin were determined by the fluorometric thiochrome procedure. Riboflavin and niacin were obtained both chemically and microbiologically. Pantothenic acid was determined microbiologically.

Section 15 of the revised *Handbook No. 8* serves as a basic reference for data on nutrients in finfish and shellfish products (USDA, 1987a). The nutritive values in this revision are based on an extensive review of the literature published since 1960. Data are presented for 92 raw and 82 processed or prepared finfish and shellfish products. Fewer items appear in this revision than in the 1963 edition of the handbook because many items in the previous edition are now of limited commercial importance, and, in some cases, several items are grouped under one listing to give a more complete nutrient profile. Thiamin was determined chemically by the thiochrome procedure or by a microbiological method. Thiaminase, a thiamin antagonist, is a heat-labile enzyme present in some finfish (carp, mackerel, and sardines) and in shellfish. Since some finfish and shellfish are eaten raw, the amount of available thiamin will be less than the value given. Fluorometric or microbiological methods were used to measure riboflavin. Niacin data were obtained either chemically or microbiologically and do not include the niacin that could be contributed by tryptophan, a niacin precursor. Pantothenic acid was determined microbiologically.

(ii) Abbreviated Version, Data Base for Standard Reference

Agriculture Handbook No. 456 (AH-456), 1975 edition (USDA, 1975), has served as a basic reference on nutrients in common household measures and market units of food. Data in the computerized AH-456 data series have recently been replaced by the Abbreviated Version of the USDA Data Base for Standard Reference, a subset of the Standard Reference data base (USDA, 1988a). It contains data for all food items on the Standard Reference file, but is limited to 21 nutrients and food components. Data are presented as 100 gram edible portions, one pound of food as purchased and/or an edible portion in one or two common measures. This data base is updated periodically as the Standard Reference data base is revised.

(iii) Home and Garden Bulletin No. 72

Home and Garden Bulletin No. 72 (HG-72), *Nutritive Value of Foods*, was completely revised (USDA, 1986b) as to food items, nutrients listed and nutrient values. It includes 910 food items and 19 nutrients or food components in common household units and is available in printed and computerized form.

(iv) Data base for individual food intake surveys

The USDA recently developed an automated system to create nutrient data bases for assessing the nutrient content of food intakes by individuals reported in dietary surveys (Perloff, 1985). The Human Nutrition Information Service (HNIS) used the system for the first time in early 1985 to create the nutrient data base for appraising intakes from the Continuing Survey of Food Intakes by Individuals (CSFII). It has also been used to create the data base for the 1986 CSFII and the 1987–1988 Nationwide Food Consumption Survey (NFCS). The system uses the USDA Nutrient Data Base for Standard Reference, as the major source for nutrient values, and it includes procedures for calculating the nutrient content of recipes based on nutrient data for the individual recipe components. It contains data for energy and 29 nutrients or food components, including thiamin, riboflavin, and niacin, but not pantothenic acid. Data sets and computer programs included in the system are described below.

The basic nutrient composition data are provided in a Primary Nutrient Data Set for Food Consumption Surveys (PDS), consisting of the nutrient profile of items that are basic foods or that serve as components of reported foods prepared from recipes (Hepburn, 1987a). The PDS currently contains data for over 3000 foods. Most of the data are taken directly from the USDA Nutrient Data Base for Standard Reference (USDA, 1988a), although some changes and additions have been made to reflect new analytical data to be used, but not yet published in machine-readable form or as revisions to *Agriculture Handbook No. 8*. If analytical data were not available, the added values were imputed from other forms of the foods or estimates were derived from data for similar foods. There are no missing values in the PDS.

Other data bases in the food consumption survey data system are a Table of Nutrient Retention Factors for calculating retention of 18 vitamins and minerals during cooking and a Recipe File of about 5000 recipes, which controls the generation of a survey nutrient data base using the PDS and the Table of Retention Factors. Nutrient profiles of foods reported in a survey as consumed from home recipes are generated by linking the home recipe with the corresponding recipe in the Recipe File, linking the individual recipe components to foods and nutrient data contained in the Primary Data Set, and applying yield and retention factors from the Table of Nutrient Factors. The USDA Nutrient Data Base for Individual Intake Surveys is the system's output and is the nutrient data base created for analysis of food consumption survey data. This Survey Data Base contains over 5000 different foods. All nutrient values come from the PDS, either directly or through recipe calculations. About one-half of the items are foods as eaten and are treated as single-ingredient recipes.

The source of each nutrient in each food in the PDS is documented by attaching a source code to each nutrient value (Hepburn, 1987a). These codes define the values, as published in *Agriculture Handbook No. 8*, as analytical or calculated directly from analytical data, as imputed or assumed to be zero, or as industry values calculated for nutrition labeling.

The information available in the Primary Nutrient Data Set and the Nutrient Data Base for Individual Intake Surveys, together with consumption data from the CSFII and NFCS, is being used to set priorities for foods and nutrients to be studied in analytical studies (Hepburn, 1986). Source codes in the PDS provide information on the relative strengths and weaknesses of the data; the food consumption data provide information on the importance of foods in supplying each nutrient to the daily diet.

Researchers at HNIS have examined data in the Primary Data Set to determine the degree to which values are analytical (Hepburn, 1987b). The proportion of analytical data was calculated as the percentage of total data coded as either analytical or imputed. These proportions are high for the more familiar nutrients, including thiamin, riboflavin, and niacin, that have been tracked over a longer period of time. The percentage of analytical data for each of these three B vitamins is 91%, whereas analytical data on components such as carotene, dietary fiber and α-tocopherol are below 50% for all foods, although these values improve when computed only for those foods which are 'better sources' of the specific nutrients (Hepburn, 1987b). Data for pantothenic acid content of foods are not included in the PDS.

B. Quality of Food Composition Data

The value to individual users of food composition data depends in part on the intended use for the data. Nutrition research involves too many tasks for any one data system, as users have different requirements of the data. Most public data bases are designed to provide values that represent 'normal' levels in foods; it is unrealistic to expect them to provide precise data for all components in a food, since nutrient concentrations can vary and individual assays are expensive (Stewart, 1983). However, information on the range and precision of the measurements as provided in the new *AH-8* series optimizes use of available data and informs users that not all values can be used with equal confidence.

The current status of food composition data and of methods for quantifying nutrients in foods has been recently reviewed by USDA (Beecher and Matthews, 1990). The current state of knowledge for thiamin, riboflavin, niacin, and pantothenic acid is shown in Table 14-1. These data show that, for most meat items, there is a substantial amount of data for thiamin, riboflavin, and niacin, although data are inadequate for fish and shellfish and home-prepared mixed dishes. Pantothenic acid data are inadequate for most food groups, including meats; data for dairy and egg products, cereals, and legumes, are more substantial.

The state of knowledge about nutrient composition for these B vitamins is a reflection of the adequacy of analytical methodologies for assaying the nutrients in foods (Table 14-2). The state of methodology for thiamin, riboflavin, and niacin is substantial with respect to accuracy and speed of analysis, although costs range from modest to high (Beecher and Matthews, 1990). Extraction methods need improvement, and some modification of methods is also needed. The methodologies for analysis of pantothenic acid provide conflicting results. Better analytical methods and extraction

TABLE 14-1
STATE OF KNOWLEDGE OF NUTRIENT COMPOSITION[a] FOR VITAMINS

	Vitamin B_1 —thiamin	*Vitamin B_2 —riboflavin*	*Pre-formed niacin*	*Pantothenic acid*
Baby foods	S	S	S	—
Baked products, breads	S	S	S	I
Sweet goods	S	S	S	I
Cookies, crackers	S	S	NA	I
Beverages	I	I	I	I
Breakfast cereals	I	I	I	I
Candies	I	I	I	I
Cereals grains, whole	S	S	S	S
Flour	S	S	S	S
Pasta	S	S	S	S
Dairy products	S	S	S	S
Eggs and egg products	S	S	S	S
Fast foods	S	S	S	—
Fats and oils	NA	NA	NA	NA
Fish and shellfish: raw	I	I	I	I
cooked	—	—	—	I
Frozen dinners	S	S	S	—
Fruits: raw	S	S	S	I
cooked	I	I	I	I
frozen or canned	S	NA	S	I
Infant formula	—	—	—	—
Institutional food	—	—	—	—
Legumes: raw	S	S	S	S
cooked	S	S	S	S
processed	I	I	I	—
Meat: beef	S	S	S	I
lamb	S	S	S	I
pork	S	S	S	I
sausage	S	S	S	I
veal	S	S	S	I
Mixed dishes: commercial	S	S	S	—
home prepared	I	I	I	—
Nuts and seeds	I	I	I	I
Poultry	S	S	S	I
Restaurant food	—	—	—	—
Snack foods	I	I	I	I
Soups	S	S	S	—
Vegetables: raw	S	S	S	—
cooked	I	I	I	—
frozen	S	S	S	I
canned	S	S	S	I

Source: Beecher and Matthews (1990)
[a] S—(Substantial data)
I—(Inadequate data)
— —(Little or no data)
NA—(Not applicable).

TABLE 14-2
STATE OF DEVELOPMENT OF METHODS FOR THIAMIN, RIBOFLAVIN, NIACIN, AND PANTOTHENIC ACID IN FOODS

Nutrient category	*State of methodology*			
	Adequate	*Substantial*	*Conflicting*	*Lacking*
Vitamins		Niacin	Pantothenic acid	
		Riboflavin		
		Thiamin		
Factors	*Description of methodology states*			
	Adequate	*Substantial*	*Conflicting*	*Lacking*
Accuracy	Excellent	Good	Fair	Poor
Speed of analysis	Fast	Moderate	Slow	Slow
Cost per analysis	Modest (<$100)	Modest to high	High	?
Development needs		Method modification	Method development and modification	Method development
		Extraction procedures	Extraction procedures	Extraction procedures
		Applications	Applications	Applications

Source: Beecher and Matthews (1990).

procedures are needed, and current analytical methods need improvement with respect to accuracy, speed, and cost of analysis.

The representativeness of food composition data depends upon a number of factors including the number and quality of laboratories performing food composition analyses, the number and quality of samples used, and any weighting procedures (Southgate, 1983; Stewart, 1983). Representative data reflect the nutrient composition of food products on a nationwide, year-round basis. When data are obtained from the direct analysis of samples, natural variations in food samples should be considered. Conditions which influence nutrient content include genetic variation, degree of maturity, soil conditions, fertilizer use and type, climate, availability of water, and postharvest or postmortem handling (Tannenbaum *et al.*, 1985). Techniques for analyzing samples and the values obtained often change with changes in prevailing cultivars or breeds, food products, and advances in food technology. Often, a weighting scheme is used to average nutrient values from a number of samples (Southgate, 1983; Rizek *et al.*, 1984). This makes nutrient values more representative of a national food supply and allows varieties of foods that are produced and consumed in larger quantities to be more accurately represented in the final value.

C. Production and Processing Effects

Changes in production and processing of animal products have resulted in significant changes in composition of dietary meat sources and increases in the variety of products available in the marketplace. The National Research Council, National Academy of Sciences (NRC/NAS, 1988) has recently evaluated new technologies and production methods that hold promise for improving nutritional attributes of animal products. Recent research shows that use of growth hormone in beef and pork may result in increased feed efficiency in the live animal and improved lean-to-fat ratio in the carcass. Producers may soon be using biotechnological methods to enhance growth and improve carcass quality. Processors currently apply new techniques such as restructuring, ultrafiltration, enzymatic modification, and supercritical fluid or solvent extraction in the manufacture of new animal products.

Most efforts directed toward modifying nutritional attributes of animal products are focused on decreasing fat composition, and thus cholesterol content, in relation to lean tissue, decreasing the fat and cholesterol content in milk and milk products and the cholesterol levels in eggs, lowering the sodium content in processed meats and cheeses, and increasing calcium and iron levels in animal foods and their products (NRC/NAS, 1988).

Most production techniques being proposed or used for altering the composition of animal products have little effect on nutrient composition of thiamin, riboflavin, niacin, and pantothenic acid, although lowering the fat-to-lean ratios may result in slight increases in the nutrient densities of these B vitamins. Processing of meats and meat products can, however, have significant effects on the water soluble vitamins because of their instability under different conditions of pH, heat, light, and oxygen.

All foods that undergo processing are subject to some degree of loss in vitamin content, even though the bioavailability of a nutrient is occasionally increased or some antinutritional factor is inactivated. In general, food processing is accomplished in a manner that attempts to minimize nutrient losses. In addition to losses from processing, pre-processing conditions can also influence nutrient content. These include genetic variation, degree of maturity, soil conditions, and postharvest or postmortem handling.

(i) Thiamin

Various food-processing operations may considerably reduce thiamin levels. Heat, oxygen, sulfur dioxide, leaching, and neutral or alkaline pH may all result in destruction of thiamin. Sulfur dioxide and sulfites should not be used in products containing this vitamin because they cause the molecule to break up into its two derivatives, thus destroying its activity (deMan, 1980; Lee, 1983). Thiamin has been shown to be susceptible to losses during irradiation under certain conditions, however, radiation in the frozen state greatly reduces losses of the vitamin (Karel, 1975).

Cooking of meat causes losses related to size of cut, and fat content: boiling loss is 15–40%; frying, 40–50%; roasting, 30–60%; and canning, 50–75%. Similar losses apply to fish. Losses of vitamins due to salting, curing, and smoking have been studied for meat and for fish. Smoking after curing results in 15–20% higher losses of thiamin as compared to curing alone (Rice *et al.*, 1947). These losses may be attributable to the heating effect. Dry curing followed by smoking is less destructive to the thiamin (84% retained) than wet curing (74% retained) under the same conditions (Jackson *et al.*, 1945). Thiamin losses of 2–25% have been reported on studies of 15 processed meat and sausage items (Beuk *et al.*, 1950). Smoking of haddock, cod and herring does not cause any appreciable changes in thiamin content, although loss of thiamin has been observed in smoked salmon (Taarland *et al.*, 1958). Nitrite is used to preserve meats, and it may be added as such or may be formed by microbial reduction of nitrate and can lead to the destruction of thiamin (Tannenbaum *et al.*, 1985).

Thiamin is also subject to enzymatic attack and destruction by the enzyme thiaminase, found in raw entrails of stock animals; raw, fresh or saltwater fish; crustaceans, such as lobsters; mollusks, such as clams; and certain plants (deMan, 1980; Lee, 1983). The enzyme severs the thiazole ring from the vitamin structure, thus destroying its activity. If such food items are consumed as a major part of the diet, thiamin deficiency could result. Thiamin losses in milk processing are as follows: pasteurization, 3–20%; sterilization, 30–50%; spray drying, 10%; roller drying, 20–30% (deMan, 1980).

Considerable amounts of dietary thiamin can be lost from cooked vegetables when pot liquors are drained from food. For meat, leaching of thiamin from tissues is not as significant a problem as the *in situ* destruction of thiamin during roasting. From a standpoint of food storage, thiamin losses are minimized by lower storage temperatures $\leq 0°F$ $(-18°C)$ (Zapsalis and Beck, 1985).

(ii) Riboflavin

Riboflavin is chemically stable during most food processing; but, similar to thiamin, it becomes prone to destruction under alkaline conditions. However, considerable loss of riboflavin may occur if foods are exposed to light. Sun-drying of foods will destroy most of the riboflavin. Exposure of milk in glass bottles will result in loss of riboflavin. Cooking eggs or meat in pots open to light also causes destruction. Furthermore, the vitamin sensitivity to light is enhanced by the presence of vitamin C (Cooperman and Lopez, 1984).

It appears that the wavelengths of light responsible for the destruction are in the visible spectrum below 550–520 nm (deMan, 1980). Ultraviolet light has been reported to have no destructive effect on riboflavin (Hartman and Dryden, 1965). The nature of packaging material has an important effect on the extent of riboflavin destruction. Normal photosensitivity of riboflavin should encourage the use of amber glass containers, metal cans, or opaque food-packaging materials for foods high in riboflavin (Zapsalis and Beck, 1985).

Riboflavin in meat is relatively stable during cooking, canning, and dehydration. However, since it is water soluble, some riboflavin will be found in juices and drippings of meat, as well as in the water in which meat is cooked. Riboflavin is stable in these products during storage if kept out of high-temperature environments (Cooperman and Lopez, 1984). Dry-curing and subsequent smoking of meat causes a 43% loss of riboflavin, whereas, 11% is lost during wet-curing (Jackson *et al.*, 1945). Riboflavin losses are not significant for processed meats and sausages (Beuk *et al.*, 1950). Smoking of fish exhibits no appreciable effect on riboflavin content of haddock, cod, and herring (Tarr, 1960), but losses have been reported in smoked salmon (Taarland *et al.*, 1958).

The light sensitivity of riboflavin results in losses of up to 50% when milk is exposed to sunlight for two hours. Riboflavin is stable in dry milk for storage periods up to 16 months. Processes such as pasteurization, evaporation, or condensation of milk causes only minor losses of riboflavin (deMan, 1980). Dietary antagonists to riboflavin have not been widely reported in the literature. A natural substance in the ackee nut of Jamaica may be antagonistic to normal riboflavin metabolism but is not of nutritional significance in the United States (Lambooy, 1955; Fox and Miller, 1960; Zapsalis and Beck, 1985).

(iii) Niacin

Niacin is probably the most stable of the B vitamins. It is unaffected by heat, light, oxygen, acid, alkali, or irradiation. In many foods the amount of niacin is increased by application of heat, such as in roasting or baking. This results from the change of bound niacin to the free form (deMan, 1980). The main loss of niacin resulting from processing involves leaching into process water (Zapsalis and Beck, 1985).

Niacin has been found to be very resistant to destruction when exposed to gamma radiation. Day *et al.* (1957) found no destruction of niacin in beef when exposed to gamma radiation doses of 30–40 kGray. This finding indicates that destruction of niacin is not a concern when beef is sterilized by ionizing radiation, since the 40 kGy level exceeds the dosage level considered necessary for sterilization. Generally the use of irradiation for sterilization is similar to heat processing in its effects on niacin. Storage of meat at 0°F (−18°C) for periods of about a year had no significant effect on the niacin levels (Hankes, 1984).

Dry-curing of pork followed by smoking results in 96% retention of niacin, whereas 81% retention was observed with wet-curing (Jackson *et al.*, 1945). No significant losses of niacin occurred for processed meats and sausages (Beuk *et al.*, 1950) nor for smoked fish (Tarr, 1960), except smoked salmon (Hoogland, 1953).

Virtually all of the niacin in milk and animal tissues occurs in the form of nicotinamide. Processing of milk, such as pasteurization, sterilization, evaporation, and drying has little or no effect on niacin level.

(iv) Pantothenic acid

Pantothenic acid occurs in all living cells and tissues and is, therefore, found in most food products. In animal products most of the pantothenic acid is present in the bound form, but in milk only about one-fourth of the vitamin is bound (deMan, 1980). The vitamin is stable to air and labile to dry heat at pH values above 7 or below 5. Boiling in water involves losses, which depend on the amount of water used (deMan, 1980).

Pantothenic acid has been reported to be fairly stable during ordinary cooking and storage, but there has recently been concern that the vitamin may be destroyed during food processing. The effect of sterilization and storage on the pantothenic acid content of canned foods has been studied, and losses as great as 50% reported (Hellendoorm *et al.*, 1971). Walsh *et al.* (1981a) reported a relatively low pantothenic acid content in many highly processed foods, including products made from refined grains, fruit products, and fat- or cereal-extended meats and fish. Smoking of fish does not cause any appreciable changes in the pantothenic acid content of haddock, cod and herring, but losses were observed in smoked salmon (Taarland *et al.*, 1958).

Pasteurization does not affect pantothenic acid in milk, which may be due to the neutral pH of milk. The production and storage of dried milk involves little or no loss of pantothenic acid. Manufacture of cheese involves large losses during processing, but during ripening the pantothenic acid content increases due to synthesis by microorganisms (deMan, 1980).

IV. MEAT CONSUMPTION AND HEALTH

A. Food Consumption

The information gathered in food consumption surveys has contributed greatly to the understanding of dietary levels in the population and changes in food consumption which occur over time. Survey uses have evolved beyond the traditional food and nutrition questions of measuring food consumption, the money value of the food used, and developing food plans (National Academy of Sciences, 1984). National nutrition monitoring is now essential for identifying and maintaining components of healthful diets and for improving the quality of suboptimal diets in the United States.

The US Department of Agriculture provides data on food and nutrient consumption at three levels: (1) the US food supply, (2) food use by households, and (3) food intake by individuals. The food supply data measure the amount of food that is available for consumption in the United States. More direct estimates of food consumption are provided by the USDA's Nationwide Food Consumption Survey (NFCS), conducted approximately every ten years, most recently during 1977–78 and 1987–88. This survey is the most comprehensive source of data available on the food and nutrient intake of the US population. Until the 1987–88 NFCS data are available for analysis, the 1977–78 survey provides useful data for assessing food and nutrient intakes by population segments.

The Continuing Survey of Food Intake by Individuals (CSFII), conducted by the USDA in 1985 and again in 1986, is the most recent source of data available on the dietary intake of individuals. This survey is designed to complement the decennial NFCS by providing continuous data on the dietary status of those who may be at nutritional risk. The core monitoring group selected for the survey is women 19–50 years of age and their children, ages 1–5 years.

(i) Food supply data

Analysis of food supply data, sometimes referred to as food-disappearance data, indicates that increased consumer awareness of diet and health issues has influenced food choices being made in the marketplace. Food disappearance is not a measure of actual consumption or the quantity of foods consumed but is rather an estimate of the amount of food available for human consumption in the United States. The data are more useful as indicators of trends over time than as measurement of absolute levels of consumption (USDA, 1988c).

Recent analysis of food disappearance data indicates that veal, lamb, and mutton consumption at the retail level has decreased by more than half during the last 25 years, while chicken and turkey consumption almost doubled. Fish consumption has increased but not dramatically (Fig. 14-9) (USDA, 1988c). However, the lack of any clear-cut trends for beef and pork consumption indicates that nutrition is not the only factor influencing consumer food choices, despite some negative campaigns implicating red meat in the etiology of degenerative diseases in the United States.

Meats, poultry, and fish are important sources of many essential nutrients, including the B vitamins, thiamin, riboflavin, niacin, and pantothenic acid. Given the efforts to modify animal food production and processing, along with ill-advised, negative campaigns to significantly reduce meat consumption, any attempts to maintain or improve the nutritional quality of diets for these nutrients must be based on a clear understanding of the contemporary role of animal products to the nutritional adequacy of diets.

(ii) Meat consumption

NFCS 1977–78 data (USDA, 1984) of average intakes and percentages of individuals consuming meat, poultry, and fish are presented in Table 14-3. This table also includes meat intake data (USDA, 1987b) of women ages 19–50 years who were participants in the CSFII-85 and CSFII-86, plus a comparable group of women who participated in the NFCS 1977–78. The meat, poultry, and fish group (total meat group) includes beef, pork, lamb, veal, game, luncheon meats, fish, and shellfish. Meat mixtures include

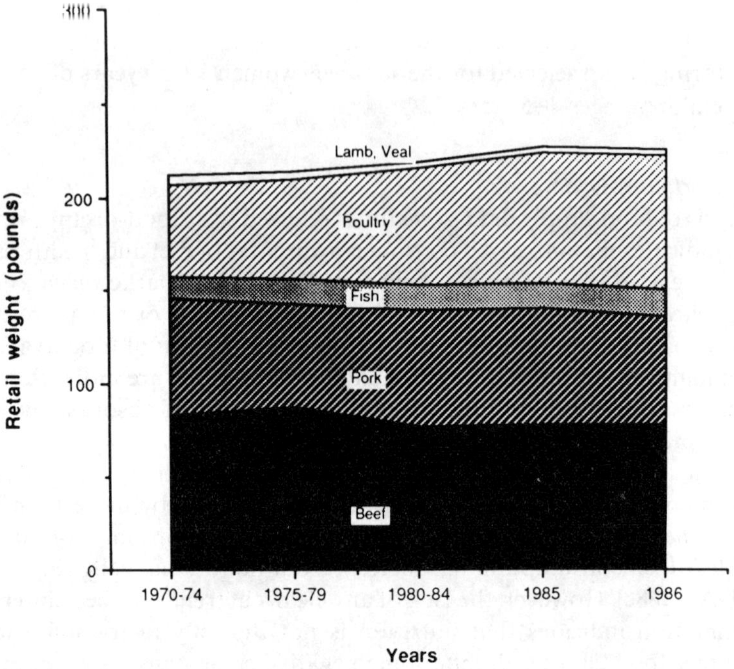

FIG. 14-9. Trends in *per capita* retail meat consumption, 1970–86.

recipes with one or more items of meat, poultry, or fish as a major ingredient.

For all individuals in the NFCS 1987–88, the average of three days of intake of foods from the meat group is 204 g. Meat mixtures provided the largest average amount (75 g), followed by beef (51 g), poultry (24 g), pork (20 g), and frankfurters, sausages, and luncheon meats (19 g). Nearly all individuals (99%) reported eating at least one item from the meat groups during the three survey days. Meat groups with the highest proportion of users are beef (68%), meat mixtures (67%), frankfurters, sausages, and luncheon meats (54%), and pork (50%) (USDA, 1984).

B. Nutrient Consumption

(i) Pantothenic acid

Data on dietary levels of pantothenic acid have not been included in national food consumption surveys, because analytical methodologies are less reliable than for other nutrients. A typical American diet of the 1940s

TABLE 14-3

MEAN DAILY INTAKES OF AND PERCENTAGE OF INDIVIDUALS USING MEATS AND MEAT PRODUCTS

Food group	Mean daily intakes (g)				% individuals using meat			
	All 1977–78[a]	Women			All 1977–78	Women		
		1977[b]	1985[c]	1986[d]		1977	1985	1986
Total meat, poultry, and fish	204	178	181	164	99	92	88	88
Meat mixtures	74	65	88	71	69	33	37	32
Beef	51	49	27	28	68	35	23	25
Frankfurters, sausages and luncheon meats	19	16	13	12	54	25	25	22
Pork	20	18	14	13	50	24	20	20
Poultry	24	24	22	23	43	18	19	20
Fish and shellfish	12	11	13	11	25	10	12	10

Source: USDA (1984; 1987c; 1988d).

[a] 1977–78 NFCS, all individuals, 4 day average.

[b] 1977–78 NFCS, women 19–50 years, 3 day average.

[c] 1985 CSFII, women 19–50 years, 4 day average.

[d] 1986 CSFII, Spring, women 19–50 years, 1 day.

was reported to contain approximately 4·9 mg pantothenic acid per 2500 kcal (Cheldelin and Williams, 1943). In the 1960s, typical American meals or self-selected diets provided between 3·4–20 mg pantothenic acid daily (Chung *et al.*, 1961; Fox and Linkswiler, 1961). Diets that met allowances for other nutrients for children 7–9 years of age provided 4–5 mg per day of pantothenic acid (Pace *et al.*, 1961). The wide range of intakes probably reflect methodological variation rather than dietary variation.

Generally pantothenic acid intakes reported from more recent studies are lower than those reported before the 1960s. Diets consumed by a group of low-income women provided about 4 mg per day (Johnson and Nitzke, 1975). In a small group of teenage, pregnant, postpartum, and nonpregnant girls, the calculated dietary intakes ranged from 1·1–7·2 mg per day (Cohenour and Calloway, 1972). Studies employing radioimmunoassays for quantifying dietary pantothenic acid found daily intakes of 2·5–9·5 mg per day, with a mean of 5·9 mg in an elderly population (Srinivasan *et al.*, 1981); average intakes of 4·80, 4·61, and 5·72 mg per day in a non-supplemented sample of control, pregnant/bottlefeeding, and pregnant/breastfeeding women, respectively (Song *et al.*, 1984, 1985); and mean intakes of 4·14 and 6·25 mg per day in female and male adolescents, respectively (Eissenstat *et al.*, 1986). Tarr *et al.* (1981) constructed 'typical' American diets based upon 1974 food-supply data and fed the diets to six male subjects ages 21–35 years in a balance study designed to determine dietary availability of pantothenic acid. The diet contained 11·5 mg pantothenate per day, of which 50%, or 5·8 mg, was found to be available.

(ii) Thiamin, riboflavin and niacin

The proportion of total intakes of thiamin, riboflavin, and preformed niacin provided by all food groups in the NFCS 1977–78 is illustrated in Fig. 14-10. The data in Table 14-4 reveal that almost one-fourth of total dietary thiamin and riboflavin and 44% of preformed niacin are provided by meats (USDA, 1984). Average daily intakes of these three vitamins (USDA, 1984) are 1·26, 1·72, and 18·2 mg (Table 14-5), or 133, 113 and 124% of the 1980 recommended dietary allowances for thiamin, riboflavin, and niacin respectively (Table 14-6).

Obviously, meats are major contributors to dietary intakes of thiamin, riboflavin, and niacin. For those in the population who frequently eat pork, this form of meat provides a dependable source of thiamin. However, total elimination of meat from the diet (without increasing intake from other food groups) would not place average population consumption of thiamin

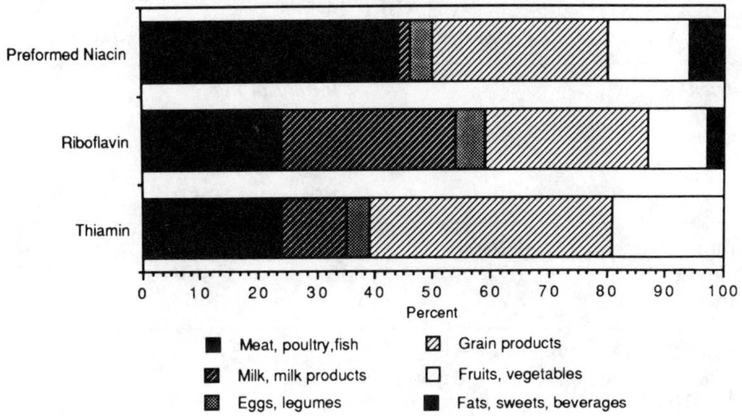

FIG. 14-10. Percentage contribution of meats and other commodity food groups to average daily intakes of thiamin, riboflavin and niacin.

and riboflavin below the RDA for these nutrients. Because 44% of preformed niacin, and undoubtedly a major proportion of niacin from tryptophan, is provided by meats, and the average intake of preformed niacin is 124% of the RDA, niacin nutriture could easily be compromised by elimination of meat from the diet.

Women of child-bearing age are one of a number of selected population groups being monitored yearly by the USDA, because this group has been

TABLE 14-4

CONTRIBUTION OF MEAT, POULTRY AND FISH TO AVERAGE PERCENTAGES OF DIETARY INTAKES OF THIAMIN, RIBOFLAVIN, AND NIACIN

Nutrient	*Percent*			
	All	*Women*		
	1977[a]	*1977–78*[b]	*1985*[c]	*1986*[d]
Thiamin	23·6	26·1	24·2	23·0
Riboflavin	24·2	28·0	24·1	23·2
Niacin	44·3	48·2	44·6	44·3

Source: USDA (1984; 1987c; 1988d).
[a] 1977–78 NFCS, all individuals, 4 day average.
[b] 1977–78 NFCS, women 19–50 years, 3 day average.
[c] 1985 CSFII, women 19–50 years, 4 day average.
[d] 1986 CSFII, Spring, women 19–50 years, 1 day.

TABLE 14-5

AVERAGE DAILY INTAKES OF THIAMIN, RIBOFLAVIN AND NIACIN

Nutrient	*Intake in mg*			
	All	*Women*		
	1977[a]	*1977–78*[b]	*1985*[c]	*1986*[d]
Thiamin	1·26	1·04	1·05	1·03
Riboflavin	1·72	1·36	1·34	1·33
Niacin	18·2	15·9	16·1	15·7

Source: USDA (1984; 1987c; 1988d).
[a] 1977–78 NFCS, all individuals, 4 day average.
[b] 1977–78 NFCS, women 19–50 years, 3 day average.
[c] 1985 CSFII, women 19–50 years, 4 day average.
[d] 1986 CSFII, Spring, women 19–50 years, 1 day.

shown to be more likely to have diets low in certain nutrients. Examination of data for women 19–50 years in the NFCS 1977–78 shows that average intakes of thiamin, riboflavin, and niacin were 1·04, 1·36, and 15·9 mg (Table 14-5), or 18, 22, and 13% lower than the sample averages for thiamin, riboflavin, and niacin, respectively. These values do not differ from those reported for comparable groups of women in the 1985 and 1986 CSFII (Table 14-5), indicating that women consume lower amounts of these

TABLE 14-6

THIAMIN, RIBOFLAVIN AND NIACIN INTAKES AS PERCENTAGES OF 1980 RECOMMENDED DIETARY ALLOWANCES

Nutrient	*Percent RDA*			
	All	*Women*		
	1977[a]	*1977–78*[b]	*1985*[c]	*1986*[d]
Thiamin	133	100	102	101
Riboflavin	113	110	108	108
Niacin	124	120	121	119

Source: USDA (1984; 1987c; 1988d).
[a] 1977–78 NFCS, all individuals, 4 day average.
[b] 1977–78 NFCS, women 19–50 years, 3 day average.
[c] 1985 CSFII, women 19–50 years, 4 day average.
[d] 1986 CSFII, Spring, women 19–50 years, 1 day.

vitamins than is average for the population. The percentages of the RDA consumed are also correspondingly lower (Table 14-6). In fact, the CSFII 1985 and 1986 report should be 50% or less of the women in the surveys consumed diets which supplied 100% or more of the RDA for thiamin and riboflavin; 33% or less consumed the RDA for niacin from preformed sources of the vitamin (USDA, 1987c, 1988d).

In 1977–78 the percentage of women 19–50 years who reported consuming meat at least once during the three days of the survey was 92%, less than the sample average of 99% (Table 14-3). Average daily intake of meat (186 g) was also lower than the sample mean (204 g). Nevertheless, the contribution of meats to total dietary intake of thiamin, riboflavin, and niacin for these women was greater than that for the total sample. As the number of women reporting daily meat consumption and the amounts consumed declined from 1977 to 1986, the contribution of meat to thiamin, riboflavin, and niacin intake obviously also decreased. Average daily intakes and percent RDA consumption have not changed significantly, indicating that women are obtaining a portion of these B vitamins from other dietary sources. But, given the numbers of women who are not meeting the RDAs and the significant contribution that meat and meat products make to thiamin, riboflavin and niacin nutriture, the effect of the trend to decrease meat intake is worthy of continued monitoring.

V. SUMMARY

A healthful diet has been defined as one that minimizes the risk of all nutrition-related diseases and problems (Hegsted, 1982). This means that the diet must provide all the essential nutrients in adequate amounts and must avoid the problems related to excessive consumption. Such a diet is not very useful, however, unless it can be provided by the available food supply and is also reasonably palatable and thus acceptable to the population that is expected to consume it. Available data indicate that meat and meat products, including poultry and fish, make a major contribution to thiamin, riboflavin, niacin and pantothenic acid intake in the US. Any major decline in consumption of these products could have an impact on the adequacy of the diet.

Although nutritionists have more recently been concerned with balance of macronutrient consumption and of intakes of cholesterol, sodium, trace elements, and B vitamins other than thiamin, riboflavin and niacin, there continues to be a need to monitor the traditional indicator nutrients, especially in population groups identified at high risk for inadequate intake of the specific vitamins or of energy. Pantothenic acid is an essential nutrient of emerging interest to nutritionists and consumers because better food composition, food consumption, and nutrient requirement data, based on improved methodologies for quantifying this nutrient in foods and biological tissues, have recently become available. As the character of the food supply changes, sound nutrition policy should involve determination of the nutritional value of available food, monitoring diets and their potential to meet nutritional needs, and educating and motivating consumers to make appropriate food choices to ensure adequacy of all essential nutrients with moderation of dietary components associated with chronic disease.

VI. ACKNOWLEDGEMENTS

The authors gratefully acknowledge the technical assistance of Patrice Isabella, MS, RD, Eileen DeLeeuw, MS, RD, and Brenda K. Tibbitts. This review is published with the approval of the Director, Utah Agriculture Experiment Station (UAES), Utah State University, Logan, Utah. Original work described here was supported by UAES Projects Nos 260 and 758 and by the National Live Stock and Meat Board.

VII. REFERENCES

Admed, F., Bamji, M. S. and Iyengar, L. (1975). Effect of oral contraceptive agents on vitamin nutrition status. *Am. J. Clin. Nutr.* **28**, 606.

Altschul, Z., Hoffer, A. and Stephen, J. D. (1955). Influence of nicotinic acid on serum cholesterol in man. *Arch. Biochem. Biophys.* **54**, 558.

American Institute of Nutrition, Committee on Nomenclature (1979). Nomenclature policy: Generic descriptors and trivial names for vitamins and related compounds. *J. Nutr.* **109**, 8.

Association of Official Agricultural Chemists (1960). *Official Methods of Analysis.* Collegiate Press, George Banta Co., Inc., Menasha, WI.

Association of Official Analytical Chemists (1980). *Official Methods of Analysis.* AOAC, Arlington, VA.

Association of Vitamin Chemists, Inc. (1966). *Methods of Vitamin Assay*, 3rd edn. Interscience Publ., Inc., New York.

Baker, H., Frank, O., Fennelly, J. J. and Leevey, C. M. (1964). A method for assaying thiamine status in man and animals. *Am. J. Clin. Nutr.* **14**, 197.

Balaghi, M. and Pearson, W. N. (1966). Metabolism of physiologic doses of thiazole-2-^{14}C-labeled thiamine by the rat. *J. Nutr.* **89**, 265.

BAMJI, M. S. (1969). Glutathione reductase activity in red blood cells and riboflavin nutritional status in humans. *Clin. Chim. Acta* **26**, 263.

BEAN, W. B. and HODGES, R. E. (1954). Pantothenic acid and pyridoxine. *Proc. Soc. Expl. Biol. Med.* **86**, 693.

BEAN, W. B., HODGES, R. E. and DAUM, K. (1955). Pantothenic acid deficiency induced in human subjects. *J. Clin. Invest.* **34**, 1073.

BEECHER, G. R. and MATTHEWS, R. H. (1990). Food composition. In *Present Knowledge in Nutrition*, 6th edn (M. Brown, Ed), International Life Sciences Institute-Nutrition Foundation, Washington, DC (in press).

BELKO, A. Z., OBARZANCK, E., KALKWARF, H. J., ROTTER, M. A., BOGUSZ, S., MILLER, D., HAAS, S. J. D. and ROE, D. A. (1983). Effects of exercise on riboflavin requirements of young women. *Am. J. Clin. Nutr.* **37**, 509.

BEUK, J. F., FRIED, J. F. and RICE, E. E. (1950). Nutritive values of sausage and other table-ready meats as affected by processing. *Food Res.* **15**, 302.

BLUM, C. B., LEVY, R. I., EISENBERG, S., HALL, M., GOEBEL, R. H. and BERMAN, M. (1977). High density lipoprotein metabolism in man. *J. Clin. Invest.* **60**, 795.

BRIGGS, M. and BRIGGS, M. (1974). Oral contraceptives and vitamin nutrition. *Lancet* **i**, 1234.

BRIN, M. (1962). Erythrocyte transketolase in early thiamine deficiency. *Ann. NY Acad. Sci.* **98**, 528.

BRZEZINSKI, A., BROMBERG, U. M. and BRAUN, K. (1952). Riboflavin excretion during pregnancy and early lactation. *J. Lab. Clin. Med.* **39**, 84.

BURSCH, J. G. (1957). Fluorometric assay of FAD, FMN and riboflavin. In *Methods in Enzymology. Vol. 3.* Preparation and Assay of Substrates. (S. P. Colowick and H. O. Kaplan, Eds), p. 960. Academic Press, New York.

CERLETTI, P. and IPATA, P. (1960). Determination of riboflavin and its coenzymes in tissues. *Biochem. J.* **75**, 199.

CHELDELIN, V. H. and WILLIAMS, R. R. (1943). Studies of the average American diet. II. Riboflavin, nicotinic acid and pantothenic acid content. *J. Nutr.* **26**, 417.

CHRISTENSEN, N. A., ACHOR, R. W. P., BERGE, K. G. and MASON, H. L. (1961). Nicotinic acid treatment of hypercholesterolemia. *J. Am. Med. Assoc.* **177**, 546.

CHUNG, A. S. M., PEARSON, W. N., DARBY, W. J., MILLER, O, N. and GOLDSMITH, G. A. (1961). Folic acid, vitamin B6, pantothenic acid and vitamin B12 in human dietaries. *Am. J. Clin. Nutr.* **9**, 573.

CLARK, B. R. (1980). Fluorometric quantification of picomole amounts of 1-methylnicotinamide and nicotinamide in serum. In *Methods in Enzymology, Vol. 66. Vitamins and Coenzymes, Part E.* (D. B. McCormick and L. O. Wright, Eds), p. 5. Academic Press, New York.

CLARK, M. F. (1940). Biological assay of riboflavin. *J. Nutr.* **20**, 133.

COHENOUR, S. H. and CALLOWAY, D. H. (1972). Blood, urine, and dietary pantothenic acid levels of pregnant teenagers. *Am. J. Clin. Nutr.* **25**, 512.

CONSOLAZIO, C. F., JOHNSON, H. L., KRZYWICKI, H. J. and WITT, N. F. (1972). Tryptophan–niacin interrelationships during acute fasting and caloric restriction in human. *Am. J. Clin. Nutr.* **25**, 572.

COOPERMAN, J. M. and LOPEZ, R. (1984). Riboflavin. In *Handbook of Vitamins: Nutritional, Biochemical and Clinical Aspects* (L. J. Machlin, Ed.), p. 299. Marcel Dekker, Inc., New York.

COOPERMAN, J. M., COLE, H. S., GORDON, M. and LOPEZ, R. (1973). Erythrocyte glutathione reductase as a measure of riboflavin nutritional status of pregnant women and newborns. *Proc. Soc. Expt. Biol. Med.* **143**, 326.

Coronary Drug Project Research Group (1975). Clofibrate and niacin in coronary heart disease. *J. Am. Med. Assoc.* **231**, 360.

Day, E. J., Alexander, H. D., Sauberlich, H. E. and Salmon, W. D. (1957). Effects of gaining radiation on certain water-soluble vitamins in raw ground beef. *J. Nutr.* **62**, 27.

de Lange, D. J. and Joubert, C. P. (1964). Assessment of nicotinic acid status of population groups. *Am. J. Clin. Nutr.* **15**, 169.

DeLuca, C. and Kaplan, N. O. (1958). Flavin adenine dinucleotide synthesis in animal tissues. *Biochim. Biophys. Acta* **30**, 6.

deMan, J. M. (1980). *Principles of Food Chemistry*, p. 330. AVI Publ. Co., Inc., Westport, CT.

DeMerre, L. J. and Brown, W. S. (1944). Effect of various lighting conditions on riboflavin solutions. *Arch. Biochem.* **5**, 181.

DeVries, W. H., Grovier, W. M., Evans, J. S., Gregory, J. D., Novelli, G. D., Soodak, M. and Lipmann, F. (1950). Purification of coenzyme A from fermentation sources and its further partial identification. *J. Am. Chem. Soc.* **72**, 4838.

DeVries, J. X., Gunthert, W. and Derig, R. (1980). Determination of nicotinamide in human plasma and urine by ion-pair reversed high phase high-performance liquid chromatography. *J. Chromatogr.* **221**, 161.

Dipalma, J. R. and Ritchie, C. M. (1977). Vitamin toxicity. *Ann. Rev. Pharmacol. Toxicol.* **17**, 133.

Einstein, N., Baker, A., Galper, J. and Wolfe, H. (1975). Jaundice due to nicotinic acid therapy. *Am. J. Digest. Dis.* **20**, 282.

Eissenstat, B. R., Wyse, B. W. and Hansen, R. G. (1986). Pantothenic acid status of adolescents. *Am. J. Clin. Nutr.* **44**, 931.

Ellestad-Sayed, J. J., Nelson, R. A., Adson, M. A., Palmer, W. M. and Soule, E. H. (1976). Pantothenic acid, coenzyme A and human chronic ulceratic and granulomatous colitis. *Am. J. Clin. Nutr.* **29**, 1333.

Ellestad, J. J., Nelson, R. A., Adson, M. A. and Palmer, W. M. (1970). Pantothenic acid and coenzyme A activity in blood and colonic mucosa from patients with chronic ulcerative colitis (Abstract) *Fed. Proc.* **29**, 820.

Elvehjem, C. A. (1940). Relation of nicotinic acid to pellagra. *Physiol. Rev.* **20**, 249.

Elvehjem, C. A., Madden, R. J., Strong, F. M. and Woolley, D. W. (1938). The isolation and identification of the anti-black tongue factor. *J. Biol. Chem.* **123**, 137.

Emmett, A. D. and Luros, G. O. (1920). Water-soluble vitamins. *J. Biol. Chem.* **43**, 265.

Falk, R. H. and Protheroe, D. E. (1979). Ventricular fibrillation following high potency intravenous vitamin injection. *Postgrad. Med. J.* **55**, 201.

Fazekas, A. P. and Kokai, K. (1971). Extraction, purification, and separation of tissue flavins for spectrophotometric determination. In *Methods in Enzymology, Vol. 17. Vitamins and Coenzymes, Part B* (D. B. McCormick and L. D. Wright, Eds), p. 385. Academic Press, New York.

Ferrenbee, J. W., Weissman, N., Parker, D. and Owen, P. S. (1942). Tissue thiamin concentrations and urinary thiamin excretion. *J. Clin. Invest.* **21**, 401.

FOOD AND NUTRITION BOARD (1980). *Recommended Dietary Allowances.* National Research Council, National Academy of Sciences. National Academy Press, Washington, DC.

FOX, H. C. and MILLER, D. S. (1960). Ackee toxin: a riboflavin antimetabolite? *Nature* **186**, 561.

FOX, H. M. and LINKSWILER, H. (1961). Pantothenic acid excretion on three levels of intake. *J. Nutr.* **75**, 451.

FRY, P. C., FOX, H. M. and TAO, H. G. (1976). Metabolic response to a pantothenic acid deficient diet in humans. *J. Nutr. Sci. Vitaminol.* **22**, 339.

FUNK, C. J. (1911). The chemical nature of the substance which cures polyneuritis in birds induced by a diet of polished rice. *Physiol.* **43**, 395.

GHOLSON, R. K. (1966). The pyridine nucleotide cycle. *Nature* **212**, 933.

GHOSH, H. P., SARKAR, P. K. and GUHA, B. C. (1963). Distribution of the bound form of nicotinic acid in natural materials. *J. Nutr.* **79**, 451.

GLATZL, D., KORNER, W. F., CHRISTELLER, S. and WISS, O. (1970). Method for the detection of a biochemical riboflavin deficieincy stimulation of $NADPH_2$-dependent glutathione reductase from human erythrocytes by FAD *in vitro.* Investigations on the vitamin B_2 status in healthy people and geriatric patients. *Internat. J. Vit. Res.* **40**, 166.

GLUSMAN, M. (1947). Syndrome of 'burning feet' (nutritional melalgia) as manifestation of nutritional deficiency. *Am. J. Med.* **3**, 211.

GOKAL, R., MANN, J. I., OLIVER, D. O., LEDINGHAM, J. G. and CARTER, R. D. (1978). Treatment of hyperlipidaemia in patients on chronic haemodialysis. *Brit. Med. J.* **1**, 82.

GOLDBERGER, J. (1916). The transmissibility of pellagra. *Public Health Rep.* **31**, 3159.

GOLDBERGER, J. and WHEELER, G. A. (1915). Experimental pellagra in the human subject brought about by a restricted diet. *Public Health Rep.* **30**, 3336.

GOLDBERGER, J. and WHEELER, G. A. (1928). Experimental black tongue of dogs and its relation to pellagra. *Public Health Rep.* **43**, 172.

GOLDBERGER, J., WHEELER, G. A., LILLIE, R. D. and ROGERS, L. M. (1926). A further study of better, fresh beef and yeast aspellagra preventives with considerations of the relation of fact P-P of pellagra (and black tongue of dogs) to vitamin B. *Public Health Rep.* **41**, 297.

GOLDSMITH, G. A. (1958). Niacin–tryptophan relationships in man and niacin requirements. *Am. J. Clin. Nutr.* **6**, 479.

GOLDSMITH, G. A., GIBBENS, J., UNGLAUB, W. G. and MILLER, O. N. (1956). Studies of niacin requirement in man. III. Comparative effects of diets containing lime-treated and untreated corn in the production of experimental pellagra. *Am. J. Clin. Nutr.* **4**, 151.

GOLDSMITH, G. A., MILLER, O. N. and UNGLAUB, W. G. (1961). Efficiency of tryptophan as a niacin precursor in man. *J. Nutr.* **73**, 172.

GRUNDY, S. M., MOK, J. Y. I., ZECH, L. and BERMAN, M. (1981). Influence of nicotinic acid on metabolism of cholesterol and triglycerides in man. *J. Lipid Res.* **22**, 24.

GUBLER, C. J. (1968). Enzyme studies in thiamine deficiency. *Internat. Z. Vitaminforsch.* **38**, 297.

GUBLER, C. J. (1984). Thiamin. In *Handbook of Vitamins: Nutrition, Biochemical and Clinical Aspects* (L. J. Machlin, Ed.), p. 245. Marcel Dekker, Inc., New York.

HALVORSEN, O. and SKREDE, S. (1980). Separation of coenzyme A and its precursors by reversed phase high performance liquid chromatography. *Anal. Biochem.* **107**, 103.

HANKES, L. V. (1984). Nicotinic acid and nicotinamide. In *Handbook of Vitamins: Nutrition, Biochemical and Clinical Aspects* (L. J. Machlin, Ed.), p. 329. Marcel Dekker, Inc., New York.

HARRIS, R. S. and LEPKOVSKY, S. (1954). Pantothenic acid. In *The Vitamins: Chemistry, Physiology, Pathology*, Vol. 2 (W. H. Sobrell, Jr and R. S. Harris, Eds), p. 591. Academic Press, New York.

HARTMAN, A. M. and DRYDEN, L. P. (1965). *Vitamins in Milk and Milk Products.* Am. Dairy Sci. Assoc., Champaign, IL.

HATANO, M. (1962). Microbiological assay of pantothenic acid in blood and urine. *J. Vitaminol.* **8**, 134.

HAWKINS, D. R. (1968). Treatment of schizophrenia based on the medical model. *J. Schiz.* **2**, 3.

HAYES, K. C. and HEGSTED, D. M. (1973). Toxicity of the vitamins. In *Toxicants Occurring Naturally in Foods.* pp. 235–53. National Research Council, National Academy of Sciences, Washington, DC.

HEGSTED, D. M. (1979). Food and nutrition policy: probability and practicality. *J. Am. Dietet. Assoc.* **74**, 534.

HEGSTED, D. M. (1982). What is a healthful diet? *Primary Care* **9**, 445.

HEIDELBERGER, C., ABRAHAM, E. P. and LEPKOVSKY, S. (1949). Tryptophan metabolism; concerning mechanism of mammalian conversion of tryptophan into nicotinic acid. *J. Biol. Chem.* **179**, 151.

HELLENDOORM, E. W., DEGROTT, A. P., VAN DER MYLL DEKKER, L. P., SLUMP, P. and WILLIAMS, J. J. L. (1971). Nutritive values of canned meats. *J. Am. Dietet. Assoc.* **58**, 434.

HELLER, S., SALKED, R. M. and KORNER, W. F. (1974). Riboflavin status in pregnancy. *Am. J. Clin. Nutr.* **27**, 1225.

HENDERSON, L. M. (1983). Niacin. In *Annual Review of Nutrition*, Vol. 3 (W. J. Darby, H. P. Broquist and R. E. Olson, Eds), pp. 289–307. Annual Reviews, Inc., Palo Alto, CA.

HENGEN, N., SEIBERTH, V. and HENGEN, M. (1978). High-performance liquid chromatographic determination of free nicotinic acid and its metabolite, nicotinuric acid, in plasma and urine. *Clin. Chem.* **24**, 1740.

HENNESSY, D. J. and CERECEDO, L. R. (1939). The determination of free and phosphorylated thiamin by a modified thiochrome. *J. Am. Chem. Soc.* **61**, 179.

HEPBURN, F. N. (1982). The USDA nutrient data bank. *Am. J. Clin. Nutr.* **35**, 1297.

HEPBURN, F. N. (1986). USDA update. In *Proc. 11th National Nutrient Data Bank Conference*, p. 1. CBORD Group, Inc., Ithaca, NY.

HEPBURN, F. N. (1987a). Managing food composition data at the national level. In *Food Composition Data: A User's Perspective* (W. M. Rand, C. T. Windham, B. W. Wyse and V. R. Young, Eds) *Food Nutr. Bull.*, Suppl. **12**, 109.

HEPBURN, F. N. (1987b). Food consumption/composition interrelationships. In *Proc. 12th National Nutrient Data Bank Conference*, p. 68. National Technical Information Service, Springfield, VA.

HILKER, D. M. and SOMOGYI, J. C. (1982). Antithiamins of plant origin: Their chemical nature and mode of action. *Ann. NY Acad. Sci.* **378**, 137.

HILLS, O. W., LIEBERT, E., STEINBERG, D. L. and HORWITT, M. K. (1951). Clinical aspects of dietary depletion of riboflavin. *AMA Arch. Intern. Med.* **87**, 682.

HODGES, R. E., OHLSON, M. A. and BEAN, W. B. (1958). Pantothenic acid deficiency in man. *J. Clin. Invest.* **37**, 1642.

HODGES, R. E., BEAN, W. B., OHLSON, M. A. and BLEILER, R. (1959). Human pantothenic acid deficiency produced by omega-methyl pantothenic acid. *J. Clin. Invest.* **38**, 1421.

HOOGLAND, P. L. (1953). The B-vitamins of cod and haddock. Fisheries Research Board Canada. *Atlantic Coast Sta. Progr. Rpt.* **55**, 11.

HOOVER, L. W. and PELICAN, S. (1984). Nutrient data bases; considerations for educators. *J. Nutr. Educ.* **16**, 58.

HORWITT, M. K. (1955). Niacin–tryptophan relationships in the development of pellagra. *Am. J. Clin. Nutr.* **3**, 244.

HORWITT, M. K. (1958). Niacin–tryptophan requirements of man. *J. Am Dietet. Assoc.* **34**, 914.

HORWITT, M. K., HILLS, O. W., HARVEY, C. C., LEIBERT, E. and STEINBERG, D. L. (1949). Effects of dietary depletion of riboflavin. *J. Nutr.* **39**, 357.

HORWITT, M. K., HARVEY, C. C., HILLS, O. W. and LIEBERT, E. (1950). Correlation of urinary riboflavin with dietary intake and symptoms of ariboflavinosis. *J. Nutr.* **41**, 247.

HORWITT, M. K., HARVEY, C. C., ROTHWELL, W. S., CUTLER, J. L. and HAFFRON, D., (1956). Tryptophan–niacin relationships in man. *J. Nutr.* **60** (Suppl. 1), 1.

HORWITT, M. K., HARVEY, D. D. and DAHM, C. H. (1975). Relationship between levels of blood lipids, vitamins C. A and E, serum copper compounds and urinary excretions of tryptophan metabolites in women taking oral contraceptives. *Am. J. Clin. Nutr.* **28**, 403.

INTERDEPARTMENTAL COMMITTEE ON NUTRITION FOR NATIONAL DEFENSE (1963). *Manual for Nutrition Surveys*, 2nd edn, p. 136. National Institutes of Health. Government Printing Office, Washington, DC.

INTERNATIONAL UNION OF NUTRITION SCIENCES, COMMITTEE ON NOMENCLATURE AND THE COMMISSION ON BIOCHEMICAL NOMENCLATURE IUPAC-IUB (1966). Tentative rules. *J. Biol. Chem.* **241**, 2987.

ISHIGURO, K. (1962). Blood pantothenic acid content of pregnant women. *Tohoku J. Expt. Med.* **78**, 7.

ITOKAWA, Y. and COOPER, J. R. (1970). Ion movements and thiamin II. The release of the vitamin from membrane fragments. *Biochem. Biophys. Acta* **196**, 274.

IVES, M. and STRONG, F. M. (1946). Preparation of samples for the microbiological assay of pantothenic acid. *Arch. Biochem.* **9**, 251.

JACKSON, S. H., CROOK, A and DRAKE, T. G. H. (1945). The retention of thiamine, riboflavin and nicacin in cooking pork and in processing bacon. *J. Nutr.* **29**, 391.

JANSEN, A. P. and JANSEN, B. C. P. (1954). Riboflavin-excretion with urine in pregnancy. *Internat. Z. Vitaminforsch.* **25**, 193.

JANSEN, B. P. C. and DONATH, W. F. (1926). Antineuritisch Vitamine. *Chem. Weekblad* **23**, 201.

JOHNSON, N. E. and NITZKE, S. (1975). Nutritional adequacy of diets of a selected group of low-income women. Identification of some related factors. *Home Econ. Res. J.* **3**, 241.

JOHNSTON, L., VAUGHAN, L. and FOX, H. M. (1981). Pantothenic acid content of human milk. *Am. J. Clin. Nutr.* **34**, 2205.

JOINT FAO/WHO EXPERT GROUP (1967). *Requirements of Vitamin A, Thiamine, Riboflavin and Niacin.* WHO Technical Report Series No. 362.

JUKES, T. H. (1941). The distribution of pantothenic acid in certain products of natural origin. *J. Nutr.* **21**, 193.

JUKES, T. H. (1947). The biological and microbiological assay of pantothenic acid. *Biological Symposia* **12**, 253.

KAMMAN, J. F., LABUZA, T. P. and WARTHESEN, J. J. (1980). Thiamin and riboflavin analysis by high performance liquid chromatography. *J. Food Sci.* **45**, 1497.

KAPLAN, N. O. and LIPMAN, F. (1948). The assay and distribution of coenzyme A. *J. Biol. Chem.* **174**, 37.

KAREL, M. (1975). Radiation preservation of foods. In *Principles of Food Science, Part II: Physical Principles of Food Preservation* (O. R. Fennema, Ed.), p. 127. Marcel Dekker, Inc., New York.

KARRER, P., SCHÖPP, K. and PENZ, F. (1935). Synthesen von flavinen IV. *Helv. Chem. Acta* **18**, 426.

KIES, C., WISHART, C., MCGEE, M., FOSS, Z., YANG, L. C., QUILLIAN, J. and FOX, H. M. (1982). Pantothenic acid levels in urine, blood serum and whole blood of adult humans fed graded levels of pantothenic acid (Abstract), *Fed. Proc.* **41**, 276.

KNOBLOCH, E. (1971). Polarography of flavins. In *Methods in Enzymology, Vol. 17. Vitamins and Coenzymes, Part B.* (D. B. McCormick and L. D. Wright, Eds), p. 305. Academic Press, New York.

KNOX, W. E. (1976). *Enzyme Patterns in Fetal, Adult and Neoplastic Rat Tissues.* S. Karger, New York.

KOCHETOV, G. A. (1982). Structure of active center of transketolase. *Ann. NY Acad. Sci.* **378**, 306.

KODICEK, E. and WILSON, P. W. (1960). The isolation of niacytin, the bound form of nicotinic acid. *Biochem. J.* **76**, 27P.

KODICEK, E., BRAUDE, R., KON, S. K. and MITCHELL, K. G. (1956). The effect of alkaline hydrolysis on the availability of its nicotinic acid to the pig. *Brit. J. Nutr.* **10**, 51.

KODICEK, E., ASHBY, D. R., MULLER, M. and CARPENTER, K. J. (1974). The conversion of bound nicotinic acid to free nicotinamide on roasting sweet corn. *Proc. Nutr. Soc.* **33**, 105A.

KOZIOL, J. (1971). Fluorometric analyses of riboflavin and its coenzymes. In *Methods in Enzymology, Vol. 43. Vitamins and Coenzymes, Part B* (D. B. McCormick and L. D. Wright, Eds), p. 253. Academic Press, New York.

KREBS-SMITH, S. M., SMICIKLAS-WRIGHT, H., GUTHRIE, H. A. and KREBS-SMITH, J. (1987). The effects of variety in food choices on dietary quality. *J. Am. Dietet. Assoc.* **87**, 898.

KUHN, R. K., REINEMUND, K., WEYGAND, F. and STRÖBELE, R. (1935). Über die synthese des lactoflavins (Vitamin B2). *Berichte*, **68**, 1765.

LAMBOOY, J. P. (1955). Riboflavin antagonists. *Am. J. Clin. Nutr.* **3**, 282.

LATNER, A. L. (1975). *Cantarow and Trumper Clinical Biochemistry*, 7th edn, p. 814. W. B. Saunders Co., Philadelphia.

LEE, F. A. (1983). *Basic Food Chemistry*, 2nd edn, p. 199. The AVI Publishing Co., Inc., Westport, CT.

LEE, S. S. and MCCORMICK, D. B. (1983). Effect of riboflavin status on hepatic activities of flavin-metabolizing enzymes in rats. *J. Nutr.* **113**, 2274.

LEKLEM, J. E., BROWN, R. R., ROSE, D. P., LINKSWILER, J. and AREND, R. A. (1975). Metabolism of tryptophan and niacin in oral contraceptive users receiving controlled intakes of vitamin B-6. *Am. Clin. Nutr.* **28**, 146.

LEWIS, C. M. and KING, J. C. (1980). Effect of oral contraceptive agents on thiamin, riboflavin, and pantothenic acid status in young women. *Am. J. Clin. Nutr.* **33**, 832.

LIGHT, L. and CRONIN, F. J. (1981). Food guidance revisited. *J. Nutr. Educ.* **13**, 51.

LIPMANN, F. (1945). Acetylation of sulfanilamide by liver homogenates and extracts. *J. Biol. Chem.* **160**, 173.

LIPMANN, F., KAPLAN, N. O. and NOVELLI, G. D. (1947). Coenzyme for acetylation, a pantothenic acid derivative. Letter to Editor. *J. Biol. Chem.* **167**, 869.

LIPMANN, F., KAPLAN, N. O., NOVELLI, G. D. and TUTTLE, L. C. (1950). Isolation of coenzyme A. *J. Biol. Chem.* **186**, 285.

LOHMAN, K. and SCHUSTER, P. (1937). Untersuchungen über die cocarboxylase. *Biochem. Z.* **244**, 188.

MATSUDA, T. and COOPER, J. R. (1981). Thiamin as an integral component of brain synaptosomal membranes. *Proc. Nat. Acad. Sci. USA* **78**, 5886.

MAYERSOHN, M., FELDMAN, S. and GIBALDI, M. (1969). Bile salt enhancement of riboflavin and flavin mononucleotide absorption in man. *J. Nutr.* **98**, 288.

MCCORMICK, D. B. (1975). Metabolism of riboflavin. *In* Riboflavin, (R. S. Rivlin, Ed.), p. 153. Plenum Press, New York.

MCCORMICK, D. B. (1988). Pantothenic Acid. In *Modern Nutrition in Health and Disease* (M. E. Shils and V. R. Young, Eds), p. 383. Lea and Febiger, Philadelphia.

MERRILL, A. H., JR, ADDISON, R. and MCCORMICK, D. B. (1978). Induction of hepatic and intestinal flavokinase after oral administration of riboflavin to riboflavin-deficient rats. *Proc. Soc. Expt. Biol. Med.* **158**, 572.

MERRILL, A. H., JR, LAMBETH, J. D., EDMONDSON, D. E. and MCCORMICK, D. B. (1982). Formation and mode of action of flavoproteins. In *Ann. Rev. Nutr.*, Vol. 1 (W. J. Darby, H. P. Broquist and R. E. Olson, Eds). Annual Reviews Inc., Palo Alto, CA, p. 281.

METZLER, D. A. (1977). *Biochemistry*. Academic Press, New York.

MILLER, D. R. and HAYES, K. C. (1982). Vitamin excess and toxicity. In *Nutritional Toxicology*. Vol. 1 (J. N. Hathcock, Ed.), pp. 81–134. Academic Press, New York.

MOFFATT, J. G. and KHORANA, H. G. (1961). Nucleoside polyphosphates. XII. The total synthesis of coenzyme A. *J. Amer. Chem. Soc.* **83**, 663.

MOSHER, L. R. (1970). Nicotinic acid side effects and toxicity: A review. *Am. J. Psychiatry* **126**, 1290.

MURATA, K. (1982). Actions of two types of thiaminase on thiamin and its analogies. *Ann. NY Acad. Sci.* **378**, 146.

NATIONAL ACADEMY OF SCIENCES (1984). *National Survey Data on Food Consumption: Uses and Recommendations.* Coordinating Committee on Evaluation of Food Consumption Surveys, Food and Nutrition Board, National Research Council. National Academy Press, Washington, DC.

NATIONAL ADVISORY COMMITTEE ON NUTRITION EDUCATION (1983). Nutrition: The changing scene. *Lancet* **i**, 9.

NATIONAL LIVE STOCK AND MEAT BOARD (1988). *Dietary Analysis and Food Comparison System.* Chicago, IL.

NATIONAL RESEARCH COUNCIL, NATIONAL ACADEMY OF SCIENCES (1988). Existing technological options and future research needs. In *Designing Foods: Animal Product Options in the Marketplace.* Committee on Technological Options to Improve the Nutritional Attributes of Animal Products, p. 115. National Academy Press, Washington, DC.

NEAL, R. A. and PEARSON, W. N. (1964). Studies of thiamine metabolism in the rat. I. Metabolic products found in urine. *J. Nutr.* **83**, 343.

NEWMAN, L. J., LOPEZ, R., COLE, H. S., BORIA, M. C. and COOPERMAN, J. M. (1978). Riboflavin deficiency in women taking oral contraceptive agents. *Am. J. Clin. Nutr.* **31**, 247.

NOVELLI, G. D., KAPLAN, N. O. and LIPMANN, R. (1949). The liberation of pantothenic acid from coenzyme A. *J. Biol. Chem.* **177**, 97.

NOVELLI, G. D., SCHMETZ, F. J. and KAPLAN, N. O. (1954). Enzymatic degradation and resynthesis of coenzyme A. *J. Biol. Chem.* **206**, 533.

PACE, J. K., STIER, L. B., TAYLOR, D. D. and GOODMAN, P. S. (1961). Metabolic patterns in pre-adolescent children. V. Intake and urinary excretion of pantothenic acid and of folic acid. *J. Nutr.* **74**, 345.

PATSCH, J. R., YESHURUN, D., JACKSON, R. L. and GOTTO, A. M. (1977). Effects of Clofibrate, nicotinic acid and diet on the properties of the plasma lipoproteins in a subject with Type III hyperlipoproteinemia. *Am. J. Med.* **63**, 1001.

PENNINGTON, D., SNELL, E. E. and WILLIAMS, R. J. (1940). An assay for pantothenic acid. *J. Biol. Chem.* **135**, 213.

PERLOFF, B. P. (1985). Recipe calculations for NFCS data base. In *Proc. the 10th National Nutrient Data Bank Conference*, p. 11. National Technical Information Service, Springfield, VA.

PINCUS, J. H., COOPER, J. R., MURPHY, J. V., RABE, E. F., LONSDALE, D. and DUNNE, H. G. (1973). Thiamine derivatives in subacute necrotizing encephalomyelopathy. *Pediatr.* **51**, 716.

PLAITAKIS, A., HWANG, E. C., VAN WOERT, M. H., SZILAGYI, P. I. A. and BERL, S. (1982). Effect of thiamin deficiency on brain neurotransmitter systems. *Ann. NY Acad. Sci.* **378**, 367.

PRASAD, A. S., LEI, K. Y., OBERIEAS, D., MOGHISSI, K. S. and STRYKER, J. C. (1975). Effect of oral contraceptive agents on nutrients. II. Vitamins. *Am. J. Clin. Nutr.* **28**, 385.

RAO, B. S., NARASINGA and GOPALAN, C. (1984). Niacin. In *Nutrition Reviews' Present Knowledge in Nutrition*, 5th edn, p. 318. The Nutrition Foundation, Washington, DC.

RICE, E. E., BEUK, J. F. and FRIED, J. F. (1947). Effect of commercial curing, soaking, storage and cooking operations upon vitamin content of pork hams. *Food Res.* **12**, 239.

RICHARDSON, P. J., FAVELL, D. J. and GIDLEY, G. C. (1978). Critical comparison of the determination of B2 in foods by HPLC. *Proc. Anal. Div. Chem. Soc.* **15**, 53.

RIZEK, R. L., HEPBURN, F. N. and PERLOFF, B. P. (1984). USDA's nutrient data bases. In *Proc. 1984 Agricultural Outlook Conference, Oct 31–Nov 3, 1983.* US Department of Agriculture, Washington, DC.

ROE, D. A., BOGUSZ, S., SHEU, J. and MCCORMICK, D. B. (1982). Factors affecting riboflavin requirements of oral contraceptive users and non-users. *Am. J. Clin. Nutr.* **35**, 495.

RUECKEMANN, H. and RANIFFT, K. (1978). Methods for determination of vitamins by means of HPLC. *Z. Lebens. Unters. Forsch.* **166**, 151.

RUSSELL, D. C. and OLIVER, M. F. (1978). Effect of antilipolytic therapy on ST segment elevation during myocardial ischaemia in man. *Brit. Heart J.* **41**, 117.

SANPITAK, N. and CHAYUTIMONKUL, L. (1974). Oral contraceptive and riboflavin nutrition. *Lancet* **i**, 836.

SARMA, P. S., MENON, P. S. and VENKATACHALAN, P. S. (1949). Acetylation in the diagnosis of burning feet syndrome—pantothenic acid deficiency. *Curr. Sci.* **18**, 367.

SATYANARAYANA, U. and RAO, B. S. NARASINGA (1977). Effect of dietary protein level on some key enzymes of the tryptophan–NAD pathway. *J. Nutr.* **107**, 2213.

SAUBERLICH, H. E. (1967). Biochemical alterations in thiamin deficiency—their interpretation. *Am. J. Clin. Nutr.* **20**, 528.

SAUBERLICH, H. E. and LOGAN, N. M. (1983). Vitamins. In *Clinical Guide to Laboratory Tests* (N. W. Tietz, Ed.), pp. 505–15. W. B. Saunders, Philadelphia.

SAUBERLICH, H. E., JUDD, J. H., NICHOLADS, G. E., BROQUIST, H. P. and DARBY, W. J. (1972). Application of the erythrocyte glutathione reductase assay in evaluating riboflavin nutritional status in a high school population. *Am. J. Clin. Nutr.* **25**, 756.

SAUBERLICH, H. E., DOWDY, R. P. and SKALA, J. H. (1973). Laboratory tests for assessment of nutritional status. *CRC Crit. Rev. Clin. Lab. Sci.* **4**, 215.

SEBRELL, W. H. and BUTLER, R. E. (1938). Riboflavin deficiency in man. *Publ Health Rep.* **53**, 282.

SHAH, J. J. (1985). Riboflavin. In *Methods of Vitamin Assay*, 4th edn (J. Augustin, B. P. Klein, D. A. Becker and P. B. Venugopal, Eds), p. 365. John Wiley and Sons, New York.

SHAIK, B., PONTZER, N. J., HUANG, S. S. and ZIELINSKI, W. L. (1977). Determination of N^1-methylnicotinamide in urine by high-performance liquid chromatography. *J. Chromatogr. Sci.* **15**, 215.

SKEGGS, H. R. and WRIGHT, L. D. (1944). The use of *Lactobacillus arabinosis* in the microbiological determination of pantothenic acid. *J. Biol. Chem.* **156**, 21.

SNELL, E. E. and STRONG, F. M. (1939). A microbiological assay for riboflavin. *Indus. Engin. Chem. Anal. Ed.* **11**, 346.

SNELL, E. E., STRONG, F. M. and PETERSON, W. H. (1937). Growth factors for bacteria. III. Fractionation and properties of an accessory factor for lactic acid bacteria. *Biochem. J.* **31**, 1789.

SONG, W. O., CHAN, G. M., WYSE, B. W. and HANSEN, R. G. (1984). Effect of pantothenic acid status on the content of the vitamin in human milk. *Am. J. Clin. Nutr.* **40**, 317.

SONG, W. O., WYSE, B. W. and HANSEN, R. G. (1985). Pantothenic acid status of pregnant and lactating women. *J. Am. Dietet. Assoc.* **85**, 192.

SONG, W. O., SMITH, A., WYSE, B. W. and HANSEN, R. G. (1990). Indirect enzyme linked immunosorbent assay of pantothenic acid: Application to plasma samples. *Nutr. Res.* (in press).

SOUTHGATE, D. A. T. (1983). Availability of and needs for reliable analytical methods for the assay of foods. *Food Nutr. Bull.* **5**, 30.

SPIES, T. D., COOPER, C. and BLANKENHORN, M. A. (1938). The use of nicotinic acid in the treatment of pellagra. *J. Am. Med. Assoc.* **110**, 622.

SRINIVASAN, V., CHRISTENSEN, N., WYSE, B. W. and HANSEN, R. G. (1981). Pantothenic acid nutritional status in the elderly—institutionalized and noninstitutionalized. *Am. J. Clin. Nutr.* **34**, 1736.

STEWART, K. K. (1983). The state of food composition data: An overview with some suggestions. *Food Nutr. Bull.* **5**, 54.

STREET, H. R. (1941). Studies on the rat growth assay method for riboflavin. *J. Nutr.* **22**, 399.

SUBBAROW, Y. and HITCHINGS, G. H. (1939). Pantothenic acid as a factor in rat nutrition. *J. Am. Chem. Soc.* **61**, 1615.

SUGERMAN, A. A. and CLARK, C. G. (1974). Jaundice following the administration of niacin. *J. Am. Med. Assoc.* **228**, 202.

SYDENSTRICKER, V. P., SEBRELL, W. H., CLECKLEY, H. M. and KRUSE, H. D. (1940). The ocular manifestations of arabinoflavinosis. *J. Am. Med. Assoc.* **114**, 2437.

TAARLAND, T., MATHEISEN, E., OVSTHUS, O. and BRAEKKAN, O. R. (1958). Nutritional values and vitamins of Norwegian fish and fish products. *Tidsskr. Hermetikind* **44**, 405.

TANNENBAUM, S. R., YOUNG, V. R. and ARCHER, M. C. (1985). Vitamins and minerals. In *Food Chemistry*, 2nd edn (O. R. Fennema, Ed.), p. 482. Marcel Dekker, Inc., New York.

TANPHAICHITR, V. and WOOD, B. (1984). Thiamin. In *Nutrition Reviews' Present Knowledge in Nutrition*, 5th edn, p. 277. The Nutrition Foundation, Washington, DC.

TAO, H. G. and FOX, H. M. (1976). Measurements of urinary pantothenic acid excretions of alcoholic patients. *J. Nutr. Sci. Vitam.* **22**, 333.

TARR, H. L. A. (1960). Effects of processing on fish products. In *Nutrition Evaluation of Food Processing* (R. S. Harris and von Loesecke, Eds), p. 283. John Wiley & Sons, New York. Reprinted by AVI Publishing Co., Westport, CT.

TARR, J. B., TAMURA, T. and STOKSTAD, E. L. (1981). Availability of vitamin B_6 and pantothenate in an average American diet. *Am. J. Clin. Nutr.* **34**, 1328.

TETREAULT, A. and BECK, I. (1956). Anaphylactic shock following intramuscular thiamine chloride. *Ann. Intern. Med.* **45**, 515.

THURNHAM, K. I. and RATHAKETLE, P. (1982). Incubation of NAD(P)H_2: glutathione oxidoreductase (EC 1.6.4.2) with flavine adenine dinucleotide for maximum stimulation in the measurement of riboflavin status. *Brit. J. Nutr.* **48**, 459.

TILLOTSON, J. A. and BAKER, E. M. (1972). An enzymatic measurement of the riboflavin status in man. *Am. J. Clin. Nutr.* **25**, 425.

TILLOTSON, J. A. and SAUBERLICH, H. E. (1971). Effect of riboflavin depletion and repletion on the erythrocyte glutathione reductase in rats. *J. Nutr.* **101**, 1459.

US DEPARTMENT OF AGRICULTURE (1963). *Composition of Foods: Raw, Processed, Prepared. Agriculture Handbook No. 8.* Agricultural Research Service. Govt. Print. Off., Washington, DC.

US Department of Agriculture (1975). *Nutritive Value of American Food in Common Units. Agriculture Handbook No. 456*. Agricultural Research Service. Govt. Print. Off., Washington, DC.

US Department of Agriculture (1979). *Composition of Foods: Poultry Products, Raw, Processed, Prepared. Agriculture Handbook No. 8-5*. Consumer Nutrition Division, Human Nutrition Information Service. Govt. Print. Off., Washington, DC.

US Department of Agriculture (1980). *Composition of Foods: Sausages and Luncheon Meats, Raw, Processed, Prepared. Agriculture Handbook No. 8-7*. Consumer Nutrition Division, Human Nutrition Information Service. Govt. Print. Off., Washington, DC.

US Department of Agriculture (1983). *Composition of Foods: Pork Products, Raw, Processed, Prepared. Agriculture Handbook No. 8-10*. Consumer Nutrition Division, Human Nutrition Information Service. Govt. Print. Off., Washington, DC.

US Department of Agriculture (1984). *Nutrient Intakes: Individuals in 48 States, Year 1977–78. Nationwide Food Consumption Survey 1977–78. Report No. 1-2*. Consumer Nutrition Division, Human Nutrition Information Service. Hyattsville, MD.

US Department of Agriculture (1986a). *Composition of Foods: Beef Products, Raw, Processed, Prepared. Agriculture Handbook No. 8-13*. Consumer Nutrition Division, Human Nutrition Information Service. Govt. Print. Off., Washington, DC.

US Department of Agriculture (1986b). *Nutritive Values of Foods*. Home & Garden Bull. No. 72. Govt. Print. Off., Washington, DC.

US Department of Agriculture (1987a). *Composition of Foods: Finfish and Shellfish Products, Raw, Processed, Prepared. Agriculture Handbook No. 8-15*. Consumer Nutrition Division, Human Nutrition Information Service. Govt. Print. Off., Washington, DC.

US Department of Agriculture (1987b). *CSFII: Women 19–50 Years and Their Children 1–5 Years, 1 Day, 1986. Nationwide Food Consumption Survey, Continuing Survey of Food Intakes by Individuals. Report No. 86-1*. Consumer Nutrition Division, Human Nutrition Information Service. Hyattsville, MD.

US Department of Agriculture (1987c). *CSFII: Women 19–50 Years and Their Children 1–5 Years, 4 Days, 1985. Nationwide Food Consumption Survey, Continuing Survey of Food Intakes by Individuals. Report No. 85-4*. Consumer Nutrition Division, Human Nutrition Information Service. Hyattsville, MD.

US Department of Agriculture (1988a). *Machine-Readable Data Sets on Composition of Foods and Results from Food Consumption Surveys*. Human Nutrition Information Service. Admin. Rep. No. 378. Hyattsville, MD.

US Department of Agriculture (1988b). *Composition of Foods: Fast Foods, Raw, Processed, Prepared. Agriculture Handbook No. 8-21*. Consumer Nutrition Division, Human Nutrition Information Service. Govt. Print. Off., Washington, DC.

US Department of Agriculture (1988c). 1988 Yearbook: Food and the Consumer. *National Food Review* **11**, 1.

US Department of Agriculture (1988d). *CSFII: Women 19–50 Years and Their Children 1–5 Years, 4 Days, 1986. Nationwide Food Consumption Survey,*

Continuing Survey of Food Intakes by Individuals. Report No. 86-3. Consumer Nutrition Division, Human Nutrition Information Service, Hyattsville, MD.

VAN DE WEEDRDJOF, J., WIERSUM, M. C. and REISSENWEBBER, A. (1973). Application of liquid chromatography to food analysis. *J. Chromatogr.* **83**, 455.

VIMOKESANT, S., KUNJARA, S., RUNGRUANGSAK, K., NAKORNCHAI, S. and PANIPAN, B. (1982). Beriberi caused by antithiamin factors in food and its prevention. *Ann. NY Acad. Sci.* **378**, 123.

VON MURALT, A. (1945). Thiamine and peripheral neurophysiology. *Vitamin. Horm.* **5**, 93.

WADA, H. and SNELL, E. E. (1961). The enzymatic oxidation of pyridoxine and pyridoxamine phosphates. *J. Biol. Chem.* **236**, 2089.

WAGNER, J. R., AXELROD, A. E., LIPTON, M. A. and ELVEHJEM, C. A. (1940). A rat assay method for the determination of riboflavin. *J. Biol. Chem.* **136**, 357.

WALKER, M. C., CARPENTER, B. E. and COOPER, E. L. (1981). Simultaneous determination of niacinamide, pyridoxine, riboflavin and thiamine in multivitamin preparations by high-pressure liquid chromatography. *J. Pharm. Sci.* **70**, 99.

WALSH, J. H., WYSE, B. W. and HANSEN, R. G. (1980). A comparison of microbiological and radioimmunoassay methods for the determination of pantothenic acid in foods. *J. Food Biochem.* **3**, 175.

WALSH, J. H., WYSE, B. W. and HANSEN, R. G. (1981a). Pantothenic acid content of 75 processed and cooked foods. *J. Am. Dietet. Assoc.* **78**, 140.

WALSH, J. H., WYSE, B. W. and HANSEN, R. G. (1981b). Pantothenic acid content of a nursing home diet. *Ann. Nutr. Metab.* **25**, 178.

WARBURG, O. and CHRISTIAN, W. (1932). Über ein neuco oxydationferment und sein adsorptionspektrum. *Biochem. A.* **254**, 438.

WARBURG, O. and CHRISTIAN, W. (1935). The yellow enzyme and its properties. *Biochem. Ztschr.* **266**, 377.

WERTZ, A. W., LOJKIN, M. E. and DIETZ, C. G. (1952). Metabolism of nicotinic acid in pregnancy. *J. Nutr.* **46**, 335.

WERTZ, A. W., LOJHKIN, M. E., BOUCHARD, B. S. and DERBY, M. B. (1958). Tryptophan–niacin relationships in pregnancy. *J. Nutr.* **64**, 339.

WILLIAMS, R. R. and CLINE, J. K. (1936). Synthesis of vitamin B_1. *J. Am. Chem. Soc.* **58**, 1504.

WILLIAMS, R. J. and MAJOR, R. T. (1940). The structure of pantothenic acid. *Science* **91**, 246.

WILLIAMS, R. R. and CHELDELIN, V. H. (1942). Destruction of riboflavin by light. *Science* **96**, 22.

WILLIAMS, R. J., LYMAN, C. M., GOODYEAR, G. H., TRUESDAIL, J. H. and HOLIDAY, D. (1933). Pantothenic acid, a growth determinant of universal biological occurrence. *J. Am. Chem. Soc.* **55**, 2912.

WINTER, S. L. and BOYER, J. L. (1973). Hepatic toxicity from large doses of vitamin B-3 (nicotinamide). *N. Engl. J. Med.* **289**, 1180.

WITTENBORN, J. R., NENNO, R., ROTHBERG, H. and SHELLEY, W. B. (1974). Pigmented hyperkeratosis among schizophrenic patients treated with nicotinic acid. *Adv. Biochem. Psychopharmacol.* **9**, 295.

WITTWER, C., WYSE, B. W. and HANSEN, R. G. (1982). Assay of the enzymatic hydrolysis of pantetheine. *Analytical Biochem.* **12**, 213.

WITTWER, C. T., BURKHARD, D., RIRIE, K., RASMUSSEN, R., BROWN, J., WYSE, B. W. and HANSEN, R. G. (1983). Purification and properties of a pantetheine hydrolyzing enzyme from pig kidney. *J. Biol. Chem.* **258**, 9733.

WOOLLEY, D. W., WAISMAN, H. A. and ELVEHJEM, C. A. (1939). Studies on the structure of the chick antidermatitis factor. *J. Biol. Chem.* **129**, 673.

WYSE, B. W. and HANSEN, R. G. (1977). Blood pantothenic acid values in the elderly as determined by microbiological and radio immunoassay. (Abstract.) *Fed. Proc.* **36**, 1169.

WYSE, B. W., WITTWER, C. and HANSEN, R. G. (1979). Radioimmunoassay for pantothenic acid in blood and other tissues. *Clin. Chem.* **25**, 108.

ZAPSALIS, C and BECK, R. A. (1985). *Food Chemistry and Nutritional Biochemistry*, p. 197. John Wiley and Sons, New York.

15

Vitamin B_6, Vitamin B_{12} and Folate

HOWERDE E. SAUBERLICH
Department of Nutrition Sciences, University of Alabama at Birmingham, Birmingham, Alabama, USA

I. VITAMIN B_6 (PYRIDOXINE)

A. Historical Background

In 1934, György established the existence of vitamin B_6 as a nutritional factor needed to prevent rat acrodynia (György, 1934, 1935, 1971; Sauberlich, 1981). The vitamin was isolated in 1938 and termed pyridoxine (György and Eckhardt, 1939). The following year, the chemical structure of pyridoxine was elucidated followed by synthesis by Harris and Folkers (1939) (Fig. 15-1). A role of pyridoxine in human nutrition was reported by Spies *et al.* (1939) as reviewed by Sauberlich (1981). Subsequently, it was

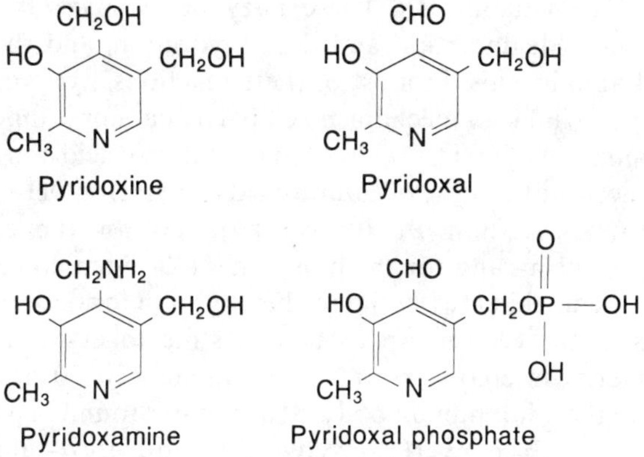

FIG. 15-1. Structures of common occurring forms of vitamin B_6.

observed that vitamin B_6 occurs in nature in three forms; namely, pyridoxine, pyridoxamine, and pyridoxal (Fig. 15-1). All three forms exist as phosphorylated derivatives. Vitamin B_6 is commonly used as a collective term for these various biologically active forms.

B. Description and Properties

Pyridoxine hydrochloride is the common commercial and pharmaceutical form of vitamin B_6. It is white and crystalline in appearance, readily soluble in water, and has a molecular weight of 205·6. Pyridoxine is quite stable to heat, but is degraded by exposure to light in alkaline or neutral solution and, to a lesser extent, in acid solution. Pyridoxal and pyridoxamine are less stable than pyridoxine. Pyridoxal-5′-phosphate is the coenzyme form of vitamin B_6. The total vitamin B_6 content of foods and biological materials is commonly measured by microbiological procedures, by using the yeast, *Saccharomyces uvarum* (Sauberlich and Canham, 1980). More recently, high performance liquid chromatography procedures have been reported for the measurement of the individual forms of vitamin B_6 (Gregory, 1988). However, their application to food analyses have been limited thus far.

C. Functions/Physiology/Biochemical Pathways

The various forms of vitamin B_6 are readily converted in the body by the action of pyridoxal kinase into the coenzyme form, pyridoxal phosphate. The coenzyme form participates in a large number and variety of enzyme system interactions almost entirely associated with protein and amino acid metabolism (Sauberlich, 1980, 1985a; Sauberlich and Canham, 1980). Well over one hundred enzymatic reactions are recognized that involve the participation of vitamin B_6. These enzymes catalyze transamination, decarboxylation, deamination and desulfhydration, and the cleavage or synthesis of amino acids. In most of these reactions, pyridoxal phosphate functions by a Schiff base mechanism. Of particular importance is its role in the transamination of amino acids, such as glutamic acid and aspartic acid, and in the decarboxylation of amino acids such as 5-OH-tryptophan to form serotonin. Vitamin B_6 is also required for the conversion of tryptophan to niacin and for the biosynthesis of δ-aminolevulinic acid, a percursor of heme that is essential for hemoglobin formation. The vitamin participates in the conversion of hemocystine to cystathionine and in glycine and serine interconversion. Approximately 20–30 mg of vitamin B_6 are present in the adult human body. Much of it is found in phosphorylase, the enzyme which converts glycogen to glucose-1-phosphate. The metabolic turnover of vitamin B_6 in the adult human is 15–20 days. The majority of the vitamin is excreted in the urine unaltered or as its metabolite, 4-pyridoxic acid.

Most of the phosphorylated forms of vitamin B_6 in the diet are hydrolyzed by intestinal phosphates before absorption (Sauberlich, 1985b, 1987). The vitamin is absorbed by a nonsaturable process. The majority of the vitamin B_6 is present in plasma as pyridoxal phosphate. The absorbed vitamin is readily taken up by the liver. The main forms of vitamin B_6 in the liver are pyridoxal phosphate and pyridoxamine phosphate. The liver serves a major role in the conversion of pyridoxine to pyridoxal and pyridoxal phosphate for use by other tissues.

D. Deficiency: Requirements

Nutrition surveys indicate that vitamin B_6 intakes may be marginal or inadequate in segments of the American population, but overt clinical deficiency of vitamin B_6 appears to be rather rare. However, a subclinical deficiency may be fairly widespread.

Vitamin B_6 deficiency in the human is manifested clinically most often by central nervous system changes and abnormal electroencephalograms. Eczema and seborrheic dermatitis may occur in the regions of the nose, ears, and mouth, in addition to cheilosis, glossitis, and angular stomatitis (Sauberlich and Canham, 1980; Sauberlich, 1981). With children, hyperirritability and convulsive seizures may occur. Occasionally hypochromic, microcytic anemia may be observed in children as well as in adults. Vitamin B_6 deficiency results in an increased excretion of xanthurenic acid due to the impaired metabolism of tryptophan. Increased excretion of xanthurenic acid may occur with pregnancy and for some users of oral contraceptive agents.

The 1989 Recommended Daily Dietary Allowances (RDA) for vitamin B_6 is given in Table 15-1. An allowance of 1·6 mg per day is recommended for women and 2·0 mg per day for men (Food and Nutrition Board, 1989). An additional allowance is recommended during pregnancy and lactation. Because of the intimate involvement of vitamin B_6 in amino acid metabolism, the requirement is partially related to the level of protein in the diet. The allowances are based on an average intake of 100 g of protein per day (Table 15-1). Lower intakes of protein may reduce the need for vitamin B_6 to 1·5 mg per day. Some women using oral contraceptive agents may have an increased requirement for vitamin B_6 supplements (Sauberlich and Canham, 1980). Also certain medications, e.g. penicillamine, cycloserine, and hydralazine, may require vitamin B_6 supplements (Sauberlich and Canham, 1980).

TABLE 15-1
RECOMMENDED DAILY DIETARY ALLOWANCES (RDA)

Group	*Age (years)*	*Vitamin B_6 (mg)*	*Folacin (μg)*	*Vitamin B_{12} (μg)*
Infants	0–0·5	0·3	25	0·3
	0·5–1·0	0·6	35	0·5
Children	1–3	1·0	50	0·7
	4–6	1·1	75	1·0
	7–10	1·4	100	1·4
Males	11–14	1·7	150	2·0
	15–18	2·0	200	2·0
	19–24	2·0	200	2·0
	25–50	2·0	200	2·0
	51+	2·0	200	2·0
Females	11–14	1·4	180	2·0
	15–18	1·5	180	2·0
	19–24	1·6	180	2·0
	25–50	1·6	180	2·0
	50+	1·6	180	2·0
Pregnant		2·2	400	2·2
Lactating		2·2	280	2·6

Adapted from the *Recommended Dietary Allowances* (1989).

Vitamin B_6 deficiency may be evaluated by blood transaminase activity measurements or by xanthurenic acid excretion following a tryptophan load. Plasma levels of pyridoxal and pyridoxal phosphate or the urinary excretion of 4-pyridoxic acid are also useful laboratory measurements (Sauberlich, 1981, 1986).

E. Food Sources: General

The majority of vitamin B_6 is present in food in the form of pyridoxine, pyridoxal phosphate, and pyridoxamine phosphate. The levels of vitamin B_6 may be reduced by light, food processing, and cooking procedures. Vitamin B_6 is widely distributed in animal and plant tissues. Poultry, fish, and other meats are a good source of the vitamin. Vegetables, including cabbage, peas, potatoes, tomatoes, carrots, and cauliflower, provide about 22% of the vitamin B_6 in the US food supply. Lesser amounts are provided by cereals, dairy items, fruits, and eggs (Sauberlich *et al.*, 1982).

Vitamin B_6 losses are high in processing and canning of meats and vegetables (Karmas and Harris, 1988; Lund, 1988; Ockerman, 1988). Losses of 50% of the vitamin may occur with processed chicken and canned salmon. With canned vegetables, losses in vitamin B_6 may be as high as 70% (Schroeder, 1971; Sauberlich, 1985b, 1987) (Fig. 15-2). The processing of cereal grain products results in large losses in vitamin B_6. For example in the milling of wheat into flour, 75–90% of the vitamin B_6 originally present is lost. Commercial foods, including grain flours, are not generally fortified with vitamin B_6.

F. Contribution of Meats and Meat Items

(i) Content of meat and meat items

The National Health And Nutrition Examination Survey (NHANES) dietary intake information indicated that on a given day 55% of the American adults consumed meat, while 33% consumed fish or poultry (Patterson and Block, 1988). Beef, pork, lamb and veal constitute about 65% of the total meat consumed in the US. Approximately 4·0 oz (112 g) of meat *per capita* per day were ingested in the US in 1987. Of that eaten, 2·46 oz (69 g) were beef and 1·45 oz (41 g) were pork. Less than 0·1 oz (2·8 g) of veal and lamb were consumed (Patterson and Block, 1988).

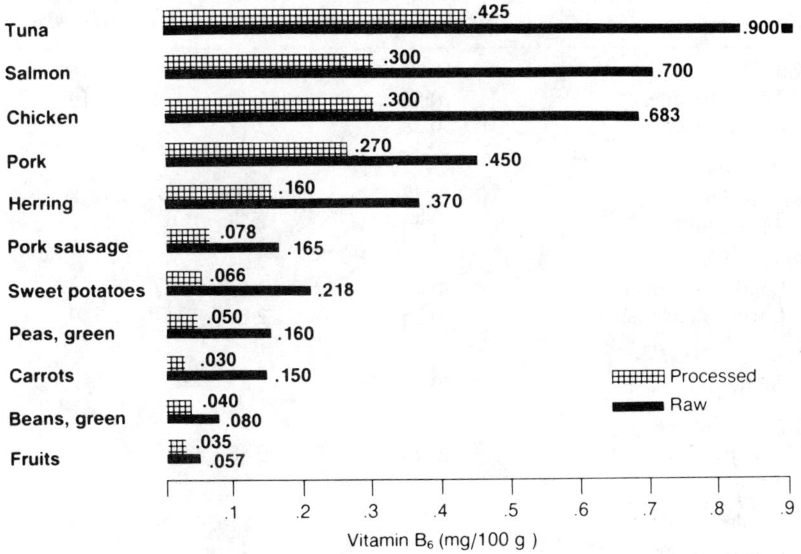

FIG. 15-2. Effect of processing or canning on the vitamin B_6 content of foods (Schroeder, 1971; Sauberlich, 1985b, 1987).

In the US, meats are the most important source of vitamin B_6. Over 40% of the vitamin B_6 in the average diet is obtained from meat. For example, a 3-oz (84 g) serving of cooked lean pork will provide 0·36 mg of vitamin B_6 representing 20% of a woman's RDA for this vitamin. A 3-oz serving of broiled beef tenderloin will provide 0·37 mg of vitamin B_6, being comparable to that provided by pork. A 3-oz cooked ground beef patty will provide about 12% of the RDA for vitamin B_6. The vitamin B_6 content of other cooked beef items are listed in Table 15-2. Marked differences in vitamin B_6 content may exist between different cuts of beef. Braised meats tend to retain less of the vitamin.

Veal is also a good source of vitamin B_6 (Table 15-3). Veal cutlets provide 0·47 mg of vitamin B_6 per 100 g of cooked meat. Lamb, however, has considerably less vitamin B_6. Roasted leg of lamb provides 0·16 mg per 100 g of prepared meat (Ono *et al.*, 1984, 1986; Breidenstein, 1987). Table 15-4 provides information as to the vitamin B_6 content of beef liver and other organ items. Beef liver is a rich source of vitamin B_6 and is largely

TABLE 15-2

VITAMIN B_6 VITAMIN B_{12} AND FOLATE CONTENT OF COOKED LEAN BEEF[a]

Item	*Vitamin B_6 (mg/100 g)*	*Vitamin B_{12} (μg/100 g)*	*Folate (μg/100 g)*
Round			
Top, broiled	0·56	2·48	12
Eye, roasted	0·38	2·17	7
Loin, broiled			
Top loin	0·42	2·00	8
Tenderloin	0·44	2·57	7
Rib			
Small end, broiled	0·40	3·32	8
Large end, roasted	0·26	2·61	9
Chuck, braised			
Blade	0·29	2·47	6
Brisket, braised			
Flat portion	0·28	2·58	8
Ground (85% lean)			
Broiled (medium)	0·27	2·71	9
Pan-fried (medium)	0·28	2·45	9

[a] Data from USDA (1986).

TABLE 15-3

VITAMIN B_6, VITAMIN B_{12}, AND FOLATE CONTENT OF COOKED LEAN LAMB AND VEAL[a]

Item	*Vitamin B_6 (mg/100 g)*	*Vitamin B_{12} (μg/100 g)*	*Folate (μg/100 g)*
Lamb (cooked, lean)[b]			
Leg, roasted (shank portion)	N/A	2·70	25·0
Rack (rib), roasted	0·16	2·15	21·0
Shoulder, chops, braised	0·14	2·65	22·0
Veal (cooked, lean)[c]			
Cutlet, pan-fry	0·47	1·73	16·3
Blade steak, braised	0·23	2·10	16·8
Sirloin chop, braised	0·35	1·73	15·6
Rib roast	0·26	1·74	14·3

[a] See Breidenstein (1987).
[b] Source: Ono *et al.* (1984).
[c] Source: Ono *et al.* (1986).

stable during cooking. A 100-g serving of pan-fried beef liver will provide 1·43 mg of vitamin B_6 or 72% of the RDA for vitamin B_6 for men. Calf liver is also a good source of vitamin B_6, but contains less than beef liver (0·54 mg/100 g).

It is estimated that pork is served in 82% of US households. In 54% of the households, pork is served at least once per two-week period (Yankelovick *et al.*, 1985). Most cuts of fresh, lean pork, when cooked, provide 0·45–0·57 mg of vitamin B_6 per 100 g (Table 15-5). Bacon and cured ham provide somewhat less vitamin B_6. Milk, cheese, and other dairy items have relatively low concentrations of vitamin B_6 (Table 15-6). Overall, dairy items contribute 11·6% of the vitamin B_6 in the food supply. Eggs contribute another 2·1%, with most of the vitamin B_6 being present in the yolk. The vitamin B_6 content of poultry meat and of most fish is comparable to beef and pork (Table 15-7).

(ii) Contribution and its importance to the diet

The level of vitamin B_6 provided by the US food supply during the past 70 years is indicated in Fig. 15-3 (Nutrition Monitoring in the United States, 1986). The highest level of vitamin B_6 provided by the food supply was 2·22 mg *per capita* per day in 1909. In the late 1950s the amount provided fell to 1·80 mg. In 1983 the food supply provided 2·02 mg *per capita* per day of vitamin B_6. Most of the increase in the vitamin B_6 food

TABLE 15-4

VITAMIN B_6, VITAMIN B_{12}, AND FOLATE CONTENT OF BEEF LIVER AND OTHER BEEF OFFAL ITEMS[a]

Item	*Vitamin B_6 (mg/100 g)*	*Vitamin B_{12} (μg/100 g)*	*Folate (μg/100 g)*
Liver			
Raw	0·94	69·2	248
Cooked (braised)	0·91	71·0	217
Cooked (pan-fried)	1·43	111·8	220
Heart			
Raw	0·43	13·7	2
Cooked (simmered)	0·21	14·3	2
Kidneys			
Raw	0·51	27·0	80
Cooked (simmered)	0·52	51·3	98
Tongue			
Raw	0·31	3·8	7
Cooked (simmered)	0·16	5·9	5
Brain			
Raw	0·26	10·9	4
Cooked (pan-fried)	0·39	15·2	6
Cooked (simmered)	0·24	8·6	7
Lung			
Raw	0·04	3·8	11
Cooked (braised)	0·02	2·6	8
Pancreas			
Raw	0·20	14·0	—
Cooked (braised)	0·18	16·6	—
Spleen			
Raw	0·07	5·7	—
Cooked (braised)	0·04	5·0	—

[a] USDA (1986).

supply is attributed to the increased use of meat, poultry, and fish. From 1909–13 to 1982, the proportion of vitamin B_6 from the meat, poultry, and fish group increased from 26 to 40% while the share from potatoes declined from 24 to 10%. The share from grain products declined from 18 to 11%.

Figure 15-4 presents the percentage contribution of the major food groups to the US food supply of vitamin B_6 (Marston and Peterkin, 1980).

TABLE 15-5

VITAMIN B_6, VITAMIN B_{12}, AND FOLATE CONTENT OF PORK ITEMS[a]

Item	*Vitamin B_6 (mg/100 g)*	*Vitamin B_{12} (μg/100 g)*	*Folate (μg/100 g)*
Ham, fresh, leg, lean			
Raw	0·50	0·71	9
Cooked (roasted)	0·45	0·72	12
Loin, fresh, lean			
Raw	0·53	0·86	5
Cooked (braised)	0·45	0·84	5
Cooked (broiled)	0·46	1·08	5
Cooked (roasted)	0·45	0·93	6
Liver			
Raw	0·69	26	212
Cooked (braised)	0·57	19	163
Bacon, cured			
Raw	0·14	0·93	2
Cooked, pan fried	0·27	1·75	5
Braunschweiger			
Cured	0·33	20·1	—
Cured, Canadian-style bacon			
Grilled	0·45	0·78	4
Cured ham, lean, fully cooked			
Unheated	0·38	0·80	3
Roasted	0·35	0·68	3

[a] USDA (1983).

The contributions were as follows: meats, 40%; dairy items, 11·6%; eggs, 2·1%; vegetables, 22·2%; cereals, 10·2%; legumes, 5·4%; and fruits, 8·2%. Thus, 53·7% of the vitamin B_6 was contributed by animal products in 1980, with little change occurring through 1985. Based on the average intake *per capita* per day in the US in 1975, meat contributed 46% of the vitamin B_6 in diet (Table 15-8). This amounted to 1·05 mg of the 2·28 mg estimated average intake of vitamin B_6 (Karmas, 1975). Contributions of vitamin B_6 by various meat items are presented in Table 15-9. The daily recommended dietary allowance for vitamin B_6 is 1·6 mg for women and 2·0 mg for men (Food and Nutrition Board, 1989). Meats, along with the other animal products (dairy items and eggs), are the major providers of

TABLE 15-6

VITAMIN B_6, VITAMIN B_{12}, AND FOLATE CONTENT OF EGGS, MILK, AND SELECTED CHEESES[a]

Item	*Vitamin B_6 (mg/100 g)*	*Vitamin B_{12} (μg/100 g)*	*Folate (μg/100 g)*
Eggs			
Whole (fried)	0·11	1·3	47
Whole (poached)	0·10	1·2	49
Yolk (raw)	0·31	3·8	152
White (raw)	0·003	0·06	16
Milk			
Whole	0·04	0·36	5
Cheese			
Cottage, 1% fat	0·07	0·63	12
Cheddar	0·07	0·83	18
Mozzarella	0·06	0·65	7
Muenster	0·06	1·47	12

[a] USDA (1976).

TABLE 15-7

VITAMIN B_6, VITAMIN B_{12}, AND FOLATE CONTENT OF POULTRY AND FISH ITEMS[a]

Item	*Vitamin B_6 (mg/100 g)*	*Vitamin B_{12} (μg/100 g)*	*Folate (μg/100 g)*
Poultry			
Turkey			
Roasted	0·46	0·37	7
Light meat, roasted	0·45	0·37	6
Dark meat, roasted	0·36	0·37	9
Chicken			
Flesh only, fried	0·48	0·34	7
Flesh only, roasted	0·47	0·33	6
Breast meat, fried	0·64	0·37	4
Fish			
Haddock, fried	0·35	1·39	—
Halibut, fried	0·40	1·37	—
Herring, kippered	0·41	18·70	—
Mackerel, fried	0·46	19·00	—
Salmon, fried	0·22	5·80	10
Sardine, canned/oil	0·17	8·94	12

[a] Data from USDA (1979, 1987).

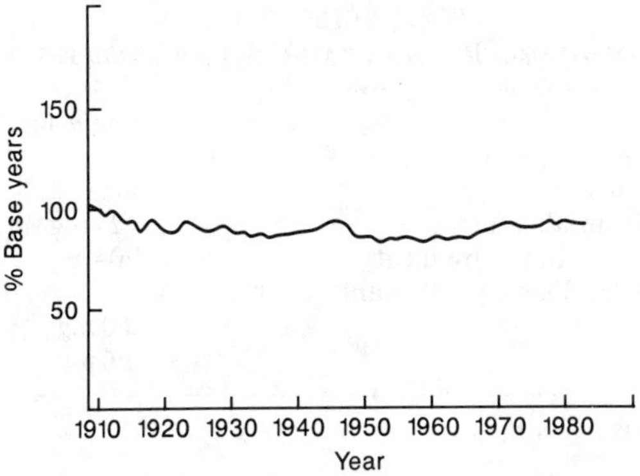

FIG. 15-3. Provision of vitamin B_6 in the US food supply as percent of base years (Nutrition Monitoring in the United States, 1986). (1909–13 = 2·17 mg vitamin B_6/*capita*/day.)

vitamin B_6 in the American diet. An average serving of meat (3·5 oz (98 g) cooked) provides 22% of the RDA for vitamin B_6 for the young adult male (National Live Stock and Meat Board, 1976; Pearson and Brooks 1978; Lofgren and Speckman, 1979; Sauberlich *et al.*, 1982). In the free-living elderly (mean age of 72·3 years), however, it has been reported from dietary intake records that only 10·8% of vitamin B_6 in their diets was obtained from beef, lamb, and pork (Vaughan and Manore, 1988). Poultry and fish contributed an additional 10·6% of the vitamin in their diet. The subjects studied were primarily those with low incomes.

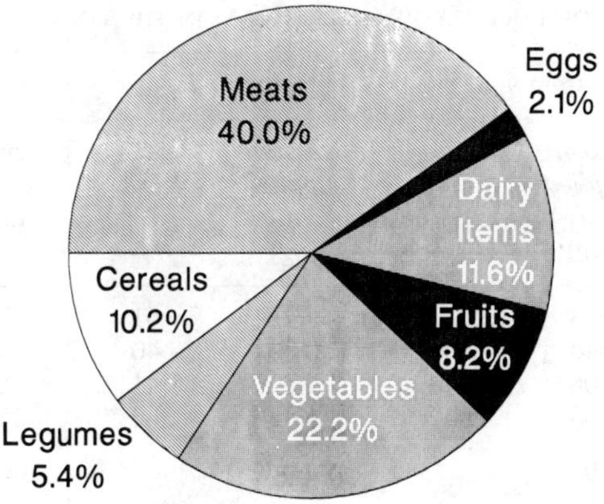

FIG. 15-4. Percentage contribution of major food groups to the US food supply of vitamin B_6. Adapted from Marston and Peterkin (1980).

TABLE 15-8

AVERAGE INTAKE OF VITAMIN B_6 AND VITAMIN B_{12} *per capita* PER DAY IN US (1975)[a]

	Vitamin B_6	*Vitamin B_{12}*
Contribution of meat	46%	77%
Average intake from all sources	2·28 mg	9·7 μg
Average intake contributed by meats	1·05 mg	7·5 μg
NAS Recommended Dietary Allowance (1989)		
Men	2·0 mg	2·0 μg
Women	1·6 mg	2·0 μg

[a] Data from Karmas (1975, 1988).

Nutrition surveys of military personnel at various locations have provided extensive information on nutrient intakes (Letterman Army Inst. Res., 1979; Sauberlich *et al.*, 1982). For example, nutrition surveys of personnel at the Naval Air Station, Alameda, California revealed a daily intake of 2·2–2·6 mg of vitamin B_6 per day. The personnel obtained 57% of the vitamin B_6 in their diets from animal products. Meats contributed 40% of the vitamin B_6 intake. A study conducted on the nutrition of the cadets at West Point Military Academy in 1979 revealed that animal products provided an average daily intake of 1·21 mg of vitamin B_6 or 61% of the RDA (Sauberlich *et al.*, 1982). Of this, meat contributed 0·85 mg.

TABLE 15-9

VITAMIN B_6, VITAMIN B_{12}, AND FOLATE CONTRIBUTED BY MEATS TO THE RECOMMENDED DIETARY ALLOWANCES (RDA) IN THE USA[a]

Meat type	*Vitamin B_6*		*Vitamin B_{12}*		*Folate*	
	Amount supplied daily (mg)	*% RDA*	*Amount supplied daily (μg)*	*% RDA*	*Amount supplied daily (μg)*	*% RDA*
Red	0·58	29	5·22	261	17·5	8·8
Poultry	0·44	22	0·80	40	5·99	3·0
Fish	0·06	3·0	0·82	41	2·10	1·0
Combined	1·08	54	6·84	342	25·59	12·8
RDA (1980)[b]	2·0		2·0		200	

[a] Sauberlich *et al.* (1982).
[b] For 19–22 year-old males.

G. Factors That Influence Contribution

(i) Bioavailability

Vitamin B_6 present in beef and fish (tuna, salmon) is considered highly available while the vitamin B_6 present in bread, soybeans, carrots, and other plant items are less available (Sauberlich, 1985b, 1987; Leklem, 1986). This relates to the presence of glycosylated forms of vitamin B_6 in cereal grains, fruits, and vegetables, but not in animal products (Gregory, 1988). Glycosylated vitamin B_6 was found to account for 3–82% of the total vitamin in cereals, fruits, and vegetables. Human studies have shown that the glycosylated forms of vitamin B_6 are poorly available as a source of vitamin B_6.

Analytical methods generally used to measure vitamin B_6 in foods would include the glycosylated vitamin B_6; hence, the analytical data used in nutrient tables may overestimate the content of nutritionally available vitamin B_6 in plant-derived foods. Thus, the contribution of available vitamin B_6 by meats and dairy products to the diet may be greater than normally indicated. Limited studies have indicated that the bioavailability of vitamin B_6 in the average American diet ranges from 61–81%.

(ii) Cooking and food processing

Since little meat is eaten raw, the effect of cooking and processing of meats on the retention of vitamins is important (Sommer and Hagen, 1981). As noted earlier, vitamin B_6 losses may be high in processed and canned meats and vegetables (Lushbough *et al.*, 1959; Orr, 1969; Adams and Erdman, 1988; Karmas and Harris, 1988; Lachance and Fisher, 1988; Lund, 1988; Ockerman, 1988). Losses in canned meats, fish, poultry, and seafoods may amount to 42–49%. Processed meats, such as luncheon meats and sausages, may have losses in vitamin B_6 of 50–75% (Schroeder, 1971). A loss of 55% in vitamin B_6 has been reported to occur with cooking of beef (Nguyen and Gregory, 1983). Regular processing of milk or spray drying produces only a slight loss in vitamin B_6 (Gregory and Kirk, 1979).

Table 15-10 presents findings on the retention of vitamin B_6 in roast beef (Reiter and Driskell, 1985). Following the initial roasting the beef contained 0·47 mg/100 g, which approximates a typical serving. After reheating and holding, the vitamin B_6 content fell progressively. After holding at 66°C, for three hours, only 31·9% of the initial vitamin B_6 was present in the roast beef, representing 0·15 mg/100 g. In this study, 62–84% of the vitamin B_6 was retained after the initial roasting. A significant amount of the vitamin was leached from the beef into the juice during cooking and holding. The percent retention of vitamin B_6 in both beef and pork is lowest when the

TABLE 15-10
RETENTION OF VITAMIN B_6 IN ROAST BEEF[a]

Roast beef	*Vitamin B_6 (mg/100 g)*[b]	*Vitamin B_6 retained (%)*
Initial	$0{\cdot}47 \pm 0{\cdot}12$	—
Reheated	$0{\cdot}26 \pm 0{\cdot}11$	55·3
Held 1 h (66°C)	$0{\cdot}22 \pm 0{\cdot}10$	46·8
Held 2 h (66°C)	$0{\cdot}20 \pm 0{\cdot}10$	42·6
Held 3 h (66°C)	$0{\cdot}15 \pm 0{\cdot}07$	31·9

[a] Data from Reiter and Driskell (1985).
[b] Approximates a typical serving.

meat is cooked by braising (Moss *et al.*, 1980) (Table 15-11). Radiation sterilization of meat produced only small losses in vitamin B_6 content, less than that of thermally processed meats (Thomas and Josephson, 1970; Thomas, 1988). Microwave cooked beef roasts retained higher amounts of riboflavin and thiamin than meat cooked by conventional means (Korschgen and Baldwin, 1978). Presumably, vitamin B_6, vitamin B_{12}, and folacin would have greater retention in meats with microwave cooking.

(iii) Storage stability

It has been long known that sterilization of canned evaporated milk and

TABLE 15-11
PERCENT RETENTION OF VITAMIN B_6, VITAMIN B_{12}, AND FOLATE IN COOKED, LEAN, FRESH BEEF OR PORK[a]

Item	*% retention*		
	Vitamin B_6	*Vitamin B_{12}*	*Folate*
Beef, fresh, lean			
Braised	46	67	72
Broiled	74	75	87
Roasted	66	72	88
Pork, fresh, lean			
Braised	52	60	65
Broiled	63	91	86
Roasted	64	82	95

[a] USDA (1983, 1986).

canned meats results in marked reduction in the content and bioavailability of vitamin B_6. Apparently during storage and heat processing, pyridoxal and pyridoxal phosphate may react to bind with ε-amino groups of proteins or peptide lysyl residues to form ε-pyridoxyl-lysine (Gregory and Kirk, 1981). This compound was found to possess only 50% molar vitamin B_6 activity. Other studies have also reported losses of vitamin B_6 with prolonged storage (Harding *et al.*, 1959; Everson *et al.*, 1964; Anderson *et al.*, 1976; Gregory and Kirk, 1978). Little loss of vitamin B_6 occurred during curing of hams (Lushbough *et al.*, 1959).

Freezing had no significant effect on vitamin B_6 content of beef steak (Lee *et al.*, 1950; Fennema, 1975, 1988). Some loss of B vitamins appears to occur in pork chops due to freezing, but the values were highly variable (Lee *et al.*, 1954). However, frozen meats on thawing give rise to the exudation of blood-like juice or 'drip'. Rapid freezing reduces the drip. Losses of vitamins in the drip of pork and beef were reported to be less than 15% (Pearson *et al.*, 1959). For most vitamins, frozen storage for up to six months produced little loss in most vitamins. However, beef lost up to 24% of its initial vitamin B_6 content according to Fennema (1975, 1988), while frozen pork lost up to 18% of its initial vitamin B_6.

II. VITAMIN B_{12}

A. Historical Background

Vitamin B_{12} has had an interesting and perplexing history (Anon., 1957). As early as 1822, an anemia was described that was considered associated with a digestive disorder. This condition became known as Addisonian pernicious anemia (megaloblastic anemia) as explained by Castle (1961). However, it was not until 1926 that a dietary component was associated with the disease. This was established by the consumption of large amounts of liver in the treatment of the pernicious anemia by Minot and Murphy (1926). Subsequently it was found that the active component could be extracted from liver and ingested to treat the anemia. In 1929, however, as described by Castle (1953) it was demonstrated that a gastric intrinsic factor was essential for the absorption of the active principle in liver.

During this period studies were being conducted on the effects of diet on the growth of animals. Early studies suggested that animal protein sources in the diet were superior to plant protein sources in promoting animal growth (Coward *et al.*, 1929). Subsequent investigations demonstrated that animal protein sources may contain a water-soluble factor that was essential for chick growth (Van der Hoorn *et al.*, 1935) and for normal growth and lactation in the rat (Mapson, 1932). This factor became known as the 'animal protein factor' (Schweigert, 1949).

The report of Shorb (1947) that a growth factor present in crude and refined liver extracts was required by the microorganism *Lactobacillus lactis* (Dorner) enhanced the isolation of the essential substance. Thus in early 1948, a crystalline substance termed vitamin B_{12} was isolated by Rickes *et al.* (1948) that required only microgram quantities to produce a positive hematologic response in pernicious anemia patients. Shortly thereafter, British investigators also purified the vitamin (Smith and Parker, 1948). Soon investigations established that vitamin B_{12} was the animal growth factor (Schweigert, 1949; Stokstad *et al.*, 1949) as well as the factor required to prevent pernicious anemia and to support the growth of the microorganisms *L. lactis* and *L. leichmannii* (Shive *et al.*, 1948). Vitamin B_{12} is commercially produced primarily by fermentation.

B. Description and Properties

Vitamin B_{12} has a complex structural formula that consists of a corrin nucleus linked through aminopropanol to a nucleotide containing dimethylbenzimidazole (Fig. 15-5). The corrin ring system contains a cobalt atom that is also attached to the dimethylbenzimidazole. In the metabolically active form of vitamin B_{12} as present in liver, the cobalt atom is attached to 5′-deoxyadenosine. In the common commercial form of vitamin B_{12}, the substituent on the cobalt atom is cyanide. Little of the cyanocobalamin form exists in nature, but this form is stable and commonly referred to as vitamin B_{12}. Other congeners of vitamin B_{12} exist in blood and tissues, such as hydroxocobalamin (—OH) and methylcobalamin (—CH_3). Vitamin B_{12} (cyanocobalamin) has a molecular weight of 1355·4, is dark red in crystal form, and is readily soluble in water. The major stored form of vitamin B_{12} in the human is the coenzyme 5′-deoxyadenosylcobalamin (Toohey and Barker, 1961).

C. Functions/Physiology/Biochemical Pathways

In the liver, vitamin B_{12} is present as deoxyadenosylcobalamin (65–75%), hydroxocobalamin (20–30%), and methylcobalamin (1–5%). The predominant form in blood is methylcobalamin. The human body stores of vitamin B_{12} range from 1–10 mg (Linnell, 1977).

The active coenzyme forms of vitamin B_{12} (5-deoxyadenosylcobalamin and methylcobalamin) function in a series of metabolic reactions. These functions include the conversion of methylmalonate to succinate, the

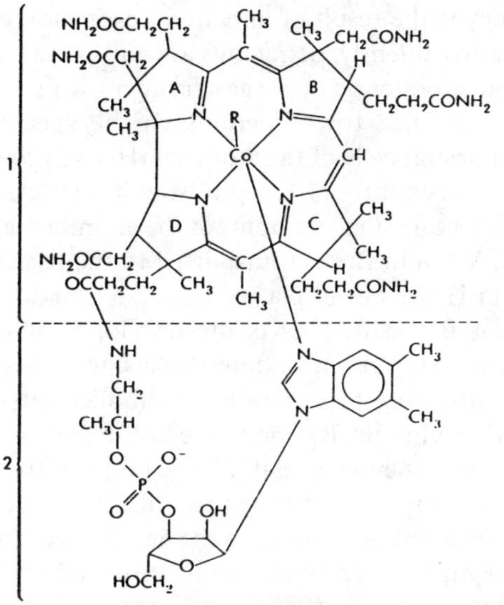

VITAMIN B_{12} CONGENERS

Permissive Name	R Group
Cyanocobalamin (Vitamin B_{12})	—CN
Hydroxocobalamin	—OH
Methylcobalamin	$—CH_3$
5′-Deoxyadenosyl-cobalamin	—5′-Deoxyadenosyl

FIG. 15-5. Structure of vitamin B_{12} and congeners. Reproduced with permission from *Goodman and Gilman's The Pharmacological Basis of Therapeutics*, Seventh Edition edited by Alfred Goodman Gilman, Louis S. Goodman, Theodore W. Rall, Ferid Murad (MacMillan, New York, 1985).

formation of methionine from homocysteine, and the maintenance of sulfhydryl groups in the reduced state. The 5′-deoxyadenosylcobalamin form is a cofactor for the mitochondrial mutase enzyme that catalyzes the isomerization of methylmalonyl coenzyme A to succinyl coenzyme A. The reaction is essential for the metabolism of odd-chain length fatty acids. The methylcobalamin form is essential for the removal of the methyl group from folate in the homocysteine–methionine transmethylation. Vitamin B_{12} deficiency results in folate being 'trapped' as metabolic non-functional methylfolate (Linnell, 1977; Herbert, 1987; Herbert and Colman, 1988). Vitamin B_{12} is involved in the transport and storage of folate in cells.

Vitamin B_{12} is essential for the normal development of red blood cells and for the normal functioning of all cells and, in particular, the nervous system, bone marrow, and intestines (Hillman, 1985). The majority of the vitamin in the body is stored in the liver.

D. Deficiency: Requirements

Since vitamin B_{12} is not present in plant foods, a deficiency in the vitamin may occur in strict vegetarians. Although dietary deficiencies of vitamin

B_{12} occur, more often a deficiency is the result of impaired absorption of vitamin B_{12} from the intestine. Consequently, pernicious anemia occurs in individuals with a deficiency in the production of the gastric intrinsic factor essential for vitamin B_{12} absorption. The intrinsic factor is a highly specific binding protein secreted by the parietal cells of the stomach (Herbert and Colman, 1988). Vitamin B_{12} is absorbed through receptor sites in the ileum which is mediated by the intrinsic factor. Small amounts of the vitamin may be absorbed by simple diffusion. Vitamin B_{12} is transported to the tissues that require it as transcobalamin II present in plasma.

The earliest sign of a vitamin B_{12} deficiency is the development of megaloblastic anemia. A deficiency may result in paresthesias, weakness, and neurologic changes. Because of their close metabolic interrelationships, a deficiency of either vitamin B_{12} or folate will result in a morphologically identical macrocytic anemia, megaloblastic bone marrow changes, and hypersegmented polymorphonuclear neutrophils. Prolonged vitamin B_{12} deficiency produces irreversible damage to the nervous system as a result of inadequate myelin synthesis. The specific role of vitamin B_{12} in this synthesis remains unclear.

Vitamin B_{12} has a relatively slow turnover in the body, probably in excess of 960 days. The amount of vitamin B_{12} required to replace the daily loss is small. Based on the body pool size, absorption efficiency, and turnover rate, the RDA for adult men and women was established at 2·0 μg of vitamin B_{12} (Food and Nutrition Board, 1989). The allowance for vitamin B_{12} was increased to 2·2 μg/day during pregnancy and to 2·6 μg/day during lactation (Table 15-1).

The most practical means to evaluate vitamin B_{12} nutritional status in patients or subjects is to measure the levels of the vitamin in serum or plasma. Microbiological assays and radioassay techniques are available for this purpose.

E. Food Sources: General

National surveys indicate that the vitamin B_{12} intake of the US population is adequate. The major sources of vitamin B_{12} in the diets are meat, poultry, and fish items, followed by dairy products. The amount of vitamin B_{12} provided by the US food supply has remained relatively constant over the past 80 years (Fig. 15-6). The *per capita* per day provision of vitamin B_{12} has fluctuated between 7·1 and 9·6 μg. This level of dietary vitamin B_{12} more than meets the Recommended Dietary Allowance (RDA) for this vitamin. The US Department of Agriculture 1977–78 Nationwide Food Consumption Survey found the vitamin B_{12} intakes of individuals

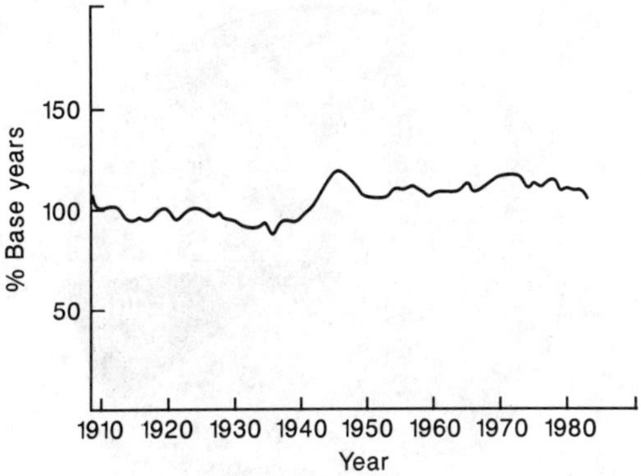

FIG. 15-6. Provision of vitamin B_{12} in the US food supply as percent of base years (Nutrition Monitoring in the United States, 1986). (1909–13 = 8·2 μg vitamin B_{12}/*capita*/day.)

averaged 260% of the RDA (Nutrition Monitoring in the United States, 1986). Intakes of vitamin B_{12} are higher for men than for women.

F. Contribution of Meat

(i) Content of meat and meat items

Animal products serve as the virtual sole source of vitamin B_{12} in the food supply. Meats contributed 69·2%, dairy items 20·7%, and eggs 8·5% (total of 98·4%). Cereals, fortified with vitamin B_{12}, provide only a small amount of the vitamin (1·6%) (Fig. 15-7).

Based on the average intake *per capita* per day in the US in 1975, meat contributed 77% of the vitamin B_{12} in the diet (Table 15-8). This amounted to 7·5 μg of the 9·7 μg estimated average intake of vitamin B_{12} (Karmas, 1975). Contributions of vitamin B_{12} by various meat items are indicated in Table 15-9. The RDA for vitamin B_{12} is 2·0 μg for men and women. Hence, meats readily provide ample amounts of vitamin B_{12} in the American diet (Table 15-2). For example, a 3-oz ground beef patty, broiled medium well-done, will contain 2·3 μg of vitamin B_{12}, which represents 114% of the RDA for vitamin B_{12}. Beef, along with lamb and mutton, has a higher content of vitamin B_{12} than that of other meats. For instance, an average 3-oz serving of lamb will provide 111% of the RDA for vitamin B_{12} while an equivalent serving of pork will provide 36%, but roast chicken will provide only 14% and flounder 47%. Table 15-3 provides information on the vitamin B_{12} content of commonly served lamb and veal items. Lamb is comparable to beef in vitamin B_{12} content, but veal generally has

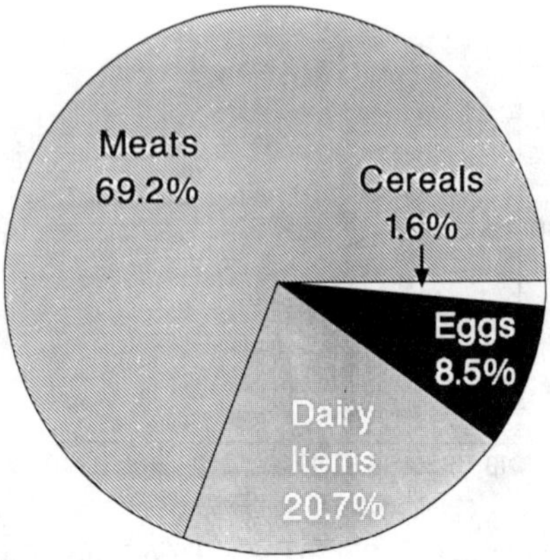

FIG. 15-7. Percentage contribution of major food groups to the US food supply of vitamin B_{12}. Adapted from Marston and Peterkin (1980).

somewhat lower levels (Table 15-3). Although pork items generally have lower vitamin B_{12} contents than beef products, pork remains a good source of the vitamin. Tables 15-5 and 15-12 provide information on the vitamin B_{12} content of a number of pork items. In comparison to broiled beef loin, broiled pork loin contains approximately 50% less vitamin B_{12} (2·00 μg/100 g of beef vs 1·08 μg/100 g of pork) as shown in Tables 15-2 and 15-5. Vitamin B_{12} content is high in pork liver and in other liver-containing

TABLE 15-12

VITAMIN B_{12} CONTRIBUTION OF CERTAIN READY-TO-SERVE SAUSAGES[a]

Item	*Common portion*	*Weight (g)*	*Percent of US RDA provided by the portion indicated*
Bratwurst	1 link	85	20
Bologna	2½ slices	57	18
Braunschweiger	3 slices	54	272
Frankfurter	1 link	57	18
Liver sausage	3 slices	54	1 155
Smoked sausage	1 link	85	32
Pork sausage	2 patties	54	24
Thuringer	2½ slices	57	66
Dry salami	4 slices	40	20
Kielbasa	1 link	85	35

[a] National Live Stock and Meat Board (1983).

items. Ham, even after curing, cooking, and roasting retains most of its original vitamin B_{12} content (Table 15-5). Beef liver is an exceptionally rich source of vitamin B_{12} (Table 15-4). Beef heart, kidneys, and other beef organ tissues are rather rich in vitamin B_{12}, which is retained quite well on cooking. A number of ready-to-eat sausages can serve as additional sources of vitamin B_{12} in the diet (Table 15-12). Liver sausage and braunschweiger because of their liver content provide high amounts of vitamin B_{12}.

As noted earlier, poultry products contain considerably less vitamin B_{12} than beef, lamb, or veal products, but only somewhat less than pork items (Table 15-7; compare with Tables 15-3 and 15-5). Fish, however, may provide to the diet vitamin B_{12} in amounts approaching or exceeding beef roasts. The vitamin B_{12} content of fish is variable depending upon the species examined. Fried salmon, for example, contains 5·8 μg of vitamin B_{12} per 100 g, while fried halibut contains 1·4 μg per 100 g (Table 15-7).

Milk, cheeses, and eggs contain significant amounts of vitamin B_{12} and provide important sources of the vitamin in lacto-ovovegetarian diets (Table 15-6). For example, an 8-oz glass of milk provides 0·8 μg of vitamin B_{12} which is equal to 38% of the RDA for vitamin B_{12}. With eggs, virtually all of the vitamin B_{12} is located in the yolk.

(ii) Contribution and its importance to the diet

Microorganisms are the source of all vitamin B_{12} in nature. Consequently, plants are devoid of vitamin B_{12} unless contaminated by microorganisms. The vitamin is absent in fruits, grains, cereal products, and vegetables unless contaminated by fecal matter. Microorganisms of the colon are capable of synthesizing considerable amounts of vitamin B_{12}, hence, feces are a rich source of vitamin B_{12} for non-ruminant animals. Ruminant animals, such as cattle and sheep, can by virtue of their ruminant miroflora produce large amounts of vitamin B_{12} that is absorbed and stored in their tissues. However, the ability of ruminants to produce vitamin B_{12} is dependent upon an adequate supply of cobalt in their diets (see Chapter 10). Hence, when deprived of a dietary source of cobalt, sheep and cattle develop a deficiency syndrome that includes a characteristic anemia. The condition can be treated with intravenous injections of vitamin B_{12} or by orally administered cobalt. Normally the vitamin B_{12} content of meats from ruminant animals is higher than that of non-ruminant animals.

During the past 80 years, the lowest level of vitamin B_{12} provided by the US food supply was during the 1930s and highest in the mid-1940s (Fig. 15-6). The higher *per capita* levels of vitamin B_{12} available during the past several decades are attributed to an increased use of the meat, poultry, and fish group and, to a small extent, to fortification of items such as grain products.

In a study with free-living elderly, meat, fish, and poultry provided a mean daily intake of 4·3 μg of vitamin B_{12} (Vaughan and Manore, 1988). Of this, 3·6 μg were contributed by red meats. These intakes amply provide the RDA for vitamin B_{12}. Military nutrition surveys have universally reported adequate sources of vitamin B_{12} in the diet, virtually all from animal products (Letterman Army Inst. Res., 1979; Sauberlich *et al.*, 1982). Personnel at the Naval Air Station at Alameda, California, had daily intakes of 11·79 μg of vitamin B_{12}, or 590% of the RDA. Meats alone provided 5·46 μg of vitamin B_{12} representing 46% of the dietary intake. Cadets at the West Point Military Academy had intakes of vitamin B_{12} from animal products that provided 308% of the RDA. Of the animal products, the meat, poultry, and fish group provide 48% of the vitamin B_{12} intake. The remainder was provided by dairy products (36%) and eggs (16%).

G. Factors that Influence Contribution

(i) Bioavailability

Few studies have been conducted on the bioavailability of vitamin B_{12} from foods. In general, vitamin B_{12} in the diet is considered highly available and absorbed by the normal person. Vitamin B_{12} in lean mutton was determined to be 60–80% bioavailable by Heyssel *et al.* (1966). Radio-label studies indicated about 60% of the vitamin B_{12} in chicken was absorbed (Doscherholmen *et al.*, 1978). In contrast, the vitamin B_{12} in eggs is poorly absorbed according to Levine and Doscherholmen (1983).

(ii) Cooking and food processing

Vitamin B_{12} contents are reduced to some extent with thermal processing of meats (Lund, 1988). Vitamin B_{12} losses during thermal processing may range from 25–45%, similar to that of vitamin B_6 and thiamin. With conventional cooking, losses of vitamin B_{12} in the range of 10–30% generally are encountered. Vitamin B_{12} is quite stable at temperatures below 250°C. Some losses may occur on the surface of roasted or fried meats. Boiling lean beef for 45 min may result in up to 30% losses of the vitamin whereas liver may lose 8% during boiling for five min. Radiation sterilization of meat produced losses of vitamin B_{12} of less than 10% (Thomas and Josephson, 1970; Thomas, 1988). Table 15-11 indicates that the retention of vitamin B_{12} in cooked beef and pork is quite high for both meats, being as high as 91% for broiled pork. Braised meats had higher losses of vitamin B_{12} than either broiled or roasted meat, with braised pork losing 40% of its B_{12} content.

Pasteurization of milk produces a loss of about 7% of the vitamin B_{12}. Boiling of milk for several minutes may cause losses of 30–75% of its vitamin B_{12} content. Flash sterilized milk loses only about 10% of its vitamin B_{12} content.

III. FOLATE (FOLIC ACID, FOLACIN)

A. Historical Background

The history of folate was confused by the fact that anemias due to a deficiency of vitamin B_{12} or of folate have the common morphological features of megaloblastic erythropoiesis. Although Addisonian pernicious anemia was recognized in 1926 as a disease associated with diet, the work of Wills (1933) in India showed that another dietary factor was associated with the megaloblastic anemia observed in pregnant women. The unknown dietary factor became known as the Wills factor. Subsequent investigations revealed that this factor was identical to an unknown substance essential for monkeys, chicks, and for certain microorganisms, such as *Lactobacillus casei*, *Leuconostoc citrovorum* (*Pediococcus cervisiae*), and *Streptococcus faecalis* R. A compound was isolated from spinach by Mitchell *et al.* (1941) that was essential for the growth of *S. faecalis* R., which they named folic acid. The structure and synthesis of folic acid (pteroylmonoglutamic acid) were reported by Angier *et al.* (1946) (Fig. 15-8).

B. Description and Properties

Folic acid is commercially produced by synthesis and extensively used for food and feed supplementation and pharmaceutical preparations. Little, if any, folic acid as such occurs naturally, but it is a stable form of the vitamin that is readily converted into physiologically active forms in the body. Folic acid has a molecular weight of 441·4, is yellow in color, only slightly soluble in water, and reasonably stable in dilute acid solution at room temperature or lower. Folic acid and its derivatives are unstable to light.

Folic acid, pteroylmonoglutamic acid, consists of a pteridine nucleus, *p*-aminobenzoic acid, and glutamic acid. Removal of the glutamic acid portion of the molecule results in pteroic acid formation. For some microorganisms, pteroic acid or *p*-aminobenzoic acid will serve as a replacement for folic acid, but they have no nutritional activity for the human. Folic acid occurs in plants and animals as numerous derivatives

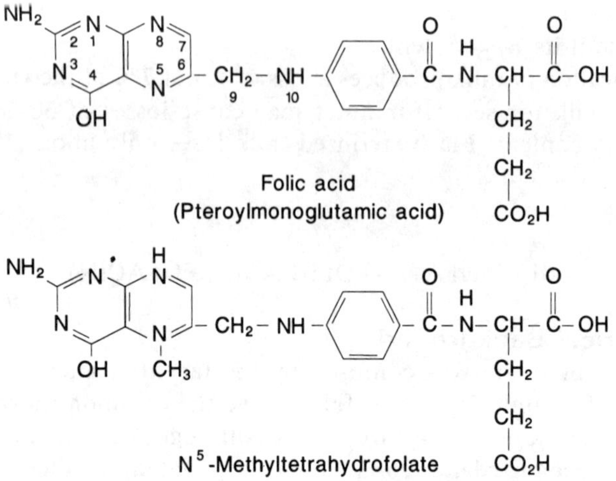

FIG. 15-8. Structure of folic acid and of N^5-methyltetrahydrofolate.

(folates), particularly as polyglutamyl peptides, with the most prevalent being the tri- and heptaglutamyl peptides. Some other forms of folate are N^5-methyltetrahydrofolate, N^5-formyltetrahydrofolate, N^{10}-formylpteroylglutamic acid, methylene tetrahydrofolate, and methenyl tetrahydrofolate.

C. Functions/Physiology/Biochemical Pathways

Folate is a B-complex vitamin essential for normal hematopoiesis. In its absence a megaloblastic anemia develops. Because of their interactive functions, a vitamin B_{12} deficiency will produce an identical megaloblastic anemia. However, in contrast to a vitamin B_{12} deficiency, a folate deficiency does not appear to produce neurological complications (Anderson and Talbot, 1981). The various 1-carbon tetrahydrofolate derivatives participate in a number of reactions which involve the transfer of single carbon groups. Thus, the vitamin participates in the synthesis of choline, of serine from glycine, formate metabolism, pyrimidine and purine biosynthesis, and the formation of methionine from homocysteine. Both folate and vitamin B_{12} are required for the formation of thymidylate that is essential for deoxyribonucleic acid (DNA) synthesis. Hence, a deficiency of either vitamin will result in a megaloblastic anemia as a consequence of the impaired cell division. Also, either deficiency will lead to hypersegmented polymorphonuclear neutrophils. Histidine is normally converted to glutamic acid through the participation of tetrahydrofolate and formiminotransferase. In a folate deficiency, the conversion is inhibited and an increased amount of formiminoglutamic acid and urocanic acid occurs.

The predominant form of folate circulating in the plasma is 5-methyltetrahydrofolate. Synthetic pteroylmonoglutamic acid (folic acid) is readily absorbed and converted by the liver to 5-methyltetrahydrofolate where it is stored primarily in the polyglutamate form. Normal individuals excrete only small amounts of intact folates in the urine, usually in the range of 5–40 μg per day. The total body pool of folate in a normal adult male is uncertain but has been estimated to range from 7·5–50 mg. The biological half-life has been estimated to be 101 days.

D. Deficiency: Requirements

Folate deficiency is relatively common and is the result of low dietary intakes, excessive alcohol consumption, pregnancy, and other influences, such as medications and oral contraceptive agents (Rose *et al.*, 1984; Roe, 1985; Sauberlich, 1990; Subar *et al.*, 1989). Nutrition surveys often indicate that the folate intake of segments of the US population is less than adequate (Sauberlich, 1990; Subar *et al.*, 1989) (Table 15-13). Therefore, measurements to assess folate status are often performed in clinical laboratories. For this purpose, folate levels in plasma and red blood cells are measured by microbiological assays, using the test organism *Lactobacillus casei*, or by radioassay procedures (Anderson and Talbot, 1981; Colman, 1981).

In addition to the megaloblastic anemia noted earlier, folate deficiency may result in clinical symptoms. They include weakness, tiredness, pallor, sleeplessness, forgetfulness, and periods of euphoria. Glossitis and anorexia may occur. The 1989 RDA for folate was established at 200 μg per day for

TABLE 15-13

MEAN DAILY INTAKE OF FOLATE AS OBSERVED IN NUTRITION SURVEYS[a]

Sex	*NHANES II*[b] (*μg/day*)	*Nutrition Canada* (*μg/day*)	*CSFII (1985)*[c]	
			Black (*μg/day*)	*White* (*μg/day*)
Men	263	192	245	307
Women	197	147	194	210

[a] From: Subar *et al.* (1989).
[b] NHANES = National Health and Nutrition Evaluation Surveys.
[c] CSFII = Continuing Survey of Food Intake By Individuals.

adult men and women (Table 15-1). During pregnancy and lactation, an additional allowance is recommended. Recent studies support the Recommended Dietary Allowances for folate (Sauberlich *et al.*, 1987).

E. Food Sources: General

Folate is present in many foods, especially green leafy vegetables (Table 15-14). Nevertheless, meats, dairy products, and eggs, provide a sizeable contribution of folate to the food supply and diets. The presence of the

TABLE 15-14

FOLATE CONTENT OF COMMON FOOD ITEMS IN THE US DIET[a]

Item as prepared for consumption	*Percent contribution to the average US diet*	*Folate content*	
		μg/usual serving	*μg/100 g*
Liver	3·07	383	428
Eggs	4·63	31	43
Veal	—	27	16
Lamb	—	35	22
Pizza	0·47	24	16
Mixed dishes with pork, veal or lamb	—	21	23
Milk (2% fat)	1·17	20	5
Beef stew, pot pie	0·49	26	10
Mixed dishes with beef	—	17	8
Orange juice	9·70	43	41
Corn	1·89	35	43
Broccoli	—	53	65
Mustard or turnip greens	0·56	36	54
Cauliflower	—	28	53
Peas	0·75	27	46
Green beans	0·80	21	28
Tomatoes	1·31	21	10
Bananas	0·70	19	19
Beef steaks, roasts (3 oz)	1·19	7	8
Hamburgers, meatloaf, cheeseburgers	1·15	38	21
Cheese, Cheddar (1 oz)	0·62	5	18
Hot dogs, ham, lunchmeat	0·42	30	30
Fried fish	0·35	3–12	4–15
Pork, roast, chops	0·30	4	5

[a] Data from Subar *et al.* (1989).

multiple forms of folate in foods has led to difficulties in estimating the folate content of foods and uncertainties about levels reported in food composition tables. Microbiological assays have been preferred for these determinations because of their sensitivity and ability to respond to most of the diverse forms of folate. The majority of the folates are present as reduced forms of polyglutamates. These forms are labile and easily oxidized. During home food preparation and food processing, as much as 50–90% of the folates initially present in foods may be lost. Folate is stable in fresh fruits and vegetables, but is oxidatively destroyed with extended cooking. Boiling with water reduces the folate contributions of vegetables. However, lightly stir-fried vegetables, as practiced with Chinese cooking, retain most of their folate.

Not all forms of folate are absorbed equally by the human. The bioavailability and absorption of folate from foods are complicated and incompletely understood (Sauberlich, 1985b, 1987; Sauberlich *et al.*, 1987). Folate absorption may be impaired with malabsorption syndromes, such as Crohn's disease and tropical sprue (Rose *et al.*, 1984). The use of some medications, such as diphenylhydantoin and sulfasalazine, may also adversely affect absorption of folate (Roe, 1985). Generally only 25–50% of the folates present in the diet are nutritionally bioavailable.

F. Contribution of Meats

(i) Content of meats and meat items

In contrast to animal products as rich sources of vitamin B_{12} and vitamin B_6, plant foods are the most abundant sources of folate. As noted in Table 15-4, orange juice, corn, broccoli, greens, peas, and cauliflower are good sources of folate with the usual serving of each item providing 27–53 μg of folate or 41–65 μg per 100 g of each prepared food item (Subar *et al.*, 1989). Nevertheless, significant contributions were made to the folate in the US diet by hamburgers, beef roasts and steaks, liver, pork, fish, and other animal products. Of the animal products, liver has the highest content of folate (Tables 15-2–15-7). Beef liver, pan-fried, provides 220 μg of folate per 100 g (Table 15-4). Comparable levels are provided by pork liver (Table 15-5). Significant amounts of folate are present in beef kidney. Lamb roast provides some folate, with a content of 22 μg per 100 g (Table 15-3). Cooked veal contains less with a content of 16 μg per 100 g. Cooked beef and pork products contain only small amounts of folate, usually in the range of 6–12 μg per 100 g (Tables 15-4 and 15-5). Except for beef liver and kidney, beef tongue and other beef offal items are very low in folate content (Table 15-5). Poultry meats are also poor sources of folate, with a content of only

4–9 μg per 100 g of meat (Table 15-7). Fish likewise do not appear to be significant contributors of folate to the diet (Table 15-7).

Although eggs contain an appreciable amount of folate, much of the vitamin appears to be of limited value in the diet because of its poor bioavailability. Cheeses contain some folate, but the low amount of cheese normally consumed in a meal would limit its contribution as a folate source (Table 15-6). An 8-oz glass of milk would provide only about 11 μg of folate.

(ii) Contribution and its importance to the diet

Until recently, data on the folate content of foods were insufficient to determine the folate intake of individuals. However, it is possible with the data available to estimate the *per capita* levels of folacin provided by the US food supply. These estimates indicate relatively low levels of folate are available in the US food supply. The major sources of folacin in the US food supply are vegetables; fruit; the meat, poultry, and fish groups; and grain products.

During the past 80 years, the level of folate provided by the US food supply was highest in 1945 (335 μg/*capita*/day) and lowest in 1964 (267 μg/*capita*/day) (Nutrition Monitoring in United States, 1986). The proportion of folate contributed to the US food supply by vegetables in 1982 was about the same as in 1909–13; namely, 27%. The proportion of folate from fruits nearly tripled during this period comprising 15% of total intake in 1982. The proportion of folate from grain products declined from 24 to 11%, and the proportion from potatoes declined from 11 to 5%. On the other hand, the proportion from the meat, fish, and poultry group increased from 10 to 14% (Nutrition Monitoring in United States, 1986). Mean folate intake in the US as estimated from dietary recall data during 1976–1980 was 241 μg per day for all adults, 263 μg per day for males and 197 μg per day for females (Subar *et al.*, 1989). Dietary contributions of folate by food groups in British households have been reported as: meats, 8%; dairy items, 9·5%; eggs, 2·6%; cereal products, 26%; vegetables, 35%; fruits, 6%; other items (e.g. juices and beverages), 13·5% (Poh Tan *et al.*, 1984).

The major contributors of folate in the US diet as observed from the 1976–1980 Second National Health and Nutrition Examination Survey (NHANES II) data are indicated in Table 15-14. In military nutrition surveys, personnel were observed to obtain 40–44% of the RDA requirements for folate from animal products, with dairy products providing about one-half of total intake (Sauberlich *et al.*, 1982). Free-living elderly obtained only 12·4% of the folate RDA from meats, with red meats providing a mere 8·8% of the folate requirement (Vaughan and Manore, 1988).

Contributions of folate by various meats are presented in Table 15-3. Red meats contribute more folate to the diet than poultry or fish. All meats combined provide daily about 26 μg of folate, representing only 12·8% of the RDA. The 1989 RDA for folate is 200 μg per day for an adult male. However, as noted, folate is provided also by other animal products (e.g. dairy items and eggs). Contributions of additional food items, including meats, are presented in Tables 15-3–15-7, and 15-10.

G. Factors that Influence Contribution

(i) Bioavailability

Over 150 different forms of folate probably exist in foods. Not all forms are absorbed equally by the human. Hence, the bioavailability and adsorption of folate in the diet are complicated (Leklem, 1986). The majority of the folates in food are present as reduced forms of polyglutamates. Before dietary folate can be absorbed from foods, the polyglutamate forms must be hydrolyzed to monoglutamate forms. This action is performed by conjugases (γ-glutamyl-carboxypeptidases) that are present in the lumen and also in the brush border of the intestine (Rose *et al.*, 1984; Sauberlich, 1985b, 1987). Much of the absorbed monoglutamate is converted to methyltetrahydrofolate and transferred into the portal circulation.

Only a few investigations have been conducted on the bioavailability of folates present in foods as consumed under normal dietary conditions (Rose *et al.*, 1984; Sauberlich, 1985b, 1987; Sauberlich *et al.*, 1987). Approximately 50% of the dietary folate appears bioavailable. Limited reports indicate that the availability of folate in individual foods as: cooked beef liver, 50%; bananas, 82%; spinach, 63%; and cabbage, 47% (Sauberlich, 1985b, 1987).

(ii) Cooking and food processing

Folates are relatively labile with as much as 50–90% of the folate present in foods being lost during food processing and home cooking. Losses of folate in commercially processed meat products are in the same range as those reported with conventional cooking. Losses of folate with conventional cooking range from 10–30%. Losses of folate in meat products with radiation sterilization or with curing and smoking are unknown although some losses would be expected.

Although one report indicated substantial losses of folate in meats as a result of cooking, more recent studies indicate less severe loss (Moss *et al.*, 1980). The effects of various types of cooking on the folate contents of various meats are indicated in Tables 15-2–15-5, 15-7, 15-11. As may be noted, the type of cooking had only a slight effect on the folate content of meats. Braised beef had a retention of 72%, in comparison to 87% for broiled beef, and 88% for roasted beef. Similar retentions were observed for pork (Table 15-11).

IV. SUMMARY

Meats and other animal products are basic to the achievement of a nutritionally adequate and balanced diet for the United States population. Meats perform a major role in providing vitamin B_{12} nutrition. Virtually all of the vitamin B_{12} in the food supply is provided by meats and other animal products. Meats contribute approximately 69% of total intake, with dairy items providing 21%, and eggs 9%. Cereals, fortified with vitamin B_{12}, provide a small amount of vitamin B_{12}.

For the American diet, meats are the most important source of vitamin B_6. Meats contribute over 46% of the vitamin B_6 present in the average diet. In addition, dairy products and eggs provide approximately 13% of the vitamin B_6 intake. Beef and pork are quite comparable in their vitamin B_6 contents. About 60–85% of vitamin B_6 is retained in beef or pork with conventional roasting.

Although folate is present extensively in vegetables and cereal products, meats, dairy items, and other animal products contribute approximately 20% of the folate in the diet. Red meats contribute more folate to the diet than poultry or fish. Of the red meats, lamb contains the highest level of folate, followed by veal. The folate content of pork and beef items is considerably less. Liver, however, is a rich source of folate.

Unique to meats is the high bioavailability of the vitamin B_{12}, vitamin B_6, and folate present. Vitamin B_{12} is considered readily available. Vitamin B_6 in meats has a high bioavailability when compared to plant sources in which the vitamin may be present in a less available bound form. Food composition tables need to be upgraded with additional data, particularly with respect to vitamin B_6 and folate contents and their relative degrees of bioavailability.

V. REFERENCES

ADAMS, C. E. and ERDMAN, J. W., JR (1988). Effects of home food preparation practices on nutrient content of foods. In *Nutritional Evaluation of Food Processing* 3rd edn. (E. Karmas and R. S. Harris, Eds), p. 557. Van Nostrand Reinhold, Co., New York.

ANDERSON, R. H., MAXWELL, D. L., MULLEY, A. E. and FRITSCH, C. W. (1976). Effects of processing and storage on micronutrients in breakfast cereals. *Food Technol.* **30**(5), 110.

ANDERSON, S. A. and TALBOT, J. M. (1981). *A Review of Folate Intake, Methodology, and Status.* Life Sciences Research Office, FASEB, Bethesda, MD.

ANGIER, R. B. *et al.* (1946). The structure and synthesis of the liver *L. casei* factor. *Science* **103**, 667.

ANON. (1957). *Vitamin B_{12} in Animal Nutrition.* Merck & Co., Inc., Rahway, NJ.

BREIDENSTEIN, B. C. (1984). Contribution of red meat to the US diet. *Food and Nutr. News* **56**, 15.

BREIDENSTEIN, B. C. (1987). Nutrient value of meat. *Food and Nutr. News* **59**, 43.

CASTLE, W. B. (1953). Development of knowledge concerning the gastric intrinsic factor and its relation to pernicious anemia. *N. Engl. J. Med.* **249**, 603.

CASTLE, W. B. (1961). A century of curiosity about pernicious anemia. *Trans. Am. Clin. Climatol. Assoc.* **73**, 54.

COLMAN, N. (1981). Laboratory assessment of folate status. *Clin. Lab. Med.* **1**, 775.

COWARD, K. H., KEY, K. M. and MORGAN, B. G. E. (1929). LXXIX. Some evidence of the existence of a further factor necessary for growth of the rat. *Biochem. J.* **23**, 695.

DOSCHERHOLMEN, A., MCMAHON, J. and RIPLEY, D. (1978). Vitamin B_{12} assimilation from chicken meat. *Am. J. Clin. Nutr.* **31**, 825.

EVERSON, G. J., CHANG, J., LEONARD, S., LUK, B. S. and SIMONE, M. (1964). Aseptic canning of foods. III. Pyridoxine retention as influenced by processing method, storage time and temperature, and type of container. *Food Technol.* **18**, 87.

FENNEMA, O. (1975). Effects of freeze-preservation on nutrients. In *Nutritional Evaluation of Food Processing*, 2nd edn (R. S. Harris and E. Karmas, Eds), p. 244. AVI Publishing Co., Westport, CT.

FENNEMA, O. (1988). Effects of freeze preservation on nutrients. In *Nutritional Evaluation of Food Processing*, 3rd edn (E. Karmas and R. S. Harris, Eds), p. 269. Van Nostrand Reinhold Co., New York.

FOOD AND NUTRITION BOARD (1989). *Recommended Dietary Allowances*, 10th edn. The National Research Council, National Academy of Sciences, Washington, DC.

GREGORY, J. F., III (1988). Methods for determination of vitamin B_6 in foods and other biological materials: A critical review. *J. Food Comp. & Anal.* **1**, 105.

GREGORY, J. F., III and KIRK, J. R. (1978). Assessment of storage effects on vitamin B_6 stability and bioavailability in dehydrated food systems. *J. Food Sci.* **43**, 1801.

GREGORY, J. F. and KIRK, J. R. (1979). Vitamin B_6 in foods: Assessment of stability and bioavailability. In *Human Vitamin B_6 Requirements* (H. E. Sauberlich and M. L. Bown, Eds), p. 72. National Academy of Sciences, Washington, DC.

GREGORY, J. F., III and KIRK, J. R. (1981). The bioavailability of vitamin B_6 in foods. *Nutr. Rev.* **39**, 1.

GYÖRGY, P. (1934). Vitamin B_2 and the pellagra-like dermatitis in rats. *Nature* **133**, 498.

GYÖRGY, P. (1935). Vitamin B_2 complex. I. Differentiation of lactoflavin and 'rat antipellagra' factor. *Biochem. J.* **29**, 741.

GYÖRGY, P. (1971). Developments leading to the metabolic role of vitamin B_6. *Am. J. Clin. Nutr.* **24**, 1250.

GYÖRGY, P. and ECKHARDT, R. E. (1939). Vitamin B_6 and skin lesions in rats. *Nature* **144**, 512.

HARDING, R. S., PLOUGH, I. C. and FRIEDEMANN, T. E. (1959). The effect of storage on the vitamin B_6 content of a packaged army ration, with a note on the human requirement for the vitamin. *J. Nutr.* **68**, 323.

HARRIS, S. A. and FOLKERS, K. (1939). Synthetic vitamin B_6. *Science* **89**, 347.

HERBERT, V. (1987). The 1986 Herman award lecture. Nutrition science as a continually unfolding story: The folate and vitamin B_{12} paradigm. *Am. J. Clin. Nutr.* **46**, 387.

HERBERT, V. D. and COLMAN, N. (1988). Folic acid and vitamin B_{12}. In *Modern Nutrition in Health and Disease*, 7th edn (M. E. Shils and V. R. Young, Eds), p. 388. Lea & Febiger, Philadelphia.

HEYSSEL, R. M., BOZIAN, R. C., DARBY, W. J. and BELL, M. C. (1966). Vitamin B_{12} turnover in man. The assimilation of vitamin B_{12} from natural foodstuff by man and estimates of minimal daily dietary requirements. *Am. J. Clin. Nutr.* **18**, 176.

HILLMAN, R. S. (1985). Vitamin B_{12}, folic acid, and the treatment of megaloblastic anemias. In *Goodman and Gilman's The Pharmacological Basis of Therapeutics*, 7th edn (A. G. Gilman, L. J. Goodman and T. W. Rall, Eds), p. 1323. MacMillan, New York.

KARMAS, E. (1975). The major food groups and their nutrient content. In *Nutritional Evaluation of Food Processing*, 3rd edn (R. S. Harris and E. Karmas, Eds), p. 11. AVI Publ. Co., Westport, CT.

KARMAS, E. (1988). The major food groups, their nutrient content, and principles of food processing. In *Nutritional Evaluation of Food Processing* (E. Karmas and R. S. Harris, Eds), p. 7. Van Nostrand Reinhold Co., Inc, New York.

KARMAS, E. and HARRIS, R. S. (1988). In *Nutritional Evaluation of Food Processing*, 3rd edn. Van Nostrand Reinhold Co., New York.

KORSCHGEN, B. M. and BALDWIN, R. E. (1978). Moist-heat, microwave and conventional cooking on round roasts of beef. *J. Microwave Power* **13**, 257.

LACHANCE, P. A. and FISHER, M. C. (1988). Effects of food preparation procedures in nutrient retention with emphasis on foodservice practices. In *Nutritional Evaluation of Food Processing*, 3rd edn (E. Karmas and R. S. Harris, Eds), p. 505. Van Nostrand Reinhold Co., New York.

LEE, F. A., BROOKS, R. F., PEARSON, A. M., MILLER, J. I. and VOLZ, F. E. (1950). Effect of freezing rate on meat. Appearance, palatability, and vitamin content of beef. *Food Res.* **15**, 8.

LEE, F. A., BROOKS, R. P., PEARSON, A. M., MILLER, J. I. and WANDERSTOCK, J. J. (1954). Effect of rate of freezing on pork quality. Appearance, palatability, and vitamin content. *J. Am. Dietet. Assoc.* **30**, 351.

LEKLEM, J. E. (1986). Bioavailability of vitamins: Applications to human nutrition. In *Food and Agriculture Research Opportunities to Improve Human Nutrition* (A. R. Doberenz, J. A. Milner and B. S. Schweigert, Eds), p. A56. Published by College of Human Resources, University of Delaware, Newark, DE.

LETTERMAN ARMY INST. RES. (1979). LAIR Institute Report No. 65. Presidio of San Francisco, California.

LEVINE, A. S. and DOSCHERHOLMEN, A. (1983). Vitamin B_{12} bioavailability from egg yolk and egg white: Relationship to binding proteins. *Am. J. Clin. Nutr.* **38**, 436.

LINNELL, J. (1977). The fate of cobalamins *in vivo*. In *Cobalamin Biochemistry and Pathophysiology* (B. M. Babior, Ed.), p. 287. Wiley, New York.

LOFGREN, P. A. and SPECKMANN, E. (1979). Importance of animal products in the human diet. *J. Dairy Sci.* **62**, 1019.

LUND, D. (1988). Effects of heat processing on nutrients. In *Nutritional Evaluation of Food Processing*, 3rd edn (E. Karmas and R. S. Harris, Eds), p. 319. Van Nostrand Reinhold Co., New York.

LUSHBOUGH, C. H., WEICHMAN, J. M. and SCHWEIGERT, B. S. (1959). The retention of vitamin B_6 in meat during cooking. *J. Nutr.* **67**, 451.

MAPSON, L. W. (1932). CXVI. Evidence of the existence of a dietary principal stimulating general growth and lactation. *Biochem. J.* **26**, 970.

MARSTON, R. M. and PETERKIN, B. B. (1980). Nutrient content of the national food supply. *Natl Food Rev. US Dept Agric., NFR-9* Winter, p. 21.

MINOT, G. R. and MURPHY, W. P. (1926). Treatment of pernicious anemia by a special diet. *JAMA* **87**, 470.

MITCHELL, H. K., SNELL, E. E. and WILLIAMS, R. I. (1941). The concentration of 'folic acid'. *J. Amer. Chem. Soc.* **63**, 2284.

MOSS, M., ONO, K., CROSS, R., HOLDEN, J. and STEWART, K. (1980). Nutrient retention in cooked retail cuts of beef. Abst. 40th Annual Mtg Inst. Food Technol. New Orleans (Abstract 292) p. 158.

NATIONAL LIVE STOCK AND MEAT BOARD (1976). *The Nutritive Value of Meat and Other Protective Food.* National Live Stock and Meat Board, Chicago, IL.

NATIONAL LIVE STOCK AND MEAT BOARD (1983). *The Nutritive Value of Meat and Other Protective Food.* National Live Stock and Meat Board, Chicago, IL.

NGUYEN, L. B. and GREGORY, J. F., III (1983). Effects of food composition on the bioavailability of vitamin B_6 in the rat. *J. Nutr.* **133**, 1550.

NUTRITION MONITORING IN THE UNITED STATES (1986). A progress report from the Joint Nutrition Monitoring Evaluation Committee. DHHS Publication No. (PHS) 86-1255, Hyattsville, MD.

OCKERMAN, H. W. (1988). Effects of agricultural practices, handling, processing, and storage on meat. In *Nutritional Evaluation of Food Processing*, 3rd edn (E. Karmas and R. S. Harris, Eds), p. 153. Van Nostrand Reinhold, Co., Inc., New York.

ONO, K., BERRY, B., JOHNSON, H. K., RUSSEK, E., PARKER, C. F., CAHILL, V. and ALTHOUSE, P. (1984). Nutrient composition of lamb of two age groups. *J. Food Sci.* **49**, 1233.

ONO, K., BERRY, B. and DOUGLASS, L. (1986). Nutrient content of some fresh and retail cuts of veal. *J. Food Sci.* **51**, 1352.

ORR, M. L. (1969). *Pantothenic Acid, Vitamin B_6 and Vitamin B_{12} in Foods.* Home Econ. Res. Rpt No. 36, US Dept of Agriculture.

PATTERSON, B. H. and BLOCK, G. (1988). Food choices and the cancer guidelines. *AJPH* **78**, 282.

PEARSON, A. M. and BROOKS, R. I. (1978). The contribution of meat to the diet of man. *Proc. Recip. Meat Conf.* **31**, 1.

PEARSON, A. M., WEST, R. G. and LUECKE, R. W. (1959). The vitamin and amino acid content of drip obtained upon defrosting frozen pork. *Food Res.* **24**, 515.

POH TAN, S., WENLOCK, R. W. and BUSS, D. H. (1984). Folic acid content of the diet in various types of British households. *Human Nutr.: Appl. Nutr.* **38A**, 17.

REITER, L. A. and DRISKELL, J. A. (1985). Vitamin B_6 content of selected foods served in dining halls. *J. Am. Diet. Assoc.* **85**, 1625.

RICKES, E. L., BRINK, N. G., KONIUSZY, F. R., WOOD, T. R. and FOLKERS, K. (1948). Crystalline vitamin B_{12}. *Science* **107**, 396.

ROE, D. A. (1985). Drug effects on nutrient absorption, transport, and metabolism. *Drug–Nutrient Interact.* **4**, 117.

ROSE, R. C., HOYUMPA, A. M., JR, ALLEN, R. H., MIDDLETON, H. M., III, HENDERSON, L. M. and ROSENBERG, I. H. (1984). Transport and metabolism of water-soluble vitamins in intestine and kidney. *Fed. Proc.* **43**, 2423.

SAUBERLICH, H. E. (1980). Interactions of thiamin, riboflavin, and other B-vitamins. *Ann. NY Acad. Sci.* **355**, 80.

SAUBERLICH, H. E. (1981). Vitamin B_6 status assessment: Past and present. In *Methods in Vitamin B_6 Nutrition* (J. E. Leklem and R. D. Reynolds, Eds), p. 203. Plenum Pub. Corp., New York.

SAUBERLICH, H. E. (1985a). Interaction of vitamin B_6 with other nutrients. In *Vitamin B_6: Its Role in Health and Disease* (R. D. Reynolds and J. E. Leklem, Eds), p. 193. A. R. Liss, Inc., New York.

SAUBERLICH, H. E. (1985b). Bioavailability of vitamins. *Prog. Food Nutr. Sci.* **4**, 1.

SAUBERLICH, H. E. (1986). Methods for the assessment of nutritional status. In *Nutritional Aspects of Aging* (L. Chen, Ed.), p. 131. CRC Press, Boca Raton, FL.

SAUBERLICH, H. E. (1987). Vitamins—How much is for keeps? *Nutrition Today* **20.**

SAUBERLICH, H. E. (1990). Evaluation of folate nutrition in population groups. In *Evaluation of Folic Acid Metabolism in Health and Disease* (M. F. Picciano, Ed), p. 211. Wiley-Liss, New York.

SAUBERLICH, H. E. and CANHAM, J. E. (1980). Vitamin B_6. In *Modern Nutrition in Health and Disease*, 6th edn (R. S. Goodhart and M. E. Shils, Eds), p. 209. Lea & Febiger, Philadelphia.

SAUBERLICH, H. E., KRETSCH, M. J., JOHNSON, H. L. and NELSON, R. A. (1982). Animal products as a source of vitamins. In *Animal Products in Human Nutrition* (D. C. Beitz and R. G. Hansen, Eds), p. 340. Academic Press, Inc., New York.

SAUBERLICH, H. E., KRETSCH, M. J., SKALA, J. H., JOHNSON, H. L. and TAYLOR, P. C. (1987). Folate requirement and metabolism in non-pregnant women. *Am. J. Clin. Nutr.* **46**, 1016.

SCHROEDER, H. A. (1971). Losses of vitamins and trace minerals resulting from processing and preservation of foods. *Am. J. Clin. Nutr.* **24**, 562.

SCHWEIGERT, B. S. (1949). The animal protein factor. *Nutr. Rev.* **7**, 225.

SHIVE, W., RAVEL, J. M. and HARDING, W. M. (1948). An interrelationship of purines and vitamin B_{12}. *J. Biol. Chem.* **176**, 991.

SHORB, M. S. (1947). Unidentified growth factor for *Lactobacillus lactis* in refined liver extracts. *J. Biol. Chem.* **169**, 455.

SMITH, E. L. and PARKER, L. F. J. (1948). Purification of antipernicious anaemia factor. *Biochem. J.* **43**, viii.

SOMMER, I. I. and HAGEN, R. E. (1981). Effects of processing, cooking and storage on nutrients in meats. In *Meat in Nutrition and Health* (K. R. Franklin and P. N. Davis, Eds), p. 19. Interstate Printers and Publishers, Danville, IL.

SPIES, T. D., BEAN, W. B. and ASHE, W. F. (1939). A note on the use of vitamin B_6 in human nutrition. *J.A.M.A.* **112**, 2414.

STOKSTAD, E. L. R., JUKES, T. H., PIERCE, J., PAGE, A. C., JR and FRANKLIN, A. L. (1949). The multiple nature of the animal protein factor. *J. Biol. Chem.* **180**, 647.

SUBAR, A. F., BLOCK, G. and JAMES, L. D. (1989). Folic acid intake and food sources in the US population. *Am. J. Clin. Nutr.* **50**, 508.

THOMAS, M. H. (1988). Use of ionizing radiation to preserve food. In *Nutritional Evaluation of Food Processing* 3rd edn (E. Karmas and R. S. Harris, Eds), p. 457. Van Nostrand Reinhold, Co., Inc., New York.

THOMAS, M. H. and JOSEPHSON, E. S. (1970). Radiation preservation of foods and its effects on nutrients. *Sci. Teacher* **37**, 59.

TOOHEY, J. I. and BARKER, H. A. (1961). Isolation of coenzyme B_{12} from liver. *J. Biol. Chem.* **236**, 560.

US DEPARTMENT OF AGRICULTURE (USDA) (1976–1987). Composition of foods: Raw, processed, prepared. In *Agriculture Handbook 8*, Vols 8-1–8-15, USDA, Washington, DC.

VAN DER HOORN, R., BRANION, H. D. and GRAHAM, W. R., JR (1935). Studies in the nutrition of the chick. II. Effect of purification of casein in simplified diet. *Poul. Sci.* **14**, 285.

VAUGHAN, L. A. and MANORE, M. M. (1988). Nutrient contributions of red meats and other flesh foods to dietary intakes of free-living elderly. *FASEB J.* **2**, A1431.

WILLS, L. (1933). The nature of the hemopoietic factor in marmite. *Lancet* **224**, 1283.

YANKELOVICK, D., SKELLY, F. and WHITE, A. H. (1985). *Consumer Climate for Meat Products.* Prepared for American Meat Institute, Washington, DC, and the National Live Stock and Meat Board, Chicago, IL.

16

The Role of Meat in Balancing Human Diets

R. GAURTH HANSEN

Department of Nutrition and Food Sciences, Utah State University, Logan, Utah, USA

AND

BONITA W. WYSE

Office of the Dean, College of Family Life, Utah State University, Logan, Utah, USA

I. INTRODUCTION

Recent USDA data indicate that the total food consumption of Americans appears to be at a relatively low level. The average caloric intake of women is about 1600 kcal a day, which is within the range of recommended intake but considerably lower than the average recommended allowance of about 2000 kcal. There are indications, however, that consumption of alcoholic beverages has been underreported and that alcohol may be providing additional calories. As much as 80% of alcoholic beverages which are reported for tax purposes and sold in the US are not accounted for by food consumption survey reports. This amounts to approximately 200 additional kcal per person per day when averaged over the US adult population.

In diets with 1600 kcal (or 1800 kcal diet with 200 kcal from alcohol), it is difficult to obtain recommended levels of all nutrients, particularly those, such as iron and zinc, which are present in relatively low concentration in foods. On the average, women need fewer calories than men, but have similar requirements for most vitamins and minerals, with the exception of iron where women of child-bearing age have significantly increased needs.

To obtain recommended allowances from a 1600–1800 kcal diet requires careful selection from food items which are nutrient dense. Lean meat is a naturally advantageous option for those people. In fact, increased consumption of lean meat is suggested in the USDA booklet *Food* as one way to improve the zinc and iron content of a diet that is low in calories. A 3 oz serving of cooked lean meat will provide a considerable quantity of B vitamins, minerals, trace minerals, especially iron and zinc, but contain only about 200 kcal.

II. CURRENT DIETARY GUIDELINES

A. 'Four-Plus-One' Concept Calls for Lean Meat

In the late 1970s, USDA updated the food group concept which has been the cornerstone of nutrition education programs for the public since the early part of this century. The revised plan was called the Four-Plus-One food plan: Four servings daily from the *Vegetable and Fruit Group* (include one good vitamin C source each day and also frequently include deep-yellow or dark-green vegetables (for vitamin A) and unpeeled fruits and vegetables and those with edible seeds (for fiber); four basic servings daily from the *Bread and Cereal Group* (select any whole-grain and enriched or fortified products); two servings daily for adults from the *Milk and Cheese Group* (2–3 servings for children under 9 years of age, 3 servings for children 9–12, 4 servings for teenagers and 3 servings for pregnant women); two basic servings from the *Meat*, *Poultry*, *Fish and Bean Group* (2–3 ounces of lean cooked meat, poultry or fish without bone is counted as a serving); and the amount of food from the *Fats, Sweets and Alcohol Group* depends on the number of calories required (it is a good idea to concentrate first on the calorie-plus nutrients foods provided in the other groups as a basis of the daily diet).

The concept is valid and helpful to consumers in making food choices that will more easily balance nutrient intake with caloric needs. The earlier Four Food Group concept also emphasized meat and related products as necessary components of a nutritious diet. Furthermore, the basic Four-Plus-One concept actively encourages the consumption of leaner meat.

B. Dietary Guidelines for Americans

The Dietary Guidelines for Americans evolved as a joint recommendation from two federal government departments (Health and Agriculture). In brief, the Guidelines are:

1. Eat a variety of foods.
2. Maintain ideal weight.
3. Avoid too much fat, saturated fat, and cholesterol.
4. Eat foods with adequate starch and fiber.
5. Avoid too much sugar.
6. Avoid too much sodium.
7. If you drink alcohol, do so in moderation.

As with other dietary guidance materials, the Guidelines are designed to help consumers make *informed* choices about food. The object is to obtain the correct balance of vitamins, minerals, and dietary fiber without overconsuming salt or calories, especially calories from fat and sugar. Whenever meat is mentioned in the Guidelines, the suggestion is that fat be trimmed, a common practice for many Americans already.

Another Guideline recommendation is: 'Choose lean meat, fish, poultry, beans, peas, as protein sources'. It is also suggested that the consumer moderate the use of eggs and organ meats. The related Guideline reference to fat, saturated fat, and cholesterol could serve its purpose as well if it referred simply to *fat*. The concern about saturated vs polyunsaturated fats and the direct linkage of dietary cholesterol to heart disease is at best an uncertain issue in scientific circles. This topic is discussed objectively in Chapter 3.

The livestock industry is using genetic and management practices to produce meat with lowered fat content. These practices have already been generally accepted by the livestock and meat industry and recognized the public interest in, and concern for, access to meat of relatively low fat content.

III. WHY FOLLOW DIETARY GUIDELINES?

The best argument for following the Dietary Guidelines lies in its sequel published by USDA *Ideas for Better Eating: Menus and Recipes to Make Use of the Dietary Guidelines* (USDA, 1981). A careful analysis of the sequel's menu ideas shows that (except for one lunch at a low calorie level) meat, poultry, or fish is included in each day's diet. *The menus approximate the amounts of beef and poultry that are now consumed by Americans on a* per capita *basis*. They include about the same total of pork but slightly more fresh and somewhat less processed pork than is consumed presently. Meat merits such inclusion in the menus for a very basic reason—meat is a very good source of trace minerals and many vitamins and it is difficult to obtain

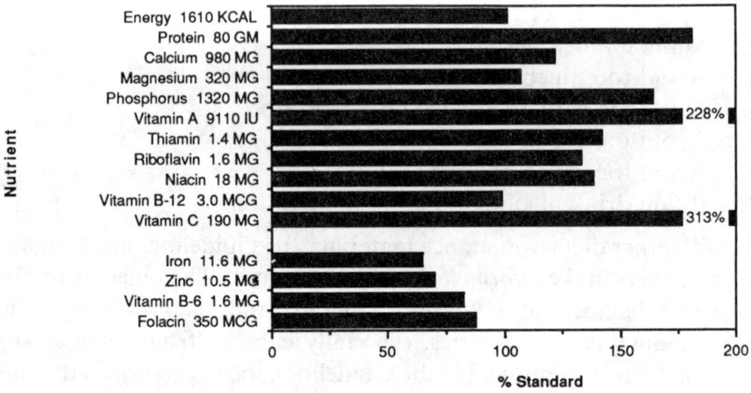

FIG. 16-1. Nutrient profile for average female intakes of 1600 kcal menus in *Ideas for Better Eating*. Standards used are for females, ages 23–50 years (USDA, 1981).

these nutrients in adequate amounts unless meat is included in the diet (Human Nutrition Information Service, 1987).

Two versions of each day's suggestions for menus are presented in *Ideas for Better Eating*. One provides 1600 kcal and the other 2400 kcal. These reflect the average amounts of energy from foods that women and men have reported consuming in recent food consumption surveys. Figure 16-1 (USDA, 1981) illustrates the average amounts of nutrients provided by the 1600 kcal menus and the percent of the Recommended Dietary Allowances for females, ages 23–50 years. The energy standard used was the lower value (1600 kcal) in the range of recommended caloric intakes for this group.

Analysis of nutrient levels provided by the menus indicates that iron, zinc, vitamin B_6, and folacin (another B vitamin) are the nutrients most difficult to obtain from a 1600 kcal diet. As calorie intake is progressively lowered from the 2400 kcal diet to 1600 kcal, these are the nutrients which become limiting.

Lean meat's contribution to these four limiting nutrients can be seen in Fig. 16-2 (USDA, 1981). Relative to the amount of calories provided, each 100 g serving supplies 1·76 and 1·55 times the recommended allowances for iron and vitamin B_6, respectively; three times the zinc allowance; and about 35% of the allowance for folacin. The calories from fat yielded by all of the menus together—including the lean meat—are less than 35% of total calories. Thus, the inclusion or substitution of lean meat in the diet would increase the levels of three of the four limiting nutrients without significantly altering the fat content.

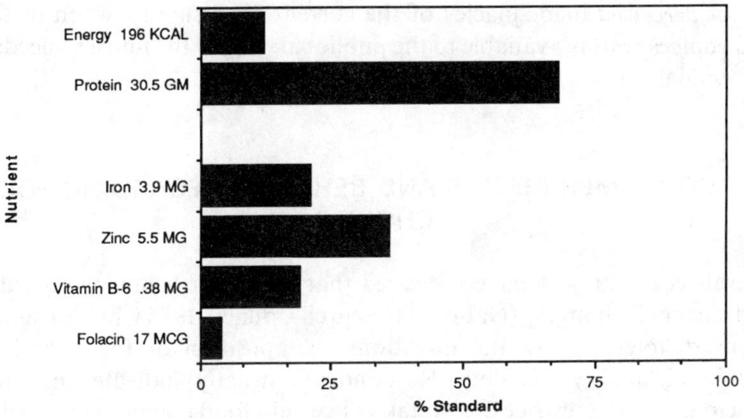

FIG. 16-2. Nutrient profile for lean beef showing contribution of iron, zinc, vitamin B_6 and folacin, 100 grams, which supplies 196 kcal of energy (USDA, 1981).

There should be no controversy over the appropriateness of meat consumption from either a scientific or public policy viewpoint. *To achieve a balanced nutrient intake from food choices that satisfy the universal standard* (*the* Recommended Dietary Allowances, *published by the National Academy of Sciences) significant amounts of meat MUST be included.* Thus, one of the Dietary Guidelines—the guideline to 'avoid too much fat'—seems to have received unwarranted attention, while the sequel menu publication, which details examples of complementary menus has been overlooked.

The USDA menu ideas illustrate some of the eating styles seen in our population, with many suggestions for adapting the menus to fit individual preferences. A variety of popular foods has been included. Some examples: hamburgers and French fries; bagel and cream cheese; pancakes and syrup; tacos; baked potato and sour cream; ham and cheese sandwich; scrambled eggs. These and many more popular foods can fit in eating patterns which meet the Guidelines.

As discussed earlier, to meet the Dietary Guidelines (which also suggest a reduced fat intake), with foods currently available in the US—taking into consideration current consumption practices—requires about as much fresh meat as Americans are now consuming in proportion to other foods. Food availability, current consumption practices, and *the ability to translate recommendations into foods which are appealing and palatable* should be important considerations when developing dietary guidance statements. Many people in the US are willing to buy food *supplements* to current perceived inadequacies of the current food supply, when in fact, food choices readily available to the public can supply the nutrient needs of the population.

IV. CONSUMER BELIEFS AND BEHAVIOR REGARDING FOOD CHOICES

Several recent surveys have indicated that consumer behavior regarding food choices is changing (National Research Council, 1985a, b). Consumers are more interested in the nutritional composition of foods and the nutritional quality of diets. Respondents usually indicate that they consciously try to restrict their intake of certain food components, such as salt, sugar, fat, and cholesterol. About two-thirds indicated that they are including other types of nutritious foods in their diet, including those high in fiber, calcium, and starch. More than one-third either were currently on a special diet or had been on one during the previous year. In many cases, they changed diets in an attempt to reduce body weight.

A. Consumer Behavior Away from Home

Consumers are changing their eating habits, '...by increasing their consumption of fruits, vegetables, or whole grains or by decreasing their consumption of refined sugar, animal fats or salt'. Consumer attitudes about nutrition persist and are not merely a passing trend (National Restaurant Association, 1986).

When respondents were asked which foods they were likely to try at a restaurant; 64% selected lean meats, 63% selected broiled/baked fish or seafood, 47% selected poultry without skin, and 36% selected food cooked without salt. There was a large increase in the demand for non-fried fish, main dish salads, rice, fruit, chicken, and Asian foods. There were also more requests for lean meat, foods prepared without sauces and butter, and foods cooked without salt.

B. Response by Restauranteurs

About 38% of the restaurant managers surveyed stated that they either feature a health or nutrition promotion or plan to do so in the future. About one-third would honor requests for reduced-calorie salad dressings, low-fat or skim milk, or salt substitutes. Nearly three-fourths reported that they would alter preparation methods upon request. Nine out of ten would serve sauce or salad dressing on the side, cook without salt, or substitute unsaturated for saturated fats to accommodate consumers. Among those who would honor requests to alter cooking methods, eight out of ten would bake or broil a food rather than fry it, and six out of ten would remove the skin from poultry before cooking (National Restaurant Association, 1986).

C. Consumer Behavior in Grocery Stores/Supermarkets

Purchases of food items are largely governed by taste, price, convenience, and healthfulness, with the relative importance of these factors changing with circumstances. About three-fourths of the public now consider nutrition in their food purchasing decisions. However, consumers will not buy a product more than once if the taste is not acceptable, even if they can save money and they know it is more healthful. New products stress convenient preparation, and some observers suggest that nutrition has replaced price as the key consideration in many food purchase decisions (Supermarket Business, 1986a, b).

Consumers are practicing what they consider to be healthier eating habits. For example, the largest increases in dollar sales in 1985 were reported for fresh and frozen poultry, fresh fruits and vegetables, fresh fish and seafood, and yogurt and fresh milk. Purchases of fresh and frozen beef, sugar, natural cheese, fresh and cured ham and pork, and bacon showed the largest decrease.

However, purchases of such items as alcoholic coolers, frozen French toast and pancakes, and potato chips also increased substantially. High-calorie, high-fat, premium foods are selling as well as some of the newer low-calorie, low-fat products. Sales of superpremium (higher in butterfat) ice cream increased by 20% in 1985, and a similar increase is expected this year. Yogurt sales increased by 18·6% in 1985. Trends in food choices are somewhat contradictory. Snack foods sales increased by more than 8% in 1985. Within this category, fruit rolls and bars showed the largest percentage change since 1984, up nearly 23%. Potato chip sales increased by more than 9% since 1984, and dollarwise comprise more than twice that of any other snack item (over $1·8 billion). Sales of popcorn, which is perceived as a healthy snack because of its low calories/high fiber content, increased by more than 18·5% from 1984 to 1985 (packages, unpopped).

Another irony is the fact that candy and gum sales increased by 3·7% in 1985, with sales totalling nearly $9 billion. Of this figure about $61 million was diet, low-calorie or sugarless candy and gum. Chocolate bar sales increased by 2·8% in 1985. Chocolate-covered nuts sales have increased by more than 14% since 1984. *Per capita* candy consumption has increased by

1 lb per year since 1982, and reached 20 lb per year in 1985. These seemingly conflicting trends may actually be signs of a new philosophy of nutrition, e.g. a balanced diet can be achieved from a variety of foods consumed over several days or even a week, compared to the more traditional standard of three 'balanced' meals a day (NRC, 1985a, b).

One study found that consumers listed price, fatness, and cholesterol as the three most important factors in their purchases of beef. Consumers perceived that retail cuts of beef that were closely or completely trimmed were more appetizing, better tasting, and more nutritious (lower in cholesterol). Some consumers showed a clear purchase preference for the Select grade, even when priced higher than the Choice grade. This study recommended that both grades of beef should be merchandised according to its attributes: Choice grade for its taste appeal and Select grade for its leanness.

In a national survey, consumers were asked to identify which grade of beef contained the least fat; 56% said Prime, 16% said Choice, 3% said Good, 11% said Standard, and 14% indicated that they did not know. In spite of these findings, 58% of those surveyed stated that US grades were helpful in making purchasing decisions. About one-third indicated that they had eaten less beef in 1986 than in 1985, and, of this group, 71% stated that they had cut down on their intake of beef for health reasons. Seventy-eight per cent indicated that they would pay more for lower-fat beef if it were available.

A survey conducted for Giant Foods, Inc., compared consumer awareness, usage, and purchase patterns of a no-roll beef equivalent to the Select grade (Giant Lean) to beef of the Choice grade. Consumers purchasing Giant Lean ranked taste, healthfulness, value, nutrition, and leanness among the most important reasons for choosing this type of beef. Those who purchased Giant Lean also bought more beef, pork, lamb, veal, and fish than those who did not buy Giant Lean. When asked to identify the grade of Giant Lean, consumers answered Prime (34%), Choice (38%), Good (14%), and Standard (4%); 9% said they did not know. These results confirm the fact that consumers are confused about the meaning of grades of meat (American Meat Institute, 1987).

D. Response by Supermarkets

Most supermarkets, grocery stores, and commodity organizations have developed consumer information programs to help shoppers identify the nutritional attributes of different food products. Food retailers have also provided more service delicatessens, in-store bakeries, fresh fish and seafood departments, and salad bars, as well as expanded the size and variety of produce departments.

In 1985, the service delicatessen achieved the largest increase in dollar sales (Supermarket Business, 1986a, b). More than 40% of US households already have microwave ovens, and 70% are expected to have them by the end of the decade. Ethnic foods, particularly Mexican, Italian, and Oriental foods, are becoming increasingly popular, as indicated by rising sales of burritos, chips, tortillas, salsas, and dips, as well as sauces and ethnic entrées. Among the best-selling food items in 1985 were Italian dishes and Oriental foods.

Frozen prepared (precooked) foods meet the consumer's preference for convenience, taste, and healthfulness, but often at premium prices. This is the best selling category of frozen food, and sales increased by 8·3% in 1985. Sales of frozen dinners increased in this category by 10·3% above 1984. Frozen pizza sales increased by 4%.

Data from the 1985 Continuing Survey of Food Intake by Individuals (CSFII) suggest that individuals eat more often throughout the day than indicated by the 1977 National Food Consumption Survey (NFCS) (NRC, 1985b). Food sales and surveys also reflect the trend toward 'grazing', snacking throughout the day, rather than eating the traditional three large meals.

V. IMPACT AND APPLICATIONS OF DIETARY GUIDELINES FOR INDUSTRY

A. Dairy Products

The new products introduced by the dairy industry indicate that it has been particularly responsive to consumer health needs and preferences. Changes in the way fluid milk is sold, are an example of a successful industry response to changing consumer preferences. In 1980, low-fat and skim milk comprised 37·3% of the *per capita* consumption of unflavored fluid milk while consumption increased to 46% in 1985. Milk with 2% fat may be more acceptable to a larger segment of the population than skim milk. Yogurt also demonstrates the variety of products developed to meet consumer demands.

Modified versions of mozzarella and ricotta cheeses (made from part skim milk) and other new cheeses are also available, as are a number of other reduced-fat/calorie dairy products. Ice cream containing 10–16% fat and ice milk with 4% fat are now available.

Some non-traditional new products have been developed to meet both the nutritional and health requirements of different groups. For example, during 1986, at least 10 newly processed milks appeared on the market, including milk fortified with calcium promoted to meet the needs of the postmenopausal woman, to low-lactose/low-fat milk (LactAid brand lactose-reduced low-fat milk, which contains 70% less lactose and 1% fat) aimed for adults and the elderly.

In 1985, a variety of non-dairy, calcium-fortified products was introduced. During the past 12 months, at least four new kinds of sour cream, all with reduced-calorie and/or reduced-fat contents, and at least eight new types of ice cream or frozen dairy-based desserts, which were also lower in fat and cholesterol than their traditional counterparts, have been introduced.

B. Beef

Beef is a nutrient-dense food, that provides a high quantity and quality of nutrients (particularly protein, the B vitamins, iron and zinc) relative to its caloric content. The nutrient composition of fresh, cooked beef differs by cut and grade. It also varies somewhat by method of preparation; most fresh beef is broiled or roasted (dry heat), or braised (moist heat). The greatest variation in nutrient value occurs because differing amounts of external and seam fat are removed during retail preparation.

The majority of US supermarkets carry the Choice grade of beef, a large number sell ungraded ('No-roll') beef, and a few also carry Prime grade beef (almost always as an alternative gourmet item). A few supermarkets sell Prime, Choice, and ungraded beef (largely Select grade but actually a composite of several grades).

There are nutritional differences between cuts of beef and grades of beef that must be considered when attempting to meet the dietary and palatability needs of consumers.

(i) Chuck blade

Even with a relatively fat cut of beef, such as chuck blade, the change in grade from Choice to Select results in a substantial reduction in total fat, saturated fat, and therefore, the percentage of calories from fat. For example, the total fat and saturated fat content of two cuts of chuck blade, both braised, one Choice grade and the other Select grade, differ by 13%; their caloric content differs by about 7%. The differences between Prime and Select grades of beef are, of course, even greater. Prime is not universally available at the retail level, but is often available in restaurants.

If Select grade chuck blade cuts were also available in restaurants, many consumers would choose the leaner cut of chuck blade that is 19·5% lower in calories and has a third less total fat and saturated fatty acids. There are similar differences between cuts of other grades.

(ii) Ground beef

Many stores carry three types of ground beef that are either packaged in the store, or purchased from packers. These types of ground beef differ in the percentage of total fat after cooking: regular (about 20% total fat), lean (about 18% total fat), and extra-lean (about 16% total fat). Ground beef is a meat product with a high fat content; even extra-lean ground beef contains more than 53% of its calories from fat and 21% of calories from saturated fatty acids. Nevertheless, substituting extra-lean ground beef for regular ground beef would decrease caloric content from fat by 9%.

The method of cooking affects percentage yield and composition of ground beef patties over a wide range of fat levels. The percentage of fat in leaner formulations increases with cooking, while the percentage of fat in ground beef patties containing more fat decreases after cooking. Of the six different cooking methods analyzed (electric broiling, charbroiling, roasting, convection heating, frying, and microwaving), microwaving produced beef patties containing the least fat and calories (Berry and Leddy, 1984).

(iii) Minimum–maximum intramuscular fat content

A minimum fat content in beef muscle of about 3% (uncooked basis) is necessary for acceptable palatability (equivalent to meat cuts that grade low Good/Select). At 7·3% intramuscular fat, the product is equivalent to meat cuts that grade high Choice.

(iv) Nutrient content of leaner beef

A change to leaner beef would have several beneficial effects on the total diet, including a higher concentration of the B vitamins, iron, phosphorus, and zinc relative to calories.

C. Pork

There has been a significant reduction in backfat and an increase in muscling (lean tissue) in US pork since 1960, but there has been little or no change in the fat content of lean tissue recognized by the grading system.

A better understanding of the genetic and nutritional effects on the composition of lean tissue can result in pork products that contain acceptable levels of fat for diet conscious consumers.

(i) Grading system for pork

There are two USDA quality designations for swine carcasses, acceptable, designated 'US', and unacceptable, designated 'US Utility'. Currently, four cutability grades are based on backfat, carcass length or carcass weight, and muscling. US No. 1 denotes the highest cutability (least fat) and US No. 4 denotes the lowest cutability (most fat). The grading system has been revised in 1955, 1968 and 1985 to reflect improvements in the leanness of swine carcasses. There is now a need to further differentiate among cutability grades to accommodate the reduction in backfat and the increase in muscling of pork. These changes would encourage packers to pay according to lean yield.

(ii) Pork quality standards

The two USDA quality grades for pork do not discriminate for differences in flavor, juiciness and tenderness of cooked pork as well as the USDA beef quality grades. Proposed pork quality grading standards for wholesale cuts would categorize the product according to differences in color, structure, firmness and degree of marbling in the lean tissue. Branded hams containing 5% or less fat must meet strict color and intramuscular fat standards. Other examples of 'quality' standardization would include packaging, shelf-life, trim, and standards for consumer oven-ready or microwave-ready fresh pork products that some companies are now marketing nationally. There is no universal identification system to help an untrained consumer select a product that is low or moderately low in fat. Identifying pork products in this manner would provide incentives to significantly reduce fat content. Pork loins are palatable, if they contain 3·5–4·5% intramuscular fat (fresh basis). Chops containing an estimated 6·7–8·5% fat are acceptable, and contain only about one-half the fat content of the lean tissue of loin cuts listed in *USDA Handbook 8-10* (Anderson, 1983). Recent research suggests that some pork carcasses may now contain only 4·3% fat (Prusa, 1987).

A more discriminating quality grading system for pork cuts would help consumers identify lean tissue with low, but acceptable, levels of intramuscular fat. Breeding and feeding programs are available to assure that intramuscular fat in pork cuts meets consumer preferences.

D. Lamb and Veal

Per capita availability of lamb and veal is about 1·5 lb (0·7 kg). Differences in the composition of lamb and veal primarily reflect age ('A' versus 'B' maturity for lambs; Bob Veal versus Special Fed Veal for bovine animals slaughtered at ages of less than 3 months).

(i) Lamb

Overall, cuts from the older lambs contain fewer calories, less total fat, and less cholesterol. For example, loin chops from 'B' maturity lambs contain 15% less fat and 5% fewer calories and 5% less cholesterol than those of 'A' maturity. Blade chops from 'B' maturity lambs contain 33% less fat, 16% fewer calories, and 12% less cholesterol than 'A' maturity lambs.

(ii) Veal

Bob Veal, which is derived from calves slaughtered at less than 4 weeks of age, tend to contain less total fat and fewer calories but more cholesterol than Special Fed Veal from calves slaughtered at about 16 weeks of age. For example, a rib roast from Bob Veal contains 64% less fat, 38% fewer calories, but 10% more cholesterol than Special Fed Veal. A Bob Veal loin chop has 67% less fat, 24% fewer calories, but 23% more cholesterol than a Special Fed Veal loin chop (Ono *et al.*, 1986).

E. Poultry

Poultry meat contributes substantial nutrients to our diets, particularly protein, niacin, vitamin B_6, and zinc. Like beef, the nutritional content can differ with the cut or part, and method of preparation. Chicken is often batter-fried, which can increase the caloric content by nearly a third and double the amount of fat compared to poultry prepared by roasting or stewing.

The leg portion and other dark meats of chicken contain more fat and calories than the breast or other white meats. The method of cooking, particularly deep-fat frying, adds more fat and calories. A roasted chicken breast contains 15·1% fewer calories, about 42% less total fat and saturated fatty acids, 32% fewer calories from fat, and 8·7% less cholesterol than a roasted chicken leg. Chicken legs and breasts contain similar levels of vitamins and minerals.

Removing the skin from roasted turkey dramatically reduces calories and fat. Roasted light meat, without skin, has 20·3% fewer total calories, 61·3% less total fat, 56% less saturated fatty acids, and 9·2% less cholesterol than light meat containing the skin. Removing the skin obviously increases the concentration of several micronutrients, including niacin, pantothenic acid, vitamins B_1, B_6, B_{12}, magnesium, phosphorus, and potassium. The concentration of all other nutrients remains about the same. Roasted dark meat without skin has about 50% more fat and about 16% more calories than roasted white meat without skin.

The effect of skin of poultry on nutritional composition is most apparent in duck meat. Roasted duck, without skin, has 40·4% fewer calories, 60·5% less total fat, 56·9% less saturated fatty acids than roasted duck with skin. The concentration of minerals, including zinc, potassium, magnesium, and phosphorus, increases from 25 to 40% when the skin is removed. The vitamin concentration increases even more from 33% to nearly 75% (for vitamin B_{12}). There are also nutritional advantages to consuming dark meat without skin since it will have 15·4% fewer calories, 37·4% less total fat, and 30·7% less saturated fatty acids than dark meat with skin.

F. Fish, Shellfish and Seafood

As a group, fish, shellfish, and seafood contribute substantial amounts of protein, niacin, vitamin B_{12}, and zinc to diet. They are an important source of the ω-3 and ω-6 polyunsaturated fatty acids. Like chicken, the nutritional composition of fish is affected by the method of preparation, including the liquid in which it is canned.

(i) Steamed or canned versus fried

Frying nearly always increases the caloric, fat and sodium contents of seafood. For example, the percentage of calories from fat can double or quadruple as a result of frying. Frying can increase the total fat content 2–13 times, depending on the type of seafood.

(ii) Canned with oil versus water or brine

Although the oil in canned seafood is usually drained prior to consumption, some is normally eaten and can influence the nutritional value. In addition, canning in oil increases the caloric content by 37–38%.

G. Convenience Meats

Many products developed by the food industry contain less fat and fewer calories than traditional products. The modified version of bologna is 39% lower in fat and 21% lower in calories than the traditional version. The modified version of corned beef (Oscar Mayer Select Slices) contains 67% less fat and 36% fewer calories, but 24% more sodium. The modified versions of pastrami are 76–92% lower in total fat, 60–72% lower in calories, but contain comparable amounts of sodium to traditional products. Modified cooked ham, available from several manufacturers, contains 36–50% fewer calories and 61–74% less fat than the traditional version (NRC, 1988).

Several different modified versions of frankfurters are available, including chicken franks, turkey franks, and modified beef franks. Chicken franks contain 18% fewer calories, 32% less total fat, 54% less saturated fatty acids, but 34% more sodium than traditional beef franks. Turkey franks and modified beef franks have 23% fewer calories and 39% less fat than traditional beef franks. Procedures for reducing the fat content of processed meats are described in Chapter 17.

H. Mixtures of Meats

Mixed meat products showed one of the largest increases from the 1977 to the 1985 surveys (NRC, 1985a, b); this includes mixtures of meat, fish, or poultry with sauces, grains, or other components. Animal products are being used more frequently as an ingredient in meals rather than as separate entrées. In 1985, frozen foods accounted for almost $14 billion in supermarket sales, and exhibited some of the largest increases in sales in 1985, showing a 10·3% increase. Sales of diet dinners grew by 3% in 1985, and reached a high of $232 million. These products attempt to meet a variety of the consumer needs, including controlled portion sizes, limited caloric intake and convenience. The consumer is often willing to pay the higher prices charged for this type of product, and accept a reduction in nutritional quality.

VI. RATIONALE FOR CONSERVATIVE APPROACH TO DIETARY GUIDANCE FOR THE PUBLIC

The report of the Lipid Research Clinics Coronary Primary Prevention Trial was released to the press as fact to be immediately applied to health guidance for all to follow. The goal seemed to be to convince the public of the validity of the findings and hence, to attempt to affect food consumption and ultimately agricultural practices. This action has had an important effect on both the press and the public which is only now being corrected with more careful and conservative interpretation. The more recent and extensive report of the Surgeon General is more cautious and states 'definitive scientific proof that specific dietary factors are responsible for specific chronic disease conditions is difficult—and may not be possible—to obtain, given available technology'. The Surgeon General suggests that 'Development of the major chronic disease conditions—coronary heart disease, stroke, diabetes, or cancer is affected by multiple genetic, environmental and behavioral factors among which diet is only one—albeit an important—component'.

Such health conscious groups as the American Heart Association have also been influenced in some of their recommendations. For example, the AHA (1986) suggestion that cholesterol intake be limited to 100 mg per 1000 calories of food. They also stated without adequate caution that 15% of the calories could come from alcoholic beverages. They ignored the fact that in 1984 we were on average consuming 44 gallons of soft drinks per person, 80% of which were sugared or 10% of calories for every man, woman and child. The soft drink industry goal is for 60 gallons per person by 1990, which they may achieve given our lifestyle and personal preferences. Dietitians find it almost impossible to balance the diet with the important minerals and vitamins if AHA recommendations are taken seriously. When our penchant for choosing so many high calorie foods is considered, a balanced diet is out of the question without careful selection of foods from all food categories including a significant component from animal products (Cleveland *et al.*, 1987).

There are some promising signs such as more recent AHA guidelines for 300 mg cholesterol intake for the general population. Since the adult average calorie intake is about 2000 calories, this in effect raises the AHA recommendation for cholesterol intake from the impossibly low 200 mg per 2000 calorie. But to date the AHA has not formally withdrawn the 1986 guidelines.

A high proportion of the population of the US is overweight. One long-term study (1959–72), which involved more than 750 000 men and women, based average weights on heights, thus avoiding the issue of what is an ideal weight. Deaths from all causes for women who were 20% above average weight for height were 1·29 times higher than average. Death rates were over 2-fold higher than normal for those 40% or more overweight. Diabetes, especially for women, had serious consequences for those who were obese. Death rates were 3·34-fold higher than normal for diabetics who were 20% overweight, and 7·9 times normal for those weighing 40% more than average. Mortality due to digestive diseases, cerebral vascular diseases, and even cancer, also increased among those who were overweight. The principal nutrition-related disease in America must certainly be consumption of calories in excess of need.

The problem in America where hundreds of new food products confront the consumer is one of enlightened choice. The quality of the choice is not greatly assisted by the new books featuring fad diets that seem to appear on the best seller lists each month. Specific medicinal properties are often attributed to certain foods, even nutritional claims of cures for terminal illness. No wonder the public is confused. The resulting commerce in 'natural foods' consumes an increasing proportion of the family food budget.

No place is the need for clarity of communication more important than that of the role of fat in the diet. One tendency of the press has been to characterize fats as either 'good' or 'bad'. For those whose caloric intake exceeds physiological need, most fats are bad because they are a concentrated source of calories. On the other hand, many fats are good because they provide essential nutritional qualities together with desirable taste. Largely on the basis of experiments with plant fats containing mostly saturated fatty acids 14 and 16 carbon atoms in length, the erroneous conclusion was made that eating fats of animal origin was unhealthy because they contained saturated fatty acids. This ignored the fact that one of the predominant saturated fatty acids in animal fats contains 18 carbon atoms. The fatty acids containing 18 carbon atoms may be metabolized quite differently than their carbon 14 and carbon 16 counterparts. Thus, animal fats which contain substantial quantities of carbon 18 fatty acids may now be categorized as 'good' fats.

In the meantime, the press attention given to preliminary findings has taken its toll on the public that now asks the question, 'Who is credible?' In spite of our expectations, there are no simple answers to complex questions of health. To understand the role which food and nutrition may have will require an educated public dependent on an attentive and responsible press. There are clear indications that the public is responsive to a choice of food lower in fat. When the choices are clearly labeled as they are on milk cartons with whole, 2%, 1% and skim milk, 2% has steadily grown in favor. In fact, more than half of the milk being consumed currently is the product intermediate in fat content. Probably the reason that skim milk, the lowest fat option, has not grown more in favor is due to the flavor. Some fat must be present for an acceptable product. Prompted by this recognized public preference for food products perceived to be more healthful, other dairy products are being developed that are lower in fat and also contain less salt, such as cheese and yogurt.

The meat industry, too, is conscious of this changing public demand for products that are perceived to be more healthy, but with beef products, there is a special problem. Prime beef, which is the top grade of commerce, is thought by many to be the grade lowest in fat. A new grading system needs to be devised that can serve consumers, packers and producers to minimize confusion, recognizing that a certain amount of fat must be present for an acceptable flavor and that does not encourage the production of animals which are too fat. There are some exciting new meat products under development that not only recognize the growing public preference for low calorie foods, but which are both appetizing and convenient to make dinner ready.

VII. SUMMARY

Food consumption patterns of Americans are analyzed and compared to recommended dietary guidelines. Among the major nutritional issues is the average total fat level of the diet, which is perceived by some that it should be lower. Thus, the consumption of food products, including meat lower in fat, is discussed. Choices from a variety of foods are deemed the most appropriate in order for a diet to include a balanced intake of nutrients. Recognizing the major nutritionally related problem in America to be overweight, foods which are low in energy-yielding nutrients relative to others should be emphasized in food selection from a variety of sources, including lean meat. Consumer perception of diet–health issues is analyzed, and the response of various segments of the food industry, especially the animal product industry, is discussed.

VIII. ACKNOWLEDGEMENT

Subject matter in this review has been drawn in part from *Designing Foods, Animal Product Options in the Marketplace*, for which one of the authors, R. Gaurth Hansen, was a panel member (National Academy of Sciences, National Research Council, 1988).

IX. REFERENCES

American Heart Association (AHA) (1986). Dietary guidelines for healthy American adults. Position statement. *Circulation* **74**, 6.

American Meat Institute (1987). Giant Lean (TM) Awareness and Usage, Research Report to the Center for Meat Marketing Research. AMI, Washington, DC.

ANDERSON, B. A. (1983). *Composition of Foods. USDA Handbook 8-10.* US Department of Agriculture. Washington, DC.

BERRY, B. W. and LEDDY, K. (1984). Beef patty composition: Effects of fat content and cooking method. *J. Am. Dietet. Assoc.* **84**, 654.

CLEVELAND, L., SHAW, A. and KREBS-SMITH, S. (1987). A system to assess the practicality of dietary recommendations. (Poster Session). Society for Nutrition Education Annual Meeting, San Francisco, CA.

HUMAN NUTRITION INFORMATION SERVICE (1987). US Department of Agriculture, unpublished data, Washington, DC.

LIPIDS RESEARCH CLINICS PROGRAM (1984). The lipid research clinics coronary primary prevention trial results: I. Reduction in incidence of coronary heart disease. *JAMA* **251**, 351.

LIPIDS RESEARCH CLINICS PROGRAM (1984). The lipid research clinics coronary primary prevention trial results: II. The relationship of reduction in incidence of coronary heart disease to cholesterol lowering. *JAMA* **251**, 365.

NATIONAL RESEARCH COUNCIL (1985a). Nationwide food consumption survey, continuing survey of food intakes by individuals. In *Designing Foods, Animal Product Options in the Marketplace*, p. 68. National Research Council, National Academy Press, Washington, DC.

NATIONAL RESEARCH COUNCIL (1985b). Nationwide food consumption survey, continuing survey of food intakes by individuals. In *Designing Foods, Animal Product Options in the Marketplace*, p. 88. National Research Council, National Academy Press, Washington, DC.

NATIONAL RESEARCH COUNCIL (1988). *Designing Foods, Animal Product Options in the Marketplace.* National Academy Press, Washington, DC.

NATIONAL RESTAURANT ASSOCIATION (1986). 1987 National Restaurant Association Foodservice Industry Forecast. National Restaurant Association, Washington, DC.

ONO, K., BERRY, B. W. and DOUGLASS, L. W. (1986). Nutrient composition of some fresh and cooked retail cuts of veal. In *Designing Foods, Animal Product Options in the Marketplace*, p. 83. National Research Council, National Academy Press, Washington, DC.

PRUSA, K. J. (1987). In *Designing Foods, Animal Product Options in the Marketplace*, p. 81. National Research Council, National Academy Press, Washington, DC.

SUPERMARKET BUSINESS (1986a). 39th Annual Consumer Expenditures Study. September, p. 69.

SUPERMARKET BUSINESS (1986b). In *Designing Foods, Animal Product Options in the Marketplace*, p. 65. National Research Council, National Academy Press, Washington, DC.

US DEPARTMENT OF AGRICULTURE (USDA) (1979). *Food.* Davis, C. A. *et al.* Home and garden bulletin no. 228. GPO, Washington, DC.

US DEPARTMENT OF AGRICULTURE (USDA) (1981). *Ideas for Better Eating: Menus and Recipes to Make Use of the Dietary Guidelines.* Science and Education Administration/Human Nutrition. GPO, Washington, DC.

US DEPARTMENT OF HEALTH AND HUMAN SERVICES (1988). *The Surgeon General's Report on Nutrition and Health.* Public Health Service. GPO, Washington, DC.

17

New Methods of Preservation and/or Reducing the Fat Content of Meat and Poultry Products

A. M. PEARSON

Department of Animal Science, Brigham Young University, Provo, Utah, USA

AND

J. I. GRAY

Department of Food Science and Human Nutrition, Michigan State University, Michigan, USA

I. INTRODUCTION

Meat and poultry processing fulfills a range of objectives including: (1) preservation, which involves reduction of food spoilage and pathogenic microorganisms by various processing methods, including application of heat and irradiation, and/or their control through lowering their water activity (a_w) by adding curing ingredients, or through inhibition of microbial growth by low temperatures (refrigeration or freezing); (2) enhancement of flavor and appearance by adding curing and flavoring agents; (3) creation of new products by using new or modified technologies to produce food products that add variety to the human diet; and (4) creation of products that meet special requirements by certain groups of consumers, i.e. low-salt or low-fat foods to meet the demands of the health-conscious individual.

In recent years concerted efforts have been directed towards developing new processing methods that fulfill special requirements towards meeting the above goals. However, like the traditional processing methods, the new procedures usually fall short in one or more respects. Pearson and Tauber (1984) have reviewed some of the new meat processing methods and their promise for future adoption by the industry. The discussion in this chapter will focus on some of the newer processing technologies with emphasis on their advantages and disadvantages.

II. REVIEW OF CONVENTIONAL METHODS OF PROCESSING

Before discussing new methods of meat processing, a short review of the principles involved in conventional meat processing will be briefly described. These include preservation by application of heat and/or smoke, preservation by removal of moisture through heating or freeze drying, and inhibition of microbial growth by addition of curing agents and/or low temperature storage.

A. Application of Heat and/or Smoke

Reduction of microbial numbers in order to control food pathogenic and spoilage organisms is commonly achieved in meat and poultry products by application of heat (cooking) and smoke. The effects of cooking and/or smoking of meat have been discussed by a number of investigators (Lowe, 1955; Gray and Pearson, 1984; Pearson and Tauber, 1984; Toth and Potthast, 1984) so will not be covered in detail. Suffice it to say that most of the meat pathogens and spoilage microorganisms are sensitive to heat so that cooking greatly reduces their numbers and extends the storage life of cooked meat. In addition, cooking decreases the a_w and helps to extend the shelf life of cooked meats (Tompkin, 1986). Thus, application of heat is commonly used for reducing the microbial load and delaying the growth of both food spoilage and pathogenic bacteria on both fresh and processed meat (Tompkin, 1986; Niven, 1987).

Sufficient application of heat will destroy pathogenic and food spoilage microorganisms and produce meat products that are commercially stable at ambient temperatures. However, these products must be protected from recontamination, which is commonly accomplished by canning or some of the newer packaging methods. In addition, the heat treatment must be sufficiently severe to not only destroy the contaminating bacteria but also certain bacterial spores, especially those of *Clostridium botulinum*. This must be accomplished by use of a retort heating schedule sufficient to injure or destroy the *C. botulinum* spores as discussed by Niven (1987).

Smoke has bacteriostatic properties, mainly due to the presence of phenolic compounds (Wilson, 1960, 1961; Wistreich, 1977; Toth and Potthast, 1984). Smoke also has some antioxidant activity (Wilson, 1960,

1961) that is also associated with its phenolic components. Smoking of meat and poultry products lowers the surface moisture content of processed meat when applied in the conventional manner (Wilson, 1960), although this may not be true when liquid smoke is applied (Toth and Potthast, 1984). However, heat is commonly applied following application of liquid smoke, which would lower the surface moisture content and help to retard bacterial growth (Pearson and Tauber, 1984).

Although application of heat will reduce the microbial load on meat and poultry products, in fresh cooked meat items heat speeds up development of rancidity. This is responsible for the rapid onset of rancidity following cooking, which is usually called 'warmed-over-flavor' (WOF). In contrast to frozen meat and poultry products that require months to develop objectionable rancid flavors, WOF develops in a matter of a few hours (Pearson *et al.*, 1977). Pearson *et al.* (1983a) have discussed some safety implications of oxidation in muscle foods. Asghar *et al.* (1988) have pointed out some procedures that can be used to stabilize muscle membranes and slow down development of oxidation and/or WOF. The addition of a nitrite also retards development of WOF so that most cured meat items normally do not develop WOF (Fooladi *et al.*, 1979; Gray and Pearson, 1984).

B. Addition of Curing Salt

Control of microbial growth can also be achieved by adding salt in order to reduce the a_w of meat and poultry products, which has been discussed by Scott (1957, 1961) and Niven (1987). Reduction of the a_w inhibits microbial growth by reducing the amount of water available. Salt, as well as a number of other substances that can lower the a_w, such as sugar, phosphates, ascorbate and nitrite, play a key role in retarding microbial growth, which has been reviewed in detail by Tompkin (1986) for a variety of meat and poultry products. The presence of salt and nitrite together can also reduce the amount of heat processing necessary to achieve either pasteurized or heat stable processed meat and poultry items that are available in commercial channels (Sofos *et al.*, 1979; Tompkin, 1986). Even though salt inhibits microbial growth, its use provides a human health dilemma to some consumers because of its effects on hypertension (Pearson and Wolzak, 1982).

Although other substances, such as sugar and/or corn syrup solids as well as spices and flavoring agents, may be added in curing, they are generally used at relatively low levels. Thus, they probably have little effect upon the microbial population (Pearson and Tauber, 1984). An exception to this may be sugar and/or other sweeteners that may be added at sufficiently high levels to alter the osmotic pressure and a_w. Even in these cases, the amounts added are rather low, although their effects may be additive to that of salt (Niven, 1987).

C. Low Temperatures

Low storage temperatures are well known procedures for delaying or retarding the growth of most microorganisms. This is true for the microbial flora present on both cured and fresh products and has been discussed by Gill (1986), Grau (1986) and Tompkin (1986). Thus, the growth of both food spoilage and pathogenic bacteria is usually delayed or else prevented by using low temperatures. While temperatures near freezing will delay bacterial proliferation, frozen storage will essentially prevent multiplication of most food spoilage and pathogenic microorganisms (Gill, 1986; Grau, 1986). Consequently, frozen storage of fresh meat products is commonly utilized if they are to be held for extended periods of time, i.e. storage beyond two to three weeks. However, temperatures just above freezing will delay microbial growth and are commonly utilized for delaying spoilage in fresh meat intended for consumption within one to three weeks post-slaughter.

III. NEW MEAT PROCESSING TECHNOLOGIES

Several relatively new methods of processing meat and poultry products have evolved since the end of World War II. These include the marketing of fresh meat in vacuum packages, controlled atmosphere packaging, radiation, restructuring and development of low-fat meat products. Each of these processes will be briefly reviewed herein.

A. Marketing of Fresh Meat Under Vacuum

Packaging of fresh meat under vacuum is a relatively recent development that has been widely used by the industry for retarding microbial spoilage. It was first used for primal beef cuts, but has more recently been utilized for pork and lamb.

(i) Beef

Although most fresh beef was marketed in the carcass form until the end of World War II, since then some 80–85% of all beef intended for use as fresh beef in supermarkets is now distributed as primal and subprimal cuts (J. Knutson, personal communication). The cuts are placed in oxygen–moisture-proof bags and a vacuum is drawn. This favors the growth of lactic acid-producing bacteria and selectively changes the microbial flora to largely eliminate problems from the common spoilage and pathogenic bacteria (Tompkin, 1986; Niven, 1987). The vacuum-packaged cuts are then packed in boxes and distributed. The entire process is commonly referred to as 'boxed beef' and has largely replaced the use of side or carcass beef at retail markets. The selective growth of lactic acid-producers prevents the outgrowth of the pseudomonads and other spoilage bacteria as well as that of pathogens. Boxed beef is held at refrigerated temperatures by the packers during distribution, and by the retail stores after arrival until removed, cut and prepared for display.

Vacuum-packaged beef can be held for four to eight weeks under proper refrigeration without any problem from spoilage, although most boxed beef is sold within four weeks post-slaughter (G. D. Wilson, personal communication). Boxed beef is usually removed from the bag, cut and repackaged at the retail store level. However, less skilled labor is required for preparation of the cuts at the store than is the case where sides or carcass beef are broken down into retail cuts by the meat department. The major advantage of boxed beef, however, is the fact that only the cuts which can be merchandised effectively are purchased. A large portion of the bone and fat is removed by the wholesaler, who has the capability of being able to market these by-products more advantageously than the retailer. For example, most of the fat removed at retail stores must be used for inedible rendering, whereas, that removed by the packer can generally be used to produce edible tallow. In addition, the cuts in less demand can either be marketed as such to other purchasers or else boned out and sold to processors by the packer.

(ii) Pork

In a recent development, fresh wholesale pork cuts have been marketed in vacuum bags. Loins, boneless loins and tenderloins are now being distributed in the boxed form. They have the same advantages as boxed beef. Some fresh pork cuts are now being marketed in consumer packages of retail cuts, containing a controlled atmosphere of carbon dioxide and/or other gases, which are wrapped ready for distribution, but are placed in vacuum bag overwraps (G. D. Wilson, personal communication). The CO_2 atmosphere prevents the outgrowth of pathogens and meat spoilage organisms (Gill, 1988). When the retailer wishes to display the cuts, the packages are removed from the overwrap and are then immediately placed in the fresh meat case. Obviously, this method eliminates any cutting and requires even less skilled labor at the retail store. Controlled atmospheric storage will be discussed later in more detail in the next section of this chapter. Single-portion fresh pork cuts are also being packaged under vacuum and distributed by several major meat packers.

B. Controlled Atmospheric Packaging

A more recent innovation in controlling bacterial spoilage and meat pathogens is the use of controlled atmosphere packaging. Although the success of controlled atmosphere packaging was referred to earlier in this chapter, it is still in the developmental stages. Gill (1988) and Gill and Penney (1986, 1988) have recently described work on packaging beef under CO_2 in order to extend its storage life.

Gill and Tan (1980) demonstrated that in aerobic systems of display packs of meat, atmospheres containing 20–30% of CO_2 inhibited the pseudomonad-dominated spoilage floras. However, increasing the level of CO_2 beyond 30% had little additional inhibitory effect. In anaerobic systems, which may be used to extend the storage life of meat before being displayed, on the other hand, CO_2 was shown to be a more effective inhibitor of bacterial spoilage.

The recent studies of Gill and Penney (1988) suggest that the full effects of CO_2 addition to gaseous meat packs can only be achieved if added in quantities in excess of that needed to saturate the meat. The quantity of CO_2 required for saturation was found to be between one and two liters per kilogram of meat. Gill (1988) reviewed some of the calculations that would be required for determining the quantity of CO_2 needed to saturate meat at different pH values, temperatures and fatty tissue levels. Using beef, it was shown that 1250 ml of CO_2 per kg of meat would be required for saturation under standard pressure at $-1{\cdot}5$°C (about 31°F).

Although the data on the conditions for achieving a satisfactory CO_2 concentration have not yet been published, fresh-packaged lamb chops can be stored for periods of up to six months in CO_2-modified atmospheres under good temperature control (N. Penney and C. O. Gill, personal communication). With this storage life, it should be possible to market fresh meat in almost any part of the world. However, both proper control of temperature and CO_2-modified atmospheres are necessary to achieve such long-time control of microbial growth. Thus, controlled atmospheric packaging of meat and poultry offers a most promising future for use in marketing of fresh meat.

C. Preservation by Radiation

Perhaps no area of research has elicited so much publicity, both favorable and unfavorable, as radiation. The use of radiation as a means of preserving meat and other foods has been extensively investigated since its potential for preservation was first recognized. It is doubtful if any other method for food preservation has been so intensively tested as radiation, with extensive studies having been carried out on not only the absence of toxic by-products from the process but also on the effects of radiation on the stability of the nutrients. Two recent reviews have discussed the potential use of radiation for preserving foods (Morrison, 1986; Roberts, 1986) which readers may wish to examine further.

(i) The radiation process

Radiation can be accomplished either by ionizing or nonionizing treatment as explained by Urbain (1982, 1986). However, only ionizing radiation possesses a level of energy capable of destroying microorganisms. Ionizing radiation, on the other hand, carries sufficient energy to penetrate the nucleus of an atom and may lead to induced radioactivity. In practice, this means that radiation of foods must utilize sources with energy levels insufficient to penetrate the nucleus so that the foods do not become radioactive. Therefore, radiation of foods is limited to using of X-rays and radioactive cobalt (^{60}Co). Thus, in irradiation of foods, the process makes use of energy levels only up to 5 MeV for gamma rays or only up to 10 MeV for X-rays (Urbain, 1986; Urbain and Campbell, 1987).

The lethal effects of ionizing radiation on microorganisms are due to chemical changes, which lead to the impairment of biological functions in all living organisms, and ultimately to death as explained by Urbain (1986). The unit of dosage for the irradiation process is expressed as Gray (Gy), which equals the absorption of one joule per kg. In the earlier literature, dosage was expressed in terms of rads (Wolin *et al.*, 1957), in which 100 rads was equal to 1 Gy.

If radiation is used to produce a commercially sterile product that will allow storage at ambient temperatures or above, it must be sufficiently severe to damage the spores and prevent their outgrowth as outlined by Urbain and Campbell (1987). This will be referred to herein as either sterilization or radappertization. Lower dosages, which provide sufficient radiation to greatly reduce the bacterial population to a low level so that refrigerated storage can be greatly extended, is called pasteurization or radurization. The necessary dosages required to produce a number of sterilized and pasteurized meat products are given in Table 17-1, which also

TABLE 17-1
MINIMUM RADIATION DOSAGES (MRD) REQUIRED FOR RADAPPERTIZATION OF SELECTED MEAT CUTS

Product	*Irradiation*[a] *temperature (°C)*	*MRD*[a] *(kGy)*	*Threshold*[b] *dose for off-flavor (kGy)*
Bacon	5–25	25	—
Beef	−30	41	2·5
Ham	5–25	31	—
Ham	−30	33	—
Pork	5–25	43	1·75
Corned beef	−30	24	—
Pork sausage	−30	27	—
Lamb	−30	41	6·25
Chicken	−30	41	2·5

[a] Values taken from Wierbicki *et al.* (1975).
[b] Values from Sudarmadji and Urbain (1972).

presents the threshold levels for detection of irradiation-induced off-flavors in some meat and poultry products.

a. Radappertization. Radappertization involves treatment of food products with a sufficient radiation dosage to make them commercially sterile, i.e. equivalent in sterility to heat processed shelf-stable canned foods. For meat and poultry products, the level of radiation needed to produce radappertized products falls in the range of 30–40 KGy (Urbain, 1986).

Although radappertization may ultimately be used to produce commercially sterile meat and poultry products, the flavor changes induced by radiation and problems in public acceptance of irradiated foods has blocked approval of the irradiation process for most foods by governmental agencies (FDA and FSIS) in US. Some of the flavor problems, however, can be overcome by using low temperatures during radiation (Wierbicki *et al.*, 1975). Nevertheless, the food products produced by radiation are free from induced radioactivity and result in relatively low losses of nutrients in comparison to that for heat processing (Urbain and Campbell, 1987). The only nutrient that suffers any major amount of destruction during radiation is thiamin, which retains only about 9% of its activity on irradiation of ham at 5°C (41°F) according to studies by Thomas and Wierbicki (1971). However, reduction of the irradiation temperature to

−20, −40, −60 and −80°C (−4, −40, −76 and −112°F) improved thiamin retention to 53, 79, 87 and 93%, respectively. The higher values are comparable to those obtained on freezing and are superior to that for canning.

At radappertization doses irradiated meat products develop an objectionable flavor that has been described as 'wet dog' or 'irradiated flavor'. The temperature of radiation, however, has a marked effect upon the degree of irradiation flavor. Thus, radiation at low temperatures can markedly reduce the problems from off-flavors in irradiated meat as has been shown by Merritt *et al.* (1975). Lowering the temperature to below freezing apparently reduces the mobility of the primary radiolytic product and other molecules present, and thereby limits their interactions, and thus minimizes flavor changes in foods (Urbain and Campbell, 1987).

Radappertized meat and poultry must be heat treated if storage is at ambient temperature or above in order to inactivate the indigenous proteolytic enzymes (Urbain and Campbell, 1987). Lakritz and Maerker (1988) have shown that radiation causes some inactivation of the indigenous muscle proteinases, with the effect being dose responsive. In spite of the effects of radappertization on inactivating the muscle proteinases, it is doubtful if inactivation of all of the proteinases will occur and allow long-term storage of meat at ambient or higher temperatures. Radappertization may, however, destroy the proteinases that are responsible for the texture changes that occur in irradiated meat products as theorized by Lakritz and Maerker (1988).

If the public perception that irradiated foods are radioactive can be overcome, it should be possible to solve most of the flavor problems of irradiated meat and poultry products. Thus, radappertized meat and poultry products could be produced and marketed as shelf-stable items.

b. Radurization. The primary objective of radurization of foods is to extend the shelf-life through reducing the microbial population, which with meat and poultry products can be achieved by doses in the range of 1–5 kGy (Urbain and Giddings, 1972; Urbain, 1982; Urbain and Campbell, 1987). The radiation process can be applied to both fresh and processed-cured meats (Tiwari and Maxcy, 1971; Dickson and Maxcy, 1985). The effectiveness and routine usage of vacuum packaging for extending the shelf-life of processed meat and poultry products, however, usually limits the usefulness of radurization for extending the storage life of these items (Urbain and Campbell, 1987).

Roberts (1986) has suggested that radiation may find its greatest usage in

TABLE 17-2
ESTIMATED HEALTH COSTS AND WAGES LOST TO DISEASES FROM PORK, CHICKEN, AND BEEF[a]

Meat	*Estimate in million dollars (US)*	
	Low	*High*
Pork		
Trichinosis	1·5	2·8
Congenital toxoplasmosis	215	323
Chicken		
Salmonellosis	64	115
Campylobacteriosus	362	699
Beef		
Salmonellosis	209	374
Tapeworm	0·1	0·1
Total[b]	850	1 500

[a] Taken from Roberts (1986).
[b] Figures are rounded off to nearest tenth of a million.

pasteurizing dosages to control the pathogenic microorganisms in fresh meat and poultry. Table 17-2 presents estimates on the health costs and losses in wages from some meat and poultry-borne diseases in humans. The diseases, which include trichinosis and congenital toxoplasmosis from pork, salmonellosis and campylobacteriosus from chicken and salmonellosis and tapeworm from beef are estimated to cost from $850–1500 million annually in US (Roberts, 1986).

The number of cases of food-borne illnesses associated with eating of meat and poultry have been reviewed by Roberts (1986) using data from the Centers of Disease Control. She pointed out that there are about 40 000 reported cases of salmonellosis annually in US, with approximately 3800 of these being due to consumption of chicken. At an estimated cost of $1290 per case the cost would be $4·9 million annually. It is estimated that there are another 1·96 million mild cases with 9·5% of these being due to eating chicken, which at a cost of $230 per case in lost wages and medical expenses would reach a total of $42·8 million annually.

Table 17-3 presents the estimated cost per case for various food borne illnesses derived from eating pork. Data are given for trichinosis per illness and per death, for congenital toxoplasmosis (average illness), and for salmonellosis/campylobacteriosus, including mild and moderate illnesses

TABLE 17-3

ESTIMATED COST PER CASE OF FOOD-BORNE ILLNESS AND DEATH FROM EATING PORK IN US[a]

Illness	*Cost/case in US dollars*
Trichinosis	
Illness	2 485
Death	140 000–471 000
Congenital toxoplasmosis	
Average illness[b]	130 303
Salmonellosis/campylobacteriosus	
Mild illness	230
Moderate illness	1 290
Death	85 800–351 500
Tapeworm	
Illness	111

[a] Taken from Roberts (1986).
[b] Does not include fetal deaths.

and death. Costs for these two diseases were estimated to vary from a low of \$230 per illness to a high estimate of \$351 500 per death. The least severe losses occurred from tapeworms, where a single case from eating pork was estimated to cost \$111.

Roberts (1986) has estimated that irradiation of all meat at a level of 4 kGy could virtually eliminate the problems from meat and poultry pathogens. This, of course, assumes that proper handling after radurization

TABLE 17-4

COMPARISON OF COSTS–BENEFITS FOR IRRADIATION OF PORK AND CHICKEN IN US[a]

	Benefits (\$*m*)[b]	*Costs* (\$*m*)[b]	*Ratio of benefits to costs*	*Net benefits* (\$*m*)[b]
Pork[c]	186–280	80	2·3–2·5	106–200
Chicken[d]	341–653	155	2·2–4·2	186–498

[a] Taken from Roberts (1986).
[b] \$m = million dollars in US.
[c] Assuming 86% of all pork is irradiated at 0·5 kGy to prevent trichinosis and toxoplasmosis in humans.
[d] Assuming 81% of all chicken is irradiated at 2·5 kGy to eliminate campylobacteriosus and salmonellosis cases by 93%.

prevents any recontamination. Table 17-4 compares the estimated costs–benefits from radiation of the pork and chicken consumed in US. As can be seen from the data presented in Table 17-4, the net benefits would fall between \$106 and \$200 million for pork and between \$186 and \$498 million for chicken annually. These figures make a strong case for radurization of fresh pork and chicken, while a similar rationale for pasteurizing radiation of beef could be developed. Thus, radurization of meat appears to be a useful technique for reducing the incidence of human diseases that are contracted from eating meat and poultry products.

D. Reduction of the Fat Content in Meat and Poultry Products

As already indicated in Chapter 5, toxic compounds may be formed during meat processing. Aside from such toxic compounds, the nutritional attributes of processed meats may be altered by cooking/processing (Bodwell and Anderson, 1986). The nutritive value of processed meats can also be changed by altering their composition during the production of new-type products, such as low-fat and low-calorie items, which are now available to consumers (Mast and Clouser, 1988; Rust, 1988). With increases in the numbers of health-conscious consumers, the interest in reduced-fat/low-calorie meat and poultry products has resulted in considerable demand for these products.

(i) Changes in meat and poultry consumption

Bailey *et al.* (1988) have reviewed changes in consumption of meat, poultry and fish for 1970–74, 1975–79, 1980–84, 1985 and 1986 which are presented in Table 17-5. The data show that beef consumption has declined from 83·9 to 78·4 lb (38·1 to 35·6 kg) annually *per capita.* Over the same time period, pork consumption has decreased from 62·1 to 58·6 lb (28·2 to 26·6 kg). On the other hand, total fish consumption has increased from 12·1 lb (5·5 kg) *per capita* to 14·7 lb (6·7 kg). The increase in consumption of chicken and turkey has been even more dramatic, going up from 40·5 and 8·6 lb (18·4 and 3·9 kg) *per capita* in 1970–74 to 58·8 and 13·3 lb (26·7 and 6·0 kg) in 1986, respectively. Thus, total poultry consumption has increased from approximately 49·1 to 72·1 lb (22·3 to 32·8 kg) over this time period. Part of the increase in poultry and poultry product consumption in contrast to the decrease in red meats by about 10 lb (4·6 kg) *per capita* is no doubt due to the lower fat content of poultry meat. Although there has been some increase in fish (about 3 lb or 1·2 kg *per capita*) consumption, probably due in part to its lower fat content, the total amount (approximately 15 lb or 6·7 kg) is still relatively small.

TABLE 17-5

CONSUMPTION OF MEAT, POULTRY AND FISH FROM 1970–74 TO 1986[a] in lb (kg) *per capita*

	1970–74	*1975–79*	*1980–84*	*1985*	*1986*
Red meat					
Beef	83·9 (38·1)	87·8 (39·9)	78·3 (35·6)	78·8 (35·8)	78·4 (35·6)
Veal	2·0 (0·9)	2·8 (1·3)	1·6 (0·7)	1·8 (0·8)	1·9 (0·8)
Pork	62·1 (28·2)	55·8 (25·4)	63·0 (28·6)	62·0 (28·2)	58·6 (26·6)
Lamb	2·6 (1·2)	1·5 (0·7)	1·5 (0·7)	1·4 (0·6)	1·4 (0·6)
Total	150·6 (68·4)	147·9 (67·2)	144·4 (65·6)	144·0 (65·4)	140·3 (63·8)
Fish					
Fresh and frozen	7·0 (3·2)	7·9 (3·6)	8·0 (3·6)	9·0 (4·1)	9·0 (4·1)
Canned and cured	5·1 (2·3)	5·1 (2·3)	5·0 (2·3)	5·4 (2·4)	5·7 (2·6)
Total	12·1 (5·5)	12·9 (5·8)	13·0 (5·9)	14·4 (6·5)	14·7 (6·7)
Poultry					
Chicken	40·5 (18·4)	44·6 (20·3)	52·5 (23·8)	57·6 (26·2)	58·8 (26·7)
Turkey	8·6 (3·9)	9·1 (4·1)	10·9 (5·0)	12·1 (5·5)	13·3 (6·0)
Total	49·1 (22·3)	53·7 (24·4)	63·4 (28·8)	69·7 (31·7)	72·1 (32·8)

[a] From Bailey *et al.* (1988).

Marston and Raper (1987) have presented data showing that meat, poultry and fish contributed 38% of the total dietary fat in 1967–69 and 22% of the energy (calories). By 1985, the percentage of dietary fat contributed by these same products had declined to 33%, or a decrease of 5%, while their contribution to total energy was only 20%—a decrease of 2%. These data illustrate the interest of consumers in decreasing their consumption of fat from muscle foods.

There are two main ways to reduce the fat content of retail fresh meat: (1) by production of meat with a minimum of amount of fat through breeding, feeding and management, and (2) by removing excessive amounts of fat through trimming prior to marketing. Both of these procedures have been discussed by Mertz (1986) and in even greater detail by the NAS–NRC Committee (1988) in the report *Designing Foods: Animal Product Options in the Marketplace.* Although reduction of fatness can be achieved by breeding, feeding and management, progress is slow and requires time (Dikeman, 1987), while removal of excess fat at the packer/retailer level can and has been adopted, which will be discussed next.

a. Reduction of fat content by trimming and cooking. Most supermarkets and meat retailers have begun programs of trimming beef cuts to some specified maximum level of fat thickness—commonly about $\frac{1}{4}$-inch (6·4 mm). This has greatly reduced the perceived level of fatness, although many consumers had previously trimmed the fat off either before cooking or eating. The trend for reducing fatness of beef cuts is reflected by the National Beef Market Basket Survey (Cross *et al.*, 1987; Savell *et al.*, 1988), which concluded that the average external fat thickness for steaks and roasts from primal cuts (round, loin, rib and chuck) was 0·11 in (2·8 mm). The National Beef Market Basket Survey (Cross *et al.*, 1987; Savell *et al.*, 1988) concluded that today's retail beef cuts on US markets contain 27% less fat than found in USDA's *Handbook 8-13* that used $\frac{1}{2}$-in (12·7 mm) external fat thickness on all retail cuts. The National Beef Market Basket Survey (Cross *et al.*, 1987; Savell *et al.*, 1988) has also shown that ground beef contains 27% less fat than shown in USDA *Handbook 8-13.* This lower value reflects the fact that nearly 60% of all ground beef on US retail markets is composed of 'lean' or 'extra lean' grinds. Thus, the National Beef Market Basket Survey (Cross *et al.*, 1987; Savell *et al.*, 1988) clearly shows that the closer-retail trim and consumer demand for less fat have resulted in a marked reduction in the fatness of beef on retail markets.

Table 17-6 presents data taken from Mertz (1986), and shows the percentage of fat derived from a number of meat and poultry products before trimming and after trimming/cooking. The data indicate that trimming/cooking reduces the fat content of intact meat cuts (beef T-bone

TABLE 17-6

EFFECT OF TRIMMING AND COOKING ON THE PERCENTAGE OF ENERGY DERIVED FROM FAT IN DIFFERENT MEAT PRODUCTS[a]

Cut/product	*% energy from fat*	
	Before trimming	*After trimming/cooking*
T-bone steak—US choice	84 (lean only)	41·5
Pork loin—medium fat	75 (lean only)	43·5
Pork sausage—raw	92	—[c]
Various sausages	71–82	—[c]
Broiler-broiled, lean only	25	—[b]
Venison—lean	29	—[b]

[a] Data from Mertz (1986).
[b] Data not given.
[c] Cannot separate lean and fat.

steak and pork loin chops) by approximately one-half. Thus, trimming/cooking can have a major impact on the fatness of meat or more particularly upon the amount of energy derived from various meat products. It should be pointed out, however, that sausages and ground beef products are not amenable to reduction of fat content once these products are prepared.

Bailey *et al.* (1988) have reviewed changes in *per capita* fat consumption at different intervals of time from 1965 through 1985, and interestingly have divided dietary fat into visible and invisible sources (Table 17-7). Presumably, the consumer can consciously eliminate the visible fats from the diet. These include baking and frying fats (part of which are probably of animal origin), lard and tallow (all of which are derived from meat animals), margarine, butter, salad and cooking oils. The invisible fats as shown in Table 17-7 include meat, poultry and fish (which as already indicated is not made up of all invisible fats), dairy products, eggs, fruits and vegetables, soybeans including nuts and legumes, grains and miscellaneous fat sources.

The data in Table 17-7 on the contribution of various visible fat sources to *per capita* fat consumption show that baking and frying fats have increased from about 14·2 to nearly 22·9 lb (6·4 to 10·4 kg) *per capita* over the 1965 to 1985 period. Part of this increase is probably due to animal fats and part to vegetable fats. Lard and edible tallow consumption has declined by 2·6 lb (1·2 kg) over the same time period. However, the major increase in *per capita* consumption of visible fats is due to the increased use of cooking and salad oils, which has risen steadily from about 14·1 lb (6·4 kg) in 1965 to 25·2 lb (11·4 kg) in 1985. Thus, most of the increase in consumption of visible fats can be attributed to the greater use of cooking and salad oils, which increased by nearly 179% from 1965 to 1985.

The changes in *per capita* consumption of invisible fats were relatively small over the 20-year period from 1965 to 1985 (Table 17-7), amounting to 1·8 lb (0·8 kg). Most of the increase, no doubt, is due to the increased consumption of fish and poultry, as the consumption of red meat declined over the same time period (Table 17-5).

Further support for data presented by Mertz (1986) showing the effects of trimming off excess fat from retail cuts is given in Table 17-8, which presents the percentage of calories from fat in a 3 oz (85·2 g) serving of trimmed cooked meat from several beef, pork, lamb and veal cuts. The percentage of calories from fat varies from 23% for veal cutlets up to 45% for fresh ham from pork. These values are in essential agreement with the values given by Mertz (1986) for trimmed cooked cuts from beef and pork. It is interesting to note that a number of trimmed cooked cuts (top round steak, pork

TABLE 17-7
SOURCES AND AMOUNTS OF VISIBLE AND INVISIBLE FATS IN THE US *per capita* DIET FOR 1965–1985[a]

	Changes in per capita *fat consumption*[a] *in lb (kg)*			
	1965	*1974*	*1980*	*1985*
Visible fats				
Baking and frying fats	14·2 (6·4)	16·9 (7·7)	18·2 (8·3)	22·9 (10·4)
Lard and edible tallow[b]	6·3 (2·9)	3·2 (1·4)	3·7 (1·7)	3·7 (1·7)
Margarine	7·9 (3·6)	9·1 (4·1)	9·2 (4·2)	8·6 (3·9)
Butter	5·2 (2·3)	3·7 (1·7)	3·7 (1·7)	4·0 (1·8)
Salad and cooking oils, etc.	14·1 (6·4)	19·9 (9·0)	22·6 (10·3)	25·2 (11·4)
Total	47·7 (21·7)	52·8 (24·0)	57·4 (26·1)	64·4 (29·3)
Invisible fats				
Meat, poultry and fish	43·6 (19·8)	46·9 (21·3)	47·5 (21·6)	46·1 (21·0)
Dairy products	16·7 (7·6)	15·0 (6·8)	14·7 (6·7)	15·7 (7·1)
Eggs	4·0 (1·8)	3·5 (1·6)	3·4 (1·5)	3·2 (1·4)
Fruits and vegetables	0·8 (0·3)	0·9 (0·4)	1·0 (0·4)	1·2 (0·5)
Soybeans, nuts and legumes	3·6 (1·6)	3·8 (1·7)	3·2 (1·4)	3·8 (1·7)
Grains	1·7 (0·8)	1·6 (0·7)	1·7 (0·8)	1·8 (0·8)
Miscellaneous[c]	1·8 (0·8)	1·8 (0·8)	1·5 (0·7)	2·2 (1·0)
Total	72·2 (32·8)	73·5 (33·4)	73·0 (33·2)	74·0 (33·6)
Grand Total	119·9 (54·5)	126·3 (57·4)	130·4 (59·3)	138·4 (62·9)

[a] Taken from Bailey *et al.* (1988).
[b] Excludes use in margarine and shortening (baking and frying fats).
[c] Includes chocolate, cocoa, coffee, tea and spices.

tenderloin, veal cutlet and veal blade steaks) that are shown in Table 17-8 fell below less than 30% of their total calories from fat. There are also a number of fresh poultry and fish items that no doubt fall within this range, but their calorie contents are not readily available. These cuts could be used in low-fat diets, which have been discussed by DeWys (1986), Levy and Ernst (1986) and Allen (1987). It should be remembered, however, that the recommendation of 30% of the total calories from fat applies to the entire meal and not to a single food or even a single cut of meat.

The results presented herein show that the number of calories from fat in fresh cooked meat and poultry products can be greatly reduced by trimming and cooking. Although different methods of cooking can be utilized to reduce the fat content of cooked fresh poultry and meats, more

TABLE 17-8

CALORIE AND FAT CONTENT FOR 3 oz (85·2 g) OF VARIOUS CUTS OF COOKED AND TRIMMED MEAT[a]

Species/cut	*Calories*	*% of calories as fat*
Beef		
Top round steak	162	29
Eye round steak	155	32
Sirloin tip roast	162	36
Sirloin steak	177	38
Pork		
Tenderloin	141	26
Center cut loin chop	196	41
Fresh ham (leg) roast	187	45
Lamb		
Foreshank—braised	159	29
Leg roast—shank half	153	34
Veal		
Cutlet	155	23
Rib roast	143	35
Blade (shoulder) steak	167	26

[a] Data taken from Breidenstein (1987) and calculated to give percent calories from fat.

information on cooking methods and their effects upon the calorie and energy level is clearly needed. Nevertheless, reduction of calorie levels by trimming and cooking has already been shown to have a profound influence on the energy content of fresh poultry and meat cuts. It should not be overlooked that some minimum amount of fat is necessary in these products to produce flavorful acceptable meat as suggested in Chapter 16 and by Cole *et al.* (1960), Pearson (1976) and Hansen *et al.* (1986).

b. Production of low-fat processed meat and poultry products

1. The Cholesterol–Fat Problem. There has been a great deal of interest in producing low-fat processed meat products in order to minimize their calorie and cholesterol contents. Although Reiser (1975) and Rhee *et al.* (1982a, b) have demonstrated that fatty tissue does not contain appreciable amounts of cholesterol, it is commonly believed that fat contributes to cholesterol (Allen, 1987; Martin, 1987). It has been demonstrated by Bonanome and Grundy (1987a, b) that individual fatty acids behave differently, with oleic acid having a hypocholesterolemic effect, whereas,

palmitic acid had a hypercholesterolemic effect. These findings confirm earlier studies by Keys *et al.* (1965) and Hegsted *et al.* (1965). Since the effect of different fatty acids has been reviewed in Chapter 2, it will not be covered in more detail herein.

As discussed in Chapter 3, the effect of cholesterol in the diet and its relationship to blood cholesterol does not appear to be an important factor in coronary heart disease. Samuel and McNamara (1982), McNamara (1985, 1987) and McNamara *et al.* (1987) have concluded that dietary and blood cholesterol levels are not closely related, with only about 30% of all humans being noncompensators, so that for most humans, blood levels of cholesterol are not closely associated with dietary cholesterol. Since this relationship has been reviewed in Chapter 3, it will not be discussed further herein.

The problem of fat in meat and poultry products is more well-defined, with a number of researchers (DeWys, 1986; Levy and Ernst, 1986; Allen, 1987; Martin, 1987) having reviewed the relationship between excess fat consumption and human health. The recent report by the NAS–NRC Committee (1988) has concentrated on the problem of fat, not only in meat and poultry products, but also for other animal products including eggs and dairy products. Nevertheless, a number of workers (Pearson and Brooks, 1978; Pearson, 1981; Pearson *et al.*, 1983b; Hansen *et al.*, 1986; Schweigert, 1986) have emphasized the important nutritional contributions that meat and poultry products make to the essential nutrient intake in the human diet.

2. Contribution of Fat to Palatability. The palatability of meat and poultry is well-known and adds to their usefulness as foods. Although a number of investigations have shown that meat flavor *per se* resides in the water-soluble fraction (Kramlich and Pearson, 1958; Hornstein *et al.*, 1960, 1963; Pearson *et al.*, 1983b), it has been demonstrated that fat also contributes to meaty flavors and is responsible for the species-characteristic flavor (Hornstein *et al.*, 1960, 1963; Pearson *et al.*, 1983b).

In addition, a certain minimum amount of fat is also necessary for tenderness of meat. Wellington and Stouffer (1959) and Blumer (1963) have reported that there is a low but significant relationship between intramuscular fat content (marbling) and flavor and juiciness. Savell *et al.* (1987) have also verified a low relationship between marbling and palatability in beef loin steaks. Even though the degree of association is quite low, the evidence indicates that at least a minimum amount of fat is necessary for palatability in meat. Although such a relationship has not been reported for poultry products, it seems reasonable to assume that such an association also exists.

3. Low-Fat Processed Meat and Poultry Products. There has been a great deal of interest in reducing the fat content of processed meat and poultry products, a subject which has been reviewed by Paul and Foget (1983). There are several ways to reduce fat content, among which are restructuring of meat and poultry products and reducing the fat content of sausage products. The former can be more easily accomplished since it involves taking the muscles apart and removal of intermuscular fat and then either reforming them directly to produce sectioned and formed items or flaking and forming. These topics have been extensively reviewed by researchers working in this area (Pearson and Dutson, 1987). Thus, the subject of restructuring will not be covered herein.

The production of low-fat sausage products has not been so extensively reviewed so will be discussed in greater detail. Nevertheless, low-fat or reduced-fat products are available on the market, indicating the capability of the meat industry to produce such items, although much of the information is of a proprietary nature. The major problem in production of low-fat sausages has been the inability to produce a palatable product in the absence of about 20–25% fat (Pearson, 1976). The addition of hydrocolloids (Wallingford and Labuza, 1983) and anionic gums (Fox *et al.*, 1983; Whiting, 1984) has permitted processors to add water as the fat is reduced while maintaining the juiciness and other palatability attributes in the products.

Foegeding and Ramsey (1986) have compared the effects of adding iota- or kappa-carrageenan, guar gum, locust bean gum, xanthan gum, methylcellulose and a mixture of locust bean gum–kappa-carrageenan for producing low-fat and high-moisture sausages. Batters containing methylcellulose suffered from excessive moisture losses on heating between 60 and 70°C. Both xanthan and guar gums were found to alter the texture, while the carrageenans were effective in binding moisture and allowed a reduction in fat content without having any adverse influence on acceptability. Results demonstrated that frankfurters containing 11–12% fat could be produced by adding carrageenans and were just as acceptable as controls containing 27% fat. Thus, it is possible to produce low-fat sausages by use of carrageenans without any palatability problems. On the basis of this and other similar work USDA's FSIS (Food Safety and Inspection Service) have altered regulations to permit substitution of water for fat in sausages.

Pearson *et al.* (1987) have reviewed some procedures for reducing the fat content of processed meat, among which was the use of carrageenans and other binders including salt–dextrose and soy proteins. Some processors may add as much as 8% dextrose and 4% NaCl to give up to 12% of added substance, which can be used to produce 90–95% fat-free processed meats. However, such high salt products may meet consumer resistance because of their high sodium content (Pearson and Wolzak, 1982).

Table 17-9 presents some carrageenan-containing brine formulations for use in tumbling or pumping of low-fat poultry products. The manufacturer's claims (FMC, 1987) state that the use of the carrageenan in the brine has a beneficial effect on moisture retention, oxidation/flavor, texture, sliceability, brine viscosity, freeze–thaw stability and dispersability. It was also claimed that carrageenan enhanced mouthfeel in reduced-fat products, improved texture, aided in retention of moisture and stabilized emulsion-type products.

More recently, Lin *et al.* (1988) have demonstrated that carboxymethyl cellulose (CMC) can be incorporated into low-fat frankfurters without any decrease in emulsion stability as long as high molecular weight CMC was utilized. Although the frankfurters containing CMC were softer in texture, this could be an advantage since the all-meat low-fat controls tended to be tough and lacking in juiciness. Means and Schmidt (1986) have described the use of an algin–calcium gel as a raw and cooked binder for restructured beef steaks, but there is little published information on alginate, as a water binding agent in processed meats.

Table 17-10 gives a formulation using carrageenan for production of low-fat frankfurters. The frankfurters were tested by a 25-member consumer

TABLE 17-9

BRINE FORMULATIONS CONTAINING CARRAGEENAN FOR TUMBLING OR PUMPING OF POULTRY PRODUCTS[a]

Ingredients	*10% brine injection*	*20% brine injection*	*30% brine injection*	*% composition in total product weight*
Water (5°C)	72·5	85·0	89·0	0·0
NaCl	16·5	9·0	6·6	1·5
STPP[b]	5·5	3·0	2·2	0·5
Gelcarin carrageenan[c]	5·5	3·0	2·2	0·5

[a] FMC Corporation (1987).
[b] STPP = sodium tripolyphosphate.
[c] Gelcarin SA 911.

TABLE 17-10

COMPARISON OF CONTROL AND CARRAGEENAN FORMULATIONS FOR PRODUCING LOW-FAT FRANKFURTERS[a]

Ingredients	*Formulation (%)*	
	Control	*Carrageenan added*
Lean meat blend (3·6% fat)	20·33	35·42
Fat meat blend (48·1% fat)	52·47	24·38
Water	21·73	34·43
Salt	2·20	2·20
Seasoning	3·22	3·22
Sodium erythorbate	0·04	0·04
Sodium nitrite	0·012	0·012
Viscarin type carrageenan	—	0·30
	100·00	100·00

[a] FMC Corporation (1987).

panel and were rated significantly higher ($P < 0{\cdot}05$) for color, overall appearance and flavor than controls containing 24% fat. However, panel scores were not different for texture.

Investigations with soy proteins by Drake *et al.* (1975) and Sofos and Allen (1977) have also shown them to be useful as water binding agents for reducing the fat content of meat products. There is also evidence that caseinate can bind water in sausage products. Thus, removal of fat with substitution of water results in satisfactory low-fat meat and poultry products.

IV. SUMMARY

Discussion in this chapter has centered on the methods for preserving meat products and on techniques for reducing their fat content. First, some of the conventional methods of preservation were discussed, including the influence of heat and smoke, addition of curing salts, low temperature storage (refrigeration and freezing) and dehydration. Some new processing technologies were then reviewed, which included vacuum packaging of fresh beef and pork as well as controlled atmosphere packaging to control microbial growth. Preservation by radiation was discussed from the standpoint of both radappertization and radurization, with emphasis being given to the latter process for controlling human health hazards from pathogenic microorganisms on meat and poultry products.

Changes in meat and poultry consumption were discussed from the standpoint of human health implications. It was concluded that many consumers desire leaner products, which can be achieved by breeding, feeding and management or by removal of excess fat. The former procedure is a slow-long-time objective, but the second can and is being accomplished rapidly by trimming and cooking. Reduction of the fat content in meat and poultry products was then reviewed. The cholesterol–fat relationship was briefly covered. The last part of the chapter reviews some processing methods that can be used to reduce the fat content of meat and poultry products, with special emphasis being directed toward replacement of part of the fat by adding water-binding agents. Overall, there are many ways of processing that show promise in producing reduced fat meat and poultry products.

V. REFERENCES

ALLEN, C. E. (1987). A perspective on the implications of animal fat on human health. *Proc. Recip. Meat Conf.* **40**, 115.

ASGHAR, A., GRAY, J. I., BUCKLEY, D. J., PEARSON, A. M. and BOOREN, A. M. (1988). Perspectives in warmed-over flavor. *Food Technol.* **42**(6), 102.

BAILEY, L., DUEWER, L., GRAY, F., HOSKIN, R., PUTNAM, J. and SHORT, S. (1988). Food consumption. *Nat. Food Rev.* **11**(2), 1.

BLUMER, T. N. (1963). Relationship of marbling to the palatability of beef. *J. Anim. Sci.* **22**, 771.

BODWELL, C. E. and ANDERSON, B. A. (1986). Nutritional composition and value of meat and meat products. In *Muscle as Food* (P. J. Bechtel, Ed.), p. 321. Academic Press, Orlando, FL.

BONANOME, A. and GRUNDY, S. M. (1987a). Stearic acid does not raise plasma cholesterol. *Clin. Res.* **35**, 365A.

BONANOME, A. and GRUNDY, S. M. (1987b). Effects of dietary fats on plasma cholesterol in humans. *Proc. Recip. Meat Conf.* **40**, 89.

BREIDENSTEIN, B. C. (1987). Nutrient composition: Nutrient value of meat. *Food & Nutr. News* **59**(2), 1.

COLE, J. W., RAMSEY, C. B. and ODAM, L. O. (1960). What effects does fat content have on palatability of broiled ground beef. *Tenn. Farm Home Sci.* **36**, 5.

CROSS, H. R., SMITH, G. C. and SAVELL, J. W. (1987). *The Beef Industries Move Towards Leanness.* Meat Research Brief. Tx. Agric. Expt. Sta., Texas A&M University, College Station, TX.

DEWYS, W. D. (1986). An overview of cancer risk factors of dietary origin. *J. Anim. Sci.* **62** (Suppl. 1), 21.

DICKSON, J. S. and MAXCY, R. B. (1985). Irradiation of meat for production of fermented sausages. *J. Food Sci.* **50**, 1007.

DIKEMAN, M. E. (1987). Fat reduction in animals and the effects on palatability and consumer acceptance of meat products. *Proc. Recip. Meat Conf.* **40**, 93.

DRAKE, S. R., HINNERGARDT, L. C., KLUTER, R. A. and PRELL, P. A. (1975). Beef patties: The effect of textured soy protein and fat levels on quality and acceptability. *J. Food Sci.* **40**, 1065.

FMC CORPORATION (1986). *Processed Poultry Products.* FMC Corp., Marine Colloids Division, Application Bul. B-51.

FMC CORPORATION (1987). *Low-Fat Frankfurters.* FMC Corp., Marine Colloids Division, Application Bul. B-60.

FOEGEDING, E. A. and RAMSEY, S. R. (1986). Effect of gums on low-fat meat batters. *J. Food Sci.* **51**, 33.

FOOLADI, M. H., PEARSON, A. M., COLEMAN, T. and MERKEL, R. A. (1979). The role of nitrite in preventing development of warmed-over flavor. *Food Chem.* **4**, 283.

FOX, J. B., ACKERMAN, S. A. and JENKINS, R. K. (1983). Effect of anionic gums on the texture of pickled frankfurters. *J. Food Sci.* **48**, 1031.

GILL, C. O. (1986). The control of microbial spoilage in fresh meats. *Adv. Meat Res.*, Vol. 2. Elsevier Applied Science, London, p. 49.

GILL, C. O. (1988). The solubility of CO_2 in meat. *Meat Sci.* **22**, 65.

GILL, C. O. and PENNEY, N. (1986). Packaging conditions for extended storage of chilled dark, firm dry beef. *Meat Sci.* **18**, 41.

GILL, C. O. and PENNEY, N. (1988). The effect of initial gas volume to meat weight ratio and the storage life of chilled beef packaged under carbon dioxide. *Meat Sci.* **22**, 53.

GILL, C. O. and TAN, K. H. (1980). Effect of carbon dioxide on growth of meat spoilage bacteria. *Appl. Environ. Microbiol.* **39**, 317.

GRAU, F. H. (1986). Microbial ecology of meat and poultry. *Adv. Meat Res.*, Vol. 2. Elsevier Applied Science, London, p. 1.

GRAY, J. I. and PEARSON, A. M. (1984). Cured meat flavor. *Adv. Food Res.* **29**, 1.

HANSEN, R. G., WINDHAM, C. T., WITTWER, C. T. and WYSE, B. W. (1986). Placing the role of meat in perspective. *J. Anim. Sci.* **62** (Suppl. 1), 7.

HEGSTED, D. M., MCGANDY, R. B., MYERS, M. L. and STARE, F. J. (1965). Quantitative effects of dietary fat on serum cholesterol in man. *Amer. J. Clin. Nutr.* **17**, 281.

HORNSTEIN, I., CROWE, P. F. and SULZBACHER, W. (1960). Constituents of meat flavor: Beef. *J. Agric. Food Chem.* **8**, 65.

HORNSTEIN, I., CROWE, P. F. and SULZBACHER, W. (1963). Flavor of beef and whale meat. *Nature* **199**, 1252.

KEYS, A., ANDERSON, J. T. and GRANDE, F. (1965). Serum cholesterol in response to changes in the diet. IV. Particular saturated fatty acids in the diet. *Metabolism* **14**, 776.

KRAMLICH, W. E. and PEARSON, A. M. (1958). Some preliminary studies on meat flavor. *Food Res.* **23**, 567.

LAKRITZ, L. and MAERKER, G. (1988). Enzyme levels in raw meat after low dose ionizing radiation and extended refrigerated storage. *Meat Sci.* **23**, 77.

LEVY, R. I. and ERNST, N. D. (1986). An overview of the cardiovascular disease risk factors of dietary origin. *J. Anim. Sci.* **62** (Suppl. 1), 38.

LIN, K. C., KEETON, J. C., GILCHRIST, S. and CROSS, H. R. (1988). Comparisons of carboxymethyl cellulose with differing molecular features in low-fat frankfurters. *J. Food Sci.* **53**, 1592.

LOWE, B. (1955). *Experimental Cookery from the Chemical and Physical Standpoint*, 4th edn. John Wiley & Sons, Inc., New York.

MARSTON, R. and RAPER, N. (1987). Nutrient content of the US food supply. *Nat. Food Rev.* **10**(1), 18.

MARTIN, R. J. (1987). Lipids in human health and disease. *Proc. Recip. Meat Conf.* **40**, 83.

MAST, M. G. and CLOUSER, C. S. (1988). Processing options for improving the nutritional value of poultry, meat and egg products. In *Designing Foods: Animal Product Options in the Marketplace.* Committee on Technological Options to Improve the Nutritional Attributes of Animal Products, p. 312. NAS–NRC, National Academy Press, Washington, DC.

MCNAMARA, D. J. (1985). Predictions of plasma cholesterol response to dietary cholesterol. *Am. J. Clin. Nutr.* **41**, 657.

MCNAMARA, D. J. (1987). Effects of a fat-modified diet on cholesterol and lipoprotein metabolism in man. *Ann. Rev. Nutr.* **7**, 273.

MCNAMARA, D. J., KOLB, R., PARKER, T. S., BATWIN, H., SAMUEL, P., BROWN, C. D. and AHRENS, E. H. JR (1987). Heterogeneity of cholesterol homeostasis in man: Response to changes in dietary fat quality and cholesterol quantity. *J. Clin. Invest.* **79**, 1729.

MEANS, W. J. and SCHMIDT, G. R. (1986). Algin/calcium gel as a raw and cooked meat binder. *J. Food Sci.* **51**, 60.

MERRITT, C. JR, ANGELINI, P., WIERBICKI, E. and SCHULTS, G. W. (1975). Chemical changes associated with flavor in irradiated meat. *J. Agric. Food Chem.* **23**, 1037.

MERTZ, W. (1986). Designing animals and animal products to fit consumer needs. *J. Anim. Sci.* **62** (Suppl. 1), 55.

MORRISON, R. M. (1986). Irradiation's potential for preserving food. *Nat. Food Rev.* **33**, 1.

NAS–NRC COMMITTEE (1988). *Designing Foods: Animal Product Options in the Marketplace.* Committee on Technological Options to Improve the Nutritional Attributes of Animal Products. NAS–NRC, National Academy Press, Washington, DC.

NIVEN, C. F., JR (1987). Microbiology and parasitology of meat. 1. Microbiology. In *The Science of Meat and Meat Products*, 3rd edn (J. F. Price and B. S. Schweigert, Eds), p. 217. Food & Nutrition Press, Westport, CT.

PAUL, D. L. and FOGET, K. S. (1983). Leaner products in the meat industry. *Proc. Meat Ind. Res. Conf.* American Meat Science Association, Chicago, IL, USA, p. 23.

PEARSON, A. M. (1976). The consumer desire for animal products. In *The Fat Content and Composition of Animal Products*, p. 45. Proc. Symp. held Dec. 12–13, 1974 in Washington, DC. National Academy of Sciences, Washington, DC.

PEARSON, A. M. (1981). Meat and Health. In *Developments in Meat Science—2* (R. Lawrie, Ed.), p. 241. Appl. Sci. Publ. Ltd, London.

PEARSON, A. M. and BROOKS, R. I. (1978). The contribution of meat to the diet of man. *Proc. Recip. Meat Conf.* **31**, 64.

PEARSON, A. M. and DUTSON, T. R. (Eds) (1987). *Advances in Meat Research, Vol. 3, Restructured Meat and Poultry Products.* Van Nostrand Reinhold Co., Inc. New York.

PEARSON, A. M. and TAUBER, F. W. (1984). *Processed Meats*, 2nd edn. AVI Publ. Co., Westport, CT.

PEARSON, A. M. and WOLZAK, A. M. (1982). Salt—Its use in animal products—A human health dilemma. *J. Anim. Sci.* **54**, 1263.

PEARSON, A. M., LOVE, J. D. and SHORLAND, F. B. (1977). Warmed-over flavor in meat, poultry, and fish. *Adv. Food Res.* **23**, 1.

PEARSON, A. M., GRAY, J. I., WOLZAK, A. M. and HORENSTEIN, N. A. (1983a). Safety implications of oxidized lipids on muscle foods. *Food Technol.* **37**(7), 121.

PEARSON, A. M., WOLZAK, A. M. and GRAY, J. I. (1983b). Possible role of muscle proteins in flavor and tenderness of meat. *J. Food Biochem.* **7**, 189.

PEARSON, A. M., ASGHAR, A., GRAY, J. I. and BOOREN, A. M. (1987). Impact of fat reduction on palatability and consumer acceptance of processed meat. *Proc. Recip. Meat Conf.* **40**, 105.

REISER, R. (1975). Fat has less cholesterol than lean. *J. Nutr.* **105**, 15.

RHEE, K. S. and SMITH, G. C. (1983). Effect of cooking on cholesterol content of patties containing different amounts of beef, textured soy protein and fat. *J. Food Sci.* **48**, 268.

RHEE, K. S., DUTSON, T. R., SMITH, G. C., HOSTETLER, R. L. and REISER, R. (1982a). Cholesterol content of raw and cooked beef longissimus muscles with different degrees of marbling. *J. Food Sci.* **47**, 716.

RHEE, K. S., DUTSON, T. R. and SMITH, G. C. (1982b). Effect of changes in intermuscular and subcutaneous fat levels on cholesterol content of raw and cooked beef steaks. *J. Food Sci.* **47**, 1638.

ROBERTS, T. (1986). Irradiation's promise: Fewer food borne illnesses? *Nat. Food Rev.* **33**, 7.

RUST, R. E. (1988). Processing options for improving the nutritional value of animal products. In *Designing Foods: Animal Product Options in the Marketplace.* Committee on Technological Options to Improve the Nutritional Attributes of Animal Products, p. 278. NAS–NRC, National Academy Press, Washington, DC.

SAMUEL, P. and MCNAMARA, D. J. (1982). Differential absorption of exogenous and endogenous cholesterol in man. *J. Lipid Res.* **24**, 265.

SAVELL, J. W., BRANSON, R. E., CROSS, H. R., STIFFLER, D. M., WISE, J. W., GRIFFIN, D. B. and SMITH, G. C. (1987). National consumer retail beef study: Palatability evaluation of beef loin steaks that differed in marbling. *J. Food Sci.* **52**, 517.

SAVELL, J. W., CROSS, H. R., HALE, D. S. and BEASLEY, L. S. (1988). *National Beef Market Basket Survey.* Meat Res. Brief. Dept Animal Science, Texas A&M University, College Station, TX.

SCHWEIGERT, B. S. (1986). 1985 Human nutrition dietary guidelines and their future significance. *J. Anim. Sci.* **62** (Suppl. 1), 16.

SCOTT, W. J. (1957). Water relations of food spoilage microorganisms. *Adv. Food Res.* **7**, 83.

SCOTT, W. J. (1961). Available water and microbial growth. *Proc. Low Temperature Microbiology Symp.*, p. 89. Campbell Soup Co., Camden, NJ.

SOFOS, J. N. and ALLEN, C. E. (1977). Effects of lean meat source and levels of fat and soy protein on the properties of wiener-type products. *J. Food Sci.* **42**, 875.

Sofos, J. N., Busta, F. F. and Allen, C. E. (1979). Botulism control by nitrite and sorbate in cured meats—A review. *J. Food Protect.* **42**, 739.

Sudarmadji, S. and Urbain, W. M. (1972). Flavor sensitivity of selected raw animal protein foods to gamma radiation. *J. Food Sci.* **37**, 671.

Tiwari, N. P. and Maxcy, R. B. (1971). Impact of low doses of gamma radiation and storage on the microflora of ground red meat. *J. Food Sci.* **36**, 833.

Tiwari, N. P. and Maxcy, R. B. (1972). *Moraxella–Acinebacter* as contaminants of beef and occurrence in radurized product. *J. Food Sci.* **37**, 901.

Thomas, M. H. and Wierbicki, E. (1971). *Effect of Irradiation Dose and Temperature on the Thiamine Content of Ham.* Tech. Rpt 71-44-FL, US Army Natick Labs., Natick, MA.

Tompkin, R. B. (1986). Microbiology of ready-to-eat meat and poultry products. *Adv. Meat Res.*, Vol. 2. Elsevier Applied Science, London, p. 89.

Toth, L. and Potthast, K. (1984). Chemical aspects of the smoking of meat and meat products. *Adv. Food Res.* **29**, 87.

Urbain, W. M. (1982). Radurization and radicidation: Meat and poultry. In *Preservation of Food by Ionizing Radiation*, Vol. 3 (E. S. Josephson and M. S. Peterson, Eds), p. 1. CRC Press, Inc., Boca Raton, FL.

Urbain, W. M. (1986). *Food Irradiation.* Academic Press, Inc., Orlando, FL.

Urbain, W. M. and Campbell, J. F. (1987). Meat preservation. In *The Science of Meat and Meat Products*, 3rd edn (J. F. Price and B. S. Schweigert, Eds), p. 371. Food & Nutrition Press, Inc., Westport, CT.

Urbain, W. M. and Giddings, G. G. (1972). Factors related to market life extension of low dose irradiated meat and poultry. *Radiation Res. Rev.* **3**, 389.

USDA (1986). *Handbook 8-13. Composition of Foods. Beef Products—Raw, Processed, Prepared.* USDA Human Nutrition Information Service, US Department of Agriculture, Superintendent of Documents, US Government Printing Office, Washington, DC, USA.

Wallingford, L. and Labuza, T. P. (1983). Evaluation of the water binding properties of food hydrocolloids by physical/chemical methods in a low fat meat emulsion. *J. Food Sci.* **48**, 1.

Wellington, G. H. and Stouffer, J. R. (1959). *Beef Marbling. Its Estimation and Influence on Tenderness and Juiciness.* Cornell Univ. Agric. Expt. Sta. Bul. 941.

Whiting, R. C. (1984). Addition of phosphates, proteins and gums to reduced-salt frankfurter batters. *J. Food Sci.* **49**, 1355.

Wierbicki, E., Brywjolfsson, A., Johnson, H. D. and Rowley, D. B. (1975). *Preservation of Meats by Ionizing Radiation—Update.* 21st Europ. Mtg Meat Res. Workers—Rapporteurs Papers—No. 14. Berne, Switzerland.

Wilson, G. D. (1960). Meat curing. In *The Science of Meat and Meat Products* (Am. Meat Inst. Found., Eds), p. 328. W. H. Freeman Co., San Francisco.

Wilson, G. D. (1961). *A Summary of the Technical Aspects of Smoking Meats.* Am. Meat Inst. Found., Spec. Rpt 26.

Wistreich, H. (1977). Smoking of meats. *Proc. Meat Ind. Res. Conf.* American Meat Science Association, Chicago, IL, USA, p. 37.

Wolin, E. F., Evans, J. B. and Niven, C. F., Jr (1957). The microbiology of fresh and irradiated beef. *Food Res.* **22**, 682.

Index